BLACKWELL'S NEUROLOGY AND PSYCHIATRY ACCESS SERIES

Child and Adolescent Psychiatry

SECOND EDITION

Other books in Blackwell's Neurology and Psychiatry Access Series

David: *Child and Adolescent Neurology*, 2nd Edition
Corey-Bloom: *Adult Neurology*, 2nd Edition
Rubin & Zorumski: *Adult Psychiatry*, 2nd Edition

BLACKWELL'S NEUROLOGY AND PSYCHIATRY ACCESS SERIES

Child and Adolescent Psychiatry

SECOND EDITION

EDITED BY

Sandra B. Sexson, MD, FAACAP, FACP

Professor and Chief
Division of Child, Adolescent and Family Psychiatry
Department of Psychiatry and Health Behavior
Medical College of Georgia
Augusta
Georgia

SERIES EDITOR

Ronald B. David, MD, FAAP, FAAN

Richmond, Virginia

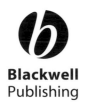

Blackwell
Publishing

© 2005 by Blackwell Publishing Ltd
Blackwell Publishing, Inc., 350 Main Street, Malden, Massachusetts 02148–5020, USA
Blackwell Publishing Ltd, 9600 Garsington Road, Oxford OX4 2DQ, UK
Blackwell Publishing Asia Pty Ltd, 550 Swanston Street, Carlton, Victoria 3053, Australia

First published 1997
Second Edition 2005

Library of Congress Cataloging-in-Publication Data

Child and adolescent psychiatry. -- 2nd ed. / edited by Sandra B. Sexson.
    p. ; cm. -- (Blackwell's neurology and psychiatry access series)
  Includes bibliographical references and index.
  ISBN-13: 978-1-4051-1768-5
  ISBN-10: 1-4051-1768-0
  1. Child psychiatry. 2. Adolescent psychiatry.   I. Sexson,
Sandra B.
  II. Series.
  [DNLM: 1. Mental Disorders--Adolescent. 2. Mental Disorders--Child.
  3. Mental Disorders--Infant. 4. Adolescent Psychiatry. 5. Child
Psychiatry.   WS 350 C535015 2005]
  RJ499.C48228 2005
  618.92'89--dc22

                                                                    2005016573

ISBN-13: 978–1–405–117685
ISBN-10: 1–4051–1768–0

A catalogue record for this title is available from the British Library

Set in 9.25/12pt Palatino by Sparks, Oxford – www.sparks.co.uk
Printed and bound in India by Replika Press PVT Ltd, Harayana

Commissioning Editor: Stuart Taylor
Development Editor: Nick Morgan
Project Manager: Kate Bailey
Production Controller: Kate Charman

For further information on Blackwell Publishing, visit our website:
http://www.blackwellpublishing.com

The publisher's policy is to use permanent paper from mills that operate a sustainable
forestry policy, and which has been manufactured from pulp processed using acid-free
and elementary chlorine-free practices. Furthermore, the publisher ensures that the text
paper and cover board used have met acceptable environmental accreditation standards.

Contents

Contributors

Ann Abramowitz, PhD is a clinical psychologist with a primary appointment in the Department of Psychology, Emory University. She also teaches in the department of Psychiatry and Behavioral Sciences. She trained at SUNY Stony Brook. Her interests include learning difficulties, behavior problems, and ADHD, with a focus on early intervention and multimodal treatment.

Dr Debbie Carter is a native of New York and graduated from Jefferson Medical College. She completed her general and child psychiatry postgraduate training at Thomas Jefferson University Hospital in Philadelphia, Pennsylvania. Dr Carter is an Associate Professor at the University of Colorado Health Sciences Center, which she joined in 1995. She is the Residency Training Director in the Division of Child and Adolescent Psychiatry and is the Medical Director of the Kempe Therapeutic Preschool in the Department of Pediatrics.

Marianne Celano, PhD is an Associate Professor in the Department of Psychiatry & Behavioral Sciences at the Emory University School of Medicine. She is a licensed psychologist specializing in clinical work with children and families. Her research interests include child maltreatment, pediatric asthma, family interaction patterns associated with childhood depression, and cultural issues in psychiatry.

Shannon Croft, MD is an Assistant Professor of Psychiatry and Behavioral Sciences at Emory University School of Medicine, and Director of Child Psychiatry at Grady Hospital in Atlanta, Georgia. He is a graduate of Emory's Medical School, where he also completed both psychiatry and child psychiatry residencies. He has recently graduated from Emory's Psychoanalytic Institute. His areas of interest include community child and adolescent psychiatry and the effects of trauma on children and families.

Michael D. DeBellis MD, MPH is a Professor of Psychiatry and Behavioral Sciences at Duke University Medical Center. He is the Director of the Healthy Childhood Brain Development Research Program at Duke. Dr DeBellis completed his medical training at the State University of New York at Downstate, his general psychiatry training at New York University, New York, and child psychiatry training at the University of Pittsburgh Medical Center, Western Psychiatry Institute and Clinic. He also completed a research fellowship at NIH. His research interests are in childhood brain and cognitive development, child maltreatment, and pediatric PTSD.

Mary Lynn Dell, MD, MTS, ThM is on the faculty of the Department of Psychiatry and Behavioral Sciences at Emory University. She completed her medical education and her general psychiatry training at Indiana University and her child and adolescent psychiatry training at Emory University. After serving on the faculties at both Emory and the University of Pennsylvania, Dr Dell was a NIMH Research Fellow. She also served on the faculty of George Washington University before returning to Emory. Her areas of special interest include pediatric psychiatry consultation and liaison, psychiatric ethics, and religion and spirituality in psychiatry.

Arden D. Dingle, MD is an Associate Professor of Psychiatry and Behavioral Sciences and the Training Director, Child and Adolescent Psychiatry, at Emory University School of Medicine in Atlanta, Georgia. She graduated from UMDNJ-New Jersey Medical School and completed a combined residency in pediatrics, psychiatry, and child and adolescent psychiatry at Mount Sinai Medical Center in New York City. Her interests include medical education, medically ill children, and community child and adolescent psychiatry.

Graham Emslie, MD is a Professor and the Chief of the Child and Adolescent Psychiatry Division at the University of Texas Southwestern Medical Center at Dallas (UTSW). He holds the Charles E. and Sarah M. Seay Chair in Child Psychiatry at UTSW. Dr Emslie completed his medical training at Aberdeen University in Scotland, his general psychiatry training at the University of Rochester, NY, and Child Psychiatry training at Stanford University. His research interests are in the psychopharmacological and psychosocial treatments of early-onset psychiatric disorders, including depression, anxiety disorders, and ADHD.

Andro Giorgadze, MD is a resident in the Child and Adolescent Psychiatry Program at Emory University School of Medicine in Atlanta, Georgia. He is a graduate of Tbilisi State Medical University and completed his psychiatry residency training also at Emory University School of Medicine. His special areas of interest are the biological underpinnings of psychotherapeutic change.

Deepa Gopalakrishnan, MD is an Assistant Professor of Psychiatry and Behavioral Sciences at Emory University School of Medicine, Atlanta, Georgia. She is the Director of the Preschool and School programs in the division of child and adolescent psychiatry. She is a graduate of Mysore Medical College, India, and completed her residencies in psychiatry at Albany Medical Center, Albany, NY and in child and adolescent psychiatry at Emory University School of Medicine, Atlanta, Georgia.

Osvaldo Gaytan MD/ PHD is a child and adolescent psychiatry resident at Emory University School of Medicine, Atlanta, Georgia. He is a graduate of the University of Texas at El Paso and received his MD/PhD from the University of Texas Medical School at Houston. He completed his residency in psychiatry at Emory University. His special area of research interest is in the effects of early life trauma on the development of psychiatric disorders.

Graeme Hanson, MD is Clinical Professor of Psychiatry and Pediatrics at the University of California, San Francisco, where he was Director of Training in Child and Adolescent Psychiatry until 2005. Dr Hanson received his MD from Harvard Medical School and completed both adult and child psychiatry residencies at Massachusetts Mental Health Center. He is Co-Chair of the Committee on Schools for the American Academy of Child and Adolescent Psychiatry. His professional interests are in child and adolescent growth and development, and in teaching and training in child and adolescent mental health.

Robert J Harmon, MD is Professor of Psychiatry and Pediatrics, University of Colorado School of Medicine; Medical Director CeDAR (Center for Dependency, Addiction, & Rehabilitation) at the Anschutz Centers for Advanced Medicine, University of Colorado Hospital; and Director, The Irving Harris Program in Child Development and Infant Mental Health, University of Colorado School of Medicine, Denver, Colorado. Dr Harmon completed his medical training – as well as his adult psychiatry and child & adolescent psychiatry training – at the University of Colorado School of Medicine. He spent three years at the National Institute of Child Health and Human Development in Bethesda, Maryland as a Research Associate in Child Development. He is a lecturer and author of more than 150 publications on infant psychiatry, infant and family development, and the effects of the death of an infant on the family.

Robert L. Hendren, DO is Professor of Psychiatry, Executive Director, MIND Institute (Medical Investigation of Neurodevelopmental Disorders) and Chief, Division of Child and Adolescent Psychiatry, University of California, Davis. Dr. Hendren took his residency in general psychiatry at the Mayo Graduate School of Medicine and his child and adolescent psychiatry fellowship at the Yale Child Study Center. His primary areas of research and publication are neuroimaging, psychopharmacology, neurodevelopmental disorders, including pervasive developmental disorder, bipolar disorder, schizophrenia spectrum disorders, and impulse control disorders.

Sarah Herbert, MD is a clinical adjunct assistant professor in the Department of Psychiatry and Behavioral Sciences at Morehouse School of Medicine in Alanta, Georgia. She is a child and adolescent psychiatrist who has had a significant interest in issues of sexuality and gender identity throughout her career. She presents on these subjects at national meetings, teaches at Emory School of Medicine as well as Morehouse, and is on the Sexual Orientation and Gender Identity Issues Committee of the American Academy of Child and Adolescent Psychiatry.

Karen Hochman, MD, FRCPC is an Assistant Professor of Psychiatry and Behavioral Sciences at Emory University School of Medicine in Atlanta, Georgia. She is a graduate of the Faculty of Medicine, at University of Manitoba, Canada and divided her psychiatry residency training between the University of Toronto and the University of Manitoba. Her research interest lies in identifying specific indicators of risk in adolescents at elevated risk of developing psychosis.

Iliyan Ivanov, MD is a clinical instructor at the division of child and adolescent psychiatry at the Mount Sinai School of Medicine in New York City. He is a graduate of the Bulgarian Academy of Medicine, and he completed residencies in psychiatry and child and adolescent psychiatry at the Mount Sinai School of Medicine in New York. He has been working in the area of psychopharmacological treatment of ADHD.

Steven L. Jaffe, MD is an Emeritus Professor of Psychiatry and Behavioral Sciences at Emory University School of Medicine and Clinical Professor of Psychiatry at Morehouse School of Medicine in Atlanta, Georgia. He attended Johns Hopkins University and the Albert Einstein College of Medicine. He completed a pediatric internship at UCLA, a psychiatry residency at the Massachusetts Mental Health Center where he was a teaching fellow at Harvard Medical School and a child psychiatry fellowship at Emory University School of Medicine. He specializes in the treatment of adolescent substance abuse disorders.

Niranjan Karnik, MD, PhD is a resident in child and adolescent psychiatry program at Stanford University Hospital & Clinics, and the Lucile Packard Children's Hospital in Palo Alto, California. He is a graduate of the University of Pennsylvania, the University of Illinois at Urbana-Champaign, and the University of Illinois College of Medicine. He was awarded his PhD in Sociology with a focus on children in vulnerable circumstances including foster, refugee, and street children. He completed his psychiatry residency training at Stanford University Hospital and Clinics. His current research interests focus on incarcerated juveniles, homeless youth, and cultural competence in medical education.

Robert A. Kowatch, MD is a Professor of Psychiatry and Pediatrics at Cincinnati Children's Hospital Medical Center and the University of Cincinnati Medical Center, of Cincinnati. He completed his internship in internal medicine at The Graduate Hospital under the auspices of the University of Pennsylvania, and his residency in psychiatry at the Hospital of the University of Pennsylvania. His research interests are in the treatment of child and adolescent bipolar disorders and the neurobiology of these disorders.

Douglas O. Lee, MD is an Assistant Professor of Psychiatry and Behavioral Sciences at the Emory University School of Medicine and is Director of the Psychopharmacology Consultation Program at the Emory Autism Center in Atlanta, Georgia. He graduated from the University of Pennsylvania and from Temple University School of Medicine. He completed his psychiatry residency at Bellevue Hospital-New York University and his child and adolescent psychiatry residency at Children's Hospital-Harvard Medical School. His interests include children and adolescents with ADHD and autism.

David J. Mullen, MD is an Associate Professor of Psychiatry in the Division of Child and Adolescent Psychiatry within the Department of Psychiatry at the University of New Mexico School of Medicine in Albuquerque, New Mexico. Dr Mullen completed his training in medicine at the University of Oklahoma and completed residencies in both general as well as child and adolescent psychiatry at the University of New Mexico. He is the Executive Medical Director of the University of New Mexico Children's Psychiatric Center, Inpatient Services. He has also provided psychiatric consultation to the Bernalillo County Juvenile Detention Center for the past 13 years. His interests include disruptive behavior disorders and mood disorders in children and adolescents.

Jeffrey Newcorn, MD is an Associate Professor of Psychiatry and Pediatrics, and the Director of Child and Adolescent Psychiatry, Mount Sinai School of Medicine. He graduated from the University of Rochester School of Medicine and did his psychiatry and child and adolescent psychiatry residencies at the Tufts-New England Medical Center. His research interests include attention deficit hyperactivity disorders and associated comorbid disorders.

Sandra B. Sexson, MD is Professor and Chief as well as Training Director of the Division of Child, Adolescent, and Family Psychiatry within the Department of Psychiatry and Health Behavior at the Medical College of Georgia in Augusta, Georgia. Dr Sexson graduated from the University of Mississippi School of Medicine and completed postgraduate training in child development (University of Mississippi), general psychiatry (University of Texas at San Antonio) and child psychiatry (Washington University in St. Louis). Prior to her present appointment, she has served as Chief of Child and Adolescent Psychiatry and Training Director at Wright State University in Dayton, Ohio, and at Emory University. Her primary professional focus has been in psychiatric education with a clinical and research focus in education, and in the emotional issues of children and adolescents with chronic medical illnesses. She is an active leader in psychiatric education in the United States.

Hans Steiner, Dr med univ, FAPA, FAACAP, FAPM is a Professor of Psychiatry and Behavioral Sciences, Child Psychiatry and Child Development at the Stanford University School of Medicine. He received his Doctor medicinae universalis from the University of Vienna, Austria, in 1972. He completed his residency in psychiatry at SUNY Upstate Medical Center and his child and adolescent psy-

chiatry residency at the University of Michigan in Ann Arbor. His research interests are in the area of aggression and its relationship to psychopathology, psychopathologies associated with trauma and victimization, and pediatric and psychiatric comorbidity.

Ayelet Talmi, PhD is an Instructor in the Department of Psychiatry at The University of Colorado Health Sciences Center (UCHSC). As a licensed clinical psychologist and neurodevelopmental infant specialist, she provides consultation and therapeutic services to infants, toddlers, and families seen at The Children's Hospital, in addition to conducting research on fragile infants' interactions with their caregivers. Dr. Talmi received her PhD in child clinical and developmental psychology from the University of Denver, completed her clinical internship at The Children's Hospital in Denver, Colorado, and was a NIMH-funded Developmental Psychobiology Postdoctoral Research Fellow at UCHSC. Dr. Talmi is also a graduate ZERO TO THREE Solnit Fellow. She is on the faculty of both the The Irving Harris Program in Child Development and Infant Mental Health at UCHSC, and at the Center for Family and Infant Interaction.

David Waller, MD is a Clinical Professor of Psychiatry at the University of Texas Southwestern Medical Center and Children's Medical Center, Dallas, Texas. He is a graduate of Harvard College and the Johns Hopkins University School of Medicine, and he completed residencies in pediatrics at Johns Hopkins University School of Medicine, in psychiatry at the Massachusetts General Hospital and in child and adolescent psychiatry at Children's Hospital in Boston. Eating disorders is an area of special interest.

Elaine F. Walker, PhD is the Chair of Psychology and the Samuel Candler Dobbs Professor of Psychology and Neuroscience at Emory University. She is a graduate of Washington University in St Louis, MO. Her research interests are in the areas of the causes of major mental disorders, for example the developmental course of schizophrenia, especially childhood precursors.

John Wilkaitis, MD is a child and adolescent psychiatry resident at Cincinnati Children's Hospital while collaborating in research with Dr. Melissa Delbello, Dr Stephen Strakowski, and Dr Robert Kowatch at the University of Cincinnati. He graduated from medical school and psychiatry residency at the University of Mississippi and has an MS in Chemistry.

Foreword

Traditional textbooks convey knowledge. It is the goal of this text in the Blackwell's Neurology and Psychiatry Access Series to convey not only essential knowledge but also the collected wisdom of its many highly regarded contributors. To achieve the goal of conveying not only knowledge but also wisdom, each book in this series is built on a structural framework that was well received by critics and readers alike in David: *Pediatric Neurology for the Clinician* and the first editions of *Child and Adolescent Neurology, Adult Neurology, Child and Adolescent Psychiatry,* and *Adult Psychiatry* (Mosby). Each volume is divided into three sections:

- tools for diagnosis
- diseases and disorders
- common problems.
  Also included to facilitate a physician's use of this book are:
- Nosologic diagnosis tables
- 'Pearls and perils' boxes
- 'Consider consultation when…' boxes
- selected annotated bibliographies
- a complete bibliography
  and (new in this edition)
- 'Key clinical questions and what they unlock.'

The Nosologic diagnosis tables are based on a discriminator model to promote clearer understanding, and are superior to a criterion-based model and others that lack similar specificity.

> Whoever having undertaken to speak or write hath first laid for themselves some [basis] to their argument such as hot or cold or moist or dry or whatever else they choose, thus reducing their subject within a narrow compass.
>
> Hippocrates

As Hippocrates has suggested, structure is the key to learning. Unless there is a structure onto which knowledge can be built, confusion and disorganization are the inevitable consequences.

Classification systems induce orderliness in thinking and enhance our ability to communicate effectively. A review of the most enduring hierarchical classification systems, particularly that of Linnaeus (that is, phyla, genera, species), makes clear the value of grouping according to discriminating features, as well as the value of simplicity, expandability, and dynamism.

The goal, whatever the classification system, is to seek the most powerful discriminating features that will produce the greatest diagnostic clarity. Discriminating features should avoid crossing domains. Much of the confusion that arises in diagnosis may be the result of the clinician who unwittingly crosses the anatomic, pathologic, pathophysiologic, phenomenologic, and etiologic classification domains used in medicine (for example, the inclusion of anatomically oriented 'temporal lobe seizures' in a phenomenologically based classification system that includes complex partial seizures). Some conditions, such as brain tumors, are classified according to their histopathology and lend themselves well to this classification system. Others, such as headaches and movement disorders, are classified phenomenologically and are therefore much less easily classified. In other cases, discriminators must encompass inclusionary, as well as, exclusionary features. At times, we can only use a criterion-based system or construct tables to compare features.

Arbitrarily, we label as consistent features those which occur more than 75% of the time. Features are considered variable when they occur less than 75% of the time. The diagnostic tables should be viewed, therefore, only as a beginning in the extremely difficult effort to make diagnosis more precise and biologically based. How well this book accomplishes the goals of identifying the most powerful discrimination features for maximum diagnostic clarity is limited by the current state of the art in child and adolescent neurology. In some areas, several features, when clustered together, serve to discriminate.

This text is designed to be pithy, not exhaustive, as there are already many available of this ilk. Each text in this series reflects appropriate stylistic differences among content editors. However, each is built upon the same structural framework, hence the value of this text to the users.

As a part of this foreword, I would like to acknowledge some of the people who have made key contributions to this effort. They include: Craig Percy, who initially saw the potential of this effort; the National Institute of Neurological Disorders and Stroke (NINDS)[1] for its support in nosolo-gic research; and the investigators who were involved with this NINDS project; Dr Grover Robinson, a long-time friend (who suggested the 'Consider consultation when…' boxes); Ms Laura DeYoung, Mr Stuart Taylor, and all the Blackwell team who made this vision a reality.

Last, but certainly not least, I would like thank Sandra Sexson who saw and shared this vision.

Ronald B. David, MD

---

[1] NINDS 1PO1NS20189–01A1 (Nosology, Higher Cortical Function Disorders in Children)

Preface to the Second Edition

When Drs Dean X. Parmelee and Ron David first asked me to edit the Second Edition of *Child and Adolescent Psychiatry*, part of the four-volume *Blackwell's Neurology and Psychiatry Access Series*, citing Dr Parmelee's inability to take on the challenge at the time, I felt what almost seemed like an obligation to see this well renowned, practical and truly accessible text updated for the twenty-first century. After all, my entire academic and clinical career in child and adolescent psychiatry has been devoted to the very goals that Dr Parmelee ascribes to this teaching text in the Preface to the First Edition. The text is designed to make available in an extraordinarily user-friendly format information regarding child and adolescent psychiatry for the physician and other health care providers devoted to caring for the whole child, and those dedicated to early identification and interventions for mental health problems that arise in the lives of children, adolescents and their families. It is within this context of the vision of Drs Parmelee and David that I eagerly accepted the challenge to edit the Second Edition.

For those who used the First Edition, the format of this text will be familiar. Many of the chapters bear the same titles, some the same authors, but all have been updated extensively. My section editors, Arden Dingle and Douglas Lee, and I have sought diligently to bring to this edition an integrated approach to the developmental, emotional and behavioral needs of children, adolescents, and their families that will provide the same utility and accessibility as that of the First Edition. It is directed primarily to the primary care physician, but should be useful to early career child and adolescent psychiatrists, general psychiatrists, and other child mental health providers. As before, contributors were chosen to share their significant clinically academic and practical expertise

The book is divided into three sections. Section One informs the diagnostic processes in child and adolescent psychiatry with an additional chapter that addresses the all-important aspects of treatment planning. Section Two again uses a DSM-IV approach to diagnostic categories in child and adolescent psychiatry with some expansions in developmental disabili-ties to include mental retardation and in the schizophrenia chapter to look at a broader range of psychotic disorders. We also moved the chapters on substance abuse and aggression into this section and added a chapter that addresses mental health disorders that may present with physical symptoms, a common challenge for the primary care physician. Finally, Section Three again addresses common problems seen in everyday practice. Changes include an expansion of the suicide chapter to include other risk taking and dangerous behaviors, the addition of a chapter highlighting the physician's role in integrating the school into the care of children and adolescents, and a greatly expanded chapter on common behavioral problems. Finally, we decided to divide the child abuse chapter into one addressing attachment issues and another on responses to trauma.

Throughout the text the reader will find the tools common to this Series – diagnostic tables when appropriate, 'Key clinical questions and what they unlock' to guide the evaluation, 'Pearls and perils' to remind the reader of important aspects as well as common pitfalls, and finally 'Consider consultation when…' to assist the physician in deciding when a formal consultation to a child and adolescent psychiatrist is indicated. These consistent features throughout the text encapsulate the quick and easy access to practically relevant information.

It is my editorial goal to continue in this Second Edition the excellent tradition established by Dr Parmelee in providing a concise, clinically relevant, practical resource for those 'most involved on a daily basis with the comprehensive health needs of children and youth' (Parmelee, 1996, xi). I am grateful to Drs David and Parmelee for offering me this opportunity. And I want to thank my Section Editors, Arden Dingle and Douglas Lee, for their considerable wisdom and counsel as we have progressed along this journey together. And, finally, a very special thanks to my family – my husband, Bill, and my children, Kristen and Ryan – whose support and incredible insights always keep me well grounded in reality.

Sandra B. Sexson, MD

Preface to the First Edition

When Dr Ron David and Mosby asked me to edit this text, I was very interested in providing a teaching text in child and adolescent psychiatry for physicians who are most involved on a daily basis with the comprehensive health needs of children and youth. It is these physicians who are in a position to identify mental health problems and to intervene at an early stage. The book reflects my commitment to those who want to help children with emotional and behavioral problems. It also reflects Dr David's commitment to creating a series of texts that foster greater diagnostic clarity and practice efficiency in our related fields of psychiatry and neurology.

The contributors were selected because of their abilities to apply clinically the findings from research in the field and experience from their busy clinical practices. Section One consists of three chapters that provide a foundation for understanding the diagnostic process in child and adolescent psychiatry. Section Two consists of chapters for each of the major diagnostic categories with current (DSM-IV) nosology and treatment approaches. Section Three presents common clinical problems and ways of managing them.

There are tools throughout the text that should help in understanding and remembering key points. Diagnostic tables highlight the discriminating, consistent, and variable features of a diagnosis. 'Pearls and perils' boxes succinctly reiterate salient facts and admonitions. The 'Consider consultation when …' feature assists the primary care physician in determining which clinical conditions and situations warrant referral to the child and adolescent psychiatrist. These tools will all help to access the information both more easily and more quickly.

Dean X. Parmelee, MD

SECTION 1

Assessment and Evaluation

Douglas O. Lee, MD

CHAPTER 1

Psychiatric Examination and Diagnosis in Children and Adolescents

Myla Harrison, MD and Jeffrey Newcorn, MD

Introduction

Psychiatric assessment of children and adolescents is a multifaceted process that includes interviewing parents, children, and families, obtaining current information and histories from other sources, assessing the severity of symptoms and overall levels of functioning, and synthesizing this information into comprehensive psychiatric formulations and treatment plans (for the American Academy of Child and Adolescent Psychiatry's practice parameters on assessment, see King, 1997; Thomas et al., 1997). The goals of this chapter are to describe the content and process of a psychiatric assessment, as well as to provide an overview of the diagnostic formulation and treatment planning process with children and adolescents. The psychiatric examination and diagnostic process are closely interwoven. Even though an accurate diagnosis depends on information collected in the psychiatric interviews and the mental status examination, knowledge regarding diagnostic categories affects the content and flow of clinical data collection. Nevertheless, for purposes of exposition, the clinical and diagnostic processes are described separately. This chapter considers assessment from the perspective of the child and adolescent psychiatrist, and it is intended for physicians who want to improve their skills in the evaluation of mental health functioning in children and youth. It also includes a section on the role of the primary care physician in psychiatric screening and assessment.

Complexities of assessment in child and adolescent psychiatry

There are several complex features of the psychiatric assessment of children that differ from the assessment of adults and that warrant special consideration. In children

and adolescents, assessment of developmental functioning is of utmost importance. The physician must understand normal development in children of different ages, genders, and sociocultural backgrounds. Children and adolescents of different ages and developmental stages differ in their physical, cognitive, and emotional capacities. Therefore, the clinician must carefully assess the ways a patient's problems reflect or deviate from normal development. The breadth of normality and the large amount of individual variation must be emphasized. For example, temper tantrums in a 2-year-old child are considered a normal part of development. However, continued temper tantrums at age 13 likely indicate a significant problem. Fears of the dark and of monsters are relatively common in children aged 4–6, and one generally does not diagnose a phobic disorder in a child of this age. In adolescents, questions regarding identity development and separation from the family are important developmental processes and should not necessarily be viewed as symptoms of psychiatric disturbance.

The fact that childhood and adolescence entail constant change also contributes to the complexities of the assessment. The presence of delays relative to peers or areas of precocious functioning should be identified, and the physician must decide whether intervention is useful or warranted. The physician must appreciate the difference between variations that fall within the "normal" or "typical" range of development and variations that indicate developmental delays (Chapters 5 and 6). When developmental delays are suspected, referral for further evaluation is recommended since developmental delays that are unaddressed can contribute to further complications (American Academy of Child and Adolescent Psychiatry, 1998).

The child is a valuable source of information for the physician, and he is interviewed as part of the assessment. However, children are vastly different in their abilities to tell the examiner about their peer and family relationships, moods, and how they conceptualize the reason for the evaluation. Many children, especially younger ones, may provide only an indirect glimpse into this material. They may be limited in their abilities to verbalize their feelings and describe their social interactions. As a result, the use of interactive play and projective techniques is often required to obtain this information. Play with dolls that represent family figures, puppets, or drawing may take on greater importance in the assessment for a younger child than for an older child. However, the verbal expression of feelings may also be difficult for an older child or adolescent, and other, less directive procedures are often helpful.

It is important to remember that the psychiatric examination assesses a child's or adolescent's functioning at a single point in time. Therefore, one cannot necessarily assume that the results of such an assessment are representative of the child's general functioning. It is possible that the physician may not see the symptoms described by the referring source in one or more evaluation sessions. Additionally, symptoms may change during the assessment process. However, even seemingly minor behaviors that may be observed during the evaluation can be highly indicative of problems in day-to-day life. For instance, some children are reluctant to participate in the individual session with the psychiatrist if it requires that their parents are left in the waiting room. Even though this degree of difficulty separating might reflect a normal degree of anxiety in an initial appointment with a young child, it could also indicate the presence of separation anxiety disorder. On the other hand, a child with oppositional defiant disorder (ODD) may be on his best behavior with the interviewer. Only by carefully listening to the child's responses to direct questions about his relationships with authority figures is it possible to develop an understanding of the problem. Because of such special considerations, a full range of information from multiple informants must be elicited and considered when formulating a diagnosis and treatment plan in children and adolescents.

The psychiatric evaluation of children further differs from that of adults in that the child can provide only a limited amount of historic information. A child cannot relate the circumstances of his birth or his developmental history. A younger child is also not cognitively capable of relating symptoms in a temporal sequence. Therefore, the physician must turn to other sources for a comprehensive picture of the child. This includes the parents, other relatives, teachers, pediatricians, guidance counselors, and camp counselors, as well as sources of objective information, such as the results of psychologic testing and rating scales. A review of the pediatrician's records can often provide information about the child's early developmental history, and school report cards can show the early cognitive and behavioral development of the child.

A complete picture of the child's strengths and the nature of the problem arises from the various sources of information. There are times when different informants provide conflicting data, and it can be difficult to know who to believe. The physician must then use his judgment to assess this information variance. It is important to remain mindful of how well the various informants know the child and to know which observers are best able to evaluate which symptoms. For instance, it is not unusual for a child to admit to mood or anxiety symptoms of which the parent is unaware. Therefore, such reports should be taken seriously even if they are not confirmed by the parent. Conversely, teachers' reports of inattention and overactivity should be given the highest priority when evaluating a child for attention-deficit/hyperactivity disorder (ADHD) because teachers see the child in a structured setting and are therefore considered the best informants regarding this behavior. A general rule is that children are essential sources for reporting internalizing symptoms such as anxiety and mood symptoms, whereas adults are often better informants about the presence of externalizing behaviors such as conduct problems. When parents and teachers differ in their accounts of a child, clinical judgment must be applied to discern the reasons for this disparity. Differences may result not only from the various perspectives of the informants but also from the child actually exhibiting different behavior in various settings.

It is important to supplement the information derived from the history and the mental status examination with additional data from rating scales, psychologic and neuropsychologic tests, and any requisite medical evaluation or laboratory tests (see Chapter 3). Clinically useful and easy-to-administer rating scales (see Chapter 2) are Achenbach's Child Behavior Checklist (CBCL) for parents and Teacher Report Form (TRF) for teachers (Achenbach and Rescorla, 2001) and the Connors rating scales for teachers and parents (Connors et al., 1998). These rating scales have been standardized and normed for age and gender, and therefore they provide comprehensive tests for the presence or absence of symptoms. They do not provide diagnosis, but rather levels of psychopathology in general. Psychologic (cognitive/educational) testing is necessary to diagnose mental retardation and learning disorders. The battery may include tests of verbal and nonverbal cognitive abilities, achievement tests (to assess academic functioning), and projective tests (to assess reality testing and interpersonal functioning). A significant discrepancy between a child's measured intelligence quotient (IQ) and his performance on a standardized academic achievement test is indicative of a learning disability. An IQ below 70 may lead to a diagnosis of mental retardation, although this requires evidence of adaptive functioning delays as well. Specific neuropsychologic tests may suggest organic pathologic conditions or localizing lesions.

The psychiatric examination

Overview

The psychiatric assessment is the comprehensive clinical evaluation used to determine whether a psychopathologic condition is present, whether treatment is indicated, and what treatment should entail. The emotional and behavioral functioning of the child are evaluated and placed in the context of the child's current developmental level and expected developmental gains.

Before the evaluation begins, the parents should be informed about the assessment process and give help to prepare the child for the evaluation. This process is normally fraught with anxiety, and if the child is not properly prepared, he may not be optimally cooperative during the interview. Therefore, it is also important to find out what the parent has told the child about the upcoming evaluation. Parents often ask for the physician's opinion regarding how to prepare a child for an evaluation. The response to this question should be at least partially related to the nature of the impairment. For example, a parent might tell the child that he is going to see a talking (or playing) doctor who will find out how to help him improve his school performance or his behavior. Typically, children are worried about needles or blood, and they are reassured if they are told that there will be no skin pricks, poking, or injections. Parents should also be given specific information about the length of the evaluation, the cost, and what they can expect when the evaluation is complete (such as a formal report or an informing session).

During the assessment, the physician gathers information about a child's problem, psychiatric history, present and past medical history, family history, current developmental status, early developmental history, school history, and mental status (see Box 1.1). When performing the assessment, the physician should consider not only the child's pathologic condition and which symptoms are present or absent, but also the areas of strength in both the child and the family. In fact, focusing on strengths may be the best way to engage the child and the family in the assessment process. When developing this profile, it is important to consider the child's age as well as his physical, cognitive, and social capabilities. The physician uses his knowledge of normal development and psychopathologic conditions to formulate a working diagnosis based on the information gathered and on the observations made. Ultimately, a treatment plan is developed (Chapter 4), and it is shared with the child and the family.

There are many approaches to the parent interview. To avoid making younger children wait excessively, it is helpful to gather a child's history from the parents in a separate appointment before the child is seen. However, regardless of the method, it is useful to have time with the parents apart

from the child and, sometimes, to interview each parent separately. In the event of divorced or separated parents, it is particularly important to have both parents participate in the assessment of the child, and it is advisable to interview each parent separately. It is often helpful to meet with the entire family together at least once during the assessment to understand what each member of the family sees as the problem and what each person sees as a realistic solution.

The parent interview provides the physician with information regarding the existing problem; the child's psychiatric, medical, and developmental histories; the family and social history; and the school history (see Box 1.1). It should include a review of past physical and emotional stresses, adjustments to school and social situations (past and current), and the patient's relationships with siblings and with each parent or caregiver. Requests for release of information from pediatricians, school personnel, and previous treatment providers should also be obtained at the time of the initial parent interview.

The reason for referral and the history of present and past problems

When beginning the psychiatric assessment, the physician needs to consider the referral source and the reason for the referral. Often, it is the parents, primary caregivers, or school officials who initiate the evaluation process, but referrals may also come from the legal or social service systems. If the referral has not come from the parents, the physician must find out whether they see a problem and if so, how they can be engaged in the treatment process.

As with the traditional medical history, the physician first determines the chief complaint and the history of the present illness, in the words of the child or a parent. There must be

---

BOX 1.1

Components of a psychiatric examination

- Reason for referral
- History of present illness
- Past psychiatric history
- Medical history
- Developmental history
- Milestones for pregnancy, birth, and the neonatal period; infancy; toddlerhood; preschool age; school age; and adolescence
- School history
- Family history
- Mental status; appearance, behavior, relatedness, speech and language, mood and affect, thought process and content, and cognitive and developmental assessment
- Formulation
- Diagnosis
- Treatment plan

descriptions of the development of the symptoms and of the historical context of the problem. The patient or a parent should also explain what has happened recently to prompt the appointment. The presenting problem may be a behavioral problem, an emotional or mood problem, a specific or a pervasive developmental disability, a psychotic disorder, a reaction to an adverse life event, or some combination of these. Many dimensions used to elucidate symptoms in the medical model are also useful for gathering information about the history of the present illness in the field of child and adolescent psychiatry. The physician should gather information about the chronology (onset, duration, periodicity, and course), quality, quantity (intensity, degree of functional impairment, frequency), setting, aggravating or alleviating factors, and associated manifestations of the problem. The course of the symptoms should be recorded, but not necessarily gathered, in chronologic order from the onset of the symptoms to the time of the evaluation. A child's level of adjustment, developmental status, and social, academic, and family functioning relative to the presenting problem are also recorded in this section. It should be noted whether a child is taking any psychotropic medications or any other medication that may affect his mental status.

The history includes information about previous psychiatric evaluations and treatment, either for the same problem or for any other psychiatric condition. Past use of psychotropic medication is highlighted, and dosages, responses, adverse effects, and duration of use are noted. If permission from the parent (and for older children and adolescents, from the patient as well) can be obtained, it is often helpful to contact physicians and therapists who have treated the patient.

When gathering the history of the presenting problem, it is important to include a "psychiatric review of systems." This allows the physician to obtain additional data that may not have been revealed spontaneously but may be relevant to the history and clinical presentation of a particular child. This information can be extremely useful in differential diagnosis and in determining whether comorbidity is present. The psychiatric review of systems includes questions regarding all major areas of function, such as the child's general level of function, developmental delays or deviations, anxiety symptoms, mood symptoms, attention or behavior problems, learning problems, somatic complaints, psychotic symptoms, elimination disorders, eating disorders, weight problems, and drug or alcohol use. Specific questions should be asked to assess the presence of suicidal or homicidal thoughts, as well as disturbances in social, academic, or family functioning.

Medical history of the child

The medical history of the child is obtained from the primary caregivers or the pediatrician. Pediatric records are also commonly available to complement the history obtained from the family. The psychiatrist should note any current or past medical conditions and previous hospitalizations (including any surgery). If there have been any major illnesses, the child's emotional and behavioral reactions should be recorded. Children who have had multiple hospitalizations for a chronic illness may show a range of developmental problems as a result of altered environmental stimulation, direct effects of the illness, or an interplay between variables involving the parent and the child. For example, bed wetting in a 5-year-old child hospitalized for asthma who had previously obtained sustained bladder continence might be viewed as an expected developmental regression in a child who was otherwise developing normally.

The use of medications to treat general medical conditions and any allergies to medications should also be noted in this section, since the behavioral symptoms presented by the family and the child in the history of the present illness may be related to prescribed medications. For example, steroids are an integral part of medical management after an organ transplantation and can have important emotional and behavioral manifestations, such as severe agitation and psychosis.

It is important to remember that the psychiatric problem may be a direct effect of a congenital or an acquired medical illness, or an indirect manifestation of the stress caused by a medical illness. Fetal alcohol syndrome is an example of a disorder that may be accompanied by psychiatric symptoms. Children with fetal alcohol syndrome have mental retardation and facial dysmorphism, and they may also have learning disorders and ADHD. Additionally, general medical conditions not directly associated with psychiatric disturbances may cause psychiatric symptoms. For example, a child with acute lymphocytic leukemia may show the symptoms of decreased energy, anhedonia, and a poor appetite disproportionate to what is normally expected from the medical illness or the chemotherapeutic agents used in its treatment. This child may possibly be suffering from a superimposed major depressive episode or an adjustment disorder with a depressed mood. As with the psychiatric history, a general medical review of systems should be included, so that the possibility that a medical condition that may be contributing to the psychiatric symptoms will not be overlooked. For example, vision or hearing deficits may be related to psychiatric or cognitive problems. Thus, if a preschool child is brought to the physician with problems in language acquisition and a history of recurrent otitis media, it is important to ask about the child's hearing and to consider obtaining additional assessments to determine whether a hearing disorder may be contributing to the language delay.

Developmental history

The child's developmental history should be gathered during the parent interview, and supplemental information should be obtained from the pediatrician. When taking the developmental history, the psychiatrist must be aware of the range of individual variations in normal development. Any delays in achieving milestones, interruptions, or setbacks in the child's expected developmental progression should be noted. This information can be especially helpful when it is compared with similar data from siblings or other peers of the same age as the patient. Parents may be unaware of developmental delays or deviations, so additional information from individuals who were familiar with the child or old family videotapes may be required to supplement the information provided by the parents.

In addition to developmental delays, areas of precocious development or unusual strengths and capacities should be noted. When writing up the developmental history, it is helpful to organize the material by developmental stage. Each of the relevant developmental stages is described in detail in the following sections.

Pregnancy, birth, and the neonatal period

Inquiring about the events preceding and surrounding the pregnancy of the mother is often a comfortable way to begin the developmental history. It is useful to learn whether the pregnancy was planned, and if so, how long it took for the parents to conceive. If the pregnancy was unplanned, what was the parents' reaction to learning about it? Ask about the nature of any medical complications during the pregnancy or after delivery, how the pregnancy was tolerated, and whether there were any complicating events in the mother's life during the pregnancy. Pertinent information about labor and delivery should be noted, and the presence of any medical complications should also be recorded. The birth weight, the APGAR scores, and the parents' feelings at the time of birth may all be revealing. The mother's use of cigarettes, alcohol, and any over-the-counter, prescription or illicit drugs taken during pregnancy should be determined, as should the presence of problems in the prenatal and postnatal periods (such as eclampsia or postpartum depression).

Infancy

Infancy is the period between birth and the emergence of language which is usually between 12 and 18 months. By the end of infancy children can walk and begin to demonstrate behaviors that indicate independence from the caregiver. It is important to know whether there were any parent-child attachment problems during this period. Such problems might occur in an infant who was in a neonatal intensive care unit for an extended period or in an infant whose mother suffered a medical or psychiatric illness after the birth of the child and was unable to provide the requisite care and attention. The presence of stranger anxiety or early separation difficulties are often important indicators of bonding. Stranger anxiety begins at approximately 8 months and often lasts several months; separation anxiety is often present

when the child is between 10 and 18 months old. Both of these behaviors are normal and expected developmental markers, but they may not be present in all children. It is also important to ask about the presence of medical problems during infancy, developmental competency in regulatory functions, such as eating or sleeping, and the presence of temperamental qualities such as irritability or avoidance. Specific areas to assess include the development of gross motor function, fine motor function, language development (not just speech), adaptive behaviors, and social skills. A variety of screening examinations can be used to assess normal development. The Denver II, a revised and re-standardized Denver Developmental Screening Test, is one screening test that is commonly used by pediatricians to estimate a child's developmental status until age 6. A child's developmental level on this test can often be obtained from pediatricians and can be used to retrospectively evaluate the presence of developmental problems. (Refer to Chapter 15 to learn more about specific issues during infancy. For practice parameters on assessing infants and toddlers, see American Academy of Child and Adolescent Psychiatry, 1997.)

Toddlerhood

Toddlerhood starts with the development of language, mobility, and other cognitive developments usually between ages 12 and 18 months and lasts until approximately 36 months. The landmarks of this stage are the development of autonomy and self-control. The toddler becomes proficient in the gross motor skills of walking, running, and climbing. He or she also masters fine motor skills such as beginning to dress and holding utensils, toys, and crayons, as well as the sometimes unwanted behaviors of opening drawers, cabinets, and medicine bottles. Speech and language development during this period should be noted carefully, as should eye contact, communication abilities (regardless of language), reciprocal interactions, and symbolic play. Problems in these areas may indicate the presence of a pervasive developmental disorder. The child should master single words before the age of 2 and should be able to combine them into short sentences by the end of the toddler period. Gender identity is clearly established during this period, usually beginning in the second year.

Other characteristic features of this stage are temper tantrums, the development of toilet training skills, and the development of fears such as specific phobias and separation problems. Normal disturbances in sleep may be related to fear of the dark. If this has been the case, it is important to discuss how the parents have handled this, as well as whether and when the child sleeps in the parents' bed. The clinician can ask in a non-judgmental way about where the child and parents sleep, how the child is put to sleep, and whether the child ever sleeps in the parents' bed. Common problems during the toddler period may involve family struggles with the toddler's newfound autonomy.

Preschool age

Preschool years typically describe the period between ages 3–5 years. Important features of development during this stage are related to socialization in school or in other out-of-home situations, and evolving cognitive capacities. Preschool development includes successful separation from parents for short periods, development of peer relationships, and the acquisition of a variety of skills such as dressing, feeding, bladder and bowel control, and being able to regulate emotional outbursts. The child's fears and capacity for impulse control should be assessed, and the presence of nightmares or other developmental problems should be noted. It is also useful to inquire about night-time bladder control, since many children continue to wet the bed during preschool years. (Enuresis is not diagnosed before a child is 5 years old.) The extent to which the preschool child is permitted or encouraged to sleep in the parents' bed varies considerably, but it may provide insight into the parent-child relationship. Therefore it is often useful to inquire about sleeping arrangements in the family.

School age

The school-age period is comprised of the ages between 6 and 11 years. This stage of development has also been referred to as the latency stage, a term derived from the psychoanalytic formulation that the sexual drive is quiescent after resolution of the Oedipus complex. However, this term is less often used at present, reflecting our current understanding that sexuality is not latent in the school-age years.

For the school-age child, the process of the history gathering often involves the child as well as the parent, although younger children in this age range are still not able to give a history. Play is an important means of communication, but there is often a mixture of talk and play. Inquiring about the school-age child's hobbies and interests is a good way to engage him in the evaluation process. Peer relationships are an important focus for school-age children. This is the time children develop "best" friends, so it is especially important to ask them about activities such as sleep-overs with friends. School-age children further develop the ability to play cooperatively with peers, and can be questioned about their involvement in after-school or team sports activities. School performance and school difficulties should be evaluated, and their effects on the child's developing sense of competence and self-esteem should be noted. Other important areas of development are related to impulse control, coordination, clumsiness, separations, and reactions to them.

Adolescence

It is often said that adolescence begins with a biologic event (puberty) and ends with a psychologic event (transition to adulthood). Thus, the duration of this stage is variable and dependent on biologic, psychologic, and life-circumstance variables. The developmental challenges in this period are negotiating puberty, developing a cohesive sense of self, and psychologically and physically forming a separation from the parents and family. More than any other stage, adolescence is affected by cultural norms and expectations. It is important to consider the impact of ethnic and cultural factors in evaluating these developmental tasks.

It is also essential to learn about the adolescent's reactions to the onset of puberty and to take a thorough psychosexual history. Sexual preference is generally well established by the adolescent period. Therefore, it is important to be mindful of the needs of homosexual as well as heterosexual adolescents in the assessment process. When taking a sexual history, the physician should remain unbiased and extremely careful not to assume the adolescent has a heterosexual orientation. Inquiry regarding sexual identity and orientation should begin in an open-ended format and proceed to direct, matter-of-fact questions. This way, the adolescent will sense that the interviewer is accepting and nonjudgmental, and the adolescent may be more comfortable sharing information about fears, worries, or alienation related to sexual identity. One can say: "Many adolescents are figuring out their own identity at your age, and this can be confusing or uncomfortable at times. How are you dealing with that?" One can also inquire: "Are you in a relationship with anyone now?" "Have you been in relationships in the past?" Or one can say: "Some kids tell me they have concerns or know that they may be attracted to kids of the same sex (one could say gay/lesbian/homosexual/bisexual). Have you had thoughts about that?"

Alcohol, tobacco, and drug usage are also key areas to include in the history of a patient in this age group. Academic or learning problems, quantity and quality of peer relationships, and symptoms of depression or identity disturbance should be noted.

The evaluation of adolescents requires less input from parents and more direct history from the adolescent. To successfully engage the adolescent and obtain an accurate history, considerable skill and experience are often required, particularly when there is resistance to participation in the assessment. An attitude that fosters openness and honesty in the dialogue is most helpful. Adolescents are much more aware of their feelings than younger children and are usually good reporters, provided they are positively engaged in the process. Depending on the specific content of the history and the goals of the evaluation, providing the adolescent with the opportunity to meet apart from the parents and the rest of the family can be very helpful in forming an alliance. Often, adolescents are seen alone as a first step in the process, with parent and family interviews coming later on. With the younger adolescent, play, in the form of drawing or table games such as cards, can help develop the relationship.

School history

The school history should be taken chronologically, beginning with organized daycare or preschool experiences and continuing through the time of the interview. Emphasis should be placed on learning, behavioral and social competencies, and problems that arise in school. Reactions of the child to separations, such as the beginning of school, and transitions to different schools should be noted. This is the section of the history in which general cognitive capacities are described. It is important to consider the child's strengths as well as his weaknesses. Note whether the child is in a special education program, has repeated a grade, or has received extra help or tutoring for any reason. Assessment of academic achievement often requires contact with the child's current teacher. Standardized reading and arithmetic tests are usually administered in school and may be available in the records. Old report cards may also be used to supplement retrospective accounts. For children of all ages, it is important to inquire about the peer group at school and the child's participation in extracurricular activities. This may include religious instruction, clubs, scouts, or school teams.

If there are school-related problems, it is important to learn how the problems began and what factors have maintained them. For example, an 8-year-old child who has attentional problems and hyperactive behavior in the third grade may be experiencing increased demands to sit, focus, and learn in school as the curriculum becomes more difficult. Therefore, the assessment should attempt to elucidate whether this child's problems are related to a learning disorder (Chapter 6), attention-deficit/hyperactivity disorder (Chapter 7), or both.

Family history

The family history section of the assessment involves obtaining each parent's personal history, including the level of education, vocation, and presence of medical and psychiatric problems. Relevant medical and psychiatric histories of the child's siblings, grandparents, the parents' siblings, and their children should also be obtained. It is helpful to ask whether there is anyone else in the family who has had similar problems to the patient.

Obtaining a sociocultural history is also important. Any migrations or relocations should be noted, and attention should be given to the impact this has had on the family and the child. Additional information of interest might include the languages spoken at home, the religion of the family, and the impact of these on the child. Cultural differences regarding child-rearing and discipline should be considered, since individuals of different ethnic groups often have different expectations regarding their children's behavior and how to manage it. The meaning of having a child evaluated by a mental health provider may also need to be explored in the context of cultural differences. It is especially important to understand the family's ideas and value judgments regarding psychiatric treatment before presenting the results of the evaluation and the treatment plan. This will prevent an otherwise good plan from being doomed to failure because it is at variance with culturally determined values.

Interview with the child or adolescent

Overview

The purpose of the interview with the child (in this section, the term child refers to both children and adolescents) is to clarify the differential diagnosis through direct observation, discussion, questioning, or play. This session is often used to confirm hypotheses generated from the parent interview or to generate additional diagnostic hypotheses, although it occasionally provides more definitive information. History-taking from the child should include questions about the present and past aspects of the child's life and overall functioning. During the child interview, the physician also attempts to learn about the child's feelings and internal states. However, this may require patience on the part of the interviewer and may not happen at the beginning of the interview.

The first task is to engage the child in the process. It is this aspect of the examination that often makes beginning child psychiatrists the most uncomfortable. Nevertheless, it is important that the beginning psychiatrist interacts with the child without conveying his sense of anxiety about the interview. In general, skills used to develop a relationship with a child in the pediatric setting are applicable. Telling the child why he is being seen and requesting his assistance is paramount, just as if the physician were seeing the child for abdominal pain. However, it is also important to indicate how this visit differs from a visit to the pediatrician. It is often useful to indicate at the outset that there will be no injections or other procedures during the evaluation. The format of the interview invariably differs with respect to the individual child and the style and temperament of the interviewer. Approaches used with the same child may also vary from session to session. The structure and flow of the child interview varies by necessity as a function of the child's age and developmental level. For example, adolescents are often seen before their parents to solidify the relationship with the interviewer and to demonstrate their centrality in the evaluation process. The preschool child is often seen with the parent present, especially if there are separation problems or questions about the parent-child interaction.

Children are often quite anxious when beginning the evaluation process. They are usually aware that they are going to the doctor because of unpleasant or unwanted feelings (such as sadness, anxiety, fear, or anger) or problem behaviors (for instance, biting other children, having tantrums, or skipping school). The physician should communicate early that he does not consider the child to be bad but that some of the child's behaviors are problematic. In this way, the interviewer distinguishes between self-worth and behavior problems. It may also be helpful to indicate that there may be different ways to behave that are more socially acceptable, and this will be determined together.

The observation of the child commonly begins in the waiting room. The physician should take note of the child's behavior, including how the child relates to his or her parents, general level of anxiety, and how he or she separates from the caregiver. Usually the child will have been told about the appointment by the parent before the interview. Ideally, the parent will have given the child information regarding the purpose of the assessment and how the child may be helped. However, it is important to review this information at the beginning of the interview. Also at the beginning of the interview, the physician should introduce him or herself to the child and tell the child what type of clinician he or she is (a psychiatrist or other health-care provider), the amount of time the child will be in the office to play or talk, and that the parents or caregivers will be in the waiting room at the conclusion of the session.

In the same way that a physician engages conversation with a new pediatric patient, the psychiatrist begins by gathering neutral data, such as who the child lives with, age, school grade, school, and his interests or hobbies. Taking an active interest in who the child is and what he or she likes to do helps reduce anxiety. It may also be reassuring to the patient if the physician shares what has been learned from the parent about the reason for the visit at that time. However, it is essential to inquire about what the child sees as the problem, and how he or she is coping. Young children should not be expected to give a factual and chronological account of their behavior; it is better to obtain this information from other sources.

When interviewing the child, it is important to interact in a manner that is appropriate to the child's level of development. Depending on the age of the child, the interview may be more or less verbally oriented. Most adolescents have no trouble speaking directly with the interviewer. However, a young child is more likely to use play as an important means of communication. It is helpful to have paper, pencil, crayons, and some age-appropriate toys available for the assessment. Family figures and a doll house can be especially useful in allowing a child to express issues about the family. The use of projective techniques with puppets and dolls can be a less threatening way for the child to convey feelings, perceptions, and means of regulating impulses. This play can be used to build rapport, as well as for diagnostic purposes. Additionally, the child may be asked to draw a picture of his or her choosing or to draw something specific, such as a person or his or her family. In either case, care must be taken not to distort the child's play

with unjustified assumptions or overly intense interpretations regarding its "true meaning." Other commonly used projective techniques are to have the child say what his or her three wishes would be if he or she could have anything in the world, or what animal he or she would like to be. Finally, it is useful to ask what the child's plans are. For example, the physician could ask what the child would like to do or be when he or she is older. This will give information about the child's sense of self, future goals, values, and concerns.

Another important aspect of the child interview is the evaluation of the child's capability to engage in a particular type of treatment. It is important to assess the child's insight into the presenting problems and his or her desire for change, as well as verbal skills and capacity for abstract reasoning. This is especially important in older children, who generally assume a greater responsibility for coming to treatment and in determining the process of treatment. Key clinical questions below illustrates the clinical questions to ask a child and what these unlock.

Mental status examination

The mental status examination is comprised of the physician's observations regarding the child's psychologic process and level of functioning, which are based on the child's overall level of relatedness and responses to specific objective and subjective questions. It is the psychiatric equivalent of the physical examination. It is important to remember that the mental status examination is a cross-sectional profile, and may vary from day to day. Examples and descriptions should be used in the write-up as much as possible.

The mental status examination contains the following domains of assessment: appearance, behavior, relatedness, speech and language, mood and affect, thought process and content, and cognitive and developmental assessment.

Appearance

The general appearance of the child is noted, and attention is given to the way he or she is dressed and groomed. The presence of any unusual physical marks or dysmorphic features should be noted. Scars or bruises may indicate accident-prone behavior or physical abuse. Dysmorphic features may indicate the presence of genetic or prenatal syndromes that may be related to the child's symptoms. Dysmorphic features should be described specifically. Examples include "low-set ears" or "a flat philtrum."

Behavior

The level of motor activity should be noted, and attention should be given to the presence of any purposeless movements such as tics, stereotypies, or other involuntary movements. Tics are involuntary rhythmic motor activities or vocalizations. Stereotypies are repetitive, nonfunctional motions such as hand waving, head banging, body rocking, or

KEY CLINICAL QUESTIONS

- *Draw a picture and tell me about it. Draw a picture of your family doing something.*

Facilitates the relationship with the clinician.

- *What do you like to do for fun? What are you good at?*

Strengths of the child.

- *Tell me about your friends.*

Social relationships.

- *Who can you count on to help you if you are upset or feeling down?*

Support systems and important relationships.

- *Do you ever feel sad, blue, or depressed? Are you generally pretty happy?*

Mood symptoms.

- *Have you ever felt so bad that you wished you were dead/never born/not alive/you could be somewhere else? Do you think about dying, ending your life, or killing yourself?*

Suicidal thoughts and further questions about suicidal behaviors are required.

- *Are you picked on in school? Do other kids call you names or make fun of you?*

Possibility of being bullied.

- *Has anything happened to you that has been so frightening or terrible it is difficult to talk or think about?*

Possibility of exposure to trauma.

- *Do people ever say that you seem not to listen to them, or that you are spacey? Do people ever say that it's hard for you to finish things you start, or to follow directions?*

Symptoms of attention-deficit/hyperactivity disorder.

- *Do you ever get into trouble because you act before you think?*

Impulsivity.

- *Do you worry about things a lot? What kinds of things do you worry about? When do you worry?*

Possibility of anxiety.

- *How have you adjusted to starting school, new schools, or new school years? How do you do in school? How are your grades? How do you get along with your teacher? How do you get along with the other children?*

School functioning and how transitions are managed.

- *If you could have three wishes for anything in the world, what would you wish for?*

Part of the child's current mental status examination and a sense of the child's stated desires.

Note: These are suggested questions, not inclusive of all problems, and should not be thought of as the only way to gather history from the child. In general, open-ended questions allow the relationship between the clinician and child to develop, and these specific questions are offered as guidance. The goal should be to let the clinical assessment flow naturally, and not to be perceived as interrogative.

hitting one's own body. Observations should be made about the child's ability to sit still, level of attentiveness or distractibility, and any mannerisms or habits that may be present, such as hand wringing, nail biting, or thumb sucking. Note whether the child can regulate his or her own behavior or whether he or she requires considerable structure.

Relatedness

When assessing the child's relatedness to the interviewer, it is important to keep in mind the level of anxiety that is often present in the initial evaluation session. However, most children make meaningful contact with the interviewer if they are given enough time. If this does not occur, it might signal the presence of a pervasive developmental disorder (PDD) or an anxiety disorder. Consider the length of time required for the child to warm up and his or her responsiveness to reassurance, both of which may constitute important temperamental features. Relatedness is described according to the child's ability to maintain eye contact, establish rapport, and engage in meaningful play or dialogue with the interviewer.

Speech and language

Speech is the actual production of words. Language is the entire process of understanding communication and expressing one's thoughts and ideas. Speech should be evaluated for stuttering or other phonologic problems. Note the volume and quality of speech and whether it is loud, soft, whining, or monotonal. Also note the child's fluency and competence in English, as well as whether he or she speaks other languages. Language has both verbal and nonverbal components. Both expressive and receptive language should be assessed (American Academy of Child and Adolescent Psychiatry, 1998). Pointing to pictures and drawing can be useful techniques in the assessment of receptive language in a child with expressive language problems.

Mood and affect

Mood is defined as the internal emotional state of a person (that is how the person feels). It is often helpful to ask the child to describe his general mood. If that does not elicit a response, providing examples of moods such as mad, sad, or happy can be helpful. With young children it may be helpful to draw or point to pictures that describe these feelings. Affect is the overall expression of the present emotional content (how the person presents himself to another individual). The description of the child's affect should include an assessment of the range of affect, its appropriateness to the situation, its quality, and its intensity. A child may look frightened or display a constricted range of affect during the early part of the interview, but as he or she relaxes, his or her affect may be more complete and appropriate.

Thought process and content

The process of thought is evaluated through the child's spontaneous verbalizations and through play. Some children may initially be reluctant to talk, but have no difficulty drawing or playing. If a child is given items such as paper and pencil or crayons, or a doll house with figures, the play that follows may be indicative of the child's inner world. The thought process is described according to the coherence, goal-directedness, logic, rate, and sequence of thoughts. In adolescents, thought process can usually be assessed directly. However, it must often be inferred from the logic and coherence of a younger child's imaginative play. For example, if a child is playing with family figures in a doll house, it is important to see whether there is an identifiable beginning, middle, and end to the story-telling or play. Of course, the child's developmental level has an impact on his ability to present a coherent story.

The content of the child's thoughts includes what he or she chooses to talk about as well as any fantasies that may be enacted. Fantasies may be inferred from the child's drawings or play, but they are best learned from what the child actually says about his or her productions. A variety of open-ended, projective techniques can be useful. For example, the physician can ask the child to describe three wishes he or she would make, or special powers he or she would want to have if the interviewer had the power to grant them. Suicidal or homicidal ideation is noted here, and all pertinent details should be asked and described, such as motive, the nature of a plan, whether any action has been taken to execute the plan if there is one. (Additional details about evaluating the suicidal child can be obtained from the practice parameters of the American Academy of Child and Adolescent Psychiatry, 2001a). If the child describes behavior or thoughts about self-harm or harm to others, safety is of paramount concern.

The child's reality testing should be assessed, and the presence of delusions or perceptual disturbances should be noted (for assessment of schizophrenia, see American Academy of Child and Adolescent Psychiatry, 2001b). There are many ways to assess reality. Children can be asked about ideas they may have that other people do not believe. They can be asked whether they feel they have special powers or whether they think that people are purposely out to get them. The presence of any perceptual disturbances, such as auditory or visual hallucinations, or any other unusual sensory phenomena should also be assessed. When asking children about hallucinations, it may be helpful to say, "Some children hear voices (or see things) that other people don't. Does that ever happen to you?" or, "Are there ever times when your eyes or ears seem to play tricks on you?" It is important to distinguish hallucinations from illusions (an illusion is a misperception of a real, bona-fide external stimulus). One can ask, "Have you ever thought you saw something but it was really something else?" Note the timing of hallucinations if they are present, and determine whether they are related to sleep, stressors, or particular events. If the child's reality testing seems impaired, question him about how firmly the beliefs are held and about the possibility that these ideas are pretend or make-believe.

However, care must be taken before labeling a child psychotic because some aspects of impaired reality testing may be developmentally appropriate. For example, it is often developmentally appropriate for children to have imaginary friends. It is also not unusual for children to have hallucinations or altered sensory perceptions upon falling asleep or awakening, referred to as hypnagogic or hypnopompic hallucinations, respectively. Finally, many children who report hallucinations have language problems and should not be viewed as psychotic. Psychotic symptoms are rare in prepubertal children.

Cognitive and developmental assessment

The evaluation of cognitive function should include an assessment of the child's general fund of knowledge, memory, reasoning ability, vocabulary, and conceptualization ability. These assessments should reflect the child's age and developmental level. A variety of techniques, such as the use of vocabulary, level of comprehension, curiosity, digit span, and drawing ability, can be used. The cognitive exam should include the evaluation of age-appropriate developmental skills. Can the child copy shapes such as a circle, square, or triangle at ages 3, 4, and 5, respectively? What is the child's fund of knowledge? Does the child know colors or body parts? How is language development proceeding? How well developed are fine and gross motor function? Psychometric tests may also provide useful information about cognition, but testing is expensive and not readily available in some settings. Additionally, whereas psychometric testing is required to accurately diagnose a learning disability (by calculating a discrepancy score), the clinical evaluation can often indicate that a learning problem is present.

Diagnostic formulation and treatment planning

Organization of data

After all the relevant informants have been contacted and interviewed, and after the history has been supplemented with appropriate reports, rating scales, and laboratory tests, the physician must synthesize the information into a working diagnosis. The physician should begin by considering whether a general medical condition that could account for the presenting problem is present before making a psychiatric diagnosis. The range of normal developmental deviation should also be considered. In children who do have a psychiatric diagnosis, symptoms of multiple conditions may be present. In such cases, all relevant diagnoses need to be recorded. For example, a child may have ADHD and a developmental reading disorder.

It is often useful to develop an initial working assessment and differential diagnosis while the history is being gathered. For example, if after talking with the parents the physician suspects that the child may have a disruptive behavior disorder, a subsequent conversation with the child's teacher can be used to ask specific questions about the child's school behavior and attentional performance. In this way, the physician can better determine whether the child meets criteria for ADHD or for conduct disorder (CD) or oppositional defiant disorder. Establishing a working diagnosis is important because it allows the physician to use deductive reasoning while taking the history or writing it up.

Formulation

The diagnostic formulation provides an opportunity to develop a comprehensive framework for understanding a child's symptomatic presentation in the context of his strengths, risk factors, and life events. Additionally, it allows the physician to describe the severity of the disorder and the level of function. As a general rule, the physician's formulation should follow the biopsychosocial model, which stresses that biologic, psychologic, and social factors all be taken into account when studying the emergence of the psychopathologic condition. The formulation section of the case summary need only be a paragraph long, but it is the only place for the physician to integrate all the information that has been gathered. The formulation should always provide a statement regarding the current developmental status, but it may also include a summary of the hypothesized source of the psychiatric problems that are observed, the coping and adaptive mechanisms of the child, and the adequacy of family and social supports.

Treatment plan

In current psychiatric practice, the cause of a disorder cannot necessarily be inferred from the diagnosis. Treatment practices are often not specific to particular diagnoses, but are becoming more so with evidence-based practices. However, the combination of the diagnosis, the overall level of functioning, and the modifying effects of risk and protective factors can be used to develop a specific treatment plan appropriate to the child's problem (see Chapter 4 which reviews treatment planning in greater detail).

The treatment plan is an individualized recommendation for care. The goal of the treatment plan is to facilitate the child's development and alleviate symptoms. For the treatment plan to succeed, both the primary caregiver and the child need to be included in the process so they understand the plan and are willing to participate in its implementation. A child's ability to participate depends on a variety of factors such as the age of the child and the nature of the plan. When constructing a treatment plan, all the relevant data from the assessment should first be incorporated into a comprehensive, multidimensional problem list. Each entry on this list should point to a target intervention; multiple treatment modalities are often required. The specifics of the plan depend on the nature and severity of the impairment, as well as a variety of mediating factors. Unfortunately, it is not always feasible for the optimal treatment plan to be enacted. There may be constraints on any one of numerous levels. These should be anticipated as much as possible when preparing the treatment plan and discussed in realistic terms with the family. Financial resources need to be considered, since treatment recommendations that do not correspond to a family's economic circumstances are not likely to be employed.

Psychiatric diagnosis in children and adolescents

The development of a comprehensive nosology for psychiatric disorders in children is a relatively recent phenomenon, although tremendous gains have been made since the publication of the *Diagnostic and Statistical Manual of Mental Disorders*, third edition (DSM-III) in 1980. DSM employs a multiaxial system consisting of five parts. It encourages the use of more than one diagnosis when appropriate and provides a format for recording information about the context of disorders and general level of impairment, as well as for the description of symptoms. Axis I is used to describe clinical syndromes such as disruptive behavior disorders, mood and anxiety disorders, specific and pervasive developmental disorders, and other conditions that may be a focus of clinical attention but do not represent a psychiatric disorder (for example, conditions such as parent-child relational problem and bereavement). Axis II is used to record mental retardation or personality disorders. (Personality disorders are often not diagnosed in children and adolescents, but there may be traits present, particularly in adolescents.) Axis III is used to code general medical conditions, and axis IV helps the physician describe the psychosocial and environmental context with respect to the illness. Examples include parental divorce or chronic medical illness in the child. Axis V is used to code the global assessment of functioning. The child is rated on a scale of 1 to 100 on social, occupational (school), and psychologic functioning, where 100 describes superior functioning and 1 signifies seriously impaired functioning. A score of less than 60–70 is most often consistent with the presence of a psychiatric diagnosis (<60 is clear evidence and <70 represents a "possible case").

As in previous editions, the fourth edition of DSM (DSM-IV TR; American Psychiatric Association, 2000) begins with a chapter devoted to disorders that begin in infancy, childhood, and adolescence. The following disorders are included in that section: mental retardation, learning disorders, motor skills disorders, communication disorders, pervasive developmental disorders (such as autistic disorder and Asperger's disorder), attention-deficit and other disruptive behavior disorders (such as conduct disorder and oppositional defiant disorder), feeding and eating disorders of infancy or early childhood, tic disorders, elimination disorders, and others such as separation anxiety disorder (SAD), selective mutism, and reactive attachment disorder of infancy or early childhood. However, many disorders described in other sections of the manual may also be present in children and adolescents. These include mood and anxiety disorders, schizophrenia, somatoform disorders, and eating disorders. Therefore, it is important that physicians who work with children and adolescents do not restrict themselves to the so-called "child disorders" section. Additionally, physicians who work with adults would be well served to familiarize themselves with the disorders that first appear in childhood, since many of these persist into adulthood. The following paragraphs briefly describe the diagnostic categories most often used with children and adolescents. Section 2 of this book reviews most of these conditions in greater detail.

Disorders of development and attachment are most often present at an early age. Examples include mental retardation, pervasive developmental disorders, and reactive attachment disorder. Mental retardation is defined as general intellectual functioning that is significantly below average. It is coded on axis II, and it is separated into mild, moderate, severe, and profound subgroups based on the degree of intellectual impairment defined by the IQ and the level of adaptive functioning. An IQ score below 65–70 (that is, two standard deviations below the mean) is the upper limit of mental retardation. Parallel impairments in adaptive functioning are also required to fulfill the criteria.

The PDDs are defined by impairments in reciprocal social interaction and communication and by a restricted range of behavior, interests, and activities (see Chapter 5). Autistic disorder, Asperger's disorder, Rett's disorder, childhood disintegrative disorder, and pervasive developmental disorder not otherwise specified (PDD-NOS) are all identified. Children with these disorders exhibit varying abnormalities of language function that may profoundly affect their abilities to communicate with others and to make their wishes and needs known. There is also a qualitative impairment in reciprocal social interaction and relatedness, even, with primary caregivers. Additionally, these children often have an inability to play symbolically, so pretend play is limited or nonexistent. Stereotyped movements such as hand flapping or head banging may be present, or there may be a fascination with parts of objects, such as the wheels on toy cars. There is often, but not always, an associated degree of mental retardation in individuals with autistic disorder (approximately two-thirds have an IQ below 70). The onset of autistic disorder is usually evident in the first years of life and, by definition, occurs before age 3.

Reactive attachment disorder is another disorder that is present in preschool children. The features of this disorder begin before a child is 5 years old with disturbed and developmentally inappropriate social relatedness (for example, a child may be overly friendly with strangers or withdrawn). By definition, the unrelatedness is associated with patho-

genic care of the child. Children who come to the physician with failure to thrive without a medical cause often qualify for this diagnosis.

There are more diagnostic categories that may apply to the school-age child. The most prominent among these are ADHD (see Chapter 7) and disruptive behavior disorders. However, a variety of cognitive and learning disorders, such as specific developmental or communication disorders, may also become apparent at this age. ADHD is a disorder characterized by a pattern of inattention and hyperactivity-impulsivity that is excessive relative to the behavior of other children of the same age and gender. Children with this disorder may have difficulty remaining seated, waiting their turn, completing assignments, sustaining attention, or organizing their work. By definition, some of these symptoms must be present before a child reaches 7 years of age, and there must be some symptoms causing impairment in more than one setting (for example, at home, at school, or in other activities). ADHD often begins in preschool years and commonly extends into adolescence or adulthood, but the largest number of cases can be found in school-age children. Individuals with this disorder are commonly both inattentive and hyperactive-impulsive, although a smaller number of children may have disturbances in only one of these domains. Many children with ADHD show symptoms of aggression and defiance; comorbid learning, behavior, mood, and anxiety disorders are often present. However, although these conditions may coexist with ADHD, they must be distinguished from it. When multiple disorders are present, they should all be diagnosed.

Oppositional defiant disorder (ODD) and conduct disorder (CD) (see Chapter 8) are the other disruptive behavior disorders listed in DSM-IV. ODD is defined by the presence of persistent minor violations of age-appropriate social norms. Children with ODD often argue with adults, lose their temper, refuse to follow rules, deliberately annoy people, and blame others for their actions. They are often angry and resentful. Exclusionary criteria for this disorder include the presence of a psychotic, mood, or conduct disorder. CD is a behavior pattern in which the basic rights of others or major age-appropriate societal norms are violated. Examples include aggression directed toward people and animals, destruction of property, deceitfulness or theft, and serious violation of rules. This diagnosis takes precedence over ODD if criteria for both diagnoses are met, since approximately 90% of children with CD also meet criteria for ODD. There is good evidence that ODD represents a developmental precursor to CD in a subgroup of children.

Learning disorders (see Chapter 6) are defined by academic functioning that is significantly below what is expected for an individual's chronologic age, measured intelligence, and age-appropriate education. These disorders may involve deficits in reading, mathematics, and written expression. The accurate diagnosis of learning disorders requires the use of standardized intelligence and achievement tests to establish a discrepancy score. (That is, the score on a standardized achievement test is below what would be expected from the level of intellectual functioning as measured on a standardized IQ test.)

The communication disorders, which are characterized by difficulties in speech or language, include expressive language disorder, mixed receptive-expressive language disorder, phonologic disorder, and stuttering. Communication disorders often appear in preschool years, but they may not be properly identified until the child is in a school setting. Expressive language disorder is characterized by lower than expected abilities in vocabulary, use of tenses, production of complex sentences, and word recall. Mixed receptive-expressive language disorder involves an impaired understanding of language and a concomitant difficulty with expressive language. Phonologic disorder consists of errors in sound production and substitutions or omissions of sounds that would be developmentally expected. Stuttering is a disturbance of the fluency and time patterning of speech.

Several types of tic disorders are listed in DSM-IV. The most common is transient tic disorder, which involves the transient presentation of single or multiple motor or vocal tics. A tic is a sudden, rapid, recurrent, non-rhythmic, stereotyped movement or vocalization. Tics may be simple or complex. Tourette syndrome is the least common but most dramatic of the tic disorders. The diagnosis is made when there is a history of multiple motor tics and at least one vocal tic. The average age of onset of tics is 7 years. Approximately 40–50% of children with Tourette syndrome in clinical samples also have symptoms of ADHD. Tourette syndrome is also often comorbid with obsessive-compulsive disorder (OCD). However, it is not clear to what extent Tourette syndrome causes impairment in nonreferred samples, since referral bias as a function of psychiatric comorbidity is not uncommon. (That is, cases with comorbidity and cases of greater impairment are more likely to be referred for treatment.)

Enuresis and encopresis comprise the elimination disorders in DSM-IV. These disorders have a minimum age threshold defined by the child's chronologic age or equivalent developmental level. Encopresis is the repeated passage of feces in inappropriate places by a child who is at least 4 years old. Enuresis is the repeated voiding of urine into the bed or clothes by a child who is at least 5 years old.

Separation anxiety disorder (see Chapter 9) is a condition in which there is developmentally inappropriate and extreme anxiety about separation from home, parents, or primary caregivers. This is the most common anxiety disorder in childhood. It can have such symptoms as school avoidance or phobia, sleep disturbance, and nightmares. This disorder commonly follows an acute life event such as the medical illness of the child or parent, the loss of a close family member, parental separation, or the birth of a new sibling. Most often, separation anxiety disorder lasts for a limited time and good return to normal function results from the use of simple behavioral measures and encouragement. However, some children develop more chronic symptoms and impairment.

Disorders that are also diagnosed in children and adolescents that are not described in the childhood section of DSM-IV include schizophrenia and other psychotic disorders, mood disorders, other anxiety disorders [such as obsessive compulsive disorder and generalized anxiety disorder (GAD)], eating disorders, substance use disorders, and gender identity disorder. Schizophrenia (see Chapter 12) is phenotypically similar in children and adults, although children may have a less pronounced onset of symptoms and may not meet the full criteria for months or years after they are first brought to a physician. Children with schizophrenia have blunted or inappropriate affect, isolation, withdrawal, auditory and visual hallucinations, and thought disorders. There is some indication that the "negative symptoms" (such as thought disorder and isolation) predominate over the "positive symptoms" (such as hallucinations and delusions). However, the only diagnostic criterion that actually differs in children is that they may fail to reach expected levels of social and academic functioning (rather than deteriorate from a predetermined level). Schizophrenia is rare before puberty and must be aggressively distinguished from the PDDs, developmental language disorders, and mood disorders (depression and bipolar disorders) when it occurs in this age group.

Since the 1980s, there has been considerable interest in the subject of mood disorders in children and adolescents (see Chapter 10). Even though it is now recognized that children of all ages can develop depression and often show the same symptoms as adults, major depressive disorder (MDD) is not as common in young children as in adolescents and adults. There are only minor differences in the diagnostic criteria for the mood disorders in children and adolescents when compared with adults. Associated changes in a depressed child or adolescent include social withdrawal, academic decline, oppositional behavior and noncompliance. A child or adolescent with MDD may have an irritable rather than depressed mood, and he may fail to make expected weight gain instead of having a significant weight loss. In children or adolescents with dysthymic disorder, the mood may again be irritable rather than depressed, and the duration of the mood need only be 1 year, as compared with 2 years for adults. Even though there are no differences in the criteria for bipolar disorder as a function of age, it can be much more challenging to diagnose bipolar disorder in children and the presentation can more typically include irritability, tantrums, and agitation. Again, whereas bipolar disorder can exist in prepubertal children, it is not often present in its typical form until after puberty.

The "adult" anxiety disorders include panic disorder, specific phobias, social phobia, obsessive-compulsive disorder, posttraumatic stress disorder (PTSD), acute stress disorder, and generalized anxiety disorder. Anxiety disorders (see Chapter 9) may be present in children and adolescents as well as in adults, and they do not appear to be particularly different in children. OCD is characterized by recurrent intrusive thoughts or behaviors. OCD symptoms often have their onset in childhood or adolescence, although the specific disorder may not be identified for several years. Common signs of OCD in children are excessive hand washing and avoidance of supposedly contaminated objects.

Adolescents may have any of the disorders that begin in childhood, or they may have the initial onset of any of the disorders commonly seen in adults. Developmental differences related to a psychopathologic condition must be considered. For example, ADHD is often seen in adolescents, but there are usually fewer hyperactivity and impulsivity symptoms than in the school-aged child. Symptoms of several of the personality disorders may become clinically apparent in the adolescent period, although they are not usually diagnosed until an adolescent reaches 18 years of age. Disorders that are common in adolescents include the eating disorders, anorexia nervosa and bulimia nervosa, and the substance-related disorders (see Chapter 14). These include disorders of drug use and abuse. They may involve the use of alcohol, cannabis, cocaine, or other substances. Substance abuse is defined as substance use that interferes with a person's capacity to meet obligations in work, school, or home that results in a physically dangerous situation, legal problems, or continued use despite recurrent problems. Substance dependence pre-empts a diagnosis of abuse. Dependence involves a long-standing pattern of abuse that shows tolerance, withdrawal, and a lack of control over the substance.

The eating disorders (see Chapter 11) involve severe disturbances in eating behavior and perceptions of body shape and weight. These disorders have received considerable attention since the late 1970s, and there has been a resultant increase in case identification. Anorexia nervosa is the refusal to maintain a minimally normal body weight accompanied by an unshakable fear of gaining weight or becoming fat. Bulimia nervosa involves repeated episodes of binge eating and purging behavior in an attempt to control weight gain. Self-induced vomiting, use of laxatives or diuretics, and compulsive exercising may all be seen. The most common age of onset of anorexia nervosa is in the mid-teenage years, and the disorder is much more common in females. Bulimia nervosa has a later age of onset and often begins in the late teens or the 20s. Both disorders may be characterized by serious medical complications and comorbid psychopathologic conditions.

Child psychiatry and the primary care physician

Recently, there has been increasing interest in the role of the primary care physician in the arena of child and adolescent mental health. This is important, because there are few child and adolescent psychiatrists relative to the number of children in need and because the vast majority of children see a primary care physician. The primary care physician is well suited for screening and early intervention in children's mental health problems (see Pearls & perils, below left). Some of these problems may also be treated by primary care physicians, although referral to specialists and collaborative case management is still the norm.

Screening is the process by which the existence of a problem becomes known. To successfully screen for mental health problems, the primary care physician must be able to understand developmentally appropriate skills and functions, recognize major difficulties a child may have in school, social, or family functioning, be aware of major psychiatric syndromes, ask about the presence of symptoms, and investigate events that are known to be stressful to the child and family. Some screening can actually be done in the waiting room by using a parent rating scale such as the Pediatric Symptom Checklist (PSC, Jellinek, 1999), CBCL or Connors parent questionnaire (see Chapter 2). These scales provide a comprehensive profile of developmentally appropriate tasks and a range of psychiatric symptoms, and they allow the physician to note any areas of past or present difficulties. Inquiries should be made at each visit about the child's mental health functioning, level of functioning in age-appropriate activities, and general sense of well-being. Specific areas of functioning to be evaluated are the child's sleep and appetite habits, social skills (such as the presence of friends and participation in groups or clubs), academic and behavioral performance in school, and relationships within the family (how the child gets along with parents and siblings). Screening questions regarding mood and anxiety symptoms, suicidal or homicidal thoughts, and hallucinations should be included in each contact and can be helpful in identifying a problem requiring referral.

PEARLS & PERILS

- Efficiently identify children who will need more intensive assessment for potential mental health concerns by using a screening instrument in a primary care physician's waiting room, such as the Pediatric Symptom Checklist.
- Engage the child and family in the mental health assessment by focusing on the whole child. Concern for the child's strengths helps with diagnostic decisions and treatment planning.
- Screening tools should not be used for diagnostic purposes, as improper conclusions and treatments may occur.
- Do not assume that the child's presenting hyperactivity is caused by attention deficit/hyperactivity disorder without identifying other potential causes or comorbidities, such as abuse, anxiety, or learning problems.

The primary care physician is also in a perfect position to make early interventions and manage risk factors when they are present. These interventions may decrease the need for an additional visit to the psychiatrist. Examples of prevention or early intervention services well suited to primary care settings include parenting classes for parents of infants and toddlers, dissemination of information regarding management of common behavior problems, and providing directive parental counseling for the management of specific problems. Teaching parents techniques they can use to manage behavior problems, such as ignoring a tantrum rather than giving in (so as not to reinforce the behavior), can be reassuring to parents, especially if techniques are discussed in a conversational and nonjudgmental manner.

There are many types of events that may place a child at increased risk for behavioral or psychiatric problems. Primary care physicians should be alerted to the possible consequences of these events. Some of the more common are parental divorce or separation, a death in the family, a move to a new home or school, a change in the parent's employment status, or a medical illness of the child or a family member. The occurrence of such events can be determined during the beginning of a routine visit by asking open-ended questions about the family's circumstances. If significant events or changes in the family are identified, more specific questions can be asked. Once a profile of risk is elicited, supportive management techniques can often help alleviate more significant problems.

There can be no simple rule about when to refer. Some pediatricians are comfortable managing certain conditions, but they are more likely to refer others to a specialist (see Consider consultation when …). The primary care physician needs to know when a problem is interfering with a child's development and functioning, as well as when early

CONSIDER CONSULTATION WHEN ...

Problem	Manifestation	Whom to consult
Developmental delays	Failure to achieve expected milestones in language, motor, social functions	Developmental pediatrician, neurologist, psychologist, language or learning specialist
Disruptions in early childhood caregiving relationships	Poor eye contact or relatedness, problems with nurturance, abnormal feeding behavior, delayed growth	Psychiatrist, psychologist, early intervention program
Exposure to trauma	Family violence, child or spouse abuse, experience of major loss	Psychiatrist, psychologist
Suicidal or self-injurious behavior	Suicidal thoughts, intent or attempts	Psychiatrist
Severe aggression, dangerous to others	Serious threats; assaultive behavior	Psychiatrist
Significant medical problems or seizure disorders	Some medical problems present with increased frequency in psychiatric patients; or must be ruled out in the case of suspected psychiatric disturbance	Medical specialist, neurologist, psychiatrist, psychologist
Significant learning/academic problems	Underachievement, poor motivation	Local department of education/special education, neuropsychologists, learning specialists, tutor
Psychotic symptoms	Paranoia, delusions, hallucinations, disordered thinking	Psychiatrist (following medical assessment)
Bullying or being bullied	Actual peer abuse or threats; school phobia	Psychiatrist, psychologist, guidance counselor
Attention problems/hyperactivity	Inability to focus, developmentally excessive motor activity, impulsivity	Neuropsychologist, neurologist, psychiatrist, psychologist, educational counselor
Disruptive behavior	Defiance of authority, rule violations, minor aggression	Psychologist, psychiatrist
Mood dysregulation	Depression, mania or hypomania, mood lability	Psychologist, psychiatrist
Anxiety	Separation problems, overanxious behavior, obsessions, compulsive behavior, social fears	Psychologist, psychiatrist

Note: All of the above behaviors and emotions exist on a spectrum that extends from normality to severe pathology. The presence of some symptomatology does not necessarily imply the presence of a psychiatric disorder or diagnosis. However, when problems are suspected, referral to a mental health specialist is often indicated. Also note that the range of mental health specialists often varies by community. Here, we specify psychiatrists and psychologists as primary mental health professionals to whom to refer. However, in some communities these functions are performed by social workers, nurse practitioners, and other professionals.

intervention has not been successful. In this case, referral for more extensive treatment is generally appropriate. Once a referral has been made, it is essential that there be collaboration between the primary care physician and the mental health specialist. This contact maximizes the likelihood that the referral will be successfully negotiated by the patient and family.

Summary

The psychiatric assessment of children and adolescents is a complex process. However, it can be made less intimidating when a basic framework is followed. The components of the examination include meeting with the parents and the child to gather a complete history, obtaining the mental status examination of the child, developing a treatment plan, and presenting the results of the evaluation to the family. Yet within this framework, it is necessary to account for individual differences in children and parents, as well as for stylistic differences among physicians. The basic issues that should be addressed in the assessment process are whether the child has a problem that significantly interferes with his normal development, whether there are problems in social, academic, or family functioning, and whether there is effective treatment that will allow the child to reach his potential free of interference from psychiatric morbidity. More effective recognition

of mental health problems in children is needed, and closer collaboration between primary care providers and mental health specialists is imperative in this regard.

Annotated bibliography

Cepeda C, MD (1999) *Concise Guide to the Psychiatric Interview of Children and Adolescents*. Arlington VA, Amer Psychiatric Pub Inc.
This comprehensive book describes interviewing children and adolescents, techniques for eliciting information, documenting the mental status examination, and developing a formulation.

King RA (1997) Practice parameters for the psychiatric assessment of children and adolescents. American Academy of Child and Adolescent Psychiatry. *J American Acad Child Adolesc Psychiatry*, 36(Suppl 10):4S–20S.
This review article highlights the state-of-the-art recommended guidelines for assessing children and adolescents.

Morrison JR, Anders TF (2001) *Interviewing Children and Adolescents: Skills and Strategies for Effective DSM-IV Diagnosis*. New York, Guilford.
This is a thorough guide that walks the clinician through the step-by-step process of evaluating the child or adolescent, with guidelines on obtaining relevant information to make a diagnosis based on DSM-IV.

Shaffer D, Lucas CP, Richters JE (eds) (1999) *Diagnostic Assessment in Child and Adolescent Psychopathology*. New York, Guilford.
This is a complete assessment book that focuses on diagnosing specific psychiatric conditions by integrating interviews, rating scales, and medical tests.

CHAPTER 2

Diagnostic Instruments

Aradhana A. Sood, MD and Donald P. Oswald, PhD

Introduction

Psychiatric assessment is both a science and an art, and it is the clinician who has to integrate the two in practice. Many assessment instruments are grounded in empirical research and have robust psychometric properties, well-validated cutoff scores, and computerized scoring and interpretation methods. Others have less of an empirical basis and are more subjective, relying on the clinician's training and experience for interpretation of the findings. Assessment is an art because it involves clinical judgment, an appreciation of the individual within an ecologic context, and the use of intuition to integrate clinical knowledge and data from various assessment instruments. Furthermore, the mere fact that the clinician chooses which assessment instruments should be used to answer specific questions that will lead to a diagnosis and treatment means that a subjective element is introduced in the assessment process. Additionally, the clinician is interested in providing an evaluation of the individual in as efficient yet effective a manner as possible.

The contents and the process of psychiatric assessment were presented in Chapter 1. The goals of this chapter are to briefly present the issues that a physician must address when selecting an instrument, to briefly discuss the various types of diagnostic instruments that are available for clinical use, and to provide an overview of the most commonly used instruments in child and adolescent psychiatry. The instruments are discussed within the context of specific disorders of children and adolescents taken from the *Diagnostic and Statistic Manual of Mental Disorders*, fourth edition (DSM-IV, 2000). They were chosen with the intention of providing clinicians and primary care physicians with a guide to instruments that are of practical use within a clinical context. Some instruments, such as intelligence, achievement, and neuropsychologic tests, are not presented here because

advanced training in psychologic measurement is required before they can be used. Psychiatric clinicians and primary care physicians are advised to refer the child or adolescent to a licensed clinical psychologist for such testing. In this chapter, the term *child* is used to include children and adolescents.

Choosing diagnostic instruments

There are several issues that a physician must consider before selecting a diagnostic instrument or a battery of instruments for use with children and adolescents. Of these, the four most important areas are practical considerations, standardization, reliability, and validity.

Practical considerations

The choice of diagnostic instruments is first and foremost dependent on practical considerations related to both the physician and the patient. Instruments that provide the best clinical picture of the child must be chosen. The usefulness of the instrument depends on the specific questions to be asked and the specific problems of the patient to be solved. Thus, there should be a good match between the selected instruments and the purpose for which they are chosen. It is also important to know whether the physician needs additional training to use the test, or whether the patient should be referred to another professional who is trained to use the instrument (as in the case of an achievement or intelligence test). If a self-report measure is to be used, the physician must be certain that the child's reading level matches the level required by the test. Furthermore, the length of each test is a consideration because time is at a premium and lengthy instruments do not necessarily provide more relevant information than shorter ones.

Standardization

The physician must be certain that the instruments being considered for use have adequate norms for the population that is being assessed. This means that a child's scores on an instrument are meaningful only if there is significant similarity between the child and the sample on which the instrument was standardized. There are three critical issues that merit consideration. First, the sample used to standardize the instrument should be representative of the population that the physician would like to evaluate. Second, the size of the sample used to standardize the instrument should be large enough to give stable estimates of the construct being tested. Small samples have the problem of random fluctuation within the group. Third, the instrument should have broad national norms as well as specialized subgroup norms. The subgroup norms may be based on a number of variables, including gender, age, race, school grade, and living environment (for example, rural vs. urban). Physicians may find that their patients match subgroups better than the overall population on which the instrument was standardized. Thus, subgroup norms may be more appropriate than the national norms for specific children. Additionally, a well-standardized instrument provides a set of administration procedures that the physician must know and adhere to closely.

Reliability

Reliability refers to the extent that the scores obtained by a child on a specific instrument remain the same when the child is tested on different occasions. In technical terms, reliability refers to the degree of stability, consistency, predictability, and accuracy of the scores obtained on diagnostic instruments. Physicians must remember that there is rarely 100% reliability because of natural variation in the child's performance on an instrument. Additionally, psychiatric and psychologic testing methods are imprecise, and many factors are inferred rather than directly measured. There are several types of reliability, including test-retest reliability (repeated administration of the same test with the same child), alternate forms (parallel forms of the same test), split-half reliability (correlation between the two halves of a single test), and inter-rater reliability (administration of the same test by two or more clinicians). Current consensual agreement is that a reliability of over 70% is acceptable, although many physicians expect about 90% reliability on pivotal tests used for making treatment decisions. Data on reliability are presented in the administration manual of an instrument.

Validity

From the psychiatrist's perspective, validity is probably the most important aspect of an instrument. That is, does the instrument measure what it purports to measure, and does it provide clinically useful information? A valid instrument reliably measures the variable that it is intended to measure. Validity is established by correlating the test scores with some external, independently observed event. There are three ways of establishing validity: content validity (how well the instrument covers the major aspects of the content area being measured), criterion validity (how well the scores on this instrument correlate with other instruments or procedures that measure the same variable), and construct validity (the extent to which the instrument measures the variable of interest). Clinicians may also be interested in incremental validity, or the ability of an instrument to produce new information.

Clinical judgment

Regardless of the scientific basis of the instruments used, it is the clinician who has to synthesize the information, and thereby the very important element of clinical judgment is introduced into the evaluation process. Astute clinical judgment is required at all phases of assessment and particularly during data gathering and data synthesis. During data gathering, it is essential that the physician develops an optimum level of rapport with the child if the data to be obtained are to be reliable and valid. Additionally, the physician should be aware of possible factors that may make a child's responses unrepresentative of his typical behavior. Such factors may include transient conditions (such as test anxiety or lack of sleep) and conscious or unconscious faking.

The physician should also be conscious of the fact that he or she is influenced by various cultural and personal factors and that the questions he or she asks during unstructured and semistructured interviews may be influenced by factors other than those related to the child. Data gathering and data analysis are interactive processes that are guided by the child's response, as well as the clinician's clinical judgment and theoretical orientation. Therefore, bias is introduced at several points, including during the choice of instruments, in the questions asked, in the initial impressions of the psychiatrist, in the level of rapport, in the psychiatrist's theoretical assumptions, and in the weight given to information obtained through different sources (for example, the child's vs. the parent's response, or direct observations vs. teacher reports).

When all the data have been gathered and analyzed, the physician has to judge what the data show. The accuracy of this judgment may be compromised if the physician fails to take into account the base rate of the disorder in question (that is, the rate at which the particular disorder occurs in the general population of children) or the developmental level of the child. Furthermore, the data must be interpreted within the ecologic and cultural contexts of the child variables that have not received enough emphasis in the past. A child's behavior does not occur in a vacuum. Thus, it is imperative that the context in which the behavior occurs (such as family, school, and community contexts) is considered in the clinical judgment. Physicians can increase the accuracy of their clinical judgments by combining different methods of data gathering (for example, interviews and formal assessment) and by following statistical interpretive rules. The fact that physicians feel confident about the accuracy of their clinical judgments does not necessarily lead to more accurate clinical judgments. Indeed, as physicians increase their knowledge and experience, they typically show less confidence in their clinical judgments.

Ecologic context of assessment

The social ecology of the child is an important consideration in psychiatric assessment because a child's behavior operates in a dynamic relationship with his environment. Inherent in this view is the emphasis that a child's behavior is shaped by and interacts with the social contexts and physical environments in which his or her behavior occurs. The general principle is the interrelatedness of all phenomena. Thus, the physician should realize that making a change in the behavior of a child inevitably leads to a change in not only other aspects of the child's behavior but also in aspects of his or her social and physical environments.

This poses a unique problem in assessment, since no battery of instruments can encompass the totality of a child's social ecology. However, an approximation can be made by using an ecobehavioral approach to assessment. This approach provides a methodology for describing the interactions and influences that occur among individuals, their internal states, their behavior, and their physical and social settings. In traditional assessment practices, these contextual conditions are often viewed as confounding variables, or noise, but our view is that greater emphasis on these variables during assessment provides a closer approximation of the nature of a child's problems.

In practice, this involves gathering a wide variety of peripherally related data on the child (such as age, race, gender, school, grade level, history of mental illness, and achievement scores) and family (for example, race, age, family income, parents' education level, family size, source of referral, area of residence, parental mental health, and an index of socioeconomic disadvantage). Similarly, if the child is in school, a number of school variables may need to be considered, including the instructional environment, a record of the child's school history, and the teacher's expectations and standards for the children in the target child's class. Although it is not possible to comprehensively characterize the child's ecologic context, physicians should attempt to gather sufficient contextual information to be able to interpret assessment findings with integrity.

KEY CLINICAL QUESTIONS

- *How anxious was your child about coming to this visit? How well rested is your child or how well did your child sleep last night? Are there any stressors at home or school? What are the expectations of your child's teachers? What are your family's expectations?*

  It is important to assess how well the information that is obtained on the rating scales corresponds to the overall clinical impression. Clinical impressions generally take precedence, but discrepancies between clinical impressions and parent or child self-reports should be carefully explored. Environmental influences must be considered when interpreting results from rating instruments. Several stressors at home or school can influence the accuracy of responses, and unstructured, chaotic environments, variable expectations, or inconsistent parenting can influence behavior as well as the accuracy of assessment instruments.

- *Does your child have any difficulty reading? Does your child have difficulty understanding what he reads? Does your child have any difficulty understanding directions?*

  The accuracy of data obtained from rating scales is dependent upon the competence and cooperation of the patient or other respondent. The accuracy of patient reports is especially important for self report instruments.

Types of instruments used with children and adolescents

The types of diagnostic instruments used with children and adolescents are the same as those used for adults: structured interviews, checklists and rating scales, direct behavioral observations, intelligence and achievement tests, physiologic tests, neuropsychologic tests, and projective personality tests. As the diagnostic criteria for psychiatric disorders have been developed and refined, diagnostic instruments are increasingly based on the International Classification of Diseases (ICD) and *Diagnostic and Statistical Manual of Mental Disorders* (DSM) diagnostic classification systems. However, there has been an unevenness in the development of instruments for assessing various psychiatric disorders. There are several types of instruments for some disorders and very few for others. Further, just because many instruments are available for a disorder, it is not necessary to use them all. Certainly, it would be an overkill to use each type of diagnostic instrument listed with any one child at any one time. The selection of instruments should be guided by the questions being asked rather than by the availability of well-validated instruments.

Diagnostic instruments suitable for use with children and adolescents may be designed to assess several disorders or a specific disorder. Furthermore, there are some measures that provide a broad range of data on sociodemographic and ecobehavioral constructs that affect the child's behavior and

Assessments

- Assessment is always undertaken within an eco-logic context; be wary of assessments that do not specify the parameters of this context.
- Assessment instruments must be chosen to answer specific questions.
- Assessment instruments must have good psycho-metric properties, such as validity and reliability, to be useful.
- Assessment instruments should have adequate norms for the target population.
- Even the best quantitative assessments can be meaningless unless they are artfully interpreted by the physician with reference to each child within his or her environmental context.
- Any assessment instrument may be culturally bi-ased; choose instruments that have been validated on the target population.
- All phenomena are interrelated and are constantly changing; an assessment is a snapshot that is an-chored in time and therefore less accurate with the passage of time. Be wary of dated assessments.

are of interest to the physician because they characterize the environmental context in which the child functions. In this chapter, we briefly discuss instruments that provide a broad range of diagnostic data, and then we discuss disorder-specific instruments.

General instruments

Diagnostic interviews

For the physician, the diagnostic interview is the most important source of data on the child. Data that are often unobtainable through formal testing can be collected efficiently with this procedure. The diagnostic interview gathers information about the nature and history of the child's problem, level of adjustment, and child and family strengths. The interview allows the physician to collect diagnostic information and to uncover unique aspects of the child's history in a natural, flexible, and open-ended manner. Even though the interview format has many strengths, it has been criticized with regard to reliability and validity, particularly when it is used as the sole basis to diagnose a child's problems. The two most important factors contributing to the lack of diagnostic reliability are differences between physicians in the amount and kind of information obtained during diagnostic interviews, and differences between physicians in their use of inclusionary and exclusionary criteria when translating interview findings into a psychiatric diagnosis. To address these problems, researchers have developed explicit criteria and classification schemes, as well as structured interviews

that include standardized questions for systematically eliciting data from both children and adults.

In a structured interview, the sequence and specific wording of questions are prescribed by the instrument. It serves as a method to obtain diagnostic information in a standardized manner. Most of the diagnosis-generating interviews – e.g. the Diagnostic Interview for Children and Adolescents-Revised (DICA-R) and the Diagnostic Interview Schedule for Children-Revised (DISC-R) – fall into this category of instruments. The advantage of using structured interviews is that a person with little or no training in mental health can be trained in a short time to reliably and inexpensively gather clinical information. Additionally, some structured interviews can be administered and scored by computer. Disadvantages of these instruments include their length and their tendency to be overinclusive.

Interviews that are semistructured by design also specify the content and items that are to be included, but they provide more flexibility in terms of wording and the sequence of the interview. They are designed to be conducted by clinicians who are well versed in diagnostic issues in children and adolescents because they allow the interviewer to probe the child to obtain more sensitive and more detailed data. Thus, semistructured interviews require some clinical judgment throughout the interview process.

While structured and semistructured interviews provide a method for gathering diagnostic information in a thorough and standardized manner, their practical use may be limited in a busy clinic. However, in some situations clinicians may choose to use specific modules from these interviews to gather data on disorders of interest, and computer algorithm scoring programs can be used for scoring.

Rating scales and behavior checklists

Rating scales have been used for a number of purposes in child and adolescent psychiatry, including the diagnosis and classification of psychiatric disorders, the measurement of severity of psychopathologic conditions, the prediction of the response to treatment, and the evaluation of treatment outcome. Furthermore, rating scales can be classified in terms of the purpose for which they were developed. For example, there are scales to measure psychiatric symptoms, clinical impairment, social functioning, family functioning, and ecobehavioral assessment. Physicians should consider the following variables when selecting a rating scale or checklist: comprehensiveness (how well the subscales cover the areas of interest); mode of administration (self-report or other-report); subgroup norms (norms by age, race, sex, and other characteristics); and psychometric characteristics (reliability and validity).

An ecobehavioral assessment includes consideration of environmental factors as well as child characteristics. Two scales that can contribute to such an assessment include The

Instructional Environment Scale and the Family Environment Scale.

Rating scales are often used to complement the information obtained through diagnostic interviews. They are particularly useful for providing a global measure of the severity of a disorder, as well as for categorizing classes of symptoms. Although a few broad-based diagnostic rating scales are available, most have been designed to provide a rapid assessment of a specific disorder or specific subsets of psychiatric symptoms. Examples of broad-based scales include the Child Behavior Checklist (CBCL), the Conners Parent Rating Scale-Revised, the Conners Teacher Rating Scale-Revised, and the Revised Behavior Problem Checklist (RBPC). Each of these rating scales contains a number of subscales derived through factor analysis that provide information on specific subsets of psychiatric symptoms.

Child Behavior Checklist

Of broad-based diagnostic rating scales, the CBCL (Achenbach and Rescorla, 2001; Achenbach and Edelbrock, 1983) is probably the best-known and most-used rating scale in child and adolescent psychiatry. It consists of 120 items that describe behavior or emotional problems, and these items can be categorized into two broad-band factors (internalizing and externalizing) and eight or nine narrow-band factors or specific scales, depending on the age group used. A recent version of the instrument derives scores on six DSM-oriented scales that address the most common child diagnoses. This is available in parent and teacher versions. The CBCL has excellent reliability and validity, and it can also be used with children from diverse cultures.

Pediatric Symptom Checklist

Recent years have seen the development of brief screening instruments designed to identify emotional and behavioral concerns in children. The Pediatric Symptom Checklist (PSC) (Jellinek, Murphy, and Burns, 1986) is one such screening questionnaire. Consisting of 35 items, the parent-report scale is designed for use in a primary care setting and can be scored quickly by clerical staff. For children whose scores exceed a cutoff, physicians are encouraged to conduct a parent interview that includes a review of major areas of child functioning in order to determine whether a referral for further evaluation is needed. Psychometric data are limited, but initial studies yielded prevalence rates comparable to national estimates.

The Instructional Environment Scale

The Instructional Environment Scale (TIES) (Ysseldyke and Christenson, 1987) was developed to help professionals systematically analyze a student's instructional environment. It can be used to describe the extent to which a child's academic and behavior problems are a function of the instructional environment.

Family Environment Scale

The Family Environment Scale (FES) (Moos and Moos, 1994) is a 90-item scale consisting of 10 subscales that measure the social-environmental characteristics of families in terms of three underlying domains: relationship, personal growth, and system maintenance. The Real Form (Form R) can be used by physicians to measure families' perceptions of their nuclear family environments. This is a widely used scale that has excellent psychometric properties. It can be used to determine the extent to which a child's behavior problems are a function of the family environment.

Self-report instruments

Self-report instruments are used to complement other sources of information, such as rating scales completed by parents and teachers and the physician's own observations. Self-reports offer the physician a peek at the child's perception of reality and conception of her problems. Self-reporting is an essential method for probing into internalized problems, such as depression and anxiety, which involve subjective emotional states of the child. Self-reports can be used to gather information on a range of behaviors or disorders, or they can be used to obtain detailed information on just one problem area. The Youth Self-Report (Achenbach and Rescorla, 2001) is an excellent example of a broad-based self-report that provides information on two competence scales and seven problem scales for adolescents ages 11–18.

The limitations of self-report instruments in general may be even more important when eliciting self-reports from children. These limitations include questions of competence and developmental level (the extent to which the reporter is able to understand and respond to the items), accuracy and social desirability (the extent to which the reporter gives responses that are accurate reflections of her perceptions of reality, uninfluenced by stigma, expectations, and self-presentation factors), and willingness to self-disclose. As a general rule, physicians should be more cautious about relying on self-reports from younger children and children with lower developmental levels. Additionally, the choice of instruments is important, and physicians should be wary of using instruments that do not have adequate psychometric properties or instruments with norms that are not current.

Disorder-specific instruments

Information obtained through diagnostic interviews and physicians' observations can be supplemented with rating scales designed to determine the presence and severity of specific psychiatric disorders. There are a large number of behavior- and disorder-specific instruments that evaluate various aspects of childhood disorders, however, they vary tremendously in terms of their psychometric properties and clinical utility. We focus on commonly used scales that are relatively easy to administer in clinical settings.

Pervasive developmental disorders

Pervasive developmental disorders (PDDs) are characterized by delayed and deviant development of social reciprocity and relatedness, impaired communication, and the presence of repetitive, ritualistic, or stereotyped behaviors. The PDDs included in DSM-IV are autistic disorder, Rett's disorder, childhood disintegrative disorder, Asperger's disorder, and pervasive developmental disorder not otherwise specified (PDD-NOS). We present instruments that focus on autistic disorder and Asperger's disorder. PDD-NOS is not uncommon but is not sufficiently well defined to have yielded structured assessment instruments. Rett's disorder and childhood disintegrative disorder are relatively rare.

CHAT and M-CHAT

The Checklist for Autism in Toddlers (CHAT) (Baron-Cohen and Gillberg, 1992) was developed in the United Kingdom for use by visiting nurses to screen young children for autism. The CHAT consists of nine parent-report items and five items that are administered by the medical professional. Initial studies of the instrument have supported its use as a screening tool. Diana Robins has produced a modified version of the instrument that is entirely parent report with language that is tailored for American consumers. Known as the Modified Checklist for Autism in Toddlers (M-CHAT) (Robins, Fein, Barton, and Green, 2001), the scale has shown promise as a screening device. The M-CHAT is not yet commercially available but is included in Robins et al., 2001.

Social Communication Questionnaire

The Social Communication Questionnaire (SCQ) (Rutter, Bailey, and Lord, 2003) is a screening instrument designed to identify children who may have autism or an autism spectrum disorder. The scale is completed by parents or caregivers and can be used with children who are 4 years of age or older. The SCQ, formerly known as the Autism Screening Questionnaire, is brief enough to use routinely in a primary care setting as a means of identifying children who need further evaluation for an autism spectrum disorder. It has demonstrated good agreement with the Autism Diagnostic Interview-Revised, the gold standard for semistructured parent interviews to diagnose autism spectrum disorders. Published by Western Psychological Services, a Spanish-language form is available.

Childhood Autism Rating Scale

The Childhood Autism Rating Scale (CARS) (Schopler, Reichler, and Renner, 1988) can be used to screen for the presence and severity of autistic disorder and is best used as part of a full diagnostic evaluation. It consists of 15 subscales or

dimensions of behavior that are rated along a seven-point scale and summarized to provide one of three classifications: not autistic, mildly to moderately autistic, or severely autistic. The CARS has good inter-rater reliability and validity in terms of concordance with clinical diagnosis. The CARS can be used in several settings and is based on a number of sources of information (such as a parent interview and direct observations in the clinic, home, and school). Novice interviewers can be trained with relative ease, or the CARS can be used by experienced physicians, teachers, or psychologists in a variety of situations.

Gilliam Asperger's Disorder Scale

The Gilliam Asperger's Disorder Scale (GADS) is a behavior rating scale intended to assist with the diagnosis of individuals in whom Asperger's Disorder is suspected. The instrument comprises 32 items associated with Asperger's disorder characteristics and eight supplemental items related to early development. Suggested uses include assessment of individuals with unique behavior problems, documentation of progress in the treatment of challenging behaviors, identification of individualized education plan (IEP) goals, and measurement of Asperger's disorder for research purposes. The 32 diagnostic characteristic items are divided into four subscales: Social Interaction, Restricted Patterns of Behavior, Cognitive Patterns, and Pragmatic Skills. A composite score, the Asperger's Disorder Quotient, is based on the sum of standard scores from the subscales. The score from the supplemental scale, Early Development, can be omitted in the computation of the Asperger's Disorder Quotient.

Anxiety disorders

Anxiety in children may be assessed through diagnostic interviews, self-report measures, parent and teacher checklists, direct behavioral observations, and physiologic measures (Myers and Winters, 2002). For example, structured and semistructured diagnostic interviews such as the DISC-R, the CAS, the ISC, and the K-SADS can be used for this purpose. We briefly discuss two new semistructured interviews and a few commonly used rating scales developed specifically to assess anxiety disorders in children. Physicians should note that although they are not widely used, parent and teacher ratings can be used to complement self-report measures of anxiety in children. The anxiety or withdrawal subscales of such instruments as the Conners Teacher Rating Scale-Revised, the CBCL, the Teacher Report Form, and the RBPC can be used for this purpose.

Revised Children's Manifest Anxiety Scale

The Revised Children's Manifest Anxiety Scale (RCMAS) (Reynolds and Richmond, 1994) is a widely used, easy-to-read self-report scale for assessing the presence of anxiety in children (ages 6–19). It provides a total score, as well as scores on three factors: physiologic, worry and oversensitivity, and difficulty with concentration. It has excellent reliability, but its validity is not well established.

State-Trait Anxiety Inventory for Children

The State-Trait Anxiety Inventory for Children (STAIC) (Spielberger, 1973) is a 20-statement inventory that consists of two self-report inventories, one for measuring anxiety proneness, or trait anxiety, and the other for measuring transitory anxiety, or state anxiety. It was originally developed for measuring anxiety in children aged 9 to 12, but it can also be used with younger children if they have adequate reading ability. The reliability and validity of the STAIC are well established, and in addition to norms for children in the general population, there are norms for children with emotional disturbance. This is a clinically useful self-report instrument for measuring anxiety in children.

Depression

Structured and semistructured interviews and self-report instruments are most often used to diagnose and assess the severity of depression in children. Peer nomination procedures and projective tests are also available but are less widely used in clinical settings. The two structured interviews (DICA-R and DISC-R) and the three semistructured interviews (CAS, K-SADS, and ISC) have modules on depression that can be used for this purpose. Physicians may find the semistructured interviews more appropriate for their needs because these incorporate clinical judgment and flexibility in the diagnostic process. We briefly present some of the commonly used self-report measures for depression in children.

Children's Depression Inventory

The Children's Depression Inventory (CDI) (Kovacs, 1985; 1992) is a 27-item self-report inventory based on the Beck Depression Inventory that was designed to measure the severity of depression in children aged 8 to 17. It is one of the easiest-to-understand self-report measures of depression because it is written at the third-grade reading level. It has good psychometric properties generally, but some research suggests that the CDI does not discriminate well between depression and other psychiatric conditions in children. Thus, physicians may wish to use the CDI only as a measure of severity of depression in children who have already been diagnosed as being depressed rather than as a diagnostic instrument.

Reynolds Adolescent Depression Scale

The Reynolds Adolescent Depression Scale (RADS) (Reynolds, 2002) is a self-report assessment designed to quickly screen adolescents (grade 7–12; ages 11–20) for significant symptoms of depression and can be used in individual or group assessment. It consists of 30 self-report items and generally takes 5–10 minutes to complete. Reliability and validity studies are adequate. The RADS can be hand scored using a scoring template.

Beck Depression Inventory

The Beck Depression Inventory (BDI) (Beck and Steer, 1993) was designed for use with adults in research and clinical practice, but it has been found to be equally useful with adolescents between the ages of 11 and 18. It has good reliability and validity. The BDI is written at the sixth- to eighth-grade reading level, which may be difficult for many adolescents. Physicians can use the BDI both as a screening instrument and as a measure of severity of depression in adolescents.

Children's Depression Rating Scale-Revised

The Children's Depression Rating Scale-Revised (CDRS-R) (Poznanski and Mokros, 1995) is a clinician-completed rating scale for children aged 6 to 12. The revised scale has good reliability and concordance with psychiatrists' global rating of depression in pediatric and psychiatric inpatients. Physicians can use the CDRS-R to complement self-report scales, especially as a measure of change during treatment.

Suicide rating scales

Suicidal behavior is often a part of Major Depressive Disorder in children and adolescents. The Suicidal Ideation Questionnaire (Reynolds, 1988) can be used to assess suicidal ideation in adolescents, and the Hopelessness Scale for Children (Kazdin, French, Unis, Esveldt-Dawson, and Sherick, 1983) can be used to measure a negative view of the future by children aged 6–13. However, the best information on suicidal behavior in children and adolescents can probably be obtained through a clinical interview. A detailed set of questions on suicidal risk to use in a clinical interview can be found in Pfeffer's 1986 book *The Suicidal Child*.

Attention-deficit/hyperactivity disorder

Structured and semistructured diagnostic interviews can be used to assess children with ADHD. However, additional information derived from other sources, such as direct observations, rating scales, and psychoeducational testing, should be sought before a diagnosis of ADHD is made. Furthermore, given that the behavior of children with ADHD varies according to the environment, it is important that assessments are undertaken in socially important contexts, such as at school and at home. To better understand the interaction between environment and child, rating scales to assess ADHD symptoms can be utilized in conjunction with broad-based ecobehavioral assessments.

Many rating scales are available to screen and measure ADHD symptoms in children and adolescents (Collett et al.,

TABLE 2.1

Commonly used scales for attention-deficit/hyperactivity disorder (ADHD)

Scale	Number of items (teacher/parent version)	Comments
ADHD Rating Scale	18	Extensive normative data. Strong psychometric properties. Easy to complete
Conners Rating Scale-Revised	58/80	Extensive normative data. Long history of clinical and research use. Strong psychometric properties. Ability to detect other externalizing disorders
Conners short-revised	27/28	Requires less time to complete than the full version
Conners abbreviated	10	Widely used in clinical settings. Short and quick, making it a very easy-to-use screening tool and treatment monitoring scale
IOWA-Conners	10	Widely used with relatively good psychometric properties. Less extensive normative data. Unique in providing overactive-inattentive subscale. Short and quick, making it appropriate for screening and treatment monitoring
SNAP-IV-long version	40 items	Long history of research use. Provides subscales for not only ADHD but also internalizing and externalizing disorders. Limited psychometric and normative data. Available online
SNAP-IV-short version/	18	Provides both ADHD and opposition defiant subscales. Easy to use
SNAP-IV MTA version	28	
Attention-deficit disorder Comprehensive Teacher Rating Scale	24	Long history of clinical use, especially in schools. Limited psychometric and normative data

2003). These rating scales are especially useful and important for measuring change with treatment (see Table 2.1). Physicians who wish detailed information on other instruments used to assess children with ADHD should consult Gordon and Barkley's chapter on 'Tests and observational measures' in Barkley's *Attention-Deficit Hyperactivity Disorder: A Handbook for Diagnosis and Treatment, Second Edition* (1998).

ADHD Rating Scale-IV

The ADHD Rating Scale-IV (DuPaul et al., 1997) is an 18-item parent- or teacher-completed rating scale that is based on all 18 DSM-IV criteria. Children aged 5–17 can be rated using this scale and two subscale scores – inattention and hyperactivity/impulsivity – can be derived from the data. This scale does not address or incorporate any frequently associated oppositional behaviors. Convergent and discriminant validity have been found, and normative data by age and gender are available.

Conners Rating Scales

The Conners Parent Rating Scale-Revised and the Conners Teacher Rating Scale-Revised (Conners, 1989; Goyette et al., 1978) are the most widely used scales for rating children (ages 3–17) with hyperactivity disorders. The 48-item parent questionnaire yields five factor scores: conduct problems, learning problems, psychosomatic, impulsive-hyperactive, and anxiety. The short revised teacher version (28-item questionnaire) and parent version (27-item questionnaire) provide Hyperactive, Inattentive-Passive, and Conduct

Problem factor scores. Both scales have good psychometric properties and norms are available for both. The Conners Abbreviated Teacher Rating Scale is a 10-item scale that is sensitive to medication response but may not detect individuals with predominantly inattentive symptoms.

IOWA-Conners Rating Scale

The IOWA-Conners Rating Scale (Pelham, Milich, Murphy, and Murphy, 1989) was developed to provide independent scores for inattention/overactivity and aggression. It is a parent- or teacher-completed scale that consists of 10 items, five of which are correlated to external measures of inattention/overactivity but not to measures of aggression. The other five are correlated to external measures of aggression but not to measures of inattention/overactivity. The scale has good validity, and normative data by age and gender are available.

SNAP-IV

The SNAP-IV (Swanson et al., 1999; 2001) is a 26-item scale to measure ADHD symptoms named after its authors (Swanson, Nolan, and Pelham). It is completed by parents or teachers, and the scale has been used extensively to assess ADHD changes with medication treatment. The first 18 items are DSM-IV-based ADHD symptoms, and the following eight items are DSM-IV-based oppositional defiant disorder items that often accompany ADHD. Subscale scores can be determined for inattention, hyperactivity/impulsivity, and opposition/defiance.

Attention Deficit Disorder Comprehensive Teacher Rating Scale

The Attention Deficit Disorder Comprehensive Teacher Rating Scale (ACTeRS) (Ullman, Sleator, and Sprague, 1997) is another commonly used teacher-report rating scale to assess children with ADHD and their responses to treatment. This scale provides scores on four subscales: Oppositional Behavior, Attention, Hyperactivity, and Social Problems. Normative data are available for 5- to 12-year-old children.

Neurocognitive tests

Neurocognitive tests are clinically administered instruments that can be used for diagnosing ADHD, as well as for assessing treatment effects in children with ADHD. These tests differ from many of the rating scales in that the child must perform specific tasks, and the results provide information on attention and impulsivity. The three most widely used instruments or procedures include the continuous performance tasks for identifying attentional problems, a matching familiar figures test for assessing cognitive tempo and impulsivity in the context of visual problem solving, and a paired associate learning task (an "effortful" task that may be related to classroom learning). Computerized versions of some of these procedures are available, but they are generally administered only in the context of a neuropsychologic evaluation.

Conduct disorder

A child with conduct disorder displays a persistent pattern of antisocial behaviors that occur beyond normative levels and cannot be controlled by parents, teachers, and significant others. These behaviors affect not only the child in terms of his or her academic achievement and interpersonal relationships but also the child's family and community. Thus, a broad-based assessment is required to fully understand a child with this disorder. Several multidimensional rating scales such as the CBCL can be used with children who have CD. Direct observations can also be used, but given the low frequency and typically covert nature of the antisocial acts of children with conduct disorder, such observations are not commonly conducted. Additionally, institutional and community records (for example, school attendance, suspensions, expulsions, contacts with police, and arrest records) can supplement other measures of antisocial behavior. We present examples of self-report and informant rating scales that have been developed to assess antisocial behavior in children.

Children's Action Tendency Scale

The Children's Action Tendency Scale (CAT) (Deluty, 1979) is a self-report scale designed to assess children's responses in forced-choice interpersonal situations. It is suitable for children between the ages of 6 and 15. The scale provides subscale scores for aggressiveness, assertiveness, and submissiveness. It has good psychometric properties and can be used for initial assessment as well as for assessing treatment effectiveness.

Self-Report Delinquency Scale

The Self-Report Delinquency Scale (Elliot, Huizinga, and Ageton, 1985) was developed as part of the National Youth Survey which is a longitudinal study of delinquent behavior, use of alcohol and drugs, and related problems in American adolescents. This is a self-report scale that provides a measure of the frequency with which an adolescent has committed offenses that are included in the Uniform Crime Reports during the previous 12 months. It is suitable for children aged 11 to 21.

Eyberg Child Behavior Inventory

The Eyberg Child Behavior Inventory (ECBI) (Eyberg and Pincus, 1999) is a 36-item inventory that was developed to provide physicians with a parental assessment of a child's behavior at home. It is suitable for assessing children age 2 to 17. The ECBI provides two scores: the number of problems the child has and the intensity of the problems. It has good reliability and validity, and it has been used extensively for research and clinical purposes. Normative data are available for children and adolescents.

Sutter-Eyberg Student Behavior Inventory

The Sutter-Eyberg Student Behavior Inventory (SESBI) (Eyberg and Pincus, 1999) is a 38-item inventory that is structurally similar to the ECBI and was developed to provide a teacher's assessment of a child's behavior at school. It is suitable for assessing children age 2 to 17. As with the ECBI, this instrument has good reliability and validity. Physicians can use both the ECBI and SESBI to obtain a good clinical picture of the antisocial behaviors of the child in two settings.

Eating disorders

Eating disorders in children and adolescents include anorexia nervosa and bulimia nervosa. Given that these disorders are multiply determined in terms of their predisposing, precipitating, and maintaining factors, physicians should ensure a broad-based assessment of various factors, such as becoming familiar with a patient's clinical and treatment history, learning the patient's current body weight and weight history, the frequency, intensity, and duration of various weight-controlling methods used, the nature and frequency of binge eating and eating behaviour, self-perceptions of weight, shape, body size, and body image, physical symptoms, and psychiatric comorbidity. Some of the information can be obtained through a detailed clinical interview and supplemented by information obtained through semistructured interviews and self-report instruments.

Eating Disorder Examination

The Eating Disorder Examination (EDE) (Cooper and Fairburn, 1987) is a semistructured diagnostic interview designed to elicit information on the clinical features and specific psychopathologic nature of anorexia nervosa and bulimia nervosa over the 4 weeks prior to the interview. It is intended for use by physicians who have experience and knowledge in the assessment and treatment of eating disorders, and it takes about an hour to complete.

Clinical Eating Disorder Rating Instrument

The Clinical Eating Disorder Rating Instrument (CEDRI) (Palmer, Christie, Cordle, and Davies, 1987) is a clinical rating scale that provides information on behavioral patterns, attitudes, and other symptoms (such as depression or self-esteem) that are associated with eating disorders. This scale has adequate inter-rater reliability, but other psychometric characteristics are yet to be determined.

Eating Attitudes Test

The Eating Attitudes Test (EAT) (Garner and Garfinkel, 1979) was designed to provide self-reported information on the symptoms of anorexia nervosa. This 26-item (EAT-26; Garner et al., 1982) measure has been used effectively as a screening instrument rather than a diagnostic instrument. Recent research shows that it is equally useful in providing information on bulimia nervosa. It gives a total score, as well as scores for three subscales: dieting, bulimia and food preoccupation, and oral control. This has been a widely used scale in both research and clinical practice.

Eating Disorder Inventory-2

The Eating Disorder Inventory-2 (EDI-2) (Garner, 1991) is another commonly used self-report measure that was designed to provide information on psychologic, attitudinal, and behavioral traits common in both anorexia nervosa and bulimia nervosa, but it is not a diagnostic instrument. The original scale (EDI) included three subscales that assessed attitudes and behavior concerning eating, weight, and shape, as well as five subscales that assessed general psychologic traits related to eating disorders. The EDI-2, consisting of 91 items, retains these subscales, but with the addition of more items it now includes three additional subscales (asceticism, impulse regulation, and social insecurity). Physicians will find the EDI-2 useful for determining the severity of eating disorders by comparing the child to the norms that are provided. Additionally, some of the subscales provide clinically useful information that can be used for planning treatment.

Mental retardation

Mental retardation is diagnosed in a child whose intellectual functioning and adaptive behavior are significantly subav-erage. Adaptive behavior deficits may include difficulties with communication, self-care, home living, social skills, community functioning, self-direction, health and safety, functional academics, leisure, or work. Mental retardation must manifest before age 18. Most physicians are rarely called on to provide a diagnosis of mental retardation. It is not unlikely, however, that a child with mental retardation will be referred for a psychiatric or pediatric consultation for the assessment and treatment of behavior problems or a psychopathologic condition.

The initial step in a diagnostic assessment is to undertake a thorough structural and functional analysis of the behavior problem (see Chapters 5 and 16). Typically, a behavioral psychologist is the professional who is trained to undertake this task. The second step is to screen for any broad-based psychopathologic disorder that the child may have and then to follow this up with disorder-specific assessments. We present a number of diagnostic instruments that can be used to determine the child's level of adaptive and maladaptive behavior, as well as instruments that screen for psychopathologic disorders. As with the other instruments described in this chapter, these scales can assist in the identification of a psychopathologic condition but, used in isolation, are not sufficient for establishing a specific diagnosis.

Scales of Independent Behavior-Revised

The Scales of Independent Behavior-Revised (SIB-R) (Bruininks, Woodcock, Weatherman, and Hill, 1997) is a caretaker-report instrument for the assessment of adaptive behavior. The instrument is made up of 14 subscales associated with common domains of adaptive behavior. Also included is a measure of maladaptive, challenging behaviors, including information about frequency and severity. The SIB-R is a recently developed instrument with excellent psychometric characteristics and standardization procedures and current norms. A short form is also available.

AAMD Adaptive Behavior Scales

The AAMD Adaptive Behavior Scales (ABS) (Nihira, Leland, and Lambert, 1993) is one of the standard instruments for assessing adaptive and maladaptive behavior in individuals with mental retardation between the ages of 3 and 69. It is an informant rating scale that is divided into two parts. Part I deals with adaptive behaviors across 10 domains, and part II deals with maladaptive behaviors across 14 domains. A school version is also available, but its psychometric properties are not robust. Data on the psychometric properties of the ABS are rather limited, but the scale appears to be clinically useful in evaluating and tracking adaptive and maladaptive behavior of specific individuals.

Vineland-II Adaptive Behavior Scales

The Vineland-II Adaptive Behavior Scales (VABS) (Sparrow, Balla, and Cicchetti, 2004) are the most commonly used adaptive behavior scales in studies of mental retardation. The instrument was designed for use with children from birth to age 18. It is an informant rating scale that is available in three versions: the Survey Form (297 items), the Expanded Form (577 items), and the Classroom Edition (244 items). The Survey and Expanded Forms are administered as semistructured interviews, and the Classroom Edition is administered as a questionnaire to be completed by a teacher. Each version includes four domains of adaptive behavior (communication, daily living skills, socialization, and motor skills). The Survey Form and the Expanded Form also include a maladaptive behavior domain. The VABS has very good psychometric properties that make it a useful tool for use with this population.

Aberrant Behavior Checklist

The Aberrant Behavior Checklist (ABC) (Aman and Singh, 1986) was designed to assess the effects of pharmacologic, behavioral, and other interventions on the behavior of individuals (age 5 and older) with mental retardation. This 58-item checklist is increasingly used to assess inappropriate and maladaptive behavior in the absence of treatment in the same population. The ABC is an informant rating scale and is available in two versions: residential and community. It had good psychometric properties, and it is the most widely used rating instrument for assessing clinical effects of medications in this population.

Prout-Strohmer Assessment System

The Prout-Strohmer Emotional Problems Scales (PSAS) (Prout and Strohmer, 1991) consists of two separate rating scales that measure emotional and behavioral problems in adolescents (age 14 and older) and adults with mental retardation. The Prout-Strohmer Personality Inventory (PSPI), a self-report instrument, and the Strohmer-Prout Behavior Rating Scale (SPBRS), an informant rating scale, provide assessments of two broad-band factors (internalizing and externalizing) and 12 clinical scales. The scales appear to have reasonably good psychometric properties and may prove useful to the physician.

Reiss Screen for Maladaptive Behavior

The Reiss Screen for Maladaptive Behavior (Reiss, 1994) is a screening instrument designed to assess the mental health status of adolescents and adults with mental retardation. It requires ratings from at least two informants, such as teachers and caregivers. The Reiss Screen provides a total score, as well as scores for each of eight subscales and six special symptoms (such as drug or alcohol abuse, self-injury, stealing, overactivity, sexual problems, and suicidal tendencies). Although the normative sample used was rather small, this scale has good psychometric properties.

Pain disorder

Pain can result from many sources, including accidents and trauma, recurrent pain syndromes (for example, recurrent headaches), physical disorders (such as juvenile rheumatoid arthritis), and medical procedures (such as bone marrow aspirations). Given that pain is a subjective experience that is affected by contextual variables (for example, culture and social ecology), pain assessment is challenging, especially in young children. However, there are a number of behavioral and self-report measures that provide physicians with systematic methods of assessing pain in children and adolescents.

Procedure Behavior Rating Scale

The Procedure Behavior Rating Scale (PBRS) (Katz, Kellerman, and Siegel, 1980) was designed to assess anxiety levels in children during medical procedures. The scale has been found to be sensitive to developmental changes in pain, i.e. the changing behavioral expressions of pain as children grow older. The Observational Scale of Behavioral Distress (OSBD) (Jay, Ozolins, Elliot, and Caldwell, 1983) is a modified version of the PBRS that includes partial-interval recording and an intensity rating of the pain. Both scales have very good psychometric properties and have been used extensively in pediatric settings. The Procedure Behavior Check List (PBCL) (LeBaron and Zeltzer, 1984) is a shorter version of the PBRS that includes two additional categories of the expression of distress in adolescents.

Children's Hospital of Eastern Ontario Pain Scale

The Children's Hospital of Eastern Ontario Pain Scale (CHEOPS) (McGrath, Vair, McGrath, Unruh, and Scjnurr, 1985) is a clinician rating scale designed to measure postoperative pain in children. Physicians rate a child's pain behavior every 30 seconds in six general categories: vocalizations, facial expression, child's verbal behavior, torso position, touch behavior, and leg position. The scale is valid and reliable for assessing pain in children age 1 to 7.

Child physical abuse and neglect

Although child abuse and neglect are not medical or psychiatric disorders, these phenomena may be the focus of clinical intervention. We briefly touch on this topic because of its increasing prevalence and the need for physicians to be aware of the breadth of the assessment that may be required for intervention. Physicians interested in the assessment of parents who engage in physical abuse and neglect of their children should consult Ammerman's chapter in the *Handbook of Child and Adolescent Assessment,* edited by Ollendick and Hersen (1993) for more details.

CONSIDER CONSULTATION WHEN ...

- The rating scales indicate multiple areas of deficits or clinical problems – the child may be experiencing complex psychiatric disorders that warrant assessment by a specialist.
- Rating scales and clinical assessment indicate little improvement or worsening with treatment. It is possible that an undetected condition may be contributing to the clinical difficulties or that additional types of treatment may be required.

Unlike childhood psychiatric disorders, which have a large number of disorder-specific instruments, there are no well-validated instruments to directly assess the emotional and psychologic consequences of physical abuse and neglect. In addition to a broad-based clinical interview with the child, the physician may use multidimensional rating scales to gather information on the child's social functioning and psychopathologic state. The CBCL and TRF are suitable for this purpose. Because children may engage in behaviors that elicit or escalate physical abuse from parents, the ECBI can be used to determine which of the child's behaviors the parents find difficult to manage. This information can be used by the physician to enhance the parents' skills in managing the child's behavior in socially accepted ways. Additionally, the physician should provide appropriate therapy to the child for the emotional and psychologic effects of physical abuse and neglect.

Summary

Even though the clinical assessment of children and adolescents will always, to some extent, remain an art, increasing numbers of diagnostic instruments are available that make this task much easier for physicians. The refinements in the diagnostic criteria of psychiatric disorders have led to the development of structured and semistructured diagnostic interviews and an explosion in the development of disorder-specific rating scales. However, even though there is a rating scale for virtually every behavior of children and adolescents that is of interest to mental health professionals, the lack of rigor in the psychometric properties of many of them should alert the physician that a cautious choice of instruments is warranted.

Annotated bibliography

Canino IA, Spurlock J (2000) Culturally diverse children and adolescents. In: *Assessment, Diagnosis, and Treatment*, 2nd edn. New York, Guilford.
This book provides an excellent introduction and practical guide to the assessment and diagnosis of children and adolescents of minority cultures. The focus is on the mental health needs of children of African-American, Latino, Asian-American, and American Indian heritage.

Ollendick TH, Hersen M (1993) *Handbook of Child and Adolescent Assessment*. Needham Heights, Mass., Allyn and Bacon.
This book presents the principles and procedures of child and adolescent assessment. It is divided into three major sections: fundamental issues and principles, specific assessment strategies, and the assessment of specific populations.

Reynolds CR, Kamphaus RW (2003) *Handbook of Psychological and Educational Assessment of Children*, 2nd edn. New York, Guilford.
This is a standard work in the field that comes in two volumes. The general areas of assessment covered include intelligence, achievement, personality, behavior, and context. This is a scholarly work that would be of interest to those who wish to read about different areas in some depth.

CHAPTER 3

Psychiatric Evaluation: Biomedical Assessment

Douglas O. Lee, MD and Thomas K. Cummins, MD

Introduction

Accurate assessment and conceptualization are cornerstones of optimal psychiatric treatment. As in other branches of medicine, skillful inquiry and history-taking and investigation provide sufficient information for an accurate diagnosis in most situations. Even though the biopsychosocial approach (Engel, 1977) yields accurate diagnoses in the majority of psychiatric conditions, definitive diagnosis can periodically be elusive.

Screening tools, diagnostic instruments, and rating scales (see Chapter 2) can provide additional data to make a diagnosis. Recent biomedical advances have ushered in a new era of understanding psychopathophysiology, and with it, the hope for improved diagnosis and evaluation. Neuroscience research has exploited molecular, endocrinologic, metabolic, genetic, and neuroimaging advances to elucidate conditions, course, and treatment response. In clinical settings, despite limited diagnostic applications, biomedical assessment can be helpful in certain conditions. These assessments are important for identifying both conditions whose symptoms may be confused with psychiatric symptoms and conditions that contribute to psychiatric symptoms. For example, individuals with hearing impairments may present with speech, language delays, or inattention, but an audiologic exam (with audiogram, tympanogram, and auditory brainstem response) can identify the potential root of the problem. Likewise, individuals with visual problems may have difficulty concentrating, but an eye examination can identify whether the child's vision needs to be corrected, and subsequently concentration could improve. This chapter addresses the role of laboratory tests, neuroimaging, and electroencephalograms (EEGs) in the psychiatric evaluation and the identification of conditions that may contribute to psychiatric symptoms.

Laboratory tests

A wide array of laboratory tests is now available to clinicians for use in the assessment of psychiatric symptoms and disease. However, a thorough and comprehensive clinical history remains the cornerstone of the evaluation and treatment of psychiatric illness in children and adolescents. In addition, a medical history and complete physical examination including a careful neurologic examination should precede the consideration of any laboratory tests.

Laboratory evaluations serve three main functions: 1) the identification of an underlying medical etiology of psychiatric symptoms, 2) the determination of baseline values of physiologic parameters that may be affected by psychotropic medications, and 3) the identification of any medical condition that may be complicated by medication treatment (Hendren and He, 2003).

Laboratory tests in the initial assessment of psychiatric symptoms

Baseline tests

The likelihood that a baseline laboratory test will influence the clinical management of a child with a normal physical examination and noncontributory medical history is minimal. Studies of the use of routine laboratory screening in adult psychiatric inpatients reveal that these tests rarely influence clinical patient management (Anfinson and Kathol, 1992; Sheline and Kehr, 1990). Therefore, no baseline laboratory assessment is absolutely necessary in these instances unless dictated by the initiation of certain psychotropic medications. If the medical history or physical examination indicates the possibility of an underlying medical condition, however, the appropriate laboratory tests should be ordered to further evaluate the possible presence of that disorder.

If baseline screening laboratory tests are ordered, a reasonable screening panel would include a complete blood count, serum electrolytes for sodium, potassium, chloride, calcium, phosphate, and carbon dioxide, and a liver function panel including aspartate aminotransferase (AST), alanine aminotransferase (ALT) and bilirubin and blood urea nitrogen (BUN). Lead levels should also be considered for children at risk for lead toxicity (Green, 2001). Hematologic measures should be considered for patients at risk for anemia, as anemia may present with symptoms including asthenia, depression, and psychosis. Electrolyte disturbances, hepatic disease, and elevated BUN may also present with multiple manifestations of mental status changes.

Thyroid function tests

Significant thyroid dysfunction can manifest with multiple psychiatric symptoms including depression, mania, psychosis, anxiety, restlessness, and mental status changes. Thyroid dysfunction is also a treatable cause of mental retardation. Therefore, screening thyroid function tests would appear reasonable with these presentations, especially if accompanied by a medical history or physical exam suggestive of thyroid disorder. Screening laboratories include triiodothyronine, thyroxine, and thyroid-stimulating hormone (Dallas and Foley, 1996). Hypothyroidism and hyperthyroidism may present with symptoms suggestive of ADHD. Additionally, an association between ADHD and peripheral resistance to thyroid function has been reported (Hauser et al., 1993). However, this condition is rare and therefore thyroid testing in ADHD is not necessary unless the family history, medical history, or physical examination are suggestive of thyroid disease in the child presenting with symptoms of ADHD (Zametkin et al., 1998).

Toxicology screening

Urine toxicology screening should be considered for adolescents at risk for or suspected of engaging in substance abuse. A positive screening urine test should be confirmed using a more sensitive serum screen (Bukstein, 1997). A drug screen should also be considered for any adolescent with new onset psychosis. Other potential indications for drug screening include new onset anxiety or depression. Ethical-legal issues must be considered when obtaining toxicology screens (Warner et al., 2003; American Academy of Pediatrics, 1996). Every effort should be made to obtain consent from the minor, and it is important to be familiar with circumstances when it may be permissible to obtain toxicology screening without consent and when it is required. For example, consent must be obtained prior to drug screening pregnant individuals (Annas, 2001).

Children at risk for exposure to heavy metal toxicity should be screened for heavy metals including lead and mercury if they present with behavioral changes (Zametkin, 1998).

Genetic testing

Behavioral genetics is starting to shed light upon the complex intertwining genetic picture that contributes to specific behavior phenotypes. Recent advances have identified polymorphisms in the serotonin transporter gene that are associated with stress-related depression in adults (Caspi et al., 2003), increased fear and amygdala activity in adults (Hariri et al., 2002), and shyness in children (Arbelle et al., 2003). Likewise, specific polymorphisms in dopamine transporter genes have been associated with ADHD (Rowe et al., 2001), medication-mediated changes in performance and cortical activity (Loo et al., 2003), and nonresponse to methylphenidate (Roman et al., 2002; Winsberg and Comings, 1999).

Genetic testing can be helpful for identifying underlying conditions that contribute to psychiatric presentations, especially conditions with multisystemic involvement and developmental delays (see below). Individuals with developmental delays – delays in cognitive, physical, or neurologic development – often have increased psychiatric morbidity (Dekker and Koot, 2003). Genetic testing in combination with a careful physical examination by an experienced clinician, such as a pediatric geneticist, can help to identify rare developmental disorders.

Despite many exciting breakthroughs in behavioral genetics, routine genetic testing, however, does not currently play a prominent role in the typical psychiatric work-up.

PEARLS & PERILS

- In most situations a psychiatric diagnosis can be made by history, so it is prudent not to rely exclusively upon lab data or neuroimaging to make a diagnosis. In complex situations, consider utilizing a biopsychosocial approach to address the domains which can be contributing to the psychiatric signs and symptoms.
- When evaluating psychiatric disorders, integrate other medical findings and consider whether an underlying condition such as acute intermittent porphyria, central nervous system tumor, or pediatric autoimmune neuropsychiatric disorders associated with streptococcal infections (PANDAS) may be contributing to the presentation. Appropriate laboratory tests can confirm the hypotheses.
- Remember that a negative study does not always rule out an underlying medical condition. This is especially applicable to conversion disorders. For example, if seizure disorder is worked up, EEG is negative, and atypical findings are present, it is still possible that the EEG was performed interictally or that the EEG leads are not detecting discharges that are deep.

Laboratory tests for specific psychiatric presentations

Psychosis

Children and adolescents presenting with new onset psychosis should be assessed for the possible presence of an underlying medical etiology of their psychotic symptoms. A full panel of screening laboratory tests including hematologic, serum chemistry, hepatic function, thyroid function, and urine toxicology tests are indicated. If these tests are negative, further tests that should be considered include anti-nuclear antibody (ANA), anti-double-stranded DNA antibody, anti-Smith antigen antibody, anti-Ro/SSA and anti-LA/SSB antibodies to screen for lupus, serologies for HIV and syphilis, and heavy metals. Assessment for Wilson disease may also be considered, especially if movement disorders are present.

Other possible tests may be conducted in cases where previous tests have been negative but a high index of suspicion for a medical etiology remains. When clinically indicated, these tests may include serum B12, folate, iron, Lyme titers, urine corticosteroids, urine anabolic steroids (Anonymous, 1997; Pipe and Ayotte, 2002), and urine porphobilinogens (to screen for acute intermittent porphyria). In addition to these laboratory tests, a neuroimaging scan should be considered for the pediatric patient with new onset psychosis depending on the history and physical exam (American Academy of Child Psychiatry, 2001).

Eating disorders

Patients engaging in binging and purging behavior are at risk for electrolyte abnormalities and should be assessed for electrolyte status, with special attention given to the possible presence of hypokalemia and hyponatremia. An electrocardiogram should be administered to patients with electrolyte disturbances to assess for possible cardiac arrhythmia. For patients with anorexia nervosa, laboratory tests are necessary to screen for medical complications of severe weight loss (Mehler, 2001; Walsh et al., 2000; Becker et al., 1999). Screening tests should include a complete blood count (CBC) to screen for leukopenia and anemia, serum electrolytes, glucose, urea nitrogen, creatinine, thyroid function tests, echocardiogram (EKG), and cholesterol screen.

Some clinicians have advocated for the use of serial amylase testing to screen for covert purging (Hendren and He, 2003), but this type of monitoring should be considered only if amylase can be fractionated to differentiate salivary amylase from pancreatic amylase. In cases of severe weight loss, patients should also be monitored carefully during the early phases of weight restoration to guard against the development of refeeding syndrome. In these cases serum potassium, magnesium, and phosphorous should be monitored weekly or even bi-weekly early in the course of weight restoration.

Pediatric autoimmune neuropsychiatric disorders associated with streptococcal (group A beta hemolytic streptococcal) infections (PANDAS)

PANDAS was first described in a 12-year-old child who had obsessive compulsive disorder that waxed and waned with the course of streptococcal infections (Giedd et al., 1996; case series, Swedo et al., 1998). Since symptoms of this rare condition are presumed to arise as a result of cross-reactivity between anti-streptococcal antibodies and basal ganglia, individuals with obsessive compulsive disorder who are suspected of having PANDAS should have throat cultures for streptococcus, and anti-strepotolysin O and anti-DNAse B titers should be obtained to confirm past infection. Decreasing serial titers can be helpful in tracking.

Multisystem disorders

Psychiatric symptoms with multisystem involvement can herald the presence of underlying contributing conditions. Psychiatric symptoms accompanied by progressive myopathy, neuropathy, epilepsy, and other multisystem involvement can be associated with mitochondrial diseases (review, DiMauro et al., 2002). Diagnosis of these relatively rare diseases can be made by identifying mitochondrial DNA mutations via DNA analysis. Neuropsychiatric lupus can present as anxiety, depression, psychosis, or confusion (Anonymous, 1999; Wyckoff et al., 1995). Peripheral and central nervous system involvement and more common arthralgia, arthritis, malaise, and rash, and anti-nuclear antibody and anti-dsDNA antibody titers can be central to diagnosis. In late adolescence, psychiatric symptoms along with episodic multisystem signs and symptoms can be indicative of multiple sclerosis (review, Diaz-Olavarrieta et al., 1999; O'Connor, 2002). The presence of cerebrospinal fluid oligoclonal IgG bands (two or more IgG bands) and lymphocyte count of less than 5×10^7 in conjunction with magnetic resonance imaging would confirm this diagnosis.

Some multisystem disorders can be associated with developmental delay. Children presenting with developmental delay should be assessed for treatable causes and their families may benefit from the results of genetic testing. Laboratory tests for reversible causes of developmental delay include thyroid function tests, screens for organic acids, quantitative urinary amino acids, and screening for heavy metals.

Inborn errors of metabolism including Wilson's disease, phenylketonuria, acute intermittent porphyria, and metachromatic leukodystrophy can produce psychiatric symptoms (Estrov et al., 2000). Mood symptoms, irritability, incongruous behavior, cognitive changes, in the context of dysarthria, movement disorder, and hepatic symptoms could suggest Wilson's disease (Dening and Berrios, 1990). Laboratory tests for Wilson's disease would include serum ceruloplasmin, and serum and 24-hour urine copper levels. A slit lamp opthalmalogic examination with the characteristic Kayser-Fleischer rings that are seen in 80% of individuals with Wilson's disease may also be beneficial in the diagnosis of Wilson's disease (review, El-Youssef, 2003). Acute intermittent porphyria can generate psychosis, depression, and confusion with accompanying abdominal pain, constipation, nausea, vomiting, tachycardia, hypertension, and extremity weakness. Elevated urine porphyrins and porphobilinogen confirm diagnosis, while hyponatremia can be a complication of the disorder. Other porphyrias are reflected by other elevated porphyrins. Lysosomal storage diseases can result in a multitude of psychiatric and neurologic presentations, and they can be diagnosed by measuring specific lysosomal enzymes or storage products (review, Wenger et al., 2003). For example, metachromatic leukodystrophy, which often results in progressive paraparesis, can be diagnosed by measuring lysosomal enzyme arylsulfatase A. Disorders of peroxisomal membranes can produce progressive neurologic decline (Gartner, 2000). Adrenoleukodystrophy can present with progressive cognitive changes (Ievers et al., 1999) and can be diagnosed by measuring serum long chain fatty acid concentrations and, more precisely, with DNA analysis. Another metabolic disorder, arginase deficiency (Prasad et al., 1997), resulting in the inability to convert arginine to urea and ornithine, seizures, and progressive gait disturbance, is diagnosed by detecting elevated serum arginine concentration.

Genetic testing can be helpful for identifying specific underlying conditions that are associated with psychiatric symptoms, but it is not routinely considered for diagnosis of primary psychiatric disorders. Genetic testing at this time includes DNA testing for fragile X syndrome, which can be associated with cognitive and hyperactive symptoms. Sequencing of the CGG trinucleotide repeats associated with the FRM1 gene enables characterization of premutations and full mutations that might otherwise be undetected via karyotype cytogenetic analysis, especially in individuals with carrier status (Anonymous, 1994; Maddalena et al., 2001). Cytogenetic analysis can be helpful in a small percentage of children with developmental delays and additional findings (Shevell et al., 2003).

Neuroimaging

Since the inception of neuroimaging, the ability to visualize the central nervous system (CNS) has increased the hope that neuroimaging would be a useful psychiatric diagnostic tool. Structural computed tomography scans have been useful for visualizing various brain structures, but it exposes children to ionizing radiation. Magnetic resonance imaging (MRI) has improved resolution while utilizing electromagnetic properties of hydrogen protons to visualize structures, and it has been useful for determining brain volume and assessing anatomy.

Functional neuroimaging provides another dimension of information – brain metabolism and, presumably, brain function. Positron emission tomography (PET) utilizes ra-

KEY CLINICAL QUESTIONS

- *Did you notice that behavioral changes occurred along with other changes such as neurologic changes (tremors, difficulties with coordination, complaints of tingling or pain)?*
  Behavioral changes that occur with systemic complaints could signal the presence of a multisystemic illness. Neurologic evaluation in conjunction with neuroimaging should be obtained. A comprehensive review of systems should be obtained to identify potential multisystem system disorders that will direct the clinician to potential additional follow-up studies such as Lyme Disease titers, ceruloplasmin, porphyrins, and porphobilinogen.
- *Has your child been identified with any developmental delays or mental retardation?*
  The presence of behavioral problems in the context of mental retardation or developmental delays should initiate an attempt to identify potential underlying conditions. A genetics testing and consultation should be considered, especially if physical stigmata are present. This can be useful for understanding potential causes of the presentation and can be important for family planning (e.g. fragile X). A metabolic work-up with amino acids, organic acids, heavy metal screen should be considered not only to understand potential causes but also to identify any treatable condition.

dioactively labeled compounds such as glucose to identify brain regions that increase or decrease their metabolism (brain function) during specific tasks. Single photon emission tomography (SPECT) measures brain perfusion to identify regions that are presumably more active. The use of PET and SPECT in children is limited significantly by the exposure to radiation. Functional MRI (fMRI), however, identifies neuroanatomic structures that reflect brain function without exposing children to radioactive isotopes.

Magnetic resonance spectroscopy is a potentially powerful tool to characterize metabolites in brain regions. There is promise that this technology can help to understand biochemical processes in various disease states. Overall, neuroimaging (review, Hendren et al., 2000) is advancing our understanding of brain functioning and brain development in pediatric psychiatric conditions.

Schizophrenia

MRI studies of children with schizophrenia find decreased cerebral volume in both hemispheres (Frazier et al., 1996). This has been replicated, and in a study with a 2-year follow-up there was a progressive decrease in cerebral and thalamic volume (Rapoport et al., 1997). Progressive decreases in cerebral volume have also been found in frontal lobes, temporal lobes, caudate and globus pallidus (Jacobsen et al., 1996,

1998a, 1998b; Rapoport et al., 1999), supporting the notion that schizophrenia is a dynamic condition.

Mood and anxiety disorders

Children with OCD have been found to have reduced striatal volume, especially putamen, but greater corpus callosum size (Rosenberg et al., 1997a, 1997b). Abnormalities in striatum are consistent with theories underlying OCD. Structural neuroimaging of children with depression has found a decreased frontal lobe/total cerebral volume ratio (Steingard et al., 1996).

ADHD

Neuroimaging in ADHD has confirmed hypotheses asserting not only the involvement of frontal and striatal regions but also other regions not previously considered. Structural imaging of boys with ADHD reveals smaller frontal volumes compared with controls (Castellanos et al., 1996; Filipek et al., 1997). Compared with controls, children and adolescents with ADHD, regardless of stimulant treatment history, have smaller global cerebral and cerebellar volumes, and in follow-up they follow a unique but parallel nonprogressive growth trajectory (Castellanos et al., 2002). A T-2 relaxometry fMRI study of methylphenidate effects on the cerebellar lobules of the cerebellar vermis found that there is a behavioral rate-dependent change in T-2 relaxation time, with increased relaxation time (presumably reflecting blood flow) in hyperactive children and decreased relaxation time in children without hyperactivity (Anderson et al., 2002). Structural MRI (Casey et al., 1997) and fMRI (Durston et al., 2003) have detected abnormalities in frontostriatal circuits, and instead of activating frontostriatal regions in typically developing children, those with ADHD utilize more diffuse regions including the posterior parietal and occipital regions. Reversed basal ganglia asymmetry with a smaller left caudate head volume (Castellanos et al., 1994) has been correlated with methylphenidate response (Filipek et al., 1997) and inhibition and externalizing behavior (Semrud-Clikeman et al., 2000). Functional imaging has revealed asymmetry of putamen glucose metabolism that correlated with intensity of ADHD symptoms (Ernst et al., 1997).

Autism

Structural neuroimaging of children with autism spectrum disorders parallels clinical observations. Total cerebral volume is increased compared with controls (Piven et al., 1995) and 3–4-year-olds have a 9.8% increase in volume over typically developing children (Sparks et al., 2002). An MRI study of children with autism spectrum disorders from age 2–5 years found that previously measured birth head circumference was correlated with smaller cerebellar gray matter volume, and head circumference at 6–14 months was later correlated with increased cerebral gray matter

and white matter, whole-brain white matter and gray matter, and whole-brain volumes, and cerebellar gray matter (Courchesne et al., 1994). fMRI has found that there are abnormalities in prefrontal and posterio cingulate activation during an executive functioning task involving spatial working memory (Luna et al., 2002).

Anorexia nervosa

Individuals with anorexia nervosa have CNS changes characterized by increases in ventricular volume, decreases in white and gray matter (Katzman et al., 1996). A follow-up study of adolescents with anorexia nervosa found structural abnormalities even 10–20 months after recovering from severe weight loss (Katzman et al., 1997). Ventricular volume was elevated and gray matter volume deficits persisted, while white matter volume deficits were no longer evident.

CNS tumors

Neuroimaging is especially useful for the diagnosis of CNS conditions with psychiatric sequelae. For example, pediatric tumors can produce personality changes along with other signs and symptoms. In one study, 52% of children with brain tumors had behavioral and personality changes, while vomiting was present in 65% and headache was present in 64% (Edgeworth et al., 1996). Neuroimaging can play an integral role in diagnosing CNS neoplasms (Poussaint, 2001).

In summary, neuroimaging has advanced our understanding of psychiatric disorders by tracking longitudinal brain development and identifying structures that may be related to the expression of various signs and symptoms. However, in the daily practice of making most psychiatric diagnoses, neuroimaging is not routinely employed.

Electroencephalogram (EEG)

EEGs are exceptionally important for confirming seizure activity in children. Epilepsy, one of the most common child-

CONSIDER CONSULTATION WHEN ...

- A psychiatric disorder presents in the context of "regressive" behavior and "regressive" development, a neurodegenerative disorder or CNS tumor should be considered in the differential diagnosis. Consultation with a pediatric neurologist and neuroimaging should be considered.
- Stable physical signs (or stigmata) are present with psychiatric symptoms, one might consider consulting a pediatric geneticist to work up and rule out an underlying genetic condition. Should a genetic condition be identified, genetic counseling should be incorporated when presenting findings to the family.

hood disorders, is commonly associated with psychiatric comorbidity. While evaluating behavior in an individual with epilepsy or with a high index of suspicion of having seizures, the role of epileptiform discharges, post-ictal states and medication side-effects must be considered. Seizures can contribute to psychosis (Lancman, 1999), panic (Lee et al., 1997), or confusion. However, psychiatric or behavioral conditions (such as aggression) that are directly attributable to seizure activity are relatively uncommon. Routine EEG to evaluate the presence of seizures in individuals with psychiatric symptoms usually does not yield significant findings (Bostwick and Philbrick, 2002). In contrast, video EEGs can be exceptionally useful for diagnosing nonepileptiform (pseudoseizures) seizures (Wyllie et al., 1999).

Summary

Even though biomedical testing is not routinely utilized in making most psychiatric diagnoses, it can play an important role when indicated. Biomedical testing can be indispensable for identifying underlying genetic, metabolic, and other medical conditions that can have psychiatric presentations.

Annotated bibliography

Hendren RL, De Backer I, Pandina GJ (2000) Review of neuroimaging studies of child and adolescent psychiatric disorders from the past 10 years. *J Am Acad Child Adolesc Psychiatry*, 39:815–28.
This broad review article highlights many of the seminal studies in pediatric neuroimaging.

Zametkin AJ, Ernst M, Silver R (1998) Laboratory and diagnostic testing in child and adolescent psychiatry: a review of the past 10 years. *J Am Acad Child Adolesc Psychiatry*, 37:464–72.
This review discusses some of the relevant laboratory tests that are utilized in the psychiatric work-up.

Bostwick JM, Philbrick KL (2002) The use of electroencephalography in psychiatry of the medically ill. *Psych Clin N Am*, 25:17–25.
This article highlights the rare occasions when electroencephalograms can be useful in psychiatric evaluation.

CHAPTER 4

Strategic Treatment Planning and Therapeutic Interventions

Arden D. Dingle, MD and Douglas O. Lee, MD

Introduction

A variety of interventions is available to help children and adolescents with psychiatric illness. It is essential to base treatment interventions on a comprehensive understanding of the child's and family's problems and strengths so that a multidimensional plan can be developed. Treatment requirements and issues should be considered from the beginning of an assessment so that appropriate information can be obtained, and potential impediments can be identified and managed. Involving all possible resources with coordination and communication among providers is crucial. While designing and implementing effective treatment plans can be challenging, there can be considerable benefit to the child and family. Developing a plan at the initiation of treatment that can be periodically reviewed and modified allows all involved to monitor progress. This chapter discusses issues that may affect treatment planning and implementation as well as possible approaches. Information is also provided about various interventions, agencies, and resources that may be helpful for particular children and adolescents.

Treatment planning can be a neglected component of providing for a child or adolescent with mental health needs. Planning can be more manageable if there are overall goals as well as smaller, more specific ones and if various timelines are considered. For example, treatment can be organized into categories such as short- and long-term needs or interventions for the child, caretakers, and environment. Often, the youth's needs and environment seem too overwhelming or resources appear too inaccessible. Balancing and prioritizing the needs of the youth and involved others can be demanding, especially since treatment plans should be realistic, attainable, flexible, yet comprehensive enough

to be effective. Plans can be too inclusive, with attempts to remedy everything at once, or too simple, with one aspect of the child's problems being targeted while other significant issues are not dealt with. Successful treatment strategies consider the child, family, and environment and use this information to develop a staged series of interventions that target specific difficulties with specific goals and objectives in a manner that allows periodic reassessments and adjustments. An essential element is to identify and attempt to address any barriers to the delivery and implementation of care.

Several studies have documented a significant number of children and adolescents with mental illnesses who have major difficulties accessing appropriate care. Thus, treatment planning for children and adolescents with psychiatric disorders can be constrained by financial considerations and complicated by a lack of appropriate providers and services. Depending on the community, there can be a range of interventions available, provided by both public and private (non-profit and for-profit) agencies. Generally, urban regions have a broader spectrum of services and providers than rural areas. In many areas, there is a shortage of appropriate child and adolescent psychiatric providers, especially psychologists and psychiatrists. Most insurance plans (including Medicaid) do not provide equal coverage for health and mental health services, with many plans having more restricted mental health benefits with lower provider and facility compensation. Many private practitioners do not accept Medicaid or any other form of insurance.

Health-care reform has resulted in an emphasis on short-term, problem-oriented therapies, which can be inadequate for youth with complicated, long-standing emotional disturbances. Coverage for long-term therapeutic care is often very restricted, with many insurance plans covering limited psychiatric acute inpatient and outpatient care. A small portion of the health budget is devoted to children and adolescents, so public funding for mental health interventions is limited. Depending on their financial status and disease severity, children, adolescents, and families may be eligible for social security benefits, which provide a monthly stipend as well as eligibility for Medicaid. For most young people with serious emotional disturbances, public funding for their care is necessary through the involvement of community mental health, child protective services, the juvenile justice system, and other community agencies (Zigler et al., 2002; Schreter, 2003).

Treatment for children and adolescents can be complicated by a number of other factors. Typically, caretakers, teachers, agency workers, and other adults make the decision that the young person needs psychiatric care and initiate the process. Children and adolescents rarely refer themselves for treatment or identify themselves as needing treatment. Often, the precipitating factors are related to the adults being distressed by the child's behavior rather than the child or adolescent recognizing psychologic dysfunction or impairment. A number of young people will agree they need help after being assessed, though some continue to maintain through much or all of the treatment that they do not need therapeutic interventions. Thus, engagement of the child or adolescent can be a challenge since the young person's motivation may be lacking, especially if therapy interferes with scheduled activities or is emotionally uncomfortable. Children and adolescents are also vulnerable to and dependent upon their caretakers and other aspects of their environments, over which they have little control. It can be challenging to decide what should be a focus of treatment, and some aspects of the child's world may not be amenable to interventions. A common issue in treatment can be the young person's perception and resentment that they are labeled as the problem despite malfunctioning systems or other family members needing treatment. Finally, additional barriers to treatment can include significant family or parent problems (e.g. parental psychiatric illness, parental conflict), difficult living circumstances (e.g. poverty, high stress), obstacles to attendance (e.g. lack of parent job flexibility, transportation issues), and views that treatment is too difficult, ineffective, or slow as well as relationship issues between the provider and caretakers (Kazdin, 2000a).

Treatment planning

A psychiatric assessment of a child or adolescent concludes with a summary. An essential aspect of the summary is the formulation in which the information is synthesized and integrated to provide an explanation of the child's current status, environmental issues, and possible etiologies along with the DSM-IV axis system. Formulations can be developed employing a variety of organizational models (i.e.

biopsychosocial) and theories of psychologic functioning (i.e. psychodynamic) and should provide a foundation for treatment planning. For example, using the biopsychosocial model provides information on the child's biologic, psychologic, and social functioning as well as data on the environment. Treatment planning can be organized using the same categories. Psychiatrists tend to use this model, while other professionals often use problem lists or categories such as the child, family, and environment. Thus, the information from the summary describes the child and the environment, in terms of difficulties as well as strengths, and then makes treatment recommendations based on that information. While having an identifiable psychiatric disorder informs and guides treatment, it does not provide information on an individual and environment that may modify therapy recommendations significantly.

The initial step in treatment planning is to use the assessment summary to prioritize the problems and issues so the focus and preferred outcomes of treatment can be determined. Besides including the significant problems and issues, treatment planning should cover any personal and environmental strengths, protective factors, and any other characteristics that would promote resilience. This synthesis also should include risk and causal factors as well as which features are potentially modifiable. From this information, general and specific goals can be decided upon. It is essential that outcomes be realistic and attainable. Depending on the child and the situation there can be a range of goals such as relief of suffering, acquisition of "normality," restoration of or increased functioning. The treatment aims for an adolescent with schizophrenia will differ from one with depression. At the initiation of treatment, information should be given in both verbal and written forms and all involved should participate. Issues of consent, assent, and confidentiality should be discussed initially and reviewed periodically (Rutter and Taylor, 2003).

Treatment plans should translate disorders or problems into specific thoughts, feelings, or actions, which can be targeted by particular interventions. It should be possible to describe anticipated improvements with a desired endpoint. Thus, deficits in social skills could be elaborated as difficulty making friends, as demonstrated by no age-appropriate activities with peers. Interventions could include psychotherapy exploring what happens with peer interactions and involvement in a structured program with peers. Expected behaviors could be sitting and talking with peers at school lunch, actively participating in extracurricular program activities, developing a subset of peers at the school and program with whom the patient consistently interacts. The ultimate aim could be having peers with whom the patient consistently talks and engages in activities. Obviously, describing problems as a list of specific behaviors can be difficult, and there is the risk of ending up with a list of behaviors that do not capture the essence of the difficulty.

However, without some specifics, focusing interventions and monitoring responsiveness is not feasible.

For example, using the biopsychosocial model, a treatment plan would have an overall aim with particular goals in the categories of biological, psychological, and social (see Box 4.1). Each category would have target symptoms, prioritized from most to least problematic, baseline impairment, desired level of functioning, methods and frequency of interventions, type and timing of monitoring, outcomes and tentative timelines. It can be helpful to have immediate, short-term, and long-term goals. Generally, most children and adolescents who require psychiatric care have more than one problem and require more than one intervention. Throughout treatment, it is essential to discuss progress or its lack, possible alternatives, and advantages and disadvantages of various options. Coordination of care between providers and facilities is key and should be carefully maintained throughout treatment. Good treatment plans have flexibility so that changes in functioning or environment can be incorporated and interventions modified if no longer necessary or not adequate. Plans should

---

BOX 4.1

Treatment planning example

A 14-year-old girl is referred for treatment for a depressive disorder. She has no medical problems or safety issues and was well 3 months ago.

- Biologic: Significant depressive symptoms, including insomnia, poor appetite, fatigue, decreased concentration, sadness, and major irritability with a strong family history of depression.
- Psychologic: Patient is very sad and views herself as a failure so she has not been doing her schoolwork. She no longer makes straight As. She feels worse and hopeless when her parents frequently remark about the importance of college to be successful and how all grades in high school count.
- Social: Decreased interactions with peers since depressed. History of excelling in extracurricular activities such as yearbook and volunteering. Long-term, high-functioning close friends call and invite out patient frequently and she refuses to go.
- Overall goal: Restore to previous age-appropriate functioning.

Biologic
Immediate
- *Goal:* Consider medication to target medication-responsive symptoms. Assess extent and severity of symptoms as well as evaluating the patient's and family's view of the disorder and medication.
- *Intervention:* Discuss medication with patient and family as part of a comprehensive treatment; review options in terms of immediate or delayed initiation, advantages and disadvantages of each; the patient prefers to try therapy first and her parents agree.
- *Monitoring:* Obtain information on baseline functioning, symptoms, and Children's Depression Inventory (CDI; self-report of depressive symptoms); agree that symptoms will be assessed at least weekly, more if necessary.
- *Outcome:* Agree that will try medication if not significantly better after a month of weekly psychotherapy.

Short term
- *Goal:* Start and maintain medication to target symptoms responsive to medication.
- *Intervention:* Review medication options; discuss initiation, possible length, monitoring and criteria for discontinuation of medicine; discuss and agree upon targeted symptoms; choose a medication, review its advantages and disadvantages, explain appropriate administration; obtain appropriate consent and assent.
- *Monitoring:* Obtain a baseline assessment of targeted symptoms and CDI; agree with patient and family that will monitor symptoms monthly or as needed.
- *Outcome:* Initiate medication, titrate to appropriate dose, monitor response, side-effects, and ongoing need.

Long term
- *Goal:* Resolution of depressive symptoms, first with medication and eventually without.
- *Intervention:* Ongoing medication along with other treatments.
- *Monitoring:* Monthly assessment of symptoms and functioning along with discussion of need for medication; discussion of possible taper and discontinuation of medication once stable and back to optimal functioning for at least 6 months.
- *Outcome:* Resolution of depressive symptoms with minimal side-effects on medication and restoration of prior functioning; maintenance of functioning and lack of significant depressive symptoms off medication.

Psychologic
Immediate
- *Goal:* Assess the patient's and family's understanding of illness and treatment. Engage patient and family in therapy.
- *Intervention:* Obtain information on patient's symptoms, level of functioning, and supports as well as data on the dissatisfaction with previous therapy and potential difficulties in participating in therapy. Discuss the general approach to therapy.

BOX 4.1 (continued)

- *Monitoring:* Ask for feedback on the initial sessions; discuss any issues or difficulties
- *Outcome:* Patient and parents agree to weekly psychotherapy.

Short term

- *Goal:* Establish agreement on a problem hierarchy and general psychotherapeutic approaches, and implement and provide ongoing therapy. Establish educational plan with adequate support and realistic expectations for patient.
- *Intervention:* Discuss various problems and agree that patient's view of herself as a failure, her expectations in terms of performance, and their effects on her schoolwork are priorities. Agree that will employ a cognitive-behavioral therapeutic approach with patient (identifying maladaptive thoughts that affect emotions and behavior and substituting more appropriate thoughts) in individual psychotherapy. Agree that parents will be included on a regular basis to work on relationship issues. Obtain consent and assent and review confidentiality. Contact teacher and obtain information on patient's functioning and school structure.
- *Monitoring:* Agree that parents will participate in monthly sessions to work on parent-child interactions, at which time the patient's self-perception will be reviewed as well as her schoolwork issues.
- *Outcome:* Initiate psychotherapy, monitor response, and periodically reassess need for different approach. Explore and decide upon options such as tutoring, modification of classes.

Long term

- *Goal:* Appropriate positive self-view and academic achievement, first with psychotherapy and educational modification and then without.
- *Intervention:* Ongoing psychotherapy along with other treatments.
- *Monitoring:* Monthly assessment of self-image and school achievement along with discussion of need for psychotherapy; discussion of taper and discontinuation of psychotherapy once stable and back to optimal functioning for at least 6 months.
- *Outcome:* Resolution of feelings of failure and their effect on schoolwork and restoration of prior functioning; maintenance of functioning and lack of significant self-worth and school issues once no longer in psychotherapy.

Social

Immediate

- *Goal:* Establish the resources available to patient for age-appropriate activities with peers.
- *Intervention:* Obtain information from patient, parent, and school on prior activities and level of participation as well as currently available opportunities. Also obtain information on patient's friends and their past and current relationships.
- *Monitoring:* Establish patient's current baseline of and interest in social activities.
- *Outcome:* Patient and parents agree to identify possible and desirable resources.

Short term

- *Goal:* Establish agreement on appropriate activities and friends for patient to increase involvement with.
- *Intervention:* Discuss and develop a hierarchy of activities, beginning with involvement with structured activities (i.e. yearbook) or planned by others (i.e. going out with friends once invited). Review and identify any obstacles (internal or external) and develop intervention strategies. Enlist the involvement of parents, friends, and school to provide opportunities and encourage patient.
- *Monitoring:* Agree that patient's activities will be reviewed weekly with assessment of progress.
- *Outcome:* Initiate process to help patient resume an appropriate level of social activities with peers, monitor progress, assess need for other interventions.

Long term

- *Goal:* Appropriate social activities first initiated by others and then by self.
- *Intervention:* Ongoing psychotherapy along with interventions by parents, friends, and school.
- *Monitoring:* Monthly assessment of social activities and interactions along with discussion of need for psychotherapy and interventions by others; discussion of possible taper and discontinuation of help by others then psychotherapy once stable and back to optimal functioning for at least 6 months.
- *Outcome:* Resolution of isolative behavior and restoration of prior functioning; maintenance of functioning once no longer initiated by others and in psychotherapy.

be reviewed on a regular basis and progress periodically assessed (Hendren and Hamaran, 2003).

Practitioners

A number of providers offer mental health care. Countries and states vary on the training programs and additional experiences required to be licensed to provide services. Generally, providers must be licensed by passing a test in their specialty, which they are eligible to take after completing a designated amount of education and supervision. States have specific requirements for practitioners to become licensed within their specialty. They vary on which providers can be licensed to provide psychotherapeutic services and medication.

Child psychiatrists are medical professionals who have been trained in general psychiatry as well as child and adolescent psychiatry. After medical school, the training (residency) generally is 5–6 years with at least 2 years devoted to working with children and adolescents. Training covers inpatient and outpatient experiences with psychotherapies and psychopharmacology. Child and adolescent psychiatrists usually are eligible for medical licensure after their first year of residency. There are child and adolescent psychiatry specialty boards, which can be taken after completion of a residency and passing the general psychiatry specialty boards. Child and adolescent psychiatrists can provide medication as well as psychotherapy.

Psychologists have received a PhD or PsyD in clinical psychology with experiences in psychotherapies and psychologic testing in a variety of inpatient and outpatient settings. A year of clinical internship is included as part of graduate school and many areas require additional training or supervision after graduation to be licensed as a psychologist. Nurses can obtain graduate training in child and adolescent psychiatry, which is a master's degree (nurse practitioner or clinical nurse specialist). They generally provide psychotherapy. Depending on their training and location of practice, they may prescribe medication under a psychiatrist's supervision. A variety of other practitioners have master's degrees (counseling, psychology, social work, substance abuse, marriage and family) that generally consist of at least 2 years of graduate work, which incorporates clinical experiences. These individuals generally provide psychotherapy. Psychologists and master-level clinicians can tailor their clinical experiences during training to work with children and adolescents.

Community systems/agencies

Mental health systems

Both private and public providers offer psychiatric and other services. Families usually find services through insurance plans, referrals from medical or educational professionals, or on their own initiative. Private practitioners and facilities generally provide care for individuals with resources or health insurance, though some have sliding-scale billing systems that are affordable for lower-income families. Facilities vary considerably and some offer a spectrum of services with a multidisciplinary staff, while others are more limited in both care and types of providers. Practitioners can also have their own practices either individually or as part of a group.

Public mental health systems usually provide a range of services from hospitals to outpatient clinics designed to provide care for the indigent. Both counties and states provide funding and maintain facilities; the organization style varies. These institutions tend to emphasize treatment for the most severely and chronically mentally ill (Weiner, 2002; Schreter, 2003). Some children and families may end up being served in public systems after their resources have been exhausted.

Educational systems

Children can attend either private or public schools. While there are private schools that provide services for children with behavioral problems, they are rare and tend to be very costly. Young people can receive special education services in the public school system for behavior problems (Schwab-Stone et al., 2002). Upon request, generally by a teacher or other school personnel but also by parents, the evaluation team can assess children with behavior problems. Usually, the assessment involves observation of the child in the classroom, collection of information from the teacher, parents, involved professionals, and psychologic testing. The team, with the involvement of the child and parents, review the information, discuss the available intervention options, and develop an individual education plan. If the child's behavior difficulties are judged to be emotional in origin and meet a level of severity, he or she can receive services. The educational plans are reviewed annually or as needed.

Federal guidelines mandate school systems to provide the necessary services to maintain children educationally in the least restrictive settings. State and local regulations determine how these guidelines are implemented and there is considerable variation. In general, services range from additional help in regular classrooms, part- or full-time placement in a self-contained class for behavior problems located in a regular school, or the most restrictive being placed at a school that is entirely for behaviorally disordered children. The schools are restricted in their use of suspension, expulsion, and other consequences if the child's behavior is thought to be due to their emotional difficulties. Nationally, there is increasing interest in limiting the rights of children who are considered emotionally disturbed and permitting school systems to use suspension and expulsion more liberally. If the child cannot be served by the school system, the educational system is required to fund services by other facilities to manage the child. However, this option usually is very difficult to obtain. If children are determined to have behavioral problems for social reasons (i.e. conduct disorder), they are not eligible for special education interventions. If the behaviors are problematic enough, these children are sent to alternative schools where they have to earn the right to attend regular schools. Alternative schools vary in the amount of structure provided, but generally expect their pupils to demonstrate motivation, responsibility, and appropriate behavior.

Family and children's services

States are required to provide a variety of services to support children, adolescents, and families in need. The state agency has two main responsibilities: providing temporary assistance for basic needs (welfare) and intervening in cases of neglect and abuse (child protective services). Temporary assistance is designed for families who are financially destitute and thus are eligible for services such as Medicaid, food stamps, childcare, and often a monthly stipend. This aid is time limited and recipients must participate in a back-to-work program unless exempted. Child protective services (CPS) is mandated to intervene to evaluate suspected cases of neglect and abuse, and if sustained to provide services to keep the child safe and prevent reoccurrence. It is helpful to remember that usually the agency's mission emphasizes reunification of the family as a means to serve the best interests of the child. Anyone can report suspected neglect or abuse of a child. A number of professionals, including physicians, are mandated reporters. Regions vary on their legal interpretation of neglect and abuse as well as their abilities to offer assessments and services. There is universal agreement that prevention and early intervention are the most effective strategies, though there is no consensus on what approaches are the most effective (Browne, 2003).

When receiving a report of suspected neglect or abuse, the CPS decides whether it warrants opening a case and then how quickly a response is needed. Open cases are investigated with a visit to the house or the school and with the child's caretakers. If the report is sustained, the agency is required to identify the needs of the child and family and help put resources in place to help. The caseworker, with the family, develops a corrective plan that targets the areas of concern and describes desired outcomes and timelines. The plan can include required activities for the adults such as requiring employment, participation in parenting programs, psychiatric or substance abuse treatment, and other recommendations. Compliance with the plan is monitored, with the ultimate goal being improved functioning of the family, appropriate care of the child, and non-involvement with CPS. For cases in which safety is an immediate concern, children may be removed from the home and placed elsewhere temporarily until there is a court hearing. Caseworkers are responsible for monitoring compliance with intervention plans and making recommendations for or against reunification. If children have been in care for a period of time and no progress has been made towards returning the child home, steps are supposed to be implemented to have the child adopted (Zellman and Fair, 2002).

Juvenile justice/juvenile court

Psychiatrically ill youth often are involved with the juvenile court or juvenile justice system. A number are first identified after contact with these systems. Most are adolescents, though some are older school-aged children. Involvement can occur due to status offenses, activities that are illegal because the offender is a minor such as truancy, unruly disobedient behaviour, and running away, as well as criminal offenses. Families become involved with juvenile court when child protective services has judged there is neglect or abuse of children and changes in custody or placement are necessary or caretakers declare their child incorrigible and request help with managing the child. The court determines whether children should remain in their homes and ultimately whether parents should retain their parental rights as well as deciding on consequences for juveniles whose behavior is problematic. The juvenile system is based on a philosophy of rehabilitation, though an increasingly punitive attitude has been developed about those who commit crimes. In the United States, most jurisdictions have laws that require young people who commit certain offenses be tried as adults unless there are extenuating circumstances (Steiner and Redlich, 2002).

While services and resources can be obtained through juvenile courts and the juvenile justice system, it can be challenging. Often, different public entities are responsible for various parts of the system. For example, the local government usually runs the court, probation, and parole services, while the state is responsible for the detention facilities. Both can run diversion programs and group homes. For adolescents committing status offenses, there usually are diversion programs that provide counseling and resource referral in an attempt to prevent further court involvement. A number of courts run truancy, anger management, mental health evaluation, and other programs. If that level of intervention fails, the adolescent and family have a court date, present before a judge, are assigned a probation officer, and are court ordered to engage in certain behaviors such as obeying adults, attending school, and keeping a curfew. The court can mandate psychiatric treatment. If the young person and family consistently fail to comply with court recommendations, the judge can detain the child, place the child in state custody, or remove the child from the home. Adolescents charged with criminal offenses undergo a process similar to that of the adult court, though the orientation is towards identifying the young person's needs and possible strategies to intervene. Depending on the crime, delinquents can be sentenced or put on probation. Those individuals who are detained go to an acute (jail) or long-term (prison) facility depending on the length of the sentence. These institutions are required to provide a spectrum of services including school, health care, and psychiatric care. After serving their sentence, the adolescents are on parole with additional requirements that can include school, work, and psychiatric treatment (Steiner and Redlich, 2002).

Treatment …

- Goals should be prioritized and realistic with appropriate timelines; it can be helpful to organize them into immediate, short-term, and long-term.
- Plans should be multidimensional and include all areas of the child's life as well as including and utilizing patient and family's strengths.
- Interventions should be indicated for particular problems or disorders and address specific, targeted problems.
- For most children and adolescents should involve some psychotherapy even if medication is indicated.
- Choice of medication should target specific symptoms.
- Involving complex presentations and multiple symptoms can make it difficult to determine which medication to start first. Prioritize which symptoms are most debilitating and try to focus on those symptoms first.
- Involving multiple potential medications should start with one medication at a time if at all possible, so if a side-effect arises or if there is a behavioral change it can be attributed to the one medication. If a shotgun approach with multiple medications is used, it is more difficult to sort out which medication is helping and which is not. Furthermore, if problems arise with multiple medications, it might be necessary to discontinue all medications, thus resulting in a return to the original situation.
- With multiple medications should involve trying to adjust one medication at a time so a behavioral change can be attributed to a specific medication.
- Can be optimized by trying tracking instruments or forms (see Chapter 2) to assess and record target symptoms. This information will be invaluable for future comparison.
- Should not neglect appropriate pediatric care.

Clinicians …

- Should have the appropriate credentials for the therapy being provided
- Maintain communication with other providers and involved individuals.

Caretakers …

- Should be involved in treatment even if individually oriented.

Psychiatric interventions

Psychotherapies

Most children with psychiatric illnesses requiring therapeutic interventions can benefit from some form of psychotherapy. Psychotherapy is a form of treatment that employs a therapeutic relationship and psychologic processes to improve psychologic or physical complaints, poor functioning in intrapersonal or interpersonal spheres, psychopathology, or developmental abnormalities. There are a number of psychotherapies that are utilized with children, adolescents, and families. They vary in their theoretical approach as well as having some differences in the identified patient and format. However, all are based on the premise that relationships between patients and therapists can provide the support and context for changes in behaviors, attitudes, and beliefs.

The focus is on some aspect of how patients feel, think, or act. These factors should be evaluated and dealt with in the context of the young person's developmental level and environment. Psychodynamic, supportive, and cognitive therapies are most commonly utilized in individual treatment where most of the intervention is with the child or adolescent, though the caretaker should have some consistent involvement. However, all these theoretical orientations can be utilized in group and family therapies, or parent training. Most behavior management is directed towards the caretakers and other involved adults, though the child participates more with increasing age. Regardless of the therapeutic approach utilized, in clinical situations, behavioral interventions are incorporated into most treatments. Play is often a component of therapy, either as a strategy to help the child talk or as a non-verbal expression of internal issues. For many psychiatrically ill children, psychotherapy alone is inadequate and at times much of the frustration with psychotherapy may be due to unrealistic expectations about potential results and the time required. For example, most 10-year-old boys in psychotherapy for oppositional and disruptive behavior also require family and other environmental interventions for improvement, regardless of the type of psychotherapy employed or the etiology of the problems.

Meta-analysis of a number of studies (a range of therapies, problems, populations) has demonstrated that psychotherapy is a helpful intervention. Many of the clinically relevant questions have not been examined adequately. Unanswered questions include the cost effectiveness of these interventions, which disorders, problems, or children are most appropriate, whether it matters which form of psychotherapy or what kind of practitioner, what is a reasonable definition of treatment effectiveness, and what time length is best. One approach to examining the usefulness of psychotherapy has advocated identifying the factors common to psychotherapies that lead to change and how these specific factors are related to change. Another approach has been to concentrate on time-limited, manual-based treatments, which focus on a particular problem or disorder in an attempt to answer questions about which therapeutic approach works for which disorder. Some of the difficulty has been developing specific research questions that can be informative, since global questions about psychotherapy have not helped with the clinical issue of which treatment is best for a given patient with a particular problem (Kazdin, 2000a, 2000b; Werry and Andrews, 2002; McClellan and Werry, 2003).

Psychodynamic psychotherapy

Psychodynamic psychotherapy is appropriate for children and adolescents who have adequate intelligence, capacity for self-observation, and language skills. They should be able to participate in a primarily verbal and reflective intervention as well as have the ability and resources to tolerate a process that may be lengthy, with progress that may seem slow and hard to measure. This type of treatment can be conducted using play with younger children. It is based on the idea that there is an unconscious mind which affects thoughts and behaviors, and that it can be examined through the relationship between the therapist and the patient. Psychodynamic theory is best described as having several theoretical views about how the mind functions and psychopathology develops.

Symptoms or problems are considered to be manifestations of underlying, internal processes. By concentrating on the actual relationship between the therapist and patient as well as the transference (patient unconsciously attributes feelings, actions, and thoughts that occurred in previous relationships onto the therapist), the therapist can bring unconscious processes into conscious awareness where they can be reviewed and altered. The basic technique is for the therapist to interpret or point out ongoing patterns of thought or behavior which are interfering with optimal function. Individuals develop difficulties when there is a problem early in development. The individual's psychological defenses (how an individual deals with unacceptable thoughts or feelings) or object representations (how an individual develops internal representations of other people) become fixed and do not progress appropriately. The idea is that behavior and beliefs can be the result of an unconscious mind where normal logic does not apply and idiosyncratic but potentially understandable connections exist between thoughts, feelings, and memories.

Freud is the individual most commonly identified with this theory. However, there have been a number of other influential theorists such as Anna Freud, Bowlby, Winnicot, and Axline who focused on work with children. Usually, this type of therapy occurs as individual treatment with a child or adolescent in conjunction with other interventions such as medication and education. This therapy targets the aspects of the young person's problems that are considered to be the result of intrapsychic conflict and regressive phenomena. Children and adolescents are helped to acquire a sense of control and understanding of their lives and learn to cope without having to use problematic strategies. There is evidence that this form of therapy is effective, though there is debate about the degree of effectiveness and efficacy compared with other psychotherapies. Recently, there has been increasing interest in developing models for short-term forms of this therapy (Ritvo and Ritvo, 2002; Jacobs, 2003).

Supportive psychotherapy

Supportive psychotherapy aims to improve patient functioning by recognizing and reinforcing patient and family strengths and decreasing the impact of stresses. The underlying premise is that the emotional support provided by a positive, caring relationship between a clinician and patient can be beneficial. There is an emphasis on nurturance, present reality, and optimizing environmental conditions. Indications for this type of therapy can include relatively healthy individuals in crisis, and severely personality disordered or psychiatrically ill patients for whom exploratory therapy would be dangerous (i.e. psychosis).

Insight by the patient and family is not a goal of treatment – the goal is to help the child and family reach their maximum level of functioning. The therapist helps the child or adolescent identify his or her existing abilities to manage difficulties and to utilize them effectively. Also, participants learn to distinguish potential stresses and how to minimize their impact. While commonly utilized in practice, there is little written on the underlying principles or specific interventions of supportive psychotherapy, especially in children and adolescents. And there is no consensus on the actual definition of this form of therapy. There are no systematic studies on this form of treatment in children and adolescents, though studies on adults indicate that it can be helpful. Generally, this form of therapy is used for short-term interventions for children in crisis or as an ongoing intervention to maintain individuals and families with significant illness (Rockland, 1989a, 1989b, 1989c; Gabbard, 2000).

Interpersonal psychotherapy

Interpersonal psychotherapy (IPT) was initially developed for adults and then modified for use with adolescents. It is a 12-session intervention during which the patient is seen weekly. The treatment is active, with a significant psychoeducation component. The focus is on identifying and improving the patient's symptoms and the current interpersonal functioning regardless of the cause. The general approach is to identify a few specific problems (significantly associated with relationships) to work on and to approach them through collaborative problem solving.

IPT has been demonstrated to be an effective treatment for depressed adolescents and is being tried in school settings and in a group format (Jacobs, 2003; Mufson and Dorta, 2003; McClellan and Werry, 2003).

Behavior management

Behavior management has been studied and demonstrated to be effective both for particular psychiatric disorders, such as phobias and attention-deficit/hyperactivity disorder (ADHD), and for specific problems such as social skill deficits and poor problem solving (Vitulano and Tebes, 2002; McClellan & Werry, 2003). Behavioral techniques and management commonly are incorporated into treatment even when other forms of psychotherapy are primary. It tends to be the major psychotherapeutic intervention for young children or those who are too impaired to participate in other forms (i.e. severe autism or mental retardation).

Behavior management approaches are predicated on the belief that human behavior is learned. The underlying belief is that changing behavior can alter how individuals feel and think. The overall aim is to identify and modify environmental influences, which elicit and maintain the behaviors of concern. Observed behavior is the focus of a directive and action-oriented treatment that uses empirically based intervention techniques. Subjective experiences such as feelings and thoughts can be incorporated into treatment if they can be connected to actual actions. Basically, these techniques attempt to alter behavior patterns by strengthening, maintaining, or developing desired behavior as well as reducing or eliminating undesired behavior. There are a number of techniques. Common ones used with children and adolescents include various forms of reinforcement, which occur when behavior is encouraged by its consequences. Providing a reward for a behavior after it occurs is positive reinforcement. An example is earning playtime by finishing one's chores. Negative reinforcement means removing an aversive stimulus that occurs subsequent to a behavior, putting one's toys away after playing means that they will not be confiscated. Both aim to increase the potential that the behavior will occur. Punishment attempts to reduce the occurrence of a behavior. Many behavior plans combine various forms of reinforcement to alter the child's behavior and may include punishment.

Another set of behavioral techniques often used is desensitization procedures to reduce fears or treat phobias by exposing the child in a variety of ways to decrease the fear associated with the stimulus. Behavioral assessment generally involves problem identification and target behavior selection, choice and design of intervention, periodic measurement of results, and evaluation of final outcome.

Two fields related to behavior management are hypnotherapy (hypnosis) and biofeedback. Hypnotherapy is a modality that employs an altered state of consciousness as part of the treatment. Generally, it is easier to hypnotize children and adolescents than adults. It can be helpful for pain, habit control, managing medical procedures, headaches, stress reduction, and as an adjunct to behavioral therapy. There are no controlled studies on its efficacy (Vitulano and Tebes, 2002; Williams, 2003). Biofeedback uses physiologic feedback instrumentation to train individuals to regulate their body responses such as muscle tone, heart rate, blood pressure, and cortical brain activity. There has been interest in using it as an intervention with disorders such as encopresis and attention-deficit/hyperactivity disorder, though no systematic studies exist documenting consistent benefit (Vitulano and Tebes, 2002).

Cognitive therapy

Cognitive behavior therapy (CBT) is probably the best-known cognitive therapy used with children and adolescents and is one of the best-studied psychosocial treatments. Generally, this approach has been utilized for children and adolescents who are motivated and can benefit from a limited number of sessions to work on specific, defined problems. It has been demonstrated to be effective for a number of psychiatric disorders such as depression, anxiety, obsessive-compulsive disorder, posttraumatic stress disorder, and conduct disorder. There have been inconsistent results with ADHD (Kazdin, 2000d; McClellan and Werry, 2003).

CBT emphasizes changing behavior and feelings through altering thought patterns in a defined number of sessions, usually 16–20. It is an integrative approach, which includes identifying and reducing underlying cognitive distortions that influence behaviors and developing more adaptive thinking with reflective problem solving and self-control skills. Generally, the idea is to identify distorted thinking and its association with particular behaviors and then to practice activities that promote more adaptive behaviors. A number of models exist, though the basic strategies are similar and many interventions integrate several. Verbal self-instruction training involves learning and practicing skills for interpreting situations, guiding behavior, and solving problems. Interpersonal cognitive problem solving attempts to improve problem solving skills in interpersonal situations. Children and adolescents also learn self-evaluation and management skills so they can accurately recognize, label, and modify their internal states and behaviors (Petti and Kronnennberger, 2002).

Family therapy

Family therapy involves the relevant members of a family unit and attempts to alter the interactional patterns within this unit to improve the functioning of the individual members. It is utilized as the primary treatment when the family is motivated and individual members are functional enough to participate effectively. While there often is an identified patient (often the child), the focus is on the unit and its impact on individual members as well as their contribution to the family's overall functioning. Family therapy may be the sole form of psychotherapy or an adjunct to other interventions. It is an appropriate choice of treatment when ongoing family interactions appear to be a significant factor in symptom development or maintenance and enough of the relevant family members are able to participate effectively. Conceptually, family therapy is predicated on the idea of the family as a system in which symptoms are manifestations of system issues that can cause difficulties for children or are important elements in maintenance of the family's current functioning. There are a number of schools of family therapy with different theoretical orientations, but none has been shown to be more efficacious than any other. Historically, practitioners of family therapy and child and adolescent psychiatry often have had different philosophies on mental illness, with family therapists being less interested in identifying specific psychiatric disorders (Josephson, 2002).

Current practice with children and adolescents and their families tends to blend systems, individual psychodynamic, and behavioral concepts. Generally, therapy involves identifying problematic interactions or behaviors, their impact, and developing strategies to implement more adaptive ways of acting. Often family treatment in some form is a component of other types of therapy practiced with children and adolescents, since the family is an essential aspect of the young person's environment, and even individual psychotherapy is not effective unless there is some involvement or contact with important family members. Family therapy has been utilized for a spectrum of disorders, problems, and family constellations. Contraindications can include uninvolved key family members, lack of interest by the adults in examining or changing family patterns, or family instability such that focus on the unit will cause harm. Several reviews of the literature on family therapy have reported that it is an effective treatment (McClellan and Werry, 2003). Much of the work related to children and adolescents has been on the usefulness of this treatment for externalizing disorders. There is general agreement that family therapy has been demonstrated to be beneficial in the treatment of schizophrenia (adolescents), conduct disorder, and substance abuse (Josephson, 2002).

Group therapy

Group psychotherapy is an approach in which a small number (usually up to 10–12) of individuals with between one and three therapists meet for a set time on a regular basis to work on particular themes. Benefits can include mutual support, shared or common difficulties, provision of hope, opportunity to help others, acquisition of knowledge and skills, learning to manage behavior in a group setting, catharsis, or corrective emotional experiences (Malekoff, 1997). Basically, the group interacts either through an activity or verbally, with the therapists providing feedback, structure, and modeling. Often, it is an adjunct to individual psychotherapy. It has been used for a variety of psychiatric disorders, ages, and problems. Appropriateness of group therapy for an individual depends more on a particular group's characteristics such as the goals, approaches, other group members, setting, and therapist/member ratio than the young person's age, problems, or diagnosis. Even children and adolescents who are aggressive or with low intelligence can benefit if the group is designed properly.

Group therapy has had applications in outpatient practices as well as being a component of a multimodal, integrated treatment in inpatient, residential, school, and outpatient programs. Group theoretical approaches are varied, with increasing emphasis recently on shorter-term, more manualized approaches. Psychodynamically oriented groups tend to be longer term with the aim of character changes. Shorter-term groups tend to focus on a particular problem (i.e. aggression) or psychiatric disorder (i.e. depression) and attempt to change behavior through approaches such as cognitive behavior therapy or psychoeducation. Self-help and mutual-support groups are essential aspects of many therapeutic and substance abuse programs. Groups can be heterogeneous or homogeneous in terms of ages, diagnosis, or target behaviors.

Meta-analysis of the research on this type of therapy reveals that it is cost effective and efficient. Advantages of group therapy can include therapist observation of behavior with peers in a safe, structured setting, use of peers to promote reciprocal exchange of thoughts and feedback, learning that others have similar problems, and the ability to practice skills in an environment that approximates some aspects of reality. Children's groups tend to be activity based, with adolescent groups more likely to be primarily verbal psychotherapy. Parent groups tend to focus on education or behavioral approaches (Cramer-Azima, 2002).

Parenting

Parenting work generally is a component of most treatment interventions for children and adolescents. This intervention has been utilized with diverse groups of parents, youth, and disorders, usually in conjunction with other interventions (Armbruster et al., 2002). Parenting work consists of therapeutic interventions designed for caretakers based on the premise that poor parenting is contributing to the child's or adolescent's problematic behavior by creating, maintaining, or exacerbating the symptoms. Most of these approaches are based on ideas that inadequate parenting is often due to a lack of education on how to be a good parent, replication of previous patterns (i.e. parents' relationships with their parents), or displacement of other issues (i.e. job stress). A variety of theoretical orientations including psychodynamic, cognitive behavioral, and behavioral have been employed. There is a body of literature and consensus that working with parents helps children and adolescents with psychiatric disorders. Studies examining specific programs for particular groups or problems have demonstrated effectiveness (Kazdin, 2000c; McClellan and Werry, 2003).

Multimodal interventions

Multiple intervention strategies, which utilize aggressive case management, comprehensive psychiatric services, and targeted family interventions, have been demonstrated to have positive outcomes with young people with conduct disorder, substance abuse, or in psychiatric crisis. For example, multisystemic therapy (MST) focuses on the systems that influence or interact with adolescents and their families and attempts to alter these systems in concrete ways that improve current behavior and risk factors (Kazdin, 2000d; McClellan & Werry, 2003). Combined medication and intensive psychosocial behavioral interventions demonstrated benefits for ADHD, particularly with associated problems with mood, anxiety, and behavior, social skills, and academic performance. School-based programs with interventions designed for multiple groups (children, teachers, parents) have shown to be helpful. Additional interventions can include identify-

---

BOX 4.2

Examples of various psychotherapeutic approaches

A 9-year-old boy is in treatment for anxiety. He continues to have problems in school, with daily teacher reports documenting disruptive behavior in class. In the office, he describes a recent episode where he was reprimanded for blurting out the correct answer to the teacher's question despite another student being called upon. The parents state that this behavior is frequent and that shaking, nail biting, and sweaty palms accompany these episodes. During this incident, the boy did think about the teacher's potential response. The patient tried to contain himself by counting to 10; however, his anxiety continued to increase and his behavior worsened.

Psychodynamic psychotherapy

- Exploring further the boy's actions, thoughts, and feelings.
- Comparing to similar behavior in the office with the therapist.
- Admission by the boy that he worries that adults will think he is not intelligent.
- Learning that his father frequently makes disparaging remarks about his performance at home and often talks about how only smart boys like his brother are successful.
- Learning that the boy believes that his father thinks he is stupid.
- Connecting of his worry about adults' perception to this belief.
- Clarifying of the differences between his father and other adults.
- Reinforcing examples of the teacher's positive regard with the boy.

Supportive psychotherapy

- Positively reinforcing the boy's attempts to modify his behaviour.
- Identifying similar situations where the boy's behavior was appropriate and the strategies employed during those incidents.
- Discussing with the boy other times when his behavior was appropriate and what strategies he used.
- Developing a plan to use previously successful strategies when the situation recurs.

Behavioral management

- Identifying the positive (i.e. teacher aware patient knows answer) and negative consequences (i.e. bad progress report) of behavior.
- Discussing situations where behavior was appropriate and what reinforcements helped the boy in managing his behavior.
- Developing a plan to reinforce appropriate behavior with rewards (i.e. being the teacher's helper).
- Make a chart to help the boy to monitor his progress.

Cognitive behavioral therapy

- Exploring further the boy's thoughts and feelings.
- Learning that the boy was worried that the teacher would think that he did not know the answer and would decide that the boy was not smart.
- Connecting the maladaptive thought to the behavior.
- Substituting the thought with more appropriate thoughts (i.e. "The teacher knows I'm smart because she just gave me an A").
- Developing a plan to substitute appropriate thoughts for maladaptive ones when similar situations occur.

ing problems such as parental psychiatric illness or substance abuse, lack of basic resources such as housing, or need for additional services at school and utilizing appropriate resources for these issues (Adnopoz, 2002).

Psychopharmacotherapy

Psychopharmacotherapy is the use of medication to decrease psychiatric signs and symptoms with the goal of improving functioning. Medication treatment is effective, especially when used as part of a multimodal treatment approach. Complementary non-medication approaches can be useful, especially when a medication may not be immediately effective (such as while medication is being titrated or when there is a delay in onset of action). Multimodal treatment is utilized in numerous clinical situations such as when symptoms improve faster when a multimodal approach is used or when symptoms may be only partially ameliorated by pharmaceutical interventions. Collaboration and communication among the professionals involved in providing the various interventions is essential to ensure that treatment goals and techniques are complementary and efficacious. Studies have demonstrated that integrated therapies have been effective for children and adolescents with various problems such as ADHD, obsessive-compulsive disorder (OCD) and school refusal (March and Wells, 2003).

Prior to initiation of medication treatment, it is important to engage the child's parents or family. Often, education about the diagnosis, information about the condition and treatment options will provide parents with an understanding of the rationale behind medication treatment. Information about the medication, what it is expected to do, what it cannot do, how much medication adjustment most likely will be required, the duration of medication treatment, side-effects, and what to do if side-effects arise can provide individuals with direction and guidance. It is also important to emphasize that the medication should be administered by adults, that consistent compliance should be a goal of treatment, that medication monitoring and follow-up visits will be important, that feedback from teacher and parents will be important in monitoring the medications, and that medication treatment does not replace other treatments that may be necessary. Questions should be encouraged so that concerns and potential myths can be addressed. An exchange of information as medication treatment is being contemplated can not only provide a thorough informed consent but potentially avert surprises.

Psychopharmacotherapy strategies

Accurate diagnosis and conceptualization are cornerstones of optimal psychopharmacotherapy. Clearly defined treatment goals should include target symptoms to be treated and diagnosis, when possible, that is contributing to target symptoms.

Defining target symptoms

Well-defined target symptoms are important for treatment, and in some situations the focus of treatment will be target symptoms alone (e.g. aggression). In most situations, however, understanding target symptoms in the context of a diagnosis is important, since individual target symptoms such as hyperactivity can represent multiple conditions such as ADHD, bipolar disorder, or psychosis, for which medication approaches differ significantly. Clearly defined target symptoms (e.g. hand-washing compulsion of OCD, excessive talking in ADHD, lack of enthusiasm associated with major depression) aid in the most appropriate selection of medication. Equally important, clearly defined, observable, concrete target symptoms help parents to focus on pertinent behaviors that will be important for assessing medication effectiveness, and help the clinician to track and document changes during the treatment. If target symptoms are vague and subjective ("not looking right," "being bad") it can be difficult to determine whether the treatment is beneficial.

Anticipating pharmacokinetic and pharmacodynamic properties

Familiarity with the pharmacokinetic and pharmacodynamic properties can help the clinician anticipate variations in response. For some medications, absorption can vary depending on diet (e.g. dextroamphetamine absorption may be hindered by certain food; Auiler et al., 2002). For other medications, half-life may vary depending on whether another ingested food or medication is inhibiting metabolic pathways such as the cytochrome p-450 systems (Nemeroff et al., 1996).

Familiarity with the clinical response profile enables one to anticipate the timing of clinical changes. Onset may be quick (e.g. stimulants, antipsychotics) or delayed (e.g. antidepressants). Duration may be short (e.g. immediate-release stimulants), long (e.g. long-acting stimulants), or constant (e.g. many antidepressants). Knowledge about duration enables one to anticipate when benefits may abate and target symptoms return. For example, if a child were to do homework 8 hours after taking one dose of immediate-release methylphenidate, most likely there would be very little remaining therapeutic benefit, so it would probably be difficult to complete the homework. However, if this child received a long-acting stimulant, the longer duration of benefit could still enable them to complete the homework.

Familiarity with side-effect profiles is essential to maximize safety, minimize noncompliance, assess clinical response, and decide titration strategies. Some side-effects may contribute to clinical confusion. For example, despite the associated benefits in mood, anti-epileptic medications can actually contribute to irritability and an increase in dose could exacerbate the situation (Loring and Meador,

2001). Similarly, stimulant "rebound irritability" that can arise as the medication benefit wanes can appear like intense ADHD (Carlson and Kelly, 2003). An increase in stimulant dose could exacerbate this "rebound" phenomenon. Education of parents about potential side-effects is essential for obtaining an informed consent, but also for identifying potential problems. In short, we can minimize potential pitfalls by being familiar with each medication's profile.

Assessing the baseline

Prior to initiating pharmacotherapy the clinician should obtain an informed consent and perform a baseline assessment. Characterizing baseline target symptoms enables subsequent comparison and assessment. Most often, target symptoms are characterized by repertoire, intensity, frequency, duration, and pattern of appearance. In fact, many rating scales and instruments can be helpful to characterize the baseline clinical presentation (see Chapter 2). One must be mindful of the source of baseline data, as well as when or where the observations were obtained. Additionally, depending on the medication that is selected, appropriate laboratory tests should be obtained both to identify contraindications for medication initiation and to establish a baseline value.

Titrating and monitoring

Titration, monitoring, and medication maintenance are also important. Starting with a low initial medication dose can be advantageous so as to minimize side-effects and potentially maximize compliance. As medication is increased, assessment of target symptoms can help clinicians determine whether further titration is required. Assessment instruments (see Chapter 2) can be pivotal in this assessment. It is important to appreciate that "therapeutic" doses are very individualized, so doses can vary from person to person. It is equally important to note that poor response can often be due to subtherapeutic dosing (Elia et al., 1991). Poor therapeutic response can also be attributed to a delayed onset of benefit, e.g. benefits of an antidepressant may not be noticeable for weeks after initiation. Just as psychiatric assessment should be continued during maintenance treatment, so should appropriate laboratory testing. Monitoring of side-effects is essential, especially as medications are being adjusted. For example, some antidepressant medications may contribute to suicidal behavior within days of adjusting dosage.

When more than one condition or spectrum of symptoms exists, multiple medications may be required (Woolston, 1999). More than ever, it is important to have clearly defined target symptoms and goals, since the presentation can be complex and confusing when multiple conditions exist. Additionally, it is important to prioritize which condition needs to be stabilized first. When multiple medications are prescribed, adjustment of one medication at a time can minimize confusion, especially should an adverse reaction arise. One also needs to be familiar with potential medication-medication interactions. And if a medication has equivocal or no response, one should consider discontinuing it.

Commonly used medications

Stimulants (for attention-deficit/hyperactivity disorder)

Since Bradley's discovery of the behavioral benefits of stimulants, stimulant treatment has become widely studied and established as the gold standard of attention-deficit/hyperactivity disorder pharmacotherapy (Spencer et al., 1996; Elia et al., 1999; The MTA Cooperative Group, 1999; Pliszka et al., 2000a, 2000b; Schachter et al., 2001; Greenhill et al., 2002). The mechanism of action for stimulants includes direct release and reuptake inhibition of dopamine and norepinephrine, resulting in their increased availability. Stimulants – methylphenidate and amphetamine isomers – have been rigorously studied in more than 150 controlled trials (Spencer et al., 1996), and result in improvement in inattentive, hyperactivity-impulsive, and oppositional symptoms. Fidgetiness, difficulty sitting, blurting out, excessive talking, interrupting, difficulty concentrating, distractibility, difficulty completing tasks, and forgetting are among the ADHD target symptoms that stimulants can treat. Efficacy has been supported for short-acting immediate-release Ritalin, Adderall, intermediate-release Metadate CD, Ritalin LA, and extended-release formulations such as Concerta (Pelham et al., 2001; Wolraich et al., 2001) and Adderall XR (Biederman et al., 2002; McCracken et al., 2003). In the landmark MTA study, stimulant treatment was surprisingly robustly superior to behavior treatment, and there was little overall difference between stimulant treatment alone and combined medication-behavior treatment (The MTA Cooperative Group, 1999). In fact, stimulant medication is a first-line medication treatment for ADHD (Pliszka et al., 2000a, 2000b).

Commonly tolerated side-effects include stomach-aches, headaches, decreased appetite, weight loss, insomnia, exacerbation of tics, and rebound irritability (Carlson and Kelly, 2003). In some individuals with comorbid bipolar disorder, stimulants may exacerbate irritability, and some individuals with psychosis may experience exacerbation of psychotic symptoms. Previously used magnesium pemoline was associated with severe hepatotoxicity.

Stimulant treatment of ADHD has been described in detail (American Academy of Child and Adolescent Psychiatry, 1997; Greenhill et al., 1999, 2002; Pliszka et al., 2000a, 2000b). Medication recommendations and algorithms often incorporate several similar approaches: start low and go slow, titrate and monitor progress with rating scales, monitor side-effects and titrate to minimize impairment.

TABLE 4.1

Stimulants for the treatment of attention-deficit/hyperactivity disorder

Medication	Preparation and dosage (mg)	Dose (mg)	Duration of benefit (hr) S (short) I (intermediate) L (long)
Methylphenidate:			
Focalin	2.5, 5, 10 tablet	Start: 2.5bid Max: 20mg/d	S 3–5
Methylin	5, 10, 20 tablet	Start: 5mg 2x/d Max: 60mg/d	S 3–5
Ritalin	5, 10, 20 tablet	Start: 5mg 2x/d Max: 60mg/d	S 3–5
Metadate ER	10, 20 tablet	Max: 60	I 6–8
Methylin ER	10, 20 tablet		I 6–8
Ritalin SR	20 tablet		I 6–8
Metadate CD	20 capsule	Max: 60	I 8
Ritalin LA	20, 30, 40 capsule	Max: 60	I 8
Concerta	18, 27, 36, 54 tablet	Max: 54	L 12
Amphetamine:			
Adderall	5, 7.5, 10, 12.5, 15, 20, 30 tablet	3–5yr:Start 2.5qd or 2x/d 6+yr: 5 qd or 2x/d Max: 40mg/d	S 4–6
Dexedrine	5 tablet	3–5yr:Start 2.5qd or 2x/d 6+yr: 5 qd or 2x/d Max: 40mg/d	S 4–6
Dextrostat	5, 10 tablet	3–5yr:Start 2.5qd or 2x/d 6+yr: 5 qd or 2x/d Max: 40mg/d	S 4–6
Dexedrine Spansule	5, 10, 15 capsule	6+yr: 5 qd or 2x/d Max: 40mg/d	I 6–8
Adderall XR	5, 10, 15, 25, 30 capsule	6+yr: 5 qd or 2x/d Max: 30mg/d	L 10–12

With an increasing number of medications from which to choose (see Table 4.1 adapted from American Academy of Child and Adolescent Psychiatry, 1997; Greenhill et al., 1999, 2002; Pliszka et al., 2000a, 2000b), it is important to realize that any stimulant has the potential of improving ADHD symptoms (Elia et al., 1991). However, one may compare short-acting stimulants with long-acting stimulants. Short-acting stimulants tend to have a quick onset and quick off-set. This property may be advantageous when administered at certain times of the day such as in the evening so that sleep is not affected. Unfortunately, if given during the course of the day, several doses will be required, potentially resulting in rebound irritability, trips to the nurse's office, embarrassment, and decreased compliance. In contrast, the long-acting stimulants require only one dose in the morning and provide relatively continuous coverage, thereby minimizing rebound irritability and maintaining privacy.

Stimulants can be initiated at low starting doses, and improvement can potentially be apparent immediately (see Table 4.1). However, in most cases follow-up visits will be required to adjust medication doses. Follow-up visits should include assessment of side-effects, assessment of clinical progress, and height/weight measurements. Validated rating scales for ADHD (see Chapter 2 for scales such as the ADHD rating scale, Abbreviated Conners, or SNAP-IV) are an essential part of medication assessment, and the degree of improvement in hyperactivity-impulsivity and inattention should be assessed at each visit. Often, the short versions of rating scales provide the quickest information and the highest probability that a parent or teacher will complete it. Feedback from both parent and teacher in the form of completed rating scales as well as verbal reports can provide essential information, and can help the clinician determine whether additional adjustment is required. Titration and feedback can occur as often as 1-week intervals, as in the Texas Children's Medication Algorithm Project (Pliszka et al., 2000b). If an individual does not improve on the stimulant, the clinician should assess compliance and the time frame when the feedback (rating scale) was provided. If the rating scale was completed after the medication's benefits had worn off, there could be a perceived treatment failure when in fact the medication provided benefit earlier in the day. On the other hand, if the initial selection of stimulant was ineffective, the clinician should consider trying a different stimulant in another class, since there is a possibility that it could improve ADHD symptoms (Elia et al., 1991). If no stimulants provide benefit, the clinician should consider a nonstimulant, either to augment or to be tried in lieu of a stimulant.

Nonstimulants (for ADHD)

Nonstimulants for ADHD treatment include atomoxetine, clonidine, guanfacine, and bupropion. Nonstimulants, with the exception of atomoxetine, predominantly affect norepinephrine transmission. Many case reports and studies exist for the use of nonstimulants in ADHD (Spencer et al., 1996). Of nonstimulants that are used for ADHD, atomoxetine, a norepinephrine reuptake inhibitor that results in increase in frontal cortex norepinephrine and dopamine, has the most extensive database and controlled studies (Michelson et al., 2001, 2002). Unlike other nonstimulants, atomoxetine has been shown to improve both inattention and hyperactivity-impulsive symptoms, and it has relatively long clinical effects with once-daily dosing. Commonly tolerated side-effects include decreased appetite, transient weight loss, mild increase in heart rate and blood pressure, but unlike tricyclic antidepressants (TCAs) there are no cardiac conduction delays or associated adverse effects (Wernicke and Kratochvil, 2002).

Atomoxetine can be initiated either as qd or bid dosing. For some the qd dosing may be administered at night if sedation or fatigue is experienced, and clinical benefits will be apparent in the morning. The initial dose is 0.5mg/kg for the initial 3 days, then it is increased to the therapeutic 1.2mg/kg/d dose. However, if side-effects arise the increase from 0.5mg/kg/d to 1.2mg/kg/d can be deferred until side-effects improve. Follow-up visits should also include assessment of side-effects, assessment of clinical progress with ADHD rating scales (Chapter 2), and height/weight measurements. Vital signs should be obtained at follow-up, although there are no direct cardiac effects associated with atomoxetine.

Alpha-2 agonists, clonidine or guanfacine, are medications which are often used off-label to address hyperactive-impulsive symptoms of ADHD. Many individuals benefit especially at night to address insomnia. These medications are generally second-line medications that either augment stimulants or are used in lieu of stimulants. Even though

the American Cardiology Association (Gutgesell et al., 1999) does not make any recommendations regarding cardiac work-up for use of these medications, there has been cautious initiation of these medications ever since the isolated reported deaths of children who received clonidine in combination with methylphenidate (Popper, 1995). No definitive link between clonidine and the deaths was ever established, and no definitive conclusion was ever drawn. Nevertheless, many clinicians consequently obtain baseline vital signs and EKG. Generally, these medications are started at low doses (clonidine 0.05mg qd or bid; guanfacine 0.5mg qd or bid) to minimize sedation and fatigue. Follow-up titration can occur within 2–4 weeks with additional increase in frequency to tid or qid dosing. Follow-ups should include assessment of side-effects, assessment of clinical progress with ADHD rating scales (Chapter 2), and vital signs. Maximal improvement in hyperactivity-impulsivity may not be apparent for 4 weeks, and further adjustment may be required several months later even after optimal dosing has been achieved. When clonidine or guanfacine are discontinued, a 2-week taper should be instituted to minimize the risk of rebound hypertension.

Selective serotonin reuptake inhibitors

With the increasing awareness of pediatric anxiety and mood disorders (see Chapters 9 and 10), treatment with selective serotonin reuptake inhibitors (SSRIs) has become increasingly important. SSRIs are widely used for the treatment of anxiety disorders (Velosa and Riddle, 2000). Target symptoms that can be controlled with these medications include excessive worries, fear, phobias, obsessions and compulsions, and panic attacks. Prior to the introduction of SSRIs, controlled studies found that tricyclic antidepressants (TCAs) were effective in treating separation anxiety disorder (Bernstein, Garfinkel and Borchardt, 1990; Gittelman-Klein and Klein, 1973; Klein et al., 1992). As expected, SSRIs were found to be effective in controlled studies with fluoxetine (Birmaher et al., 2003) and fluvoxamine (The Research Unit on Pediatric Psychopharmacology Anxiety Study Group, 2001) for generalized anxiety disorder, separation anxiety disorder, and/or social phobia.

SSRIs have also been found to be effective in pediatric obsessive-compulsive disorder. Previously controlled pediatric OCD studies with clomipramine (Flament et al., 1985; DeVeaugh-Geiss et al., 1992), a TCA with potent serotonin reuptake inhibition, were positive. More recently, controlled trials of fluoxetine (Riddle et al., 1992), fluvoxamine (Riddle et al., 2001), and sertraline (March et al., 1998) were also effective in pediatric OCD. In a meta-analysis of pediatric OCD studies including SSRIs and clomipramine, all SSRIs were found to be comparably effective, but clomipramine was superior (Geller et al., 2003).

Antidepressant treatment of pediatric major depressive disorder (review, Birmaher et al., 1996) has been a long-standing practice, yet meta-analysis of controlled trials of previously prescribed TCAs (desipramine, imipramine, amitriptyline, nortriptyline) found them to be ineffective in contrast to their benefits to adults (Hazell et al., 1995). Unlike TCAs, SSRIs have been effective in the treatment of pediatric major depressive disorder. In double-blind placebo-controlled studies of fluoxetine (Emslie et al., 1997, 2002), paroxetine (Keller et al., 2001) and sertraline (Wagner et al., 2003), SSRI treatment of major depression in children was superior to the placebo. Optimal duration of treatment has not been determined definitively. However, preliminary recommendations based on review of controlled studies suggest that if significant clinical improvement has occurred, a medication-free period should be tried after 1 year of treatment. Any taper of SSRI should occur during a stress-free period, and should signs or symptoms of relapse appear, the SSRI should be reinitiated (Pine, 2002). Overall, in a short period of time SSRI treatment has become integrated into the pharmacologic treatment strategy for major depression (American Association of Child and Adolescent Psychiatry, 1998; Hughes et al., 1999).

Frequently encountered side-effects including headache, gastrointestinal upset, and insomnia are generally well tolerated (Leonard et al., 1997). Other more concerning adverse effects associated with SSRIs include toxicity, irritability, nervousness, induction of mania, serotonin syndrome, and SSRI withdrawal. Induction of mania can occur when SSRIs are being used to treat depression during a depressive phase of manic depression (bipolar disorder). Resulting symptoms can include increased energy, decreased need for sleep, increased fast talking, distractibility, and grandiose thoughts. In contrast to TCAs, there is little concern for anticholinergic, antihistaminergic, or quinidine-like effects.

The use of SSRIs has not been without occasional controversy. In 2004, the US Food and Drug Administration (FDA) issued a health advisory regarding withdrawal as well as suicidal thoughts (Oransky, 2003; Connor, 2004). Even before the advisory, there had been periodic concerns about withdrawal symptoms upon sudden discontinuation of some SSRIs (Tonks, 2002; Anonymous, 2003). This discontinuation syndrome consists of dizziness, paresthesia, nausea, headache, lethargy, asthenia, and insomnia.

Concerns have been raised regarding SSRIs and associated increased suicidal thoughts or self-harm (Committee on Safety of Medicines, 2003). Even though associated suicidal thoughts are uncommon, the precise prevalence is unknown and the mechanism of such a potential side-effect is poorly understood. Some individuals who receive SSRIs may appear to have a sudden worsening of depression without the suicidal ideations. The time of most concern for suicidal thoughts is shortly after initiation, increase, or decrease of SSRIs.

To understand the risk of SSRI-related suicidal thoughts, the FDA conducted two meta-analyses of 24 published and unpublished pediatric studies involving SSRIs. Results of these meta-analyses consistently revealed that there was an approximately two-fold increase in risk of suicidal thinking or behavior. However, no individuals committed suicide in those studies. Consequently, the FDA published new guidelines and information on its website (US Food and Drug Administration, 2004). A black-box warning was mandated on package inserts regarding potential clinical worsening in addition to the increased risk of suicidal thinking and behavior. Families were recommended to be aware of new thoughts or attempts of suicide, worsening of depression/anxiety/irritability, agitation/restlessness, panic attacks, insomnia, aggression/impulsiveness, hyperactivity, increased talking, or any other behavioral changes. Regular follow-ups were recommended after initiating the medication or changing the dose (once a week for 4 weeks, then every 2 weeks for the next month and finally at the end of their 12th week taking the drug).

As a result of concerns, only fluoxetine has been recommended for continued use in children in the UK. This may in part be due to its long half-life as well as its metabolite's exceptionally long half-life. Definitive conclusions and recommendations regarding the controversial association with suicidal thoughts have been difficult to make, and the need for more uniform methodology for eliciting safety data in pediatric psychopharmacological studies is highlighted (Greenhill, 2003). Despite the clinical benefit of SSRIs in children, clinicians should be aware of sudden clinical changes especially shortly after any change in SSRI dosage.

Standard starting doses of SSRIs are conventionally less than those for adults (see Table 4.2). Often a dose for a child is less than 50% of the adult starting dose, and the degree to which it is tolerated is very individualized. Liquid preparations provide more flexibility in initiating and titrating SSRIs. Prior to initiating SSRI treatment, it is important to discuss potential side-effects, especially potential irritability, nervousness, and activation. Follow-up for the first 4 weeks after starting the medication should include evaluation of response and side-effects as well as careful evaluation of suicidal ideation. If the clinical presentation seems to worsen, the clinician should check to see whether there are any symptoms of withdrawal or manic activation. When discontinuing SSRIs it is prudent to taper the medicine gradually, usually over 2 weeks.

Mood stabilizers
As the presence of mood disorders in children and adolescents has been increasingly accepted and recognized over the past two decades, the use of mood stabilizers has been on the rise (for a review of mood stabilizers, see Ryan et al., 1999). Mood stabilizers have most often referred to lithium, valproic acid, and carbamazepine, but more recently they have often included the new-generation anti-epileptic med-

TABLE 4.2

Selective serotonin reuptake inhibitors

	Preparations and dosages	Common starting doses
Escitalopram (Lexapro)	10mg, 20mg, liquid (1mg/1ml)	5mg
Citalopram (Celexa)	10, 20, 40mg liquid (2mg/1ml)	10mg
Fluoxetine (Prozac)	10mg, 20mg liquid (5mg/20ml)	5–10mg
Fluvoxamine (Luvox)	25mg, 50mg, 100mg	12.5mg
Paroxetine (Paxil)	10mg, 20mg, 30mg, 40	10mg
Paroxetine (Paxil CR)	12.5mg, 25mg, 37.5mg	12.5mg
Sertraline (Zoloft)	50mg, 100mg, 150mg	25mg

ications (topiramate, tiagabine, gabapentin, lamotrigine, levetiracetam). This category of medications has been used in children and adolescents more frequently for the treatment of bipolar disorder (for the American Academy of Child and Adolescent Psychiatry Practice Parameters for bipolar disorder, see McClellan and Werry, 1997), aggression, and conduct disorder, despite the paucity of definitive clinical data in these age groups (Jensen et al., 1999). The paucity of clinical evidence for efficacy in treating bipolar disorder is most apparent for the new-generation anti-epileptic medications, and in some instances they continue to be used even when there is evidence that some are no better than the placebo (Pande et al., 2000). In some individuals, the profound functional impairment requires multiple mood stabilizers to see improvement and achieve clinical stability, so the issue of polypharmacy and potentially increased side-effects must be considered (for example, should a second augmentative mood stabilizer be required, a slow titration of the second agent may help to minimize side-effects) (Freeman and Stoll, 1998).

Given the challenges and limitations, it is incumbent upon the clinician to appreciate the potential significant benefits that can be offered to patients while acknowledging limited clinical and research data. With a significant knowledge gap between clinical research and practice, the informed consent becomes perhaps even more important.

Lithium

Lithium has been long used in adults as a mood stabilizer, with established efficacy in the treatment of bipolar disorder (reviews: Baldessarini et al., 2000; Schou, 1997) and it is one of the few interventions shown to reduce suicide risk (Baldessarini et al., 2001). Even though the literature on lithium use in children and adolescents is less extensive compared with that of adults, there is growing information (for a review, see Alessi et al., 1994). Review of the child literature finds that there are few controlled studies in children and adolescents (Geller et al., 1998). The majority of

studies examining the efficacy in children and adolescents have been open studies (Kowatch et al., 2000; Strober et al., 1988). The largest open study to date has consisted of 100 adolescents, ages 12–19 years (Kafantaris et al., 2003). In that study, rapid lithium titration resulted in therapeutic lithium levels at the end of week 1, and 63% of individuals responded to lithium treatment as defined by >33% improvement in Young Mania Rating Scale after 4 weeks. Age of onset, severity of comorbid manic symptoms, psychosis (even when treated with antipsychotic medication), depression, or ADHD did not influence response. Lithium has also been studied in individuals with conduct disorder and aggression. A double-blind placebo controlled study of inpatient children and adolescents responded to lithium treatment. However, more than 50% of individuals experienced nausea, vomiting, and urinary frequency (Malone et al., 2000).

Lithium initiation and maintenance require periodic but regular assessment and monitoring (McClellan and Werry, 1997). Prior to initiating lithium, baseline laboratory tests including serum creatinine, blood urea nitrogen, electrolytes, thyroid-stimulating hormone should be obtained. Higher lithium levels and elevated baseline thyroid stimulating hormone (TSH) have been associated with subsequent elevated TSH levels with lithium treatment, and an appreciable number of children (up to 24%) who took lithium in conjunction with valproic acid developed hypothyroidism within 3 months (Gracious et al., 2004). These findings underscore the importance of regular monitoring. Common side-effects (Silva et al., 1992) that include stomach-ache, nausea, vomiting, loose stools, fine tremor, enuresis, fatigue, and acne are important to monitor. If polyuria becomes problematic, urine osmolality should be obtained to rule out diabetes insipidus. Often if lithium is taken with food, if the dose is titrated gradually or if slow-release preparations are administered, side-effects can be minimized. Maintenance monitoring should include lithium level (12 hours after last dose), blood urea nitrogen, creatinine, and thyroid function tests every 3–6 months. EKGs and urine analysis can be obtained as clinically indicated.

Valproic acid

Of all anti-epileptic medications, valproic acid has had the greatest clinical use and effectiveness in stabilizing mood. Open-label studies (Kowatch et al., 2000; Wagner et al., 2002; West et al., 1994) and controlled studies (DelBello et al., 2002) with valproic acid have supported efficacy in reducing manic symptoms. Kowatch et al.'s study comparing valproic acid, lithium, and carbamazepine found that valproic acid had the largest effect size (1.63 compared with 1.06 for lithium and 1.00 for carbamazepine) as well as the highest response rate (53% as compared with 38% for either lithium or carbamazepine).

Baseline evaluation and subsequent monitoring are important (McClellan and Werry, 1997). Prior to starting valproic acid, it is important to obtain laboratory tests including hepatic function, coagulation indices, and complete blood counts. Maintenance labs should include trough valproic acid levels in addition to hepatic function and hematologic indices, and these should be obtained every 3–6 months.

Relatively common side-effects include nausea, vomiting, fatigue, and sedation. Rare but serious side-effects have included hepatic and pancreatic failure. Unfortunately, hepatic testing does not predict whether these complications will arise. Thrombocytopenia can develop with valproic acid treatment. Since the early reports of polycystic ovary syndrome associated with valproic acid in individuals with epilepsy (Isojarvi et al., 1993) there has been much debate over this potential relationship (Eberle, 1998; Johnston, 1999). It is not clear to what degree observations in the epilepsy literature can be generalized to females with mood disorders, and unfortunately without further rigorous studies addressing this concern, definitive recommendations are elusive. Nevertheless, if young females require valproic acid it has been suggested that the clinician monitor menstrual cycles and irregularities (Garland and Behr, 1996).

With very promising efficacy and the potential to benefit many, several clinical questions wait to be addressed.

Carbamazepine

Another anti-epileptic medication that has been prescribed for bipolar disorder is carbamazepine. Very few reports on the use of carbamazepine in children are available. A case series of three children with mania describes improvement with carbamazepine (Woolston, 1999b). Kowatch et al.'s (2000) open-label comparison of three mood stabilizers found that carbamazepine was very effective in treating bipolar disorder.

Baseline evaluation should include complete blood count and hepatic function tests (McClellan and Werry, 1997).

Maintenance labs should include trough carbamazepine levels in addition to complete blood count and hepatic function tests. Common side-effects include nausea, sedation, and dizziness, and rare but potentially serious side-effects include leucopenia, agranulocytosis or aplastic anemia, hepatic failure, and Stevens-Johnson syndrome.

Oxcarbazepine, a compound related to carbamazepine, has advantages of decreased side-effects and lower incidence of hematologic effects. However, there is even less data related to its use in children.

Atypical antipsychotics

Antipsychotic use in children (review, Campbell and Rapoport, 1999) has targeted both specific target symptoms and psychotic disorders, and their role in the treatment of various disorders is becoming increasingly recognized. These medications have been useful for treating delusions, hallucinations, mania, severe impulsivity, and aggression. New-generation "atypical" anti-psychotic medications which include risperidone, quetiapine, olanzapine, ziprasidone, and aripiprazole (see Table 4.3) have combined serotonin and dopamine receptor-blocking action that result in improved side-effect profiles compared with the "conventional," older-generation antipsychotics (e.g. haloperidol, chlorpromazine, perphenazine, fluphenazine). Recent data derived from examining 11 studies that utilized antipsychotics for 1 or more years found that atypical antipsychotics were associated with a lower 0.8% annual incidence of tardive dyskinesia versus the 5.4% annual incidence associated with haloperidol (Correll et al., 2004). Controlled studies with antipsychotics have found efficacy for controlling aggression (Pappadopulos et al., 2003; Schur et al., 2003) and disruptive behavior-disordered children with suboptimal cognition (Aman et al., 2002) and autism (McCracken et al., 2002). Additionally, antipsychotics have been effective or recommended for conduct disorder (Snyder et al., 2002; Findling et al., 2000) and schizophrenia (American Academy of Child and Adolescent Psychiatry, 2001), and there is preliminary evidence that antipsychotics may be beneficial as adjunctive treatment of mania (Kafantaris et al., 2001).

Side-effects include sedation, extrapyramidal symptoms (EPS, i.e. dystonia, Parkinsonism, akathisia), tardive dyskinesia, neuroleptic malignant syndrome (Silva et al., 1999), hyperprolactinemia, diabetes (Koller et al., 2001), and weight gain (Ratzoni et al., 2002). In general some side-effects may be more associated with specific antipsychotics (Pappadopulos et al., 2003), and the side-effect profile may influence medication selection. Weight gain and sedation are least associated with risperidone and ziprasidone but more associated with olanzapine and clozapine. Extrapyramidal symptoms are more associated with risperidone and less associated with other atypical antipsychotics. Tardive dyskinesia (TD) is a potentially irreversible, involuntary

TABLE 4.3

Atypical antipsychotic dosing

	Preparation/dosages (mg)	Starting doses (mg)	Target doses (mg)
Aripiprazole (Abilify)	Tablets (5, 10, 15, 20, 30)	5 qd	5–30
Clozapine (Clozaril)	Tablet (25, 100)	6.25–25	150–300
Olanzapine (Zyprexa)	Zyprexa tablet (2.5, 5, 7.5, 10, 15, 20) Zyprexa ZYDIS dissolvable tablet (5, 10, 15, 20)	2.5 bid	10–20
	Zyprexa injectable (2.5, 5, 7.5,10)	2.5 bid	
Risperidone (Risperdal)	Risperdal tablet (0.25, 0.5, 1, 2, 4)		1–3
	Risperdal M-Tab (0.5, 1, 2)	0.25 bid	
	Risperdal liquid (1mg/ml)	0.25 bid	
	Risperdal Consta injectable long acting	0.25 bid	
Quetiapine (Seroquel)	Tablet 25, 100, 200, 300	50 bid	400–800
Zisprasidone (Geodon)	Capsule (20, 40, 60, 80) injectable	20 bid	80–160

muscle movement disorder that most often presents with choreic or athetoid movement in the face and mouth. TD may be associated with pre- and perinatal injury, duration of antipsychotic treatment, and female sex (Campbell et al., 1997), and there are even reports of tardive dyskinesia with atypical antipsychotics despite the lower incidence compared with "conventional," older-generation antipsychotics (Demb and Nguyen, 1999; Kumra et al., 1998). Ziprasidone potentially delays conduction, resulting in elevated QTc, so a baseline EKG is recommended. Clozapine is considered a very effective atypical antipsychotic, but it has unique, potentially serious side-effects including seizure, leucopenia, and agranulocytosis that consequently require weekly white blood cell counts. For that reason, clinicians may prefer to initiate treatment with other atypical antipsychotics. Even though the most concerning side-effects associated with atypical antipsychotics are relatively rare, it is important for clinicians to be familiar with signs and symptoms for effective monitoring and detection. Additional long-term side-effects are unknown.

Treatment with antipsychotic medication should include the requisite informed consent, complementary psychosocial interventions, and a thorough baseline evaluation (American Academy of Child and Adolescent Psychiatry, 1997, 2001). This evaluation should include a psychiatric diagnostic assessment with clearly defined target symptoms. The importance of the psychiatric assessment cannot be emphasized enough, since identification of an underlying primary condition that is producing the presenting symptoms may require treatment other than antipsychotic therapy. A thorough medical assessment should be performed, taking special note of any pre-existing dyskinesias

and dystonias. Before starting antipsychotic medication, the clinician should also obtain baseline information that would be relevant if weight gain or diabetes were to become problematic in treatment. The American Diabetes Association (2004), in conjunction with the American Psychiatric Association, American Association of Clinical Endocrinologists, and North American Association for the Study of Obesity, issued recommended baseline data prior to starting antipsychotics: family history of diabetes, vital signs, weight, waist circumference, and laboratory tests. The pertinent laboratory tests should include fasting plasma glucose and fasting lipid profile. Additionally, a baseline assessment of involuntary movements should be performed using the Abnormal Involuntary Movement Scale (AIMS; Guy, 1976).

Several antipsychotic medications are available, but atypical antipsychotics should be chosen over the "conventional" antipsychotics because of the more favorable side-effect profile (American Academy of Child and Adolescent Psychiatry, 1997; Pappadopulos et al., 2003). Antipsychotic medication can be started at low doses but increased every 3–4 days until target symptoms improve (see Table 4.3; Pappadopulos et al., 2003; Schur et al., 2003). Dosing guidelines for children are not yet well defined and may differ depending on the age and size of the child, the severity, frequency, and nature of the target symptoms. However, a general approach of starting low and titrating slow should be followed.

With initiation of antipsychotic treatment, monitoring of the target symptoms and side-effects is essential. Assessment of side-effects at follow-up should include evaluation of any extrapyramidal symptoms: dystonia, Parkinsonism, or akathisia. Should dystonia or Parkinsonism appear, diphenhydramine 25–50mg or benztropine

0.5–1mg can be given to alleviate symptoms. Follow-up visits every 4 weeks for the first 12 weeks should include vital signs, especially weight. Thereafter, weight should be obtained quarterly (American Diabetes Association, 2004). AIMS should be performed every 3–6 months (American Academy of Child and Adolescent Psychiatry, 1997, 2001). If dyskinesias are detected, a gradual reduction of dose is recommended.

Off-label use of medications

Many medications which are used to treat pediatric and psychiatric disorders lack associated pediatric clinical trials data and indications (American Academy of Pediatrics Committee on Drugs, 1996). This "off-label" use of medications that have been approved for other uses is common in children with psychiatric conditions. In one study of physicians prescribing psychotropic medications, off-label prescribing occurs in approximately 40% (Efron et al., 2003). Additionally, with the rising identification of comorbidity, the prevalence of combined psychopharmacotherapy has risen along with potential unknowns (Woolston, 1999). In this uncharted territory, it is incumbent upon the physician to be aware of the properties, benefits, and limitations of medications. Despite a growing database of evidence-based pharmacologic treatments, future trials are needed to assess safety and efficacy (McClellan and Werry, 2003; Vitiello and Jensen, 1997).

Other therapies

Various other interventions have been tried for children and adolescents with mental illness. Alternative and complementary medicine increasingly has become an option sought by patients and their families for medical and psychiatric disorders, despite limited information on their use and effectiveness in children and adolescents. Examples include herbs, vitamins, massage, acupuncture, aromatherapy, and homeopathy (Gardiner and Wornham, 2000). A recent survey of caretakers of children and adolescents being treated for ADHD or depression found that a significant number of patients had taken herbal remedies, most without the knowledge of their psychiatrist, pediatrician, or pharmacist (Cala et al., 2003).

Dietary strategies (primarily exclusion of particular foods and substances) have been promoted as effective interventions for psychiatric disorders without significant empirical support. For example, the Feingold's hypothesis that salicylates, synthetic dyes, and preservatives have toxic effects and are responsible for hyperactivity, autism, and mental retardation has been tested and found to be false. A similar idea based on the belief that sugar or food dyes can worsen behavior of certain predisposed children has had inconclusive evidence. Two challenge studies have found that certain children with ADHD have worsening behavior symptoms when exposed to specific foods. The studies were small with highly selected children and the problematic foods varied with each child. The behaviors seem to be related to irritability and non-compliance rather than specific aspects of ADHD and the mechanism of action is unknown. The diets are difficult to maintain and resisted by children and adolescents (Kazdin, 2000c; Heyman and Santosh, 2003; Waslick and Greenhill, 2003).

Electroconvulsive therapy/transcranial magnetic stimulation

Electroconvulsive therapy (ECT) is considered to be a treatment modality for adults and some adolescents with severe, life-threatening psychiatric illnesses. Generally, for ECT to be a treatment option, an adolescent must have a severe and persistent mood (depression, bipolar) disorder, catatonia, or neuroleptic malignant syndrome. The symptoms must be severe, persistent, and disabling. They often are life-threatening. ECT usually is considered in situations where symptoms have failed to respond adequately to medication or patients who cannot tolerate medications, cannot take medication, or will be in life-threatening states while waiting for a psychopharmacologic response. It has been utilized in the acute phase of illness as a short-term intervention with pharmacology and other treatments employed for maintenance therapy since ECT does not have a permanent effect. Use in adolescents is uncommon since it tends to be a treatment of last resort. The treatment consists of causing a seizure by the application of a brief electric current through the brain, via scalp electrodes. There is insufficient data and clinical experience on the use of ECT in school-age or younger children. The data on adolescents indicates that ECT can be an effective treatment intervention, which is well tolerated. There are a few studies, but no controlled ones. The use of ECT, particularly in children and adolescents, though also in adults, continues to be controversial with the public and many professionals. Countries and states have various laws about the use of ECT, with some having limitations on its use in children and adolescents or requirements for independent second opinions (American Academy of Child and Adolescent Psychiatry, 2002; Walter et al., 2003).

Transcranial magnetic stimulation (TMS) is a developing treatment for psychiatric illness that involves passing a current through an insulated coil held in contact with the patient's head. A magnetic field then passes into the few first millimeters of the patient's cortex. A specific area of the brain is stimulated. The procedure does not require general anesthesia and a seizure does not occur. Studies in adults have suggested that TMS may be an acceptable, effective treatment with few adverse effects, particularly for depression. One published study on a small number of adolescents with mood and psychotic disorders suggests similar results (Walter et al., 2003).

Inpatient care

Psychiatry has experienced the same trends and reform that have affected pediatric care. There has been an increasing emphasis on outpatient community-based care with fewer resources devoted to inpatient care. Acute psychiatric care currently is based on a model of very short stays for emergency situations with the goals of treatment being crisis intervention, stabilization, assessment, initiation of treatment, resource identification, and referrals. Typical treatment modalities include medication, milieu therapy, family work, and individual psychotherapy. A multidisciplinary team consisting of a psychiatrist, nurses, social workers, and activity therapists provides care. Most hospital and insurance systems have screening procedures that require prior approval before any child or adolescent can be hospitalized. Usually, the length of stay is days to 1–2 weeks (Woolston, 2002).

Partial hospitalization/day treatment programs/ intensive outpatient programs

Partial hospitalization programs are designed to provide short-term crisis stabilization services as an alternative to inpatient care or as a step down from an inpatient stay. Day treatment programs are a longer-term option that provides psychiatric care as well as an educational program for those children and adolescents who require an ongoing intensive level of services. Both of these types of programs offer similar services as inpatient units but the patients live at home. Intensive outpatient or therapeutic after-school programs are designed for young people who can manage in a school

---

CONSIDER CONSULTATION WHEN ...

- Major psychiatric problems are present.
- Education and basic behavioral interventions are ineffective or caretakers need more help than basic education or parenting.
- Psychotherapies other than behavioral management or supportive psychotherapy are necessary.
- Treatment interventions require multiple, extended visits and specific expertise.
- Treating with more than one psychiatric medication is being considered.
- Initial medication trials fail to result in significant improvement. A child psychiatrist may provide diagnostic clarification, assessment of medication regimen and dosing, or recommendations regarding medication options.
- Unexpected or "paradoxical" responses occur with medication or other interventions.
- Coordination is required between multiple agencies.
- Patient may require therapeutic out-of-home placement.
- Caretakers have significant psychiatric illnesses.

---

setting but continue to need a psychiatric setting on a daily or frequent basis. The staff is multidisciplinary and a variety of therapeutic modalities are utilized such as milieu activities, individual, group, and family psychotherapies, medication management, and coordination with community agencies (Kiser et al., 2002).

Community services

General

Comprehensive treatment plans should include maximum use of existing community resources as appropriate. For many children and adolescents, providing structured and supervised activities during non-school time can be very beneficial. After-school and weekend programs can include tutoring, additional academic work, general activities, or sports. Schools, churches, community agencies (YMCA, Boys and Girls Club, recreational centers, sports leagues), and universities offer programs. Group (Scouts) or individual (Big Brother/Big Sister) mentoring and activity programs can be valuable. Summer camp, school, or work programs can provide similar benefits. In many areas, there are similar programs designed with therapeutic components for children and adolescents who cannot manage in regular programs. There should be someone on the treatment team designated to coordinate and collaborate with these programs and assist with any adjustment or transition issues.

In-home services

Home-based services generally are provided to children and families who are identified to be at risk for home disruption and are in crisis. Many of the programs are targeted at family preservation or early intervention for children at risk for abuse and are sponsored by child protective services. Additional services have arisen from community mental health and are provided as part of a spectrum of care designed to support seriously emotionally ill children either to prevent out-of-home placement or to transition back from out-of-home placements. Another targeted population has been delinquent adolescents who are sponsored by the juvenile justice system either to prevent further involvement with juvenile court or to transition back home after being incarcerated. These services usually are time limited, with master's-level clinicians visiting the children and families at home frequently with the goals of identifying needs, providing immediate support and intervention, and helping with access to longer-term services. Support is available 24 hours a day, 7 days a week. There has been little study of the efficacy or outcome of these programs, though several programs have incorporated research on outcome into their design, such as multisystemic therapy.

Home-based services can be a very helpful component of treatment if the goals of the intervention are reasonable (i.e. assessing and intervening with acute problems, identifying long-term needs, and arranging access to appropriate care), the family is appropriate, and the providers are competent (Adnopoz, 2002).

Wraparound

Wraparound services also are based on the belief that the child and family can be served best if the child remains in the home. This intervention tends to be longer term than in home services. The identified population tends to be families with chronic problems. The underlying concepts are that the family's strengths should be built upon, and that interagency and community collaboration can provide enough help to manage seriously emotionally disturbed children on an ongoing basis with the ultimate goal of greater self-sufficiency. Generally, the family and involved agencies identify the needs and potential resources. The family has an assigned caseworker (usually a bachelor's-level social worker) who helps arrange and follow through with utilization of community services. Types of services include personnel to help at the home with the child (i.e. model appropriate parenting), weekend and after-school programming, and respite care on weekends. Respite care is designed to be temporary and can be considered a version of therapeutic foster care (Adnopoz, 2002).

Out-of-home placements – basic and therapeutic

A number of facilities provide out-of-home placements. All have therapeutic versions that are designed for children and adolescents with serious emotional disturbances who cannot live at home or in basic placements. The children generally are required to be in mental health treatment, the caretakers are specially trained, the number of children in each placement is limited, the caretakers receive additional support, and the young person may receive other services such as therapeutic extracurricular activities or special school placements. Often, to be eligible for public funding for a variety of therapeutic or community services, the young person must have some involvement with community mental health, child protective services, or the juvenile justice system.

Children are placed out of their home for a variety of reasons, usually by child protective services. Short-term removals often are related to investigations of allegations of abuse or neglect or provision of temporary relief such as respite. Placement is conceptualized as a temporary remedy, with the expectation that most young people will and can return home. Unfortunately, many children and adolescents remain in care for longer periods of time than initially anticipated, though ultimately most children return to live with their families. Longer-term removals tend to be related to substantiation of abuse or neglect, failure of the caretakers to rectify identified problems in the home, or ongoing problems with the management of the young person in the home despite intervention services.

Basic foster care and group home placements are predicated on the belief that the young person does not have additional needs beyond a place to live with reasonable adults who provide structure and supervision. They attend public school and extracurricular activities as available. Foster care is usually one of the first placements utilized for children and adolescents who cannot live at home either temporally or permanently. If possible, the placement is with a relative or individual with a pre-existing relationship with the family. This type of placement is based on the belief that children and adolescents will do better when given the option of living in a family environment where the potential for new attachments and relationships can be developed. Foster home care is arranged through child protective services and the home must be licensed and approved. Foster parents must go through some initial orientation training but are not required to have any specific training in working with children. There is a chronic shortage of homes and multiple children may be placed in one home. Foster home placements often fail, requiring multiple placements for the child.

Older school-aged children and adolescents may be placed in a group home if foster care is not available or is not appropriate. Adolescents and some older school-age children may do better in a setting that does not require family-like behavior and relationships. These facilities range in size and services, though most emphasize small groups with consistent staff. Group home placement can be a better choice for young people who will have difficulty with the intimacy and relationship expectations in foster care. Adolescents also may be placed at group homes sponsored by the juvenile justice system. Other possible placements include emergency children's shelters designed for young people needing temporary housing before returning home or going into foster or group care, youth shelters for runaway or street adolescents, and family or women's shelters that have children. These facilities vary on the services provided and the length of time that individuals stay (Grigsby, 2002; Rushton and Minnis, 2003).

Residential treatment facilities provide residential care in conjunction with mental health treatment services for children and adolescents with serious emotional disturbances. These institutions serve mostly adolescents. Regardless of the size of the facility, most have the adolescents living in small groups with consistent staff. The facilities have psychiatrists, psychologists, nurses, social workers, and recreational therapists on staff. There are intermediate and intensive-level institutions with intensive-level facilities having more staff and their own schools. At intensive placements, young people can receive all of their care and treatment on site (Lewis et al., 2002).

KEY CLINICAL QUESTIONS

Identification of the essential aspects of treatment
- *What problems is this treatment plan addressing?*
- *How does this intervention help this problem?*
- *What are the goals of this treatment?*
- *Who is responsible for implementing and monitoring the treatment?*
- *Who is responsible for which aspects of care?*
- *How is care going to be coordinated/communicated?*
- *Who is going to be responsible for coordination/communication?*

Identification of any medical aspects of treatment
- *What are the child's medical needs?*
- *Who are the medical providers?*

Identification of medication issues
- *What can account for apparent non-response after pharmacotherapy has been started?*
  Several factors can contribute to "apparent non-response." One of the most common reasons for non-response is subtherapeutic dosing. Another common factor for non-response is medication wear off prior to parental observation (e.g. the teacher may see the benefits of stimulant treatment, yet the parents may see their child long after the stimulant has worn off). Evaluation that is made prior to onset of medication will also appear like "non-response" (e.g. SSRI benefits may not be realized before 1 or 2 weeks of treatment). Of course, in complex clinical scenarios, where the correct diagnosis may be in question or significant psychosocial stressors are present, lack of medication response might not be surprising.
- *What can contribute to a worsening of symptoms after pharmacotherapy was initiated?*
  One must consider whether the exacerbation is related to or independent of the treatment. Family, social or academic stressors, environmental and schedule changes, physical illness or the natural course of some illnesses may affect the child's presentation. One must also consider whether other factors including diagnostic accuracy, iatrogenic behavioral side-effects, whether the medication may be exacerbating the underlying disorder or whether medication interactions may be contributing.

All of these therapeutic placements require specific funding. Young people must go through an application process, be approved, and have their need for services reviewed on a regular basis. For most of these children and adolescents, public funding supports these levels of care. The standard of care is that these children and adolescents will be periodically assessed with the idea that with improvement they will require less intensive care and ultimately be able to function without them.

Summary

There is a spectrum of interventions – biological, psychologic, and environmental – that can be employed to help children and adolescents with psychiatric illnesses. Often, the situations and problems seem overwhelming and too difficult to manage. A key aspect of effective utilization is developing a treatment plan that considers the child's and family's difficulties and strengths with overall and specific goals as well as priorities. Having defined aims then permits the identification and implementation of targeted interventions, with the opportunity to monitor progress and modify the plan depending on the improvement or lack of it. Another essential component is having someone in charge of monitoring the overall plan and ensuring communication between all of the involved individuals. Integrating various therapies and services to provide effective care for children and their families is gratifying and productive. With reasonable and realistic goals and timelines, improvement can occur even in very difficult situations.

Annotated bibliography

Kazdin AE, Weisz JR (eds) (2003) *Evidence-Based Psychotherapies for Children and Adolescents.* New York, The Guildford Press.
Overview of the research in psychotherapy effectiveness with children and adolescents with discussion of the major issues and suggestions for future exploration.

Lewis M (ed) (2002) *Child and Adolescent Psychiatry: A Comprehensive Textbook,* 3rd edn. Philadelphia, Lippincott, Williams & Wilkins.
Major textbook of child and adolescent psychiatry with a number of individual chapters on various psychotherapies, therapeutic interventions, and institutions involved with children, adolescents, and families.

Martin A, Scahill L, Charney DS, Leckman JF (eds) (2003) *Pediatric Psychopharmacology: Principles and Practices.* New York, Oxford University Press.
Overview of psychopharmacology and associated issues in children and adolescents.

SECTION 2

Diagnostic Categories

Arden D. Dingle, MD

Developmental Disabilities: Mental Retardation and Pervasive Developmental Disorders

Douglas O. Lee, MD and Deepa Gopalakrishnan, MD

Introduction

Developmental disabilities (DDs) are a "diverse group of physical, cognitive, psychological, sensory, and speech impairments that begin anytime during development up to 18 years of age" as defined by the Centers of Disease Control. Heterogeneous and often complex in nature, DDs are more common than many realize, and the prevalence ranges from 1.49% for severe DDs (Larson et al., 2001) to 16.8% for the entire spectrum of DDs during childhood (Boyle and Decoufle, 1994). Two commonly encountered DDs that come to the physician's attention are mental retardation (MR) and pervasive developmental disorder (PDD). Physicians inevitably encounter individuals with these conditions not only because of the prevalence but also because of the associated spectrum of behavioral and emotional complications. Taken as a whole, DDs are often associated with social, educational, cognitive and psychiatric concerns resulting in the challenges that persist throughout the lifespan.

Physicians often can observe similarities between MR and PDD, underscoring the heterogeneity and overlap of both developmental conditions. These similarities can also contribute to diagnostic confusion, so appreciation of contrasting characteristics can help to distinguish these conditions. Both conditions can involve cognitive delays, and the majority of individuals with PDD have co-existing MR. Both conditions result in deficits in adaptive functioning. However, the most significant distinguishing feature is the social deficit associated with PDD.

The classification of MR and PDD differs significantly. Subtypes of MR are usually characterized by level of cognitive functioning, whereas subtypes of PDD are classified by clinical characteristics. The etiology of MR and PDD is heterogeneous. No single cause has been or will likely be identified to explain the development of either condition, and it is generally accepted that multiple causes contribute to the development and presentation of the various forms of MR or PDD.

Mental retardation

Mental retardation is a unique disorder, both a symptom as well as a syndrome, which falls under the broad rubric of neurodevelopmental disabilities (for a review, see King et al., 1997; State et al., 1997). A multidimensional "state of functioning" and a heterogeneous framework of etiology, presentation, course and outcome laced with biologic and psychosocial underpinnings characterize it. The term "mental retardation" carries diverse labels internationally including "general learning disorder," "mental handicap," "learning disability," "intellectual handicap," and "intellectual disability" (Haveman, 1996). The last two decades have witnessed tremendous change in the form of de-institutionalization and a shift to community care in parallel with breakthroughs in genetic discovery and incremental expansion of knowledge that has raised the level of awareness as well as imposed on the physician an increasing responsibility for awareness of and ability to treat and manage the psychiatric issues associated with MR.

The DSM-IV (American Psychiatric Association, 1994) diagnosis of mental retardation requires the presence of significantly subaverage intellectual functioning in conjunction with notable impairment in adaptive functioning and onset of these deficits before the age of 18 years. The diagnosis is coded on axis II in the multi-axial classification system of the DSM-IV (see Table 5.1).

Mental retardation presents with global delays in cognitive and adaptive functioning. Based on cognitive and adaptive functioning, MR is categorized as mild, moderate, severe, and profound (see Table 5.2). When considering this diagnosis, it is important for physicians to be familiar with

Table 5.1 Mental retardation

Discriminating features

1. Significantly subaverage intellectual functioning.
2. Concurrent deficits or impairments in present adaptive functioning.

Consistent features

1. An IQ of approximately 70 or below on an individually administered IQ test.
2. Impairments in adaptive functioning in at least two of the following skill areas: communication, self-care, home living, social-interpersonal skills, use of community resources, self-direction, functional academic skills, work, leisure, health, and safety.
3. Onset before age 18 years

Variable features

1. Prevalence is higher in males.
2. Stereotypies and self-injurious behaviors are often found in the moderate to severe forms of MR.
3. Often accompanied by other psychiatric disorders.

The "nature vs. nurture" etiologic debate about MR has persisted for years. Twin and adoption studies indicate that heritable factors account for 45–80% of variability in IQ scores (Plomin and Defries, 1980). Environmental factors contribute significantly to the etiology of many of the idiopathic forms of mild retardation. A lack of appropriate stimulation early during development is thought to be the significant environmental issue. The impact of the environment is further supported by the decreasing incidence of mild MR in older individuals as adaptive skills improve and environmental expectations are better matched to abilities. The ultimate phenotype for a particular individual depends on the influence of psychosocial factors on the biologic genotype.

The most common causes for mental retardation are Down syndrome, fragile X syndrome and fetal alcohol syndrome that together account for about 30% of all identified causes of mental retardation (Batshaw, 1993). The etiology is unclear in 30–40% of cases. Causes may be classified on the basis of origin into prenatal, peri-natal, and postnatal etiologies (see Table 5.3). Inborn errors of metabolism can also contribute to MR (Kahler and Fahey, 2003).

age-appropriate developmental milestones, especially during the formative years. It is also important for physicians to be mindful that ultimate functioning can vary significantly and be influenced by individual strengths, community, and family support.

Mental retardation is one of the most prevalent of the DDs, occurring in approximately 1–3% of school-aged children and often estimated to be 2.5% (Hagberg and Kyllerman, 1983). The prevalence is greater in males as compared to females by a ratio of 1.5: 1 (Silka and Hauser, 1997). While the incidence is equal in all socioeconomic groups for biologic causes, the incidence increases in lower socio economic groups for non-biologic causes, which mostly result in milder forms of retardation. The more severe forms of retardation are identified earlier due to the severity of the apparent global deficits, while the less severe forms are most often diagnosed at school age.

Pervasive developmental disorders

Physicians were familiar with the clinical picture of developmental disorders, but it was not until 1980 that the DSM-III (APA, 1980) coined the term "pervasive developmental disorder" (PDD). PDD is not a diagnosis in itself, but is rather a category of disorders (Piven et al., 1997), also referred to as autism spectrum disorders (ASD) or multisystem developmental disorder (MSDD; Greenspan and Wieder, 1997). This category of disorders has been the focus of many reviews (Rapin, 1997; Wing, 1997; Tanguay, 2000). While there is an increasing trend to use ASD to describe these disorders and emphasize the association of these disorders, PDD will be used in this chapter to conform to DSM-IV (APA, 1994). Pervasive developmental disorders are comprised of several conditions that most likely have multiple etiologies but have many common characteristics.

TABLE 5.2

Mental retardation: categorization and ultimate functioning

	Mild MR	Moderate MR	Severe	Profound
Intelligence quotient	55–70 (50–55 to 65–70)	35–55 (35–40 to 50–55)	20–35 (20–25 to 35–40)	<20 (20–25 & below)
Incidence	85%	10%	4%	1%
Socioeconomic class	Low	Low	No difference	No difference
Developmental year	7–11	3–7	1–3	<3
Academic level	6th grade	2nd grade	1st grade and below	Preschool
Learning	Educable	Trainable	Basic skills	Non-trainable
Living	Community	Sheltered	Require supervision	Require supervision

TABLE 5.3

Causes of mental retardation

Prenatal	Perinatal	Postnatal
Genetic abnormalities • Tuberous sclerosis • Phenylketonuria	Infections • Encephalitis	Infections • Encephalitis • Meningitis
Chromosomal abnormalities • Down syndrome • Fragile X syndrome • Prader-Willi	Delivery • Neonatal asphyxia • Extreme prematurity	Toxins • Lead poisoning
Brain malformations • Neural tube defects	Other • Blood group incompatibility with hyperbilirubinemia	Trauma • Head trauma
Infections (maternal) • HIV • Rubella • Toxoplasmosis • Cytomegalovirus • Syphilis		Inborn errors of metabolism • Phenylketonuria • Galactosemia Endocrine • Hypothyroidism
Toxins • Fetal alcohol syndrome • Anticonvulsants		Psychosocial causes • Malnutrition • Sociocultural deprivation • Low parental IQ • Poor parenting skills

The characteristic triad of PDD signs and symptoms includes delays/abnormalities in communication, difficulties in social interactions, and stereotypic, inflexible behaviors (APA, 1994). Speech, language, and communication problems are profound, and up to 50% of individuals will not develop adequate speech to communicate daily needs (Wing and Attwood, 1987). Despite the severity of various delays, many have argued that the distinguishing hallmark of PDD, the "core feature," is the delay in the ability to socially interact with others (Klin et al., 2002a; Waterhouse et al., 1996). In fact, some describe PDD as a disorder of social interaction. The delay may be manifested by decreased affection, diminished interest in what others are doing, decreased desire to participate, reduced reciprocity of interaction, or decreased social preferences in activities. Despite the delay in social interactions, individuals with PDD are not devoid of social relationships. Rather, they spend less time interacting with others, have poorer quality of interactions, initiate fewer interactions, and respond less to others (Sigman and Ruskin, 1999). Some have argued that individuals with PDD are socially isolated mainly because of the quality of the interactions rather than solely the quantity (Sigman, 1994).

PDDs include autism, Asperger syndrome, Rett syndrome, childhood disintegrative disorder and PDD not otherwise specified (NOS) (APA, 1994). Many have asserted that the various PDDs fall on a continuum or are part of a spectrum (Piven et al., 1997; Wing, 1997), hence the phrase "autism spectrum disorder" to describe the entire broad range of PDD. Consequently, the variations in clinical presentations can be obvious or subtle, potentially leading to diagnostic confusion. Additionally, as research has shed light on these conditions, the ability to identify PDD has become more refined, simultaneously requiring several revisions of diagnostic criteria. Together, these factors can occasionally contribute to the challenge in making the diagnosis of PDD.

Autism, a term coined by Eugene Bleuler in 1912 meaning "aloneness," was adopted in 1943 by Leo Kanner who first described this condition. Autism is often considered the prototypic PDD since it is characterized by significant delays in all three domains of communication, social interactions, and aberrant behavior (see Table 5.4). The intensity of symptoms in three domains can vary immensely. Autism is often associated with only the most severe symptoms. However, the intensity of each domain falls on a continuum. Some individuals are able to speak and communicate their needs, while others are nonverbal. Some are able to have friends based solely on common interests, while others are exclusively aloof and indifferent. Some individuals have more flexibility, less stereotypies, fewer preoccupations, while others must follow specific routines, rituals and have very well circumscribed interests. Despite frequent publicity of

DIAGNOSIS

Table 5.4 Autism

Discriminating features

1. Difficulties with social interactions.
2. Marked impairment in the use of nonverbal behaviors, such as eye-to-eye gaze, facial expression, body postures, and gestures to regulate social interaction.
3. A decrease or lack of spontaneous seeking to share enjoyment, interests, or achievements with other people.
4. Decreased or lack of social or emotional reciprocity.
5. Failure to develop peer relationships appropriate to developmental level.

Consistent features

1. Impairments in communication.
2. Delay in or total lack of development of spoken language.
3. In individuals with adequate speech, marked impairment in the ability to initiate or sustain a conversation with others.
4. Stereotyped and repetitive use of language or idiosyncratic language.
5. Lack of varied, spontaneous make-believe play or social imitative play appropriate to developmental level.

Variable features

1. Restricted, repetitive, and stereotyped patterns of behavior, interests, and activities.
2. Encompassing preoccupation with one or more stereotyped and restricted patterns of interest that is abnormal either in intensity or focus.
3. Apparently inflexible adherence to specific, nonfunctional routines or rituals – stereotyped and repetitive motor mannerisms (e.g. hand or finger flapping or twisting or complex whole-body movements).
4. Persistent preoccupation with parts of objects.

savant abilities, areas of specific exceptional proficiency and skill are relatively rare, accounting for only 1–10% of individuals with autism (Rimland, 1978).

Asperger syndrome (AS) is characterized by difficulties in social interactions, decreased flexibility, restricted interests, stereotypic behaviors but includes areas of typical development: intact language development and average or above average cognition as measured by IQ. The intact language milestones and IQ may contribute to the later age of diagnosis. Despite the ability to communicate, there are often obvious atypical variations in language such as a very formal, "professorial," pedantic, style of talking with unusual intonation and inflexion. Pragmatic speech, the general ability to make conversation, appreciate cues and keep conversation flowing, is often very limited or scripted. There may be strengths related to academic performance or knowledge about a specific area of interest. It is thought those individuals with AS have little difficulty in life since they have language and intellectual abilities, however, the

social difficulties often impair functioning. Some consider Asperger syndrome to be a type of PDD-NOS.

PDD-NOS is a condition that is characterized by key features of PDD but insufficient criteria to fulfill a diagnosis of autism or other PDDs. PDD-NOS category reflects the broad PDD spectrum and its numerous variations, though the difficulties in social interactions continue to be the primary deficit.

In the past, PDD was once thought to be a relatively static condition, perhaps contributing to the belief that nothing could be done and the philosophy of institutionalization for affected individuals. However, follow-up studies (Mesibov et al., 1989; Rutter et al., 1967; Rumsey et al., 1985) indicate that for some individuals with autism, symptoms may improve and individuals may not fulfill DSM criteria for autism in later years. While PDD characteristics persist for most, behaviors and symptoms improve (Nordin and Gillberg, 1998). For most individuals, many of the bizarre behaviors improve while social impairment continues. Even though individuals with autism tend to make progress, some individuals regress as a result of seizure activity.

In lower functioning individuals with autism, IQ predicts adaptive functioning, whereas in higher functioning individuals, language and verbal memory are predictive (Liss et al., 2001). To date, the two most accurate prognostic indicators have been verbal ability and level of cognitive functioning (Nordin and Gillberg, 1998). In some studies, flexibility and the ability to shift cognitively correlates with better social outcome. A minority of children with autism, most of whom are high functioning, will lead independent lives. In higher functioning individuals with autism, often the complications will not become a problem until they are older and social demands increase (Fombonne, 2003). Repetitive and ritualistic behaviors have been reported to persist more than the communication and social deficits in individuals with autism and high IQ (Piven et al., 1996).

Rett syndrome is the only PDD that occurs predominantly in females. Onset of delays occurs after normal prenatal and perinatal development. Usually, abilities that are lost or fail to develop are in the social and language domains. In addition there is a deceleration in head growth and loss of hand skills/acquisition of stereotypical hand movements after age 5 months and poor coordination or trunk movements.

Childhood disintegrative disorder is a relatively rare condition. Typically, there is normal development during the first two years, but a loss of functioning by age 10 years in two areas including language, social skills, continence, play, or motor skills. Characteristically, the hallmark characteristic triad of PDD symptoms is apparent.

Autism was once thought to be exceptionally rare, with a prevalence of two to four per 10,000 children. However, over the past decade the prevalence of diagnosed autism and other PDDs has risen significantly (Fombonne, 1999; Wing and Potter, 2002). In 2000, the British Medical Research Council reported the prevalence of autism to be one per 1000, but other studies have reported the prevalence of PDDs to be as high as 6.26 per 1,000 (Chakrabarti and Fombonne, 2001). Despite the increased prevalence, there continues to be a male predominance with a ratio of 4:1. Other forms of PDD are generally rarer. Rett syndrome is relatively rare with a prevalence of only 1/10,000–1/15,000 female births (review, Jellinger, 2003). Childhood disintegrative disorder has a prevalence of 1.7 per 100,000 (Fombonne, 2002).

The reason for the rise in the diagnoses of autism and PDD is not fully understood, but it most likely involves multiple factors (Prior, 2003). Epidemiological methodology has changed as researchers have started to examine the prevalence of the broader spectrum of PDD rather than just autism alone (Charman, 2002). Changes in diagnostic criteria and conceptualization have resulted in a greater number of individuals who may not have previously met criteria. Greater awareness and screening has contributed to the increased numbers found in educational settings. The ability of health professionals to identify and diagnose may have contributed as well as the recognition that autism is associated with numerous other conditions. Additionally, many believe that an environmental factor has also increased the risk of developing PDD, however, no specific toxins have been identified. From data examining the effects of thalidomide, it is suggested that PDD symptoms can result from toxin-related disruption in development. At this time, there is speculation and ongoing research to determine whether toxins such as mercury may have a role in the development of PDD. Studies looking into the relationship of measles mumps rubella (MMR) vaccine and autism have not found any correlation, however (Wilson et al., 2003; Madsen et al., 2002; Taylor et al., 2002; Kaye et al., 2001; Taylor et al., 1999; Halsy et al., 2001).

PDD can be associated with medical conditions. Even though tuberous sclerosis is relatively rare (1/10,000) up to 60% will have autism (Hunt and Shepherd, 1993). Of individuals with fragile X, which has a prevalence of 1/1000–1/4000, up to 25% may have autism (Bailey et al., 1998). Approximately 2–5% of individuals with autism have fragile X (Bailey et al., 1993). In Down syndrome, up to 7% may have autistic spectrum disorders (Kent et al., 1999). Approximately 10% of individuals with cerebral palsy have autism spectrum disorder (Nordin and Gillberg, 1996). Autism also can be associated with untreated phenylketonuria or Williams syndrome.

The etiology of PDD is currently unclear, which most likely represents not only the complexity but also the heterogeneity of these conditions. Early theories of autism asserted that the cold emotional interaction between parent and child contributed to the development of autism ("the refrigerator mother"). This idea has not been supported by research and has been rejected. Epidemiologic data support a genetic risk factor (Bailey et al., 1995; Folstein and Sheidley, 2001; Piven et al., 1997; Szatmari et al., 1998). While the prevalence of autism in the general population is 0.1%, it jumps to 5% if one child in a family already has autism, a risk of 50–100 times greater than the general population (Bolton et al., 1994). In fact, 5% of families with at least one child with autism have more than one child with the disorder. Concordance rate of autism is approximately 90% in monozygotic twins, while the rate is <10% in dizygotic twins.

Ongoing genetic research has looked at candidate genes, and studies have suggested that a multigene diathesis most likely contributes to PDD (Gillberg, 1998; International Molecular Genetic Study of Autism Consortium, 1998; Szatmari et al., 1998). One genetic breakthrough is the identification of the gene associated with Rett syndrome. In 1999, Amir et al. isolated a mutation(s) associated with Rett syndrome in the MECP2 gene that codes for the methylcytosine binding protein 2, an important transcriptional repressor. Neuroimaging research has helped to identify structures of interest (Cody et al., 2002; Rumsey and Ernst, 2000). Computed tomography (CT) and magnetic resonance imaging (MRI) structural imaging show that brain volume is increased in individuals with autism, which is consistent with the increased head circumference in childhood and adulthood. Temporal, parietal, and occipital lobes are increased, while frontal lobe volumes are unchanged. The increased volumes are consistent with theories that diminished dendritic pruning exists in autism. Functional imaging studies have shown that individuals with PDD process information very differently. For example, research (Schultz et al., 2000; Grelotti et al., 2002) found that individuals with PDD process faces and expressions differently without involving brain structures such as the fusiform gyrus that are usually required. This information in part can help to explain why there may be social difficulties such as interpreting and responding to message emotion.

Postmortem histopathologic examinations of individuals with autism reveal cellular aberrations in limbic system and cerebellum (Kemper and Bauman, 1998). There was cellular disorganization and increased cell packing in limbic structures and less Purkinje cells in the cerebellum. A striking fact was that there was no gliosis, suggesting that the cell loss occurred probably prior to 30–32 weeks. In short, there is evidence of familial, genetic, and early prenatal developmental factors that may contribute to the CNS and social functioning that is characteristic of individuals with PDD.

Psychiatric comorbidity

Individuals with MR or PDD commonly have comorbid psychiatric symptoms or conditions. Up to 75% of children with autism have comorbid mental retardation (Fombonne, 1999; Freeman et al., 1985). Epidemiologic studies have found that hyperactivity, anxiety, agitation, aggression directed at others and oneself are common. Taken together, these symptoms can create a psychiatric presentation that can often be overwhelming, leaving the physician with the question of where to start to stabilize the individual. Usually, the psychiatric complications can be broken down into separate components to be targeted for treatment.

Attention and activity disorder (ADHD) symptoms
Individuals with MR and PDD often have ADHD symptoms, and ADHD symptoms are some of the most common symptoms in individuals with PDD. Even though individuals with MR or PDD may not be able to complain about these symptoms, multiple informants can provide information to diagnose ADHD. It is important for the physician to distinguish ADHD from situation-specific inattentiveness, such as at school when expectations exceed abilities.

Disruptive behaviors
"Noncompliance and disobedience" are common, and they should be interpreted in the context of the cognitive inability to understand rules, difficulty in comprehending expectations and varying intent and motives. Aggression is common in individuals with PDD. In fact, a significant number of individuals with PDD have aggression that can be directed at others or oneself (self-injurious behavior; SIB). In some studies, self-injurious behavior is present in up to 52% of individuals with autism (Poustka and Lisch, 1993).

Mood symptoms
Individuals with both depression and MR have been described as having symptoms of apathetic facial expressions, withdrawal, aggressive behavior, dwelling on the subject of death, dysphoria, sadness, changes in motoric activity, irritability and changes in sleep and appetite (Dosen, 1990; Sovner and Lowry, 1990).

Mood disorders are common in individuals with PDD (Lainhart and Folstein, 1994), and the increased family history of depression may increase the risk of mood disorder in individuals with autism. Adolescents with Asperger syndrome often become depressed. Depression could likely be the most common psychiatric disorder in PDD (Ghaziuddin et al., 2002).

Anxiety symptoms
Anxiety symptoms in the form of obsessions, compulsions, fear, panic, and worrying are common. A distinction needs to be made between repetitive behaviors and "compulsive behaviours" that are performed to reduce anxiety or anxiety related obsessions.

Feeding problems
The incidence of pica and rumination increases in direct proportion to the severity of MR. The presence of an underlying medical condition like reflux should be ruled out.

Psychotic symptoms
Psychosis is relatively rare, but individuals with DD are at increased risk through early adulthood. Since the diagnosis often relies on the ability to report delusions or hallucinations, it is difficult to diagnose this condition in children with impaired language skills. A change from baseline behavior including decline in or loss of activities of daily living/self-care, accusatory behavior, response to imperceptible stimuli or increased agitation can suggest the presence of a psychotic process. The presence of grossly disorganized behavior and profound loss of motivation, lack of responsiveness or other 'negative' symptoms may also help in diagnosing psychosis.

Syndrome-associated disorders

Down syndrome
Down syndrome (trisomy 21) is the most common chromosomal abnormality leading to mental retardation, most often arising due to nondisjunction of chromosome 21 (State et al., 1997). The prevalence is approximately one in 800 live births. The phenotype may include a round, flat face, low-set nose, flat nasal bridge, short stature, microcephaly, small mouth, macroglossia, upward slanting eyes, epicanthal folds, hypotonia, small, misshapen ears, small, wide hands, simian crease, malformed fifth finger, wide space between the big and the second toes, unusual creases on the soles of the feet, overly flexible joints (sometimes referred to as being double-jointed) and shorter than normal height. Other associated features include atrial septal defect, ventricular septal defect, tetralogy of Fallot, duodenal atresia, hearing loss, an increased incidence of leukemia and Alzheimer's dementia. The cognitive status typically ranges from mild to moderate retardation. Socialization is relatively preserved. Rates of psychiatric and behavioral problems are higher than in the general population but less than in other groups of mental retardation. Problems typically include difficulties with attention, impulsivity, hyperactivity and aggression (Dykens and Kasari, 1997; Cuskelly and Dadds, 1992; Pueschel et al., 1991; Gath and Gumley, 1986).

Fragile X syndrome
Fragile X syndrome is the second most common genetic abnormality leading to mental retardation arising due to a "full mutation" involving the FMR-1 gene on the X chromosome where the trinucleotide sequence expands up to 3000 repeats from a normal of 5 to 50 repeated cytosine-guanine-guanine (cgg) residues (Fu et al., 1991; Snow et al., 1993). The prevalence is roughly one in 1000 males. Mental retardation is more frequently seen in males (95%) than females (approximately 50%) (Baumgardner et al., 1995; Rousseau et al., 1991). The phenotype comprises a long and narrow face,

prominent jaw, prominent ears and/or macro-orchidism. Other occasional characteristics include unusual hand mannerisms (hand flapping or hand biting), whirling, spinning, autism, frequent ear and sinus infections, nearsightedness and lazy eye, trouble with sucking, seizures, loose joints with resultant joint dislocations, a curvature in the spine, flat feet, and/or mitral valve prolapse. A decrement in IQ from latency to puberty has been noted (State et al., 1997). ADHD is highly prevalent in this population.

Prader-Willi syndrome

Uniparental maternal disomy, due to either a deletion in or nonfunctional paternal chromosome 15, has been postulated to be the cause for Prader-Willi syndrome (PWS). The PWS phenotype consists of short stature, obesity, hypogonadism, and/or hyperphagia. Children with PWS may present with a wide range of psychiatric problems including temper tantrums, emotional lability, mood symptoms, anxiety, skin picking, and/or obsessive-compulsive symptomatology (Dykens and Cassidy, 1996). This condition is associated with MR or PDD. Chromosome 15 and the savant abilities associated with PWS are thought to be linked to the savant abilities in some individuals with PDD (Nurmi et al., 2003).

Angelman's syndrome

The cause for Angelman's syndrome (AS) has been found to be uniparental paternal disomy (due to either a deletion or nonfunctional maternal chromosome 15). Children with AS may have severe MR, absence of speech, bouts of laughter, seizures and/or ataxia (Moldavsky et al., 2001). Hyperactivity, aggression, temper tantrums and stereotyped behavior have been reported (Summers et al., 1995).

Williams syndrome

Deletion in the elastin gene of chromosome 7 has been noted to cause elfin like facies, starburst iris, infantile hypercalcemia, growth deficiency, supravalvular aortic stenosis and hypertension, features that form part of a syndrome called Williams syndrome. Distinctive features include loquacious, pseudo mature communicative style referred to as cocktail party speech (Meyerson and Frank, 1987) and a remarkable ability to recognize facial features (Udwin and Yule, 1991; Wang et al., 1995). A relative weakness in visuo-spatial skills and visuo-motor integration has been noted (Bellugi et al., 1990; Udwin and Yule, 1991).

Fetal alcohol syndrome

The incidence of fetal alcohol syndrome is about 2.5–10% among alcoholic women (Sokol et al., 1980). Maternal ingestion of large quantities of alcohol during pregnancy leads to either the full-blown syndrome that is termed fetal alcohol syndrome or a milder variant, fetal alcohol effects. Children are born with any or some of the following features: short stature, low birthweight, poor weight gain, microcephaly, small eye openings, epicanthal folds, broad bridged nose, hypoplastic philtrum, thin upper lip, small chin, cleft palate, congenital heart defects, strabismus, hearing loss, defects of the spine and joints, alteration of the hand creases, small fingernails, and toenails. The cognitive and behavioral hallmarks include inattention, hyperactivity, poor motor skills, and slow language development. Approximately 72% have major psychiatric disorders (Famy, 1998; Streissguth et al., 1991).

Tuberous sclerosis

Tuberous sclerosis (TS) is a multisystem genetic disorder that is characterized by central nervous system tubers and nodules, dermatological, cardiac, and renal involvement (Bolton and Griffiths, 1997). Autism has been associated with TS, and the risk of autism is up to 1000 times greater in an individual with TS than in those without TS. Brain scans have found that a significantly higher number of tubers exist in TS individuals with MR and autism than those without those conditions. However, there is no characteristic distribution of tubers associated with autism in these individuals.

Phenylketonuria

Untreated phenylketonuria (PKU) has been associated with autism but it is relatively rare (Baieli et al., 2003). In a cohort of infants with PKU who were diagnosed early, none were diagnosed with autism. In another cohort of children who were diagnosed with PKU at a later age some were diagnosed with autism, but only 5.71% fulfilled full criteria for PKU.

Assessment

The assessment of a child with possible MR or PDD can be complex and should incorporate a multidisciplinary and biopsychosocial approach (Volkmar et al., 1999). The assessment commonly includes a biomedical appraisal, the diagnostic evaluation and assessment for presence of comorbidity, which together guide the formulation of a relevant individualized treatment plan. The general workup (Chapter 1) should include a careful history of prenatal, perinatal, developmental, medical, social, and educational information. The emphasis should be on obtaining information on delays in development, communication/language skills, bizarre behavior, and interactions with others (see Key clinical questions). A family psychiatric history can also provide invaluable information that can enable the physician to appreciate potential psychiatric risk factors. Physical and neurologic examinations are also important to identify physical stigmata and hearing or vision impairment. Work-up should incorporate a multimodal, multisystem approach and often includes psychiatric, psychologic/cognitive, educational, speech and language, medical, neurologic, and allied health evaluations (AACAP 1999a, b; Filipek et al., 2000).

The nature and extent of the laboratory investigation for MR or PDD is determined in part by the history and physical examination. Routine laboratory tests (Chapter 3) consisting of complete blood count (for anemia secondary to inborn

errors in metabolism), electrolytes, thyroid function tests (for hypothyroidism), folate levels, B2 levels and syphilis serology can be considered. Clinical history and information usually dictate whether additional laboratory tests are required, and a routine shotgun approach with multiple screening panels is not part of the routine work up due to the low yield (Curry et al., 1997). However, if the clinical presentation and physical exam warrant further evaluation to rule out specific conditions additional tests should be considered: chromosomal and DNA analysis (fragile X, Down syndrome), FISH probes (Prader-Willi and Angelman's syndromes), lead (pica), metabolic labs for plasma amino acids (phenylketonuria), urinary organic acids, urinary mucopolysaccharides and oligosaccharides (to screen for lysosomal storage diseases; Wenger et al., 2002), leukocyte enzyme activity (to diagnose lysosomal storage disease) and very-long-chain fatty acids, are indicated. Metabolic and genetics assessments can be exceptionally complex, and an experienced pediatric geneticist can provide invaluable consultation for work-up and diagnosis (for a review on evaluation of MR, see Curry et al., 1997; review on metabolic disorders and MR, see Kahler and Fahey, 2003).

A radiologic assessment including brain MRI or head CT scan is indicated when abnormalities are detected on neurologic examination or when calcifications due to TORCH infections (i.e. toxoplasmosis, other infections, rubella, cytomegalovirus, herpes simplex), tuberous sclerosis or craniosynostosis are suspected. Electrophysiologic studies such as an EEG should proceed as clinically warranted.

Additional evaluations are recommended. Audiologic testing should be performed for all children with these developmental disabilities who have speech difficulties. Testing should include audiometry, middle ear assessment, and auditory brainstem response. Vision should be evaluated to ensure that acuity is not contributing to difficulty in focusing, coordination or reading. Speech and language evaluation is crucial to assess strengths and to recommend the most appropriate means of developing communication. Occupational therapy is important to assess gross and fine motor coordination as well as sensory abnormalities that are commonly encountered in PDD. A psychologist, preferably who is familiar with developmental disorders, should perform cognitive and educational testing to identify strengths and limitations, help understand the child's cognitive processing style and formulate educational plans to be implemented. A psychologist also can assess adaptive and behavioral functioning and screen for additional behavioral conditions that may need to be addressed. Neuropsychologic testing can also be helpful to track specific cognitive changes over time. In short, multiple evaluations are required once the diagnosis of MR or PDD has been made. Case management can be essential to coordinate multiple systems and resources, many of which may be limited depending on community resources.

Presenting the diagnosis can be difficult not only for the family but also for the physician. Parents may feel devastation, guilt, and shame and be reluctant to entertain the diagnosis. This diagnosis can be devastating for many, since the lay connotations and perceptions are often very negative, and expectations of the idyllic family are difficult to relinquish. Parents as well as physicians may express resistance to "label" a child with a diagnosis. In individuals with high functioning autism, resistance to accepting the diagnosis is very common. Often there is a desire to only accept a diagnosis that holds a more auspicious prognosis. In presenting the diagnosis to families, it is important to provide information, to offer support, to emphasize that further work-up and evaluation will aid in providing optimal treatment.

Mental retardation

The diagnostic assessment for MR requires the measurement of cognitive functioning and an evaluation of adaptive skills. A variety of measures are used for the measurement of cognition (see Table 5.5). The Vineland Adaptive Behavior Scales (VABS) (Sparrow et al., 1984) is a semi-structured interview of the child's caregiver that obtains information on domains of communication, socialization, daily living, and motor skills. The Vineland Adaptive Behavior Scales can be used from birth to adulthood. Deficiencies in at least two areas of adaptive skills are required to meet the MR diagnostic criteria. See Chapter 2 for additional scales.

The DSM-IV framework upon which the diagnosis of most psychiatric disorders is based is subject to limitations in its use with children and adolescents with MR. Sovner (1986) and Menolascino (1983) described limiting factors including intellectual distortion (diminished ability to communicate abstractly and intelligibly), psychosocial masking (impoverished social skills due to the effects of the cognitive limitation on psychiatric symptoms), cognitive disintegration (proneness to disorganization under emotional stress) (Menolascino, 1983) and baseline exaggeration (amplification of cognitive deficits and maladaptive behaviors). A thorough and sensitive delineation of symptomatology within the context of existing cognitive and adaptive deficits is essential, considering the increased incidence of psychopathology in this population as reflected in epidemiologic studies (Corbett, 1985; Gostason, 1985).

Pervasive developmental disorders

Because of the high prevalence of MR in individuals with PDD, many of the cognitive assessments for diagnosing MR can be helpful for assessing individuals with PDD. However, these assessments alone may not be adequate enough to make a diagnosis of PDD.

TABLE 5.5

Cognitive measures

Test	Age	Description
The Bayley Scale of Infant Development (Bayley, 1993)	8 weeks to 3 years	Motor, mental and behavior scores
The Stanford Binet Intelligence test: Fourth Edition (SB: FE) (Thorndike et al., 1986)	2 years to 23 years	Mental age Relies on language abilities
The Wechsler Preschool and Primary Scale of Intelligence-Revised (WPPSI-R) (Wechsler, 1989)	3 years to 7 years	Verbal and nonverbal intelligence scores
Wechsler Intelligence Scale for Children-III (WISC-III) (Wechsler, 1991)	6 years to 16 years	Verbal and nonverbal intelligence scores
Wechsler Adult Intelligence Scale-Revised (WAIS-Revised) (Wechsler, 1981)	16 years and above	Verbal and nonverbal intelligence scores
The Hiskey Nebraska Test of Learning Aptitude	Deaf/hard of hearing 3 to 17 years	Instructions given by pantomime and practice exercises. A "learning age" is generated (Keele, 1984)
The Leiter International Performance Scale (Leiter, 1948)	Children with aphasia, articulation errors, other language difficulties or hearing problems	Nonverbal
The Columbia Mental Maturity Scale (Burgemeister et al., 1972)	Children with cerebral palsy	

The shotgun medical approach to work up PDD is of limited clinical utility, but selective tests can be useful (Rapin, 1999; Voigt et al., 2000). Genetic testing for fragile X is commonly obtained due to the relatively high prevalence of autism in individuals with fragile X (Bailey et al., 1998). Should genetic testing be performed, accompanying genetic counseling is recommended (Simonoff, 1998). Some metabolic disorders may be associated with autism (Page, 2000), but routine metabolic testing is not customary without evidence of an underlying metabolic condition such as lethargy, seizures, vomiting, dysmorphic features, and mental retardation (Filipek et al., 2000; Rapin, 1999; Voigt et al., 2000). Lead screening should be performed especially in the presence of pica. Routine head MRI and EEG are not usually performed, since they do not add diagnostic information or change patient treatment (Voigt et al., 2000).

As pronounced and apparent as PDD symptoms may be, diagnosis can be challenging for several reasons. Significant heterogeneity, complexity of symptoms, and varying severity of PDD symptoms can contribute to an almost endless number of variations. Diagnostic criteria for PDDs (DSM-IV) emphasize prototypic clinical presentations. Unfortunately, these criteria do not always describe signs and symptoms seen early in development, as demonstrated by clinical observation and research (Lord, 1995). And some symptoms may not be apparent at early developmental stages in youngsters, e.g. echolalia in a child who has not yet developed verbal abilities. This problem may contribute to early under-diagnosis. Appreciation of atypical characteristics or aberrations is very important because early identification, diagnosis, and intervention have prognostic implications (Harris and Handelman, 2000), further underscoring the potential of screening (Baird et al., 2001). When disabilities are not so apparent, a delay in making a diagnosis can occur. Children with autism are diagnosed at an average age of 5.5 years, while children with Asperger syndrome are not diagnosed until age 11 years (Howlin and Asgharian, 1999). In most situations, parents will note signs and symptoms associated with PDD as the child develops, often as early as infancy. A lack of responsiveness, molding to parent cradling, and stiff response to holding often alert parents to a problem.

Within the first year, early signs of autism can be identified by analyses of videos (Osterling et al., 1994, 2000, 2002; Werner et al., 2000). In studies of infants, videos revealed four behaviors at the first birthday that distinguished children with autism from those without: deficits in eye contact, pointing to objects, showing objects to others, and responding to their name. These findings have been noted when comparing these individuals with typically developing and retarded individuals (Osterling et al., 2002). These data are consistent with the finding that individuals with autism do not establish as much eye contact. They tend to look at people's mouths instead of eyes and look at objects more than people (Klin et

al., 2002b). Prospective studies involving the development of the Checklist for Autism in Toddlers (CHAT) found that if two symptoms (lack of social interest, lack of pointing, lack of joint attention, lack of social play, or lack of pretend play) were present at 18 months, autism could be predicted at age 30 months (Baron-Cohen et al., 1992).

General developmental questionnaires that can be used in pediatric settings such as the Ages and Stages Questionnaire, BRIGANCE screens, Child Development Inventories and Parents' Evaluations of Developmental Status have the sensitivity and specificity to detect developmental disabilities (Filipek et al., 1999). These questionnaires can confirm parental or physician concerns. In contrast, the widely used screening instrument, the Denver Questionnaire, lacks the sensitivity and specificity for screening conditions such as PDD (Glascoe et al., 1992).

If general developmental questionnaires are positive, follow-up screening with more specific instruments for PDD screening is recommended. Baron-Cohen's newly developed Checklist for Autism in Toddlers (1992, 2000) has enabled primary health-care physicians to screen for autism in infants as young as 18 months. It has been found to have a sensitivity of 85% and specificity of 100% in children age 2 years. This instrument focuses on behaviors that are typically present by age 18 months, specifically joint attention and pretend play (Aylward, 1997).

In older children, DSM-IV criteria are more applicable to make diagnoses. Individuals with Asperger's or high functioning autism may be screened using the Autism Spectrum Screening Questionnaire (Ehlers et al., 1999). Other rating scales and questionnaires that can be useful in the office setting to complement information derived from the history include: the Social Communication Questionnaire, the Childhood Autism Rating Scale (CARS), and Gilliam Autism Rating Scale (see Chapter 2). For the office practice, the Social Communication Questionnaire (Berument et al., 1999) is an appropriate screening tool. It is easy to answer with "yes" or "no" responses, and it is based on and well correlated with the lengthier Autism Diagnostic Interview. The CARS is a scale that is based on direct observation, but its accuracy can be limited by the experience of the rater. Even though the Autism Diagnostic Interview and Autism Diagnostic Observation Schedule are the benchmark research diagnostic instruments, they require much time and may not be ideal for office settings. See Chapter 2 for additional instruments.

Differential diagnosis

Individuals with MR or PDD can sometimes be confused with other conditions, especially in those with higher cognitive functioning. Individuals with hearing or visual impairment may be misdiagnosed with MR or PDD, but simple vision and hearing screen can distinguish these individuals.

Children with specific learning disabilities or communication difficulties, including problems with articulation or aphasia, may be confused with MR. Application of all the three diagnostic criteria and assessment of skills in multiple domains help differentiate these disorders from MR.

A common challenge in making the diagnosis of PDD often includes distinguishing PDD from MR without PDD (Fombonne, 1999; Freeman et al., 1985). Fifty per cent of those with PDD have an IQ of < 50; 20% have an IQ between 50 and 70. Both conditions have delays in language and both may have stereotypies. However, the manner in which the child socially interacts will be the main feature that distinguishes these conditions. The social interactions of individuals with MR are delayed, but they are able to interact socially to a degree consistent with their developmental and cognitive level. Social interactions of individuals with PDD are delayed, atypical, and often lack reciprocity.

Individuals with Aspergers sometimes have idiosyncratic behaviors and flat affect that may mimic prodromal symptoms of schizophrenia or schizotypal personality. However, PDD is not characterized by hallucinations, and social perception is poor in PDD.

PDD can resemble symptoms of anxiety disorders. Individuals with social anxiety may have a similar decrease in social engagement and even mutism that resembles language delay. However, in familiar settings social interactions are usually normal. Many individuals with PDD have obsessions and compulsions that resemble obsessive-compulsive disorder (OCD). However, in PDD the obsessions and compulsions are often very unusual and atypical of OCD. Furthermore, individuals with OCD do not have the difficulties with social perception and interaction.

Frequently, PDD can present as reactive attachment disorder (RAD). Both conditions can have developmental delays and abnormal attachment. However, RAD is remarkable for a history of deprivation, and, after placement into a nurturing environment, significant growth and development ensue.

Treatment

Not surprisingly, the psychiatric difficulties often receive the greatest attention since they can affect others and they hinder functioning in school and home. Behavioral, psychotherapeutic as well as pharmacologic approaches can be used to address numerous problems, but unfortunately there is no cure for the core disorders. It is important to identify the behavior(s) and characterize the behavior by onset (i.e. 11 weeks ago), pattern (i.e. only at school), setting (i.e. noisy, stimulating environment), precipitants (i.e. demands, requests), frequency, duration of episode, consequences (i.e. time out) and consistency of others' responses. Often, a behavioral log or diary is helpful in gathering this information.

This information can be useful in determining the nature of the behavioral difficulties.

The goal of treatment for individuals with MR and PDD is not merely to lessen symptoms, but to help the individual achieve the maximally feasible quality of life (Stark and Goldsbury, 1990). Treatment must be integrated, synergistic, and occur in the least restrictive setting with the primary medical provider working alongside and with child psychiatrists, social workers, teachers, counselors, speech and occupational therapists and educational and workshop consultants in a collaborative, multidisciplinary team approach (see Pearls & perils).

The most common reasons for presentation to emergency rooms include aggressive behavior, self-injurious behavior,

PEARLS & PERILS

- If a family mentions that their child does not seem to respond to them and is aloof, that their child is too laid back, cooperative, quiet, or difficult to engage, consider the possibility of PDD.

- If you notice that a child is minimally responsive to social prompts but the family denies any problems with their child, continue to consider the possibility of PDD. A family's denial often contributes to minimizing the presence of any developmental problems, which can be too devastating for a family to acknowledge. However, an organized and systematic treatment plan can help allay anxiety.

- Even though families often do not want to "label" their child with a PDD diagnosis, knowing the diagnosis can enable families to read about the condition, find out more about treatment experiences of others and access resources that otherwise might not be available. Early intervention services can be pivotal to development.

- Multiple problems are commonly present in children with PDD. It is important to prioritize the problems. Keep in mind the different treatment domains that can be addressed concurrently: neurologic treatment, educational planning, behavioral modification, medication treatment, speech therapy, occupational therapy, and physical therapy.

- Keep in mind the presence of associated or comorbid conditions when MR or PDD has been diagnosed. Genetic assessment such as fragile X should be considered.

- Multisystem treatments can result in multi-appointment schedules. The stress associated with multiple medical and therapy visits as well as coping with disappointment, frustration, finances, and comorbid behavioral difficulties can place tremendous stress on couples and families. Remember to inquire about how well parents are dealing with stressors. Supportive counseling, support groups, and respite services can provide support for parents.

medication side-effects, and mental status changes including psychotic symptoms, sleep difficulties and behaviors indicating physical illness including constipation, infection, and pain. It is important for physicians to evaluate the context in which help is sought. In many instances, effective interventions involve environmental manipulation rather than psychotropic medications. For example, agitation can occur with stressors such as changes in routines, family illness or miscommunication. The indications for hospitalization include imminent danger to self or others, failure of outpatient treatment and/or inability to function and take care of self.

Any emergency evaluation should incorporate and address the four functions of the problem behavior as described by Lowry and Sovner (1991): socio-environmental control (inadvertent reinforcement or reward of the problem behavior), communication of discomfort or needs, modulation of physical discomfort, (i.e. pain) and modulation of emotional discomfort (i.e. depression or anxiety).

Psychopharmacologic treatment

Pharmacologic treatment (Santosh and Baird, 1999; Tsai, 1999; for additional information for psychopharmacologic treatment, see Chapter 4) can effectively decrease specific target symptoms and behaviors associated with autism as well as MR. Many case reports have described effective medication treatment. However, few controlled studies have been performed to provide definitive treatment direction.

These individuals commonly have multiple symptoms, so it is advantageous to prioritize treatment of target behaviors by severity and degree of impairment, and then systematically treat each behavior. Medications should be directed at specific target symptoms rather than used indiscriminately for non-specific reasons (e.g. sedation to keep an individual quiet or for the convenience of caregivers). The rule of thumb is to use the lowest dose of medication that can provide the desired effect. Once symptoms stabilize, it is strongly recommended to re-evaluate the medication so as to avoid continuous use of medications such as antipsychotic medications.

An effort should be made to understand the specific target symptoms and the context in which they occur. Environmental factors that exacerbate symptoms should be identified and addressed. Often, once the environmental stressor has passed, medications can be reduced or tapered. Dose reduction and discontinuation should be considered from time to time with attention to withdrawal symptoms and symptom exacerbation. The use of medications in individuals with MR is guided by knowledge of specific drug interactions, unusual behavioral effects in patients with MR and close monitoring for side-effects due to the patient's inability to report them.

The most common target signs and symptoms include attention-deficit/hyperactivity disorder (ADHD) spectrum, anxiety, mood, and aggressive symptoms. In most situations, standard medications that are typically used to control these target symptoms can be utilized. Double-blind placebo efficacy data in individuals with autism and MR are increasing, but most information at this time is derived from open studies or studies with small cohorts.

Most standard medications that are used to treat ADHD can be used to treat attention and activity symptoms in individuals with autism and MR. Stimulants (methylphenidate and amphetamine isomers) and nonstimulants can potentially improve these target symptoms. A double-blind placebo controlled study with methylphenidate involving 10 individuals with PDD demonstrated efficacy of stimulants to decrease ADHD symptoms in a small number of individuals (Quintana et al., 1995). Reports of stimulant related side-effects are mixed, with some reports of increased tics and irritability (Campbell et al., 1976), but other reports of relatively good tolerability (Quintana et al., 1995). Nonstimulant trials including clonidine (Jaselskis et al., 1992), haloperidol (Campbell et al., 1978), risperidone (McCracken et al., 2002), and naltrexone (Campbell et al., 1993; Komen et al., 1995) have resulted in decreased hyperactivity in individuals with PDD.

Anxiety in the form of obsessions, compulsions, phobias, and transition related stress can be treated pharmacologically. Various selective serotonin reuptake inhibitors (SSRIs) including fluoxetine, sertraline, fluvoxamine, citalopram, and paroxetine have been reported to decrease anxiety. Anecdotally, some have reported that lower starting doses have been better tolerated in individuals with PDD. Since many individuals with autism require multiple medications to address numerous target symptoms, the drug-drug interactions must be considered, and the profile of cytochrome p-450 inhibition for each SSRI must be considered. Paradoxical and disinhibiting reactions to benzodiazepines have been described, but there are few definitive data to guide clinical use.

Many individuals with PDD and MR have comorbid mood symptoms, including irritability. For depressive symptoms, SSRIs have traditionally been used, but few controlled data using SSRIs in MR and PDD are available. Symptoms related to bipolar disorder must also be considered. Standard mood stabilizers such as sodium valproate, lithium, and carbamazepine have traditionally been used to control manic symptoms, but controlled studies in PDD and MR have focused on treating aggression rather than bipolar disorder. For acute treatment, atypical antipsychotics can also be used, and in controlled studies risperidone has effectively decreased irritability (McCracken et al., 2002).

Aggression in MR and PDD is a common target behavior. Antipsychotic efficacy in the treatment of aggression in PDD has been supported by controlled studies, and haloperidol was the first and best-studied antipsychotic medication (Campbell et al., 1978). A double-blind placebo controlled study of children with risperidone showed improvement in aggression (McCracken et al., 2002). The potential risk of antipsychotic associated dyskinesias has been a concern, so risks and benefits must be considered carefully (Campbell et al., 1997), but there are few data on newer atypical antipsychotics regarding this issue. SSRIs have been reported to decrease aggression in some individuals with PDD. A double-blind placebo controlled study of adults with fluvoxamine was positive, with improvement in aggression as well as repetitive thoughts and maladaptive behavior (McDougle, 1996). However, few controlled data in children exist. Open label treatment with sertraline (Hellings et al., 1996; McDougle et al., 1998) has resulted in improvement in aggression or self-injurious behavior, however, further treatment for some was precluded by the development of agitation. Controlled studies with clomipramine (Gordon et al., 1993), clonidine (Frankhauser et al., 1992; Jaselskis et al., 1992), and pimozide (Naruse et al., 1982) have also reported improvement in aggression. The atypical neuroleptics are being widely used for the treatment of psychosis, stereotypies, and self-injurious behaviors in this population. The incidence of tardive dyskinesia and akathisia with older typical antipsychotic agents is higher in individuals with MR (Gualtieri et al., 1984, 1986).

Psychosocial treatments

Behavioral therapy

Behavioral modification is effective for the treatment of pica, self-injurious behavior, and stereotypies in individuals with MR and PDD. Behavior modification should be generalizable, consistent, and focus on replacing maladaptive behaviors with adaptive prosocial skills. General principles of behavioral therapy can be successfully applied to individuals with PDD and MR (for a review see Campbell, 2003; Matson et al., 1996). This approach is especially important to help shape behavior in individuals who have limited ability to utilize psychotherapeutic approaches, individuals with literal concrete cognitive styles or limited cognitive abilities. Change is effected via training parents and adults to provide structure and reinforce behaviors (i.e. parent training). Once target behaviors have been identified, they should be specifically described. In assessing target symptoms for behavioral therapy, the evaluation of the behaviors must be evaluated as previously discussed. One must evaluate precipitants or triggers of the behavior, responses (consequences) of others, and response to consequences. Continuity and consistency are important to maintain across caregivers and settings. If responses are inconsistent, behaviors will be difficult to change. Positive reinforcement, negative reinforcement, and redirection should be considered. Often parents can keep journals to track the patterns of behavior and the child's response to interventions. Parents and physicians must be aware of environmental effects, such as noise, light, crowds,

smells, on behavior. Transitions and even subtle changes in routine, schedules, routes, and furniture placement can result in significant behavioral changes.

Studies of individuals with PDD have found that behavioral therapy is most successful when principles of applied behavioral analysis are incorporated (Campbell, 2003; Pelios et al., 1999). Functional behavioral assessment and functional behavioral analysis seek to examine the "function" of a behavior, thereby elucidating the cause of or motivation behind the behavior. Functional behavioral assessment can be accomplished by either using rating scales or observation (behavioral assessment). This assessment can provide information on antecedents (triggers), behaviors (target behaviors), and consequences (response of caregivers), thereby providing data on potential patterns that may perpetuate behavior. Functional analysis incorporates manipulating or changing the environment to effect behavioral changes. The power of this approach is further reflected by the recommendation of the Individuals with Disabilities Education Act [1997; IDEA; Public Law 105–17, Sections 614(b) (2) (C), 614(d) (3) (B) and 615(k) (1) (B)] to incorporate functional behavioral assessments for students who have behavioral problems.

Social interaction interventions

Facilitating social skills has been a component of treatment for children with MR or PPD. This area of intervention has been explored especially for individuals with PPD, given the hallmark core delays in social development. There has been considerable interest in developing social skills interventions for the preschool and elementary years. There are well proven established data supporting the efficacy of interventions designed to improve social interactions, and the age of intervention can influence the success of treatment (Gresham and MacMillan, 1998; Harris and Handleman, 2000; Rogers, 1998). Of the various facets of social interaction, interventions have been found to improve initiation of social interaction, greeting of others, responding to peers, perpetuating interaction, taking turns, and sharing. Individuals with autism can be taught social interactions, learn to use social interactions, and generalize social interactions.

Many different approaches are currently used and being studied. These interventions include changing the environment, developing "collateral skills," developing "child-specific" skills, and training peers. "Collateral skills" training focuses on the development of activities that subsequently result in improvement in social interactions. Studies find that individuals with PDD who are taught how to play/sociodramatic play or how to ask questions can increase social interaction in other situations. "Child-specific" interventions, which include social skills training, focus on developing social skills, teaching how to initiate and sustain social interactions, and reinforcing social behavior. This form of intervention has been more effective in increasing the social initiation than sustaining the interaction. Peer-mediated training interventions focus on training peers at home and at school to initiate interactions with children with autism, to engage and interact with children, and to increase communication. This powerful approach has produced increased social interaction, but it is unclear how well the benefits can be generalized in the absence of trained peers. Together, these approaches provide evidence that social behavior can be taught, and that individuals with PDD can learn to interact with others.

Even though these interventions differ in approach, all of these interventions have common characteristics that may contribute to their efficacy. Thorough training of adults, instructors or peers on how to facilitate and promote social initiation is essential. Structure of the environment and reinforcement are also important. Data support that inclusion in classrooms with typically developing students is effective. However, inclusion alone will not produce improvement in social interaction. This finding underscores the importance of active involvement and training. To date, studies have not yet determined the most effective approaches or the duration of the intervention. Unfortunately, many of these interventions are not yet commonly used in the community.

Psychotherapy

The goal of therapy is alleviation of problem symptoms. Therapy needs to be individualized, directive, structured, flexible, and concrete commensurate with the child's cognitive status and language abilities.

Individual psychotherapy incorporates the objective of symptom relief with cognitive strategies to help the child understand his/her disability, recognize strengths, have realistic expectations, recognize and alter maladaptive behavior patterns, attain age appropriate social skills, develop a positive self-image, and discern emotional feeling states. An exploratory approach may be used in persons with mild MR. Rescue fantasies need to be avoided. Despite very limited data on psychotherapy with individuals with PDD, individuals with insight, a desire to understand their difficulties with others, and reasonable verbal abilities may benefit from various psychotherapeutic approaches. Commonly, as individuals with Aspergers syndrome or high functioning autism become more aware of their social differences and isolation, depression may arise. Supportive therapy can be one modality to help address mild depressed mood and various stressors.

Psychotherapeutic approaches can also be important to consider for families. Often family stress can arise with the initial shock and concern about the child's diagnosis, maladaptive behavior, cognitive difficulties, social interaction difficulties, limited independence, and potential future as well as the challenges of finding adequate treatment, coordination of multiple appointments, and financial demands. Family therapy should attend to guilt feelings, recognition of patient strengths, cultivation of realistic expectations, education about the disability and available resources, advocacy, empathy, and concrete behavioral management programs.

Group therapy is useful with adolescents and can include social skills training. Multiple family group therapy has been described by Szymanski and Kiernan (1983) to be useful and supportive.

Non-traditional treatments

Several alternative approaches have been reported to help individuals with autism. In some situations, the reports have been anecdotal and in other reports the claims have been unambiguously refuted. One alternative approach that garnered much attention is facilitated communication (FC). Facilitated communication was an approach that was initially heralded as a means by which an individual with PDD could express him or herself. With FC, a "facilitator" was required to guide the individual's hand so that he or she could type a message on a typewriter or keyboard. Scientific studies, however, could not replicate findings, and the facilitator introduced significant bias (review, Mostert, 2001).

Another intervention approach that has received some attention is auditory integration training (AIT). With AIT (review, Mostert, 2001), an individual with PDD receives an initial audiogram and attends 20 half-hour sessions which consist of listening to computer-modified music. Interestingly, individuals in a control group who listened to music, as well as those receiving AIT, benefited. Whether PDD symptoms improve awaits randomized, blinded and controlled studies. The American Academy of Pediatrics (Anonymous, 1998) does not recommend either AIT or FC for routine treatment in individuals with autism.

Dietary approaches have been reported to help in some instances. Gluten- and casein-free diets have been purported to improve symptoms of autism (Knivsberg et al., 2002). However, there is little available blinded data to help elucidate or recommend these interventions at this time. The ketogenic diet has been effective for treating certain forms of epilepsy (Kossoff et al., 2002), and Evangeliou et al. (2003) have reported that the ketogenic diet improves certain aspects of autism. These findings must be repeated with large numbers of participants in a randomized, blinded and controlled study. B12 and folate therapy has also been reported to help, but these approaches have not yet been found to be effective in improving behavior (Lowe et al., 1981).

Anecdotal reports asserting efficacy of various medications are common. For example, secretin, a polypeptide hormone that is produced in the gastrointestinal tract, was reported to dramatically improve symptoms of autism. However, multiple double-blind placebo controlled studies have found no significant difference between placebo and secretin (Coplan et al., 2003; Levy et al., 2003; Carey et al., 2002; Molloy et al., 2002; Unis et al., 2002). No improvement in aberrant behaviors or core autistic behaviors could be identified with secretin treatment.

Many of these approaches have not yet been readily embraced because of their anecdotal nature. In general, reports and studies that are open (unblinded), uncontrolled and involving very few participants should be interpreted cautiously and critically.

Other interventions

By the nature of most PDDs and MR, multimodal treatment is more the rule than the exception. In addition to psychiatric treatment, treatment of additional symptoms is also common. Individuals with fine motor coordination difficulties such as difficulty buttoning, coloring or writing can benefit from occupational therapy. Dystonias, dyskinesias, and poor motor coordination can contribute to gross motor difficulties, which can be addressed in part through physical therapy. Individuals with difficulty speaking or communicating will benefit from speech and language evaluations and treatment. Underlying neurologic problems including generalized seizures warrant concurrent neurologic evaluation and treatment. And for some individuals, social skills training or groups can be helpful.

Many social and behavioral interventions can be carried out in the school setting. It is important for families to be familiar with their child's educational and legal rights. Public law 94–142, enforced through the Education for all Handicapped Children Act of 1975, states that all children with handicaps including mental retardation, learning disabilities, serious emotional disturbance, and speech and language impairment are entitled to a free and public education and related services, the need for which is assessed and meted out using an "individualized educational plan" in the "least restrictive environment." The law was further amended in 1991 and the new statute "Individuals with Disabilities Act (IDEA)" defined its purpose to protect rights of children and adolescents with disabilities, to provide assistance and early intervention opportunities.

Accurate educational information about MR and autism can be important not only for the immediate family but also the extended family. Organizations such as the Autism Society of America can provide much information not only for the physician but also for families. Some universities with autism programs have websites with information about diagnoses and treatment. And many national organizations have local chapters for families such as the National Autistic Society (www.nas.org.uk) and the Autism Society of America (www.asa.org). The Arc of the United States (www. thearc.org) provides parents of individuals with MR with support, information, and advocacy.

Summary

Individuals with pervasive developmental disorders, mental retardation, and other developmental disabilities comprise a significant proportion of children. Early identification of delays in cognition, communication, and social development is important so that intervention can be started early. Since comorbid psychiatric presentations are exceptionally common in these individuals, awareness and early identifi-

CONSIDER CONSULTATION WHEN ...

- Parents express concern about their young child's expressive language, receptive language, fine and gross motor skills, or general cognitive skills, consider referring for a speech-language evaluation and/or psychoeducational evaluation. Additionally, referral to an audiologist to assess hearing is essential, and a vision test is recommended. Psychologic testing can be pivotal for identifying MR or PPD and providing recommendations.

- A cognitive delay is suspected in a school age child, or when the child is having academic difficulties, a psychoeducational consultation should be made. A consultation should be requested for educational/cognitive testing to determine both strengths and areas that need to be improved. A psychologist, preferably with experience with developmental disabilities, should perform cognitive testing. Recommendations can help the child develop learning strategies that work.

- The diagnosis is unclear, when parents continue to assert that something is wrong, "odd," or "different" about their child, or that their child is not interacting with other children, a referral should be made to a child psychiatrist or psychologist who is experienced with evaluating children with autism. If possible, a referral to a center that specializes in diagnosing autism could provide specialized diagnostic testing. Often, a child psychiatry department within a university medical school will be able to provide consultation and referrals. The earlier the consultation, the sooner interventions can be initiated and the higher the likelihood of a better outcome.

- There is stereotypic aggression accompanied with unresponsiveness, a neurologic consultation should be considered to rule out seizures. There is a higher risk of grand mal seizures in individuals with autism, and post-ictal states may present with stereotypic agitation or decreased responsiveness/confusion.

- If MR or PDD is accompanied by other physical or neurologic findings; one should consider the possibility of an underlying genetic condition. A consultation with a pediatric geneticist can be especially useful for diagnosis and further evaluation.

cation of psychiatric problems and treatment can potentially reduce morbidity. Psychiatric treatment should incorporate a biopsychosocial approach to provide the most comprehensive treatment.

Annotated bibliography

Attwood A (1998) *Asperger's Syndrome: A Guide for Parents and Professionals.* London, Jessica Kingsley Publishers.
A "guide" for physicians and parents that covers diagnosis, detailed description, and practical approaches for individuals with Asperger syndrome.

Dosen A, Day K (2001) (eds) *Treating Mental Illness and Behavior Disorders in Children and Adults with Mental Retardation.* Washington DC, American Psychiatric Press.
The definitive text on psychiatric issues in individuals with mental retardation.

Volkmar FR, Wiesner LA (2004) *Healthcare for Children on the Autism Spectrum. A Guide to Medical, Nutritional, and Behavioral Issues.* Bethesda, Woodbine House.
An excellent book to introduce physicians and parents to problems that arise in children with PDD and practical solutions.

Volkmar FR (ed) (1998) *Autism and Pervasive Developmental Disorders.* Cambridge Monographs in Child and Adolescent Psychiatry. Cambridge, New York, Cambridge University Press.
A comprehensive textbook on autism that is written by authorities in the field.

CHAPTER 6

Developmental Disabilities: Learning Disorders

Ann Abramowitz, PhD

Introduction

The DSM-IV states that learning disorders (LD) are diagnosed when the individual's academic achievement in reading, mathematics, or writing is substantially below what would be expected for age, schooling, and intellectual ability (APA, 1994). The *Diagnostic and Statistical Manual of Mental Disorders* (DSM) also provides a category, Not Otherwise Specified (NOS), for which no criteria are given, but where the example given is of an instance where all three areas are affected but none to the required degree. To meet DSM criteria, learning problems must significantly interfere with achievement at school or the performance of activities in daily life that require reading, mathematics, or writing skills. The DSM-IV definition goes on to state, albeit erroneously, that the usual discrepancy required between intellectual ability and achievement is more than two standard deviations (Box 6.1). As detailed below, the measurement of discrepancy, and the requirement that discrepancy be present are fraught with problems, and within the United States the amount of discrepancy required by the public schools, and the way it is measured, vary greatly from state to state. However, from a purely psychometric standpoint, requiring a discrepancy of two standard deviations is an exceedingly stringent criterion, and is seldom obtained on psychoeducational tests, even when assessing individuals with marked learning disabilities. In general, either one standard deviation, or slightly over one standard deviation, is used. As described below, however, research has failed to support IQ-achievement discrepancy as a valid or useful criterion for LD diagnosis.

In addition to the definition included in the DSM, the most commonly used definition of learning disabilities in the United States is that of the federal government, first written in 1967 by the National Joint Committee on Handicapped Children and adopted as part of the 1975 Education of the Handicapped Act, PL 94–142, which defined the categories of handicapping conditions for which public school systems would be required to provide special education services. This definition states:

> Specific learning disability means a disorder in one or more of the basic psychologic processes involved in understanding or in using language, spoken or written, which may manifest itself in an imperfect ability to listen, think, speak, read, write, spell, or to do mathematical calculations. The term includes such conditions as perceptual handicaps, brain injury, minimal brain dysfunction, dyslexia, and developmental aphasia. The term does not include children who have learning problems, which are primarily the result of visual, hearing, or motor handicaps, of mental retardation, of emotional disturbance, or of environmental, cultural, or economic disadvantage. (U.S. Office of Education, 1968, p. 34)

Since the passage of the federal law, each state has been required to develop guidelines to comply with the law, and to oversee the provision of mandated services within school districts. Learning disabilities comprise one category of special education services. Others, which sometimes overlap with learning disabilities, but sometimes preclude them, include emotional/behavioral disorders, mental disability, preschool handicapping conditions, sensory (hearing and vision) problems, and health problems. This original law, PL 94–142, underwent a revision in 1983 that provided for some

---

BOX 6.1

DSM-IV diagnostic issues
- DSM indicates that significant discrepancy between intelligence and achievement is required.
- DSM incorrectly states the amount of discrepancy that is generally required.

expansion of services. In 1997, the law was again revised, becoming the Individuals with Disabilities Educational Act (IDEA). It is undergoing revision at the time of the writing of this chapter. At the present time, the House of Representatives and the Senate have passed separate versions, and a final compromise version must now be developed. It is expected that some of the most important changes will be to bring the definition more in line with research, as well as to reduce some of the excessively burdensome administrative tasks entailed in the present version. In the meantime, efforts have been made to update the broad definition of learning abilities, perhaps best represented by the following, from the National Joint Commission on Learning Disabilities:

> Learning disabilities is a general term that refers to a heterogeneous group of disorders manifested by significant difficulties in the acquisition and use of listening, speaking, reading, writing, reasoning, or mathematical abilities. These disorders are intrinsic to the individual, presumed to be due to central nervous system dysfunction, and may occur across the lifespan. Problems in self-regulatory behaviors, social perception, and social interaction may exist with learning disabilities but do not by themselves constitute a learning disability. Although learning disabilities may occur concomitantly with other handicapping conditions (for example, sensory impairment, mental retardation, serious emotional disturbance) or with extrinsic influences (such as cultural differences, insufficient or inappropriate instruction), they are not the result of those conditions or influences (NJCLD, 1988, p. 1).

Lyon et al. (2003) point out that this definition addresses the issues of heterogeneity, persistence, intrinsic etiology, and comorbidity. However, similar to the federal definition, it is vague and overly broad. At the current time, there is an increasing consensus that a single definition is not the best approach to address learning disabilities, and that separate definitions for each of the areas that can be affected is a more sensible solution.

Learning disorders unquestionably are common in children and adolescents. The DSM-IV provides a prevalence estimate at 2–10% of the population, but prevalence is a function of whatever criteria and cutoffs are used. Certainly, more than 10% of school children have significant academic difficulties, although some of those cases fail to meet criteria for learning disabilities because they meet exclusionary criteria. Exclusionary criteria include a variety of causes of academic problems, including substandard or inconsistent schooling, psychosocial stressors, sensory handicaps and other medical conditions that interfere with learning, mental retardation or low intellectual ability, and various psychiatric disorders. Assuming that learning disabilities constitute a subset of all youngsters with academic problems, specify-

ing the boundaries of this population has been, and continues to be, a great challenge, with considerable disagreement among educators, psychologists, parents, and others. Learning disabilities are reported in the DSM and elsewhere to be about four times more common in males than females, although this ratio probably is based on clinic and school settings that reflect referral bias associated with externalizing behavior problems (see Barkley, 1997; Shaywitz et al., 1992). Numerous studies indicate that learning disabilities actually are equally prevalent in males and females (e.g. DeFries and Gillis, 1991; Flynn and Rahbar, 1994; Shaywitz et al., 1992). Reading disorders constitute the greatest proportion of youngsters identified with learning disabilities, probably 80–90%. Individuals frequently have more than one learning disability, and all three areas of learning can share some cognitive underpinnings. In addition, written expression inevitably is affected in an individual with a reading disorder, whether or not writing is affected beyond the contribution from associated reading skills. Learning disabilities tend to run in families.

A fundamental assumption is that learning disabilities result from neurologic impairment affecting specific brain functions (Torgesen, 1998). This assumption stems from similarities between the performance of affected people and that of individuals with known brain lesions. However, in the vast majority of cases of learning disorders, no known brain lesion is found, and in some cases, no processing disability is found either. But the correlation between processing disabilities and learning disorders is strong enough to support the usefulness of organicity as a fundamental component of our understanding of learning disorders. Considerable research has explored the etiology of learning disabilities, particularly

---

PEARLS & PERILS

- Evaluation of learning problems includes individual testing of intellectual ability, academic achievement in all areas, and relevant areas of cognitive processing.
- Evaluation also should include assessment of attention, behavior and emotional well-being.
- Vision, hearing, and health problems should be ruled out.
- Group standardized tests administered by schools are useful for reading and mathematics screening but do not evaluate written expression.
- Written expression disabilities are often not recognized.
- Many learning disabled youngsters may not meet eligibility requirements for learning disabilities services.
- Learning disabilities are common in youngsters with ADHD and other developmental disorders.
- The primary care physician should play a key role in facilitating assessment and communicating with the school as necessary.

reading disorders. The strongest evidence of a biologic basis comes from studies of genetic transmission of reading disorders. As summarized by Torgesen (1998), approximately 50% of all variability in the phonologic processes that cause specific reading disability can be attributed to genetic factors. Various investigators have explored the brain basis for these problems, with the most interesting findings obtained largely through the use of four types of neuroimaging techniques: positron emission tomography, fMRI, magnetic resonance imaging (MRI), and magnetic resonance spectroscopy. While findings are preliminary given the newness of this type of research, it appears likely that in children with reading disorders, the functional connections between brain areas account for differences in brain activation, as opposed to there being one or more specific area(s) of the brain where reading disorders can be localized (Lyon et al., 2003).

Background

The field of learning disabilities, and the efforts to define them, emerged on two fronts. First was the desire by researchers to gain a scientific and clinical understanding of individual differences in learning among children and adults who, although intellectually normal, displayed specific deficits in spoken or written language. The other was the practical need to provide services to youngsters exhibiting these patterns (Lyon et al., 2003). Beginning in the latter part of the 19th century, medical professionals and other investigators interested in language disorders and reading problems wrote descriptively of their patients, postulating a neurologic basis for the observed difficulties (e.g. Wernicke, 1894; Broca, 1863). Several 20th-century researchers laid the groundwork for the field of learning disabilities, as we know it today, as well as for many of the key remediation strategies that are used. Samuel Orton is well known for his work in the 1920s and 1930s with children who exhibited letter and word reversals, among other difficulties. He theorized that a lack of left-hemispheric dominance for the processing of linguistic symbols underlay the disorder (Orton, 1937). While neither his theory nor the centrality of reversals to the disorder has stood the test of time (Torgesen, 1991), his influence on the field has been tremendous.

It was not until after the Second World War that learning disabilities received recognition from the educational standpoint. Initially, and for the most part to this day, they have been seen as a phenomenon whereby otherwise intelligent individuals inexplicably have difficulty learning to read, perform mathematics, or put their thoughts in writing. On the practical front, parents and professionals struggled with the issue of youngsters who, despite seeming bright (and attaining average or higher scores on intelligence tests), exhibit difficulty learning. The emphasis in the field became the identification and remediation of the deficient learning processes that underlay each child's learning difficulties.

The assumption was that learning disabilities were associated with, or caused by, neurologic dysfunction. In particular, emphasis was placed on perceptual-motor functioning, and remedial approaches were developed that focused on this area with the expectation that reading skills would improve. A movement also grew whereby presumed underlying processes were assessed across a variety of areas of perception, visual and auditory and perceptual-motor areas. Instruction was then tailored to the individual's pattern of strengths and weaknesses in these areas. This approach has failed to be supported by research, and those early tests of processing have been gradually replaced by more theoretically and psychometrically sound tests based on advances in neuropsychology. In the 1950s and 1960s, in addition to the work on assessment and remediation of perceptual processes, research began to examine environmental factors. Since many of these youngsters exhibited distractibility and short attention span in addition to learning difficulties, many specialists in the field emphasized reducing stimulation in the classroom environment (e.g. Cruickshank et al., 1961). This avenue, too, failed to gain research support, and has largely been abandoned.

Conceptualization issues

Since the 1970s, the field of learning disabilities has gradually responded to research involving the specific deficits involved in reading, written expression, and mathematics. Increasingly, assessment and remediation have targeted the specific academic areas of need via direct instruction, as opposed to focusing on the remediation of underlying processes, and the field now stresses optimally delivered academic instruction rather than instruction tailored to a particular student's pattern of processing strengths and weaknesses. For reading, this strategy has meant phonetically based reading instruction and task analytically derived instruction in all areas. Optimal instruction is based on a careful analysis of the component skills of reading, written expression, and mathematics. Instruction should be presented via a carefully developed sequence, with the goal being mastery of each skill prior to presentation of the next.

The aforementioned changes in the conceptualization of learning disabilities have been reflected in the successive versions of the DSM. Consistent with the perspective of most professionals in the field of learning disabilities, the category of "Learning disorders" in the DSM-IV does not state that they are attributable to minimal brain dysfunction, as was the case with earlier versions of the DSM. However, both the current federal definition of learning disabilities, as well as the DSM-IV definition, are flawed and in need of revision. In addition to the federal definition and that of DSM-IV, there have been, and continue to be, many definitions of learning disabilities. Besides the exclusions noted, most definitions have proposed that intellectual ability be at least average, a requirement that has been incorporated into federal definition of LD in the United States. However, considerable research has indicated that this requirement is unsupportable, for both psychometric and educational reasons. Consistent with the expectation of at least average intellectual functioning, most LD definitions require that a significant discrepancy be evident between intellectual ability and academic achievement, in order for the academic problem to qualify as an LD. This requirement, too, has not been supported by research. Lyon et al. (2003) provide an excellent review of the research concerning both the average IQ requirement and the discrepancy requirement. This research is summarized here. However, given the extent to which research findings challenge conventional wisdom and the DSM and federal definitions of LD, the reader is encouraged to read a full review of the topic (e.g. Lyon et al., 2003). It should be noted that the majority of the research has dealt with reading disabilities, but emerging results in the areas of mathematics and written expression yield similar findings.

The notion that learning disabilities must involve a discrepancy between intellectual ability (as measured by an IQ test) and academic achievement was integral to the birth of the field. The awareness of otherwise normal individuals who struggled academically was fundamental to the conceptualization of these disorders, and to the intense advocacy efforts that led to the establishment of this as a category within federal law. Unquestionably, many such individuals exist, and perhaps they constitute a group of youngsters with "classical" learning disabilities. But alongside them, and often indistinguishable in terms of their learning characteristics, are individuals who do not exhibit a measured "significant discrepancy." In understanding this issue, it is crucial to distinguish between the strong advocacy that has developed within this field, and the findings of research. Several issues are integral to this distinction. First, measurement of intelligence is fraught with complexity. IQ tests are comprised of a variety of tasks that essentially measure a broad sampling of skills, vocabulary, verbal categorical reasoning, nonverbal fluid reasoning, visual-spatial constructional, quantitative, processing speed, felt to provide an overall estimate of a person's intellectual ability. However, the same weaknesses in cognitive processing that underlie many learning disabilities also affect IQ scores, and there is considerable overlap between the skills measured on IQ tests and skills required by academic tasks. These factors act to lessen any measurable discrepancy.

Importantly, no research has shown that different instructional strategies should be applied depending on whether or not a discrepancy is present. The largest amount of research has been conducted on reading instruction, but for none of the three areas is there much question of how remediation, and for that matter initial instruction, should be conducted. It should be based on a task analysis of the skill to be taught.

Thus, it is questionable from a purely practical standpoint to separate youngsters who meet some arbitrary discrepancy criterion from those who do not, for purposes of delivering instruction.

Studies that have examined the outcomes of reading interventions have found that neither IQ-achievement discrepancy nor level of IQ predicts response to intervention, or provides information as to what type of intervention is needed (Vellutino et al., 2000). Studies that have examined whether youngsters with IQ-achievement discrepancy differ across various cognitive variables from youngsters without the discrepancy largely have found that most cognitive abilities assessed show considerable overlap between the two groups, tending to discredit discrepancy as an important factor in learning disabilities (Sternberg and Grigorenko, 2002; Hoskyn and Swanson, 2000; Stuebing et al., 2002). Further, studies generally have shown that neither IQ nor presence or absence of discrepancy predicts the developmental course of reading acquisition (e.g. Share et al., 1989; Shaywitz et al., 1999; Flowers et al., 2001; Wristers et al., 2002). Finally, neuroimaging studies, although of small sample sizes, have not demonstrated structural or functional differences between individuals with or without discrepancies. While there have been fewer studies of individuals with speech-language or math disorders, the findings have been similar.

A serious pragmatic problem also exists with the IQ-achievement discrepancy requirement, based solely on the psychometric properties of achievement tests.

Given the cumulative nature of learning problems, a significant discrepancy often will not be obtained before grade 3, even in youngsters who exhibit strong evidence of a learning disorder. This issue occurs because on standardized achievement tests even a little knowledge in an area usually causes a first or second grader's score to fall within a range that is not discrepant from an average IQ.

A related problem is the unfairness of the discrepancy requirement for youngsters who have received intervention. A youngster who has a learning disability that is characterized by an ability/achievement discrepancy will manifest symptoms of this disability earlier than the school system's LD identification process kicks into gear. Parents, alert to the learning problems that have become evident, often will work intensely with their child to overcome the difficulties, and may obtain remedial services privately. These efforts may be virtually identical to what the youngster would have received had the LD been identified and served by the school system. Thus, by the time the school system provides formal testing, a discrepancy of sufficient size may no longer be present, falsely suggesting that one was not present earlier, and disqualifying the child from services. In short, an IQ-achievement discrepancy is something that should be targeted for intervention as early as possible, but should not be considered either an enduring characteristic of LD nor essential for making the diagnosis.

Thus, regardless of whether the etiology is known, and regardless of whether the difficulties meet a state's particular criteria for learning disabilities, the topography of the problems may be the same, as may be the optimal remediation strategies. Further, many in the field now feel that little can be gained from perpetuating and refining broad definitions of, and criteria for, learning disabilities, and that greater progress in understanding these disorders will be made once narrower definitions gain general acceptance. These narrower definitions likely would be based on the specific domain of difficulty, i.e. reading, mathematics, or written expression. Currently, the DSM-IV specifies these three types of learning disorders, as well as Learning Disorder Not Otherwise Specified (NOS). This chapter will describe the various types of learning disabilities that are generally accepted by professionals in the field, including the American Psychiatric Association and the American Association for Learning Disabilities, and offer a critical assessment of current diagnostic and intervention practices.

Most definitions of learning disabilities are broad, allowing considerable flexibility in making the diagnosis, and contributing to diverse criteria that vary greatly from state to state and discipline to discipline. All professionals would agree that the diagnosis should be made after a thorough evaluation of cognitive and academic abilities as well as behavioral, medical, attentional, and psychosocial factors that may be contributing to and/or causing the difficulties. Only through such an assessment, using norm-referenced instruments, can academic deficiencies be definitively documented and can judgments about their probable cause be made. Assessment must include individually administered, up-to-date, normed tests of intellectual ability, academic skills across all areas, and any relevant areas that can shed light on the difficulties, such as receptive and expressive language, phonologic skills, sequencing ability, and various areas of executive functioning (Table 6.1). Outdated instruments and those with inadequate psychometric properties cannot be used to make diagnoses of learning disorders, although informal tests often can be helpful for understanding specific deficits in need of remediation. A school psychologist or clinical psychologist, sometimes in conjunction with an educational diagnostician trained in psychoeducational assessment, performs testing generally. Learning disorders cannot be diagnosed informally based on parent or teacher report, behavior rating scales, or review of group-administered standardized test results.

The current federal definition of LD (now under revision) and the resulting state guidelines require a significant discrepancy between intellectual ability and achievement in order for a learning disorder to be identified and served. Each state has

TABLE 6.1

Selected assessment instruments

Instrument	Skills assessed	Limitations	Helpful for
Wechsler Intelligence Test for Children, 4th edn	Intellectual ability		Learning disorders
Differential Abilities Scale	Intellectual ability and achievement screen		Learning disorders Mental retardation
Stanford-Binet, 5th edn	Intellectual ability		Learning disorders Mental retardation
Woodcock-Johnson Tests of Cognitive Ability and Tests of Achievement, 3rd edn	Academic achievement: reading, math, written expression		Learning disorders
Kaufman Assessment Battery for Children, 2nd edn	Intellectual ability		Learning disorders
Wechsler Individual Achievement Test	Academic achievement: reading, math	No measure of reading fluency	Learning disorders
Kaufman Test of Educational Achievement	Academic achievement		Learning disorders
Gray Oral Reading Test, 4th edn	Oral reading and comprehension		Reading disorder, particularly involving fluency
Comprehensive Test of Phonologic Processing	Phonologic processing		Processing problems that may underlie reading disorder
KeyMath	Math		Mathematics disorder
Test of Written Language, 3rd edn	Writing		Disorder of written expression

developed guidelines that comply with federal law, but there are large differences between states as to the actual criteria. For example, given standardized tests with a standard deviation of 15 (which characterizes the majority of instruments currently used for this purpose), one state may require a discrepancy of 20 standard score points between a measure of IQ and academic achievement, while another state may require 15. Some states take standard error of measurement and regression to the mean into account in determining discrepancy, but others do not. Some states require that average cognitive ability be present and remarkably, some states also require that average achievement be demonstrated in some academic area – that is, to qualify as having a learning disability in some area, some other area must be relatively unaffected. The result of this variability is that a youngster may qualify as having a learning disability in one state but not another. However, specialists outside of school systems who perform evaluations are not subject to these guidelines, and may diagnose learning disabilities based on evidence of academic difficulties and associated difficulties in cognitive processing, consistent with what research has shown about the relationship between intelligence tests and achievement tests. In addition to the psychologic testing component of the assessment, it is important to obtain current vision, hearing, and health evaluations to rule out any contribution from any of these areas to difficulties in learning. It is also essential to ascertain that educational factors such as inconsistent attendance or inadequate instruction do not account for the difficulties.

In summary, four key conclusions should be drawn here regarding the assessment of learning disorders. First, a learning disorder can only be diagnosed when a battery of psychoeducational tests has been performed and interpreted by a qualified psychologist, and when other causes of the problem have been ruled out (i.e. significant absences). Second, such a specialist can diagnose a learning disorder based on an appropriate interpretation of the instruments used, in combination with a comprehensive history and a medical evaluation, to rule out other causes of the learning deficiencies such as hearing impairments, diabetes mellitus, or other medical problems. Third, a child who is properly assessed and diagnosed as having a learning disorder may not qualify as learning disabled within the public school system, because of factors that have nothing to do with the accuracy of the diagnosis. Fourth, because eligibility criteria vary dramatically from state to state, many youngsters who qualify for services in one state will fail to qualify in another or vice versa.

Types of learning disorders

Reading disorders

Description
The federal definition specifies two areas of reading disabilities (Table 6.2): basic reading (word recognition) and

---

DIAGNOSIS

Table 6.2 Reading disorder

Discriminating features

1. Reading skills significantly below expectancy.

Consistent features

1. Significantly interferes with academic achievement or activities requiring reading skills.

Variable features

1. Other learning disorders may be present.
2. Cognitive processing deficits may be present.

---

comprehension. Problems with basic reading can involve fluency as well as accuracy. While word recognition, fluency, and comprehension must be considered separately, they are interrelated, and each aspect makes an essential contribution to reading competence. Accuracy sets a ceiling on comprehension, as a youngster can only be expected to understand what he or she has been able to read. Accurate and fluent decoding depends upon solid phonologic knowledge that can be readily called upon, as well as automaticity with respect to common words, and sufficient knowledge of vocabulary and other components of spoken language. There are many component skills involved in successful comprehension, and not uncommonly an individual evidences difficulty only in some of them. Difficulties in word recognition represent about 70–80% of children identified with reading disorders (Lyon et al., 2003). The largest group of those with difficulties in word recognition is the group with problems in phonologic processes underlying decoding.

Assessment
A thorough evaluation of reading difficulties should look at the full range of components separately, as well as how the youngster can use the various skills together. Within the area of decoding, skills to be assessed include the ability to read words in isolation as well as in context, and the ability to derive meaning from what is read. The reason for assessing the ability to read words out of context is that this evaluation is a purer measure of reading. The reason for assessing word reading within context is that this better approximates the demands of reading in the real world. The ability to "sound out words" by applying knowledge of letter sounds and blending must be assessed as well, as it underlies the ability to decode unfamiliar words and apply the rules of the language. Assessing this skill typically involves having the youngster read a series of "nonsense words" that can only be read via the application of phonetic principles. Reading rate should be assessed as well, because some readers are accurate but must expend extreme effort to decode, reducing their ability to derive meaning from what they have read.

Such fluency problems in an otherwise accurate reader often go undetected, yet can have an extremely detrimental effect on learning. They can cause struggles with homework and contribute to uncompleted classwork.

There are a number of ways of assessing comprehension, and more than one should be employed, since a youngster may have difficulty with some, but not all, aspects. For example, one method involves a cloze procedure, in which the child supplies a missing word to meaningfully complete a sentence. Another method involves asking the child to read a passage and answer questions that are read by the examiner. In general, however, tests of reading comprehension fail to assess how the youngster deals with the types of longer text that students encounter in actual reading.

Remediation

A large body of research on methods of reading instruction has clearly demonstrated that methods that involve early, systematic, intense emphasis on phonics are superior to methods that place heavy emphasis on sight word acquisition. Despite this large amount of evidence, and despite the great emphasis placed on reading competence by federal, state, and local educational authorities, reading instruction in American schools frequently is based heavily on sight methods. Prevalent methods emphasize the use of context while decoding, and stress content over basic phonetic decoding skills, beginning with the earliest instruction.

An emerging literature is showing that often reading disorders can be prevented through early identification of young children with weaknesses in phonologic awareness and phonologic processing. Sadly, most learning disabilities are not identified until at least the third grade, by which time the youngster has experienced considerable failure and is far behind classmates. When identified in kindergarten or early first grade, youngsters whose phonologic weaknesses warrant careful instruction in this area can become skilled readers without having had to experience failure.

Beyond using an overall approach that is supported by reading research, remediation should address deficits identified in the youngster's assessment. Weaknesses in phonics and word identification skills should be remediated by systematic direct instruction addressing these areas, with mastery of each skill before subsequent skills are introduced. Skill mastery should be measured by both adequate accuracy and rate. Weaknesses in comprehension can be harder to target for instruction, because of the many skills involved, some of which are separate from the reading process per se. Such skills include understanding the different types and formats of written material, adequate vocabulary knowledge, distinguishing more important from less important information, and the ability to draw inferences.

Mathematics disorders

Description

Math disabilities (Table 6.3) can involve difficulties recognizing numbers and symbols, memorizing facts, grasping various aspects of mathematical reasoning to solve problems, or performing computation. Concepts such as place value, fractions, percentages, and square roots can be problematic for those with a mathematics disorder. Mathematics skills are involved in understanding time, money, and measurement. Hence, these areas typically are impacted by a math disorder.

Youngsters may exhibit disabilities in mathematics alone, or they may have more generalized difficulties that impact several academic areas including mathematics. For example, memory weaknesses and deficits in the ability to employ strategies are problematic for most basic skill areas. In mathematics, they can cause difficulty with conceptualization in performing math operations, recalling math facts, learning and understanding algorithms and formulae, or solving word problems. Language and communication problems that underlie many children's reading disorders can impact on mathematics achievement as well, most obviously in the performance of word problems. For some youngsters, deficiencies in processes and strategies impact on acquisition of math skills and math performance, but not on other curricular areas.

Assessment

It is important to assess the various skills involved in mathematics performance. Some achievement tests assess computational skills alone, but not mathematical reasoning ability or the understanding of concepts that underlie computation. Needless to say, mathematics performance is comprised of several separate skills that must be integrated, and youngsters may have problems with one or more of these. In addition, because of the important roles played by immediate, long-term, and working memory, these should be assessed

---

DIAGNOSIS

Table 6.3 Mathematics disorder

Discriminating features

1. Mathematics skills significantly below expectancy.

Consistent features

1. Significantly interferes with academic achievement or activities requiring mathematics skills.

Variable features

1. Other learning disorders may be present.
2. Cognitive processing deficits may be present.

as well. Competent performance of even rote computation requires adequate graphomotor skills and is reliant at least to some degree on processing speed. Visual-spatial skills are needed at the most basic level for performing written computation, and increasingly for mastering concepts involving geometry and for understanding algebraic relationships involving time and distance. In interpreting assessment results, it is essential to consider the broad picture of the youngster's achievement in other areas and his or her cognitive and graphomotor skills, and possible relationships between mathematics deficits and those in other areas.

Remediation

In most schools systems, mathematics is taught via a "spiraling curriculum" that introduces a skill or concept, then moves to another, then to a third, and so on, returning on a "spiraling" basis to each skill, with gradually increasing complexity. Even for a given skill, several formats of problem presentation and desired response will be utilized. While this approach may eventually lead to mastery and generalization by non-disabled learners, it can be quite problematic for many youngsters with learning disabilities, who often require a greater degree of practice to master any skill and who may have difficulty retaining skills and concepts when they have not been learned to mastery. A substantial literature documents the effectiveness of drill and practice and emphasis on presentation rate on success in learning. In general, approaches that are based on learning theory, where skills are carefully sequenced, and that employ reinforcement and clear mastery criteria for each skill taught, have the best likelihood of success with youngsters having learning disorders.

In addition to careful instruction in core mathematics skills, training in metacognitive skills also has proven beneficial in the remediation of mathematics disabilities. Such training generally involves self-monitoring to check whether all steps of a problem, or all components of a task, were performed. Training is based on a checklist developed for the student based on an analysis of his or her errors. A checklist may contain tasks essential for solving a problem, e.g. lining up the numbers correctly, regrouping when needed, subtracting all numbers, and writing the solution in the correct place, and/or it may contain tasks necessary for overall successful performance, such as checking that the problem was copied correctly, checking that the right operation was selected, checking accuracy, and making sure no problems were skipped.

Disorders of written expression

Description

These disorders (Table 6.4) can involve any of several aspects of written communication: graphomotor skills, grammar and usage, spelling, or limitations on the ability to put

DIAGNOSIS

Table 6.4 Disorder of written expression

Discriminating features

1. Writing skills significantly below expectancy.

Consistent features

1. Significantly interferes with academic achievement or activities involving writing.

Variable features

1. Other learning disorders may be present.
2. Cognitive processing deficits may be present.

one's thoughts into words. Written language mechanics include punctuation, capitalization, and sentence structure. Putting one's thoughts into words involves many skills and processes, such as planning, revising, and various self-regulation strategies (Graham et al., 1998). Problems with written expression may constitute a youngster's sole area of difficulty, or they may be secondary to reading problems and/or difficulties in spoken language. In general, youngsters with learning disabilities in this area produce very brief written products that contain little detail. According to Graham et al. (1998), children with LD typically convert writing tasks into tasks of telling what they know, with little planning before or during writing. Information is put down but not organized, and there appears to be little consideration of the audience or the richness of the topic. Students with LD are less knowledgeable about writing, and tend to think about it in its simplest terms (spelling, neatness) rather than in terms of the expression of ideas and a way of communicating with others on a topic (Graham et al., 1993).

Assessment

Unlike reading and mathematics, which are regularly assessed via nationally normed measures (such as the Iowa Tests of Basic Achievement and the Stanford Achievement Tests) for all children attending public school and most attending private schools, written expression is rarely assessed and generally only inadequately so. Thus, learning disorders in written expression are routinely missed until many years of schooling have passed, if they are identified at all. Youngsters who fail to complete written work or who turn in written work of poor quality often are dismissed as lazy and unmotivated, with no recognition of the underlying learning disability. It is therefore critical that any youngster exhibiting problems performing written work be promptly and thoroughly evaluated for a learning disorder in this area. Too often, other academic skills are screened as satisfactory based on group standardized tests, and no further assessment is performed.

Unfortunately, adequate measures of written expression are few, and some of the most commonly used and best-normed individual tests of writing skills fail to comprehensively assess some of the most common areas affected by learning disabilities. For example, one of the most commonly used measures (Woodcock-Johnson Tests of Achievement, third edition, Writing Samples subtest) does not penalize for errors in spelling, punctuation or grammar, and requires only brief phrases and sentences to be written. Often, even when a youngster is being assessed for a learning disability in written expression, there is no task requiring him or her to write a composition of any length. And even on one of the most commonly used tests that does require the youngster to write a story for 15 minutes on a given topic (Test of Written Language, third edition), the scoring procedure, which relies in part on counting errors, and in part on the quality of the product, would barely penalize a youngster who managed to write only two or three sentences in that amount of time. As a result of these limitations in available individual standardized tests, a qualitative assessment of writing skills has become an essential component of the evaluation, in order to ensure that written expression disorders are not overlooked. A further caution is warranted: because of the aforementioned limitations inherent in even the best tests available, obtained scores in the average or above average range should not be interpreted as indicating that no learning disorder is present.

Remediation

Graham and colleagues have written extensively on the remediation of written expression disabilities. Their "process approach" is based on helping these students acquire the knowledge, skills and strategies that are used by more skilled writers (Graham et al., 1998). Their approach is predicated on ensuring that an adequate amount of time is devoted on a regular basis for the development of writing skills. Youngsters select topics of interest to them, and must share their work with each other, in order to obtain and make use of audience feedback. Some critics of this approach express concern that learning disabled students often must receive systematic, explicit instruction in writing skills and strategies as well as text production (e.g. Reyes, 1991). Graham and Harris acknowledge that this combination of approaches may well be optimal, but caution that explicit instruction in sentence-building skills has been shown to be ineffective and should be replaced by meaningful writing in context (Graham et al., 1998).

Learning disorder NOS

DSM-IV does not define this category, other than to suggest that it may include youngsters with learning difficulties in more than one area that do not fully meet severity criteria in any single area. Sometimes the category is interpreted as

including nonverbal learning disabilities (NVLD), which are not specifically included elsewhere in either the DSM or federal law, and are also not included in most writings on learning disabilities. Rourke, the foremost researcher in this area, posits a number of specific symptoms of NVLD, which he has grouped into three domains: neuropsychologic deficits, academic deficits, and social-emotional/adaptational deficits. Neuropsychological deficits include difficulties with tactile and visual perception, psychomotor coordination, tactile and visual attention, nonverbal memory, reasoning, executive functions, and specific aspects of speech and language. Deficits in math calculation and reasoning skills, reading comprehension, specific aspects of written language, and handwriting are the primary academic concerns. Social deficits include problems with social perception and interaction (Rourke, 1995). Remediation efforts are needed to address all three areas.

Comorbid conditions

Giftedness

Although there are varying definitions of intellectual giftedness, a generally accepted criterion is an intelligence test score two standard deviations above the mean, which would be 130 on the majority of IQ tests. When learning disabilities occur in youngsters who are intellectually gifted, the youngster's intellectual prowess may be masked by his or her difficulties with reading or written expression in particular, and perhaps even with mathematics. This situation can result in the youngster being intellectually and academically underchallenged. While disorders involving basic skills can necessitate placement in lower level classes in reading, language, arts, and mathematics, these disorders should not interfere with the youngster's receiving sufficient academic challenge in content areas such as science and social studies, providing the youngster receives the necessary accommodations.

Being intellectually gifted does not preclude having a learning disability, and vice versa. The combination of giftedness and a learning disability can result in issues that extend beyond the issues associated with either separately. First, gifted individuals' academic attainment may be well below that which might be predicted given their intellectual prowess, yet consistent enough with "grade level" performance that the learning disability is never identified. Second, both the giftedness and the learning disability may go unrecognized, much to the detriment of the individual's ultimate academic attainment. Third, a disability in written expression may result in such poor quality work that the youngster fails despite possessing considerably advanced knowledge of the material, which he or she simply cannot demonstrate. The role of accommodations while remediation is taking place, and sometimes on a permanent basis, has been stressed. In the case of gifted youngsters, accommodations can be particularly important. Providing written notes, text material on tape, oral testing, and additional time can mean the difference between placement in an advanced class for a subject area course in social studies, science, or literature and a lower level class where the content or pace of instruction and class instruction is insufficiently challenging.

Attention-deficit/hyperactivity disorder

ADHD and learning disabilities frequently co-occur (Barkley, 1998; Fletcher et al., 1999). Concordance rates range from 20% to 80% (Osman, 2000). When both conditions occur together, the youngster faces considerable challenge. Essentially, he or she has a low tolerance for sustaining effort on tasks that are difficult or not especially interesting, yet finds learning basic skills difficult and requires larger amounts of practice than non-learning disabled peers. Even in the absence of an innate learning disability, ADHD can contribute to impaired academic achievement and performance. First, ADHD can render the youngster less able to attend to, and benefit from, classroom instruction. Second, even when the youngster is making academic gains, he or she may have low grades secondary to uncompleted assignments, work completed but not turned in, behavioral issues, or general disorganization. Whenever a youngster is evaluated for a possible learning disability, the possibility of ADHD must be explored and, when present, must be addressed. Similarly, whenever a youngster is evaluated for ADHD, the possibility of a learning disability must be considered. An undiagnosed learning disability results in a youngster's inability to perform classwork with which he or she is presented. In place of this, the youngster may engage in daydreaming, fidgeting or disruptive behavior. While these behaviors would suggest ADHD, an alternative explanation, which always must be ruled out, is that the youngster is filling time in the absence of an ability to perform work. Conversely, a youngster who is experiencing academic difficulties resulting from a learning disability or from some other cause may misbehave as a way to obtain attention that cannot be obtained through academic accomplishment, appearing to have ADHD. Particularly with the predominantly inattentive subtype of ADHD, overt symptoms may not be as salient as the failure of academic skills to keep pace, but the ADHD can significantly detract from learning.

This overlap between ADHD and secondary symptoms of ADHD warrant a caution for the primary care physician. Sometimes, in its effort to identify a child's primary difficulty, the school system may cite ADHD or other behavioral difficulty as the explanatory variable for a host of difficulties he or she is having. This labeling can result in a failure to fully address the academic deficits. Additionally, sometimes school personnel state that, "the behavioral (or attentional)

issues must be addressed first," before the learning problems can be addressed. This line of reasoning is flawed. The physician should eschew the notion of "primary disability," in favor of simultaneous intervention addressing all areas of difficulty.

Other conditions

Besides ADHD, children with learning disabilities are at increased risk for a number of other disorders and adjustment problems, including depression, anxiety, adjustment difficulties, and demoralization secondary to academic failure. Tourette syndrome, epilepsy, and receptive and expressive language disorders are commonly associated with learning disabilities, and will complicate their treatment. This increased risk for a host of concomitant problems highlights the importance of a thorough evaluation when youngsters are assessed for learning disabilities, as well when they are evaluated for other disorders. When screening suggests the possibility of a mental health problem such as depression or adjustment issues, a referral should be made to a mental health professional for a thorough evaluation. Communication between professionals is essential, and the findings of the medical and psychologic evaluations must be integrated to achieve a full understanding of the difficulties the youngster is encountering.

Assessment

Learning disorders are most likely to come to the attention of the health-care professional when the parent is queried during routine physical exams. It is the health-care professional's responsibility to try to ascertain whether the youngster is experiencing problems at school. Interview (see Key clinical questions) alone will not enable the health-care professional to fully distinguish between difficulties arising from learning disorders, ADHD, or circumstances arising from the child's educational environment.

KEY CLINICAL QUESTIONS

Questions for parents

Possible educational neglect or inconsistent instruction.
- *Has the child been receiving regular schooling?*
- *Do you have any concerns about your child's school (or classroom)?*
- *What are your child's grades?*

Parents' communication with the school.
- *What have the teachers said about your child's learning?*
- *What has the school done to help?*

The school's awareness of the problems, and efforts to address them.
- *Has the Student Support Team discussed your child's learning difficulties?*

The chief responsibility of the health-care provider is to see that the school addresses the concerns. It is important for these professionals to know that federal law provides a specific procedure whereby all learning disorders and other disabilities that impact on a child's educational functioning are to be identified and served by the public school system. The exact guidelines for implementation vary from state to state, and the federal legislation is being re-worked at the time of writing this chapter, but the crucial fact is that a mechanism is in place for identification and remediation. Federal special education law established within each school a Student Support Team (SST), sometimes known as a "child study team" or by some other label, charged with the responsibility of receiving from parents or teachers referrals of students who appear to be experiencing difficulty. These referrals are handled through a multi-step process: strategies are devised and implemented within the classroom and the success of these strategies is evaluated. When it is determined that the difficulties may warrant more services than can be provided through the SST alone, and when it is felt that the youngster may be eligible for special education support, the school system provides a psychologic evaluation and convenes an eligibility committee to review the academic and psychologic data as well as any relevant medical and psychosocial data.

Youngsters who attend private schools or who are home-schooled are eligible for evaluations and services by their local school systems. In practice, it can be difficult for parents to obtain such evaluations, and difficult if not impossible to meaningfully integrate services provided by the public school system into the child's education that is provided outside the system. In such cases, parents sometimes obtain private evaluations, which are comparable to those provided by the school system, and private remediation services as well. However, the primary care physician also can be instrumental in helping parents whose children are not enrolled in public schools obtain prompt and adequate evaluation and remedial services from their public school systems.

When presented with a parent's or youngster's report of school difficulties, the primary care physician can conduct a further in-office screen, in order to determine in what direction to proceed. The physician should request from the parents the results of all group standardized tests that have been performed by the school. The parents should be able to supply this information from their own files or by requesting them from the school. These tests, while not necessarily administered annually by the schools, can be very helpful at the screening level to determine whether the child is below grade level in reading or mathematics. Often, youngsters' grades will be low because of school performance issues such as not completing work or not turning it in, but evidence from group standardized tests will reveal that skill attainment is on target – suggesting that no learning disability is present.

The primary care physician should be aware of several issues pertaining to group standardized tests, before attempting to interpret them. First, these instruments are well normed and generally provide valid information. Second, and probably most importantly, these tests do not require the youngster to write, and therefore cannot be used, even at the screening level, to rule out the possibility of a disorder of written expression. Coupled with the fact that schools use these tests to screen for learning disabilities, yet often forget that they do not screen the youngster's writing ability, the physician can help the family by reminding them that the school should screen this area carefully, even in the presence of otherwise adequate school achievement. This issue is especially important, since written expression problems are a major cause of youngsters failing to complete work. Second, standardized tests use grade-based norms, not age-based norms. This requirement means that the youngster's performance is based on a comparison with others in the same grade. However, if a youngster is either younger or older than grade-mates, the tests do not provide a true picture of his or her skills for purposes of LD screening, which needs to take into account the youngster's skills in relation to age and cognitive ability. For example, if an academically struggling youngster has been retained for 1 year or more, or if a youngster's parents waited for kindergarten entry because of immaturity, he or she is a year older than the comparison group based on grade placement. Screening conducted without this insight can result in a youngster not being tested further and therefore not being identified as learning disabled. At the same time as the physician advocates a good screening of academics, he or she can supply behavior-rating scales for parents and teachers to complete to begin the process of screening for possible ADHD and other behavioral and emotional problems, if the school has not yet provided these forms. And, the physician can help the parents initiate and facilitate the school screening process.

Interventions

Once the school has initiated Student Support Team involvement for the youngster, the physician's office can maintain contact with the chair of this group in order to keep abreast of progress toward evaluation of any learning disorders and the provision of services for these. Parents can be asked to furnish the minutes of SST meeting and the results of psychologic evaluations to the health-care provider, or can be asked for written consent so that the health-care provider can request them. In this way, the child's educational progress, and special needs therein, can be considered as part of the overall health and well-being of the youngster. For those youngsters also receiving medication for ADHD, where it is crucial for the prescribing physician and the school to have regular communication, the SST can facilitate this process as well.

CONSIDER CONSULTATION WHEN ...

- Child or adolescent exhibits behavior problems in addition to learning problems.
- Anxiety or depression are suspected.
- The family needs more extensive help.

In addition to considering child and adolescent psychiatric or other mental health referrals, always work with the school to ensure that academic concerns are properly addressed.

Two key points must be made. First, while the DSM and federal law specify various exclusionary criteria, including educational deprivation, vision and hearing problems, emotional disturbance and health problems, it must never be the case that only those who qualify for learning disabilities services should receive the necessary academic remediation. It is a fundamental underpinning of IDEA and other laws that youngsters whose academic distress stems from other factors should receive the services that are most appropriate for their particular needs. Research has convincingly shown that straightforward academic instruction, conducted in a systematic and explicit fashion, is the best remediation for academic problems, whatever the cause. Second, each of the conditions that constitute exclusions can co-exist with a learning disability, and often it is impossible to know with absolute confidence whether a learning disability is present in addition to one or more of the exclusionary factors. Both these points have important implications for the role of the primary care physician, who should be a key participant in the process of gaining an understanding of the youngster's academic problems and advocating for effective and appropriate educational services.

Summary

The DSM and federal special education law identify three learning disorders (disabilities): reading, mathematics, and written expression. The DSM also provides a category, Not Otherwise Specified, for which no criteria are given. While most definitions specify average intelligence and an IQ-achievement discrepancy, neither criterion is supported by research. In most cases, etiology is unknown, although learning disabilities have a strong genetic component. A syndrome involving nonverbal learning disabilities also has been described. Identification of learning disabilities requires thorough psychoeducational assessment and consideration of all possible contributing factors. Learning disabilities cannot be diagnosed based on low achievement alone. Written expression disorders in particular may escape diagnosis. Youngsters being evaluated for possible learning disabilities must also be evaluated for possible physical and mental health problems that may be associated with the manifested learning problems. Current evidence-based approaches to remediation feature direct, systematic instruction, as opposed to remediation of underlying processes. Primary care physicians can play an important role in the identification of learning disorders, and in conducting follow-up as part of an overall continuing appraisal of the youngster's well-being.

Annotated bibliography

Lerner JW (2002) *Learning Disabilities: Theories, Diagnosis and Teaching Strategies.* NY, Houghton Mifflin.
Informative discussion of the historical and conceptual basis of the field – assessment, remediation, and characteristics of learning disabled children, adolescents and adults.

Lyon GR, Fletcher JM, Barnes MC (2003) Learning disabilities. In: Mash EJ, Barkley RA (eds) *Child Psychopathology*, 2nd edn. NY, Guilford Press, pp. 520–586.
Excellent and very current chapter on learning disabilities, with outstanding review of the issue of the research pertaining to discrepancy, as well as research on the etiology of learning disabilities.

CHAPTER 7

Attention-deficit/Hyperactivity Disorders

Iliyan Ivanov, MD and Jeffrey Newcorn, MD

Introduction

Attention-deficit/hyperactivity disorder (ADHD) is a highly prevalent condition that has generated considerable public interest and debate. From demonstrations at psychiatric meetings by groups concerned about the use of stimulant medication, to questions regarding the possibility of over-diagnosis and over-medication, to the formation of parents' support networks such as Children and Adults with Hyperactivity and Attention-Deficit Disorder (CHADD), the syndrome has received extensive coverage in network news and in major news magazines. The clinical observations and evidence based research data support not only the descriptive features of the syndrome, but also the now well accepted recognition that at least some features of the disorder persist into adolescence and adulthood. In addition, the evidence base for ADHD treatment is among the largest in psychiatry, with robust treatment effects that are rarely seen in other disorders. Thus, it is imperative that all physicians understand the nuances of treating this wide spread condition.

Descriptions of ADHD date back more than 100 years. By the First World War, observers noted that children with von Economo's encephalitis subsequently developed a hyperkinetic behavioral syndrome. The first published report documenting the potential role of psychostimulant medications for this condition came in 1937 (Bradley, 1937). These two discoveries provided the foundation for theories linking some form of brain disease and the observed behavioral pathology. An association between complications of pregnancy and a range of neurologic sequelae led to new postulates. Whereas severe brain damage led to overt neurologic disease, mild damage seemed to create a predisposition towards behavioral difficulties. The recognition that many children with mental retardation also showed hyperactive behavior led further to the supposition that if a child has excessive motor activity, there must be some component of brain damage. This hypothesis was encapsulated in the concept of minimal brain damage, MBD (Rutter, 1982). The term began to lose meaning in the 1960s when it was understood that hyperactive behavior could occur in the absence of organicity. Therefore, the term minimal brain damage was modified to minimal brain dysfunction.

In 1980, DSM-III (APA, 1980) first described the syndrome we now call ADHD, or attention-deficit disorder with hyperactivity. This new definition arose from an appreciation that key factors in this disorder included inattention, impulsivity, and hyperactivity. The syndrome was further subdivided into attention-deficit disorder with and without hyperactivity. DSM-III-R (APA, 1986) maintained the ADHD category, but eliminated the domain specific item lists and replaced them with a single, polythetic item list incorporating features from all three domains. In addition, DSM-III-R eliminated the inattentive subtype, on the grounds that there was insufficient evidence to support its existence. DSM-IV (APA, 1994) re-established distinct item lists for inattention and hyperactivity-impulsivity (linking the latter two based on evidence that they are highly correlated), reinstated the inattentive subtype, and added a predominantly hyperactive/impulsive subtype. The latest revision of the diagnostic manual, DSM-IV TR (APA, 2000), has not introduced any changes in the criteria or the subtypes of the disorder. Thus, it is essential to know which DSM diagnostic criteria are being used when evaluating research on ADHD.

Diagnostic criteria

The essential features of ADHD continue to include the triad of inattention, impulsivity, and hyperactivity (Table 7.1). There are three subtypes: the predominantly hyperactive-impulsive type, the predominantly inattentive type, and the combined type. For purposes of clarity in this chapter, ADHD refers to the combined type, and ADHD-PI refers to the predominantly inattentive type. There are too few data

DIAGNOSIS

Table 7.1 Attention-deficit/hyperactivity disorder

Discriminating features

1. The symptoms of significant inattention and hyperactivity are present before age 7.

Consistent features

1. Symptoms are pervasive and occur in two or more settings.
2. The impairment of academic/social functioning cannot be accounted for by the presence of psychotic/mood/anxiety or developmental disorder.

Variable features

1. Occurs more frequently in boys with a 4:1 ratio.
2. Family history of ADHD.
3. Presence of comorbid oppositional deficit disorder or conduct disorder.
4. Aggressive behaviour.
5. Impulsivity.
6. Subtype – combined, inattentive or hyperactive.

They may also show a more lethargic tempo, even drowsiness at times, as well as higher levels of learning problems. These differences have led to the notion that this syndrome is a unique disorder rather than a subtype of ADHD. To date, data have not been conclusive as to whether this hypothesis is in fact the case.

Clinical features

The prevalence of ADHD is generally listed as 3–5%, although recent epidemiologic data yield rates as high as 7% or even higher in school-age children (Rowland et al., 2002; Pineda et al., 1999). ADHD is generally reported to be more common in boys than in girls, with ratios raging from 4:1 to 9:1. It is possible that the preponderance of male cases is artifactual, based on both gender bias and the more frequent occurrence of disruptive behavior in boys. More recent publications have revised the estimated gender ratio to 2–4:1 (Safer and Malever, 2000). Nevertheless, on standardized behavior ratings, fewer symptoms are observed in girls than boys at any given age. Ratings also decline with increasing age for both sexes. Boys with ADHD are typically more aggressive than girls, which tends to raise parents'/teachers' concerns and no doubt results in more frequent referrals for evaluation. It is also speculated that girls may more often exhibit predominantly inattentive symptoms, and that these are more often unrecognized, leading to under-diagnosis in girls relative to boys. There also appear to be differences in boys and girls with regard to monoamine function, which may suggest that boys are at increased biologic risk for the disorder.

One of the hallmarks of ADHD is the developmental nature of the symptoms. Preschool children with ADHD are often highly impulsive and hyperactive, and frequently aggressive. Hyperactivity persists in school-age children, but more obvious inattention symptoms are seen. While hyperactivity and impulsivity may persist throughout the lifespan in more subtle forms, they tend to diminish after puberty. In contrast, impairment from inattention and disorganization remains high for affected individuals.

ADHD symptoms have now been established to be present in many countries in the industrialized world, although questions regarding the frequency of diagnosis in cross-national studies remain (Montiel-Nava et al., 2003; Danckaerts et al., 2000; Gomez et al., 1999). Traditionally, prevalence and treatment rates have been higher in US samples. However, studies that use similar systematic assessment measures in cross-national samples generally find similar prevalence rates. Recently, and consistent with the increased appreciation of ADHD outside the US, use of stimulants has also begun to increase worldwide.

on the unique predominantly hyperactive-impulsive type for extensive discussion. This group, unexpectedly identified in the DSM-IV field trials, is primarily comprised of younger children, who it is presumed will move into the combined subtype when they are presented with greater cognitive demand in school.

DSM-IV criteria indicate that symptoms are required to be pervasive, as exemplified by presentation in two or more settings. This prerequisite is important because there was concern that acceptance of symptomatology in only one setting may have resulted in over-diagnosis. Nevertheless, prevalence rates have not decreased with the shift to DSM-IV criteria. Regardless, the move to require pervasive symptomatology more clearly indicates that ADHD is not only a disorder of school function, and presents with symptoms in various settings and domains of function.

The DSM-IV criteria stipulate that symptoms must be present for at least 6 months, with onset before age 7. However, there are problems in operationalizing the age of onset criterion. Often youngsters and their families first present for assessment after age 7, so the determination of age of onset is often retrospective. This issue can be further complicated by the fact that inattention does not always result in impairment until later school years. Recent publications suggest that later age of onset occurs in a percentage of youth, particularly those with the predominantly inattentive subtype. Of course, in some cases, some symptoms of the disorder are present much earlier, even as early as toddlerhood.

There is a growing literature on the ADHD-PI subtype. These children have lower comorbidity with disruptive disorders, and higher levels of anxiety and mood disorders.

Neurobiologic basis of ADHD

Multiple theories have been advanced to explain the cause of ADHD. ADHD is more common among the first-degree biologic relatives and siblings of affected children than in the relatives of typical boys and girls or young people with other types of psychiatric disorders. Although no single genetic marker has been found, heritability is quite high, with rates that exceed most other psychiatric and medical disorders, with only a few exceptions. Studies investigating psychiatric status of parents of young people with ADHD found an increased prevalence of mood, anxiety, and substance abuse disorders (Faraone et al., 2000). The prevalence rate for ADHD in nonbiologic relatives of adopted children with ADHD is not different from controls (Thapar et al., 1999), which adds greater credence to the concept of a strong genetic contribution. Increased risk of ADHD in first-degree relatives cannot be accounted for solely on the basis of gender, social class, or intactness of the family. Studies of identical and fraternal twins suggest that genetic factors influence both behavioral and attentional aspects of ADHD (Rietveld et al., 2003).

In support of the above, recent molecular genetic studies have shown that the diagnosis of ADHD is associated with polymorphisms in specific dopamine genes (i.e. the dopamine D4 receptor gene, DRD4, and the dopamine transporter gene, DAT). The DAT is a target of stimulant action, and the DRD4 gene regulates receptor binding, therefore both may affect treatment responsiveness. The risk polymorphisms are the 10 repeat allele of DAT, and the 7 repeat allele of DRD4 (Swanson et al., 2000). Current etiologic theories suggest that ADHD stems from abnormalities in both dopaminergic and noradrenergic brainstem nuclei that act to regulate cortico-striato-thalamo-cortical networks, believed to be critical for executive functions and the regulation of behavioral responses such as arousal, attention, and inhibition (Biederman and Faraone, 2002). Noradrenergic mechanisms in ADHD are linked to the norephinephrine rich locus ceruleus (LC). Animal studies have found that treatment with stimulants reduces peripheral measures of norephinephrine, presumably via a reduction of LC firing (Mefford and Potter, 1989). Pliszka and colleagues (1996) proposed a model that recognizes the contributions of both a dopamine (DA)-mediated anterior "executive" system and a cortical posterior attentional system, each of which receives noradrenergic input. Dysfunction in the anterior system will result in executive and inhibitory control deficits, while dysregulation in the posterior system will cause inattention to sensory stimulation. Arnsten (1996) has suggested that partial denervation of postjunctional a2-receptors in the prefrontal cortex (PFC) may be an underlying cause of ADHD symptomatology. Animal research has demonstrated that a2-receptors are present on DA-containing terminals in the PFC and play an important role in the modulation of DA neurons in this brain region (Arnsten and Goldman-Rakic, 1985; Thierry et al., 1992). The strength of this model is that it incorporates the activity of multiple neurotransmitter systems in the neurophysiology of ADHD.

Various animal models of ADHD have been proposed, but none accurately captures the entire condition. Rat pups depleted of brain dopamine are more active than control rats until puberty, when the activity diminishes (Russel, 2003). However, residual cognitive difficulties in maze tasks persist. This phenomenon is attenuated with administration of stimulants. Various gene knockout models (e.g. DAT knockout, and D2 and D4 knockouts) also suggest a role for DA receptors in the regulation of activity.

Structural and functional neuroimaging techniques provide a new venue for exploring the validity of neurophysiologic theories of ADHD. Anatomical and volumetric imaging studies consistently point to involvement of the frontal lobes, basal ganglia, corpus callosum, and cerebellum (Castellanos and Acosta, 2004). Magnetic resonance imaging (MRI) studies have shown that some regions of the frontal lobes (anterior superior and inferior) and basal ganglia (caudate nucleus and globus pallidus) are smaller in ADHD patients. Anatomic and functional abnormalities, predominantly in frontal and striatal gray matter, have also been demonstrated in children with ADHD. The pattern of spatially distributed gray matter deficits, particularly in the right hemisphere (right superior frontal gyrus, right posterior cingulate gyrus, right globus pallidus and putamen) is compatible with the hypothesis that ADHD is associated with disruption of a large-scale neurocognitive network. Of note, many of the brain findings in youth with ADHD seem to normalize by adolescence, with only cerebellar size appearing different in adolescents with ADHD vs. controls (Castellanos et al., 2002).

Newer imaging techniques, such as fMRI, positron emission tomography (PET) and single photon emission computerized tomography (SPECT) allow researchers not only to study anatomic changes, but also to dynamically exam-

---

PEARLS & PERILS

Possible causes of ADHD
- ADHD is more common in first-degree relatives of affected children than in normal young people or those with other psychiatric disorders. Heritability rates of ADHD exceed most other psychiatric or medical disorders.
- Functional abnormalities in both dopaminergic and noradrenergic brainstem nuclei have been implicated in the pathophysiology of ADHD.
- Although recent neuroimaging studies strongly suggest that perturbations in prefrontal, striatal, and cerebellar circuits are involved in ADHD symptomatology, no specific abnormalities of brain structure or function are considered to be pathognomonic of ADHD.

ine receptor functions associated with behavioral and/or psychopharmacologic stimulation. An early finding of decreased regional cortical blood flow (rCBF) in adults with ADHD was not supported in an adolescent sample (Castellanos et al., 2002). Findings have more consistently suggested an asymmetry in cortical blood flow, with decreases in the left vs. right dorsolateral prefrontal cortex (DLPFC) (Spalletta et al., 2001). Recent findings using PET and SPECT methodology in adolescents suggest dysfunction in circuits linking prefrontal cortex, striatum, and cerebellum, with particular focus on right frontal-basal ganglia circuitry, possibly with modulating influence from the cerebellum and more specifically the cerebelar vermis (Overmeyer and Taylor, 2000). SPECT studies point to possible changes in the density of DAT in ADHD adults in many, but not all studies (Cheon et al., 2003; Krause et al., 2000, 2003; Martinez et al., 2001). Less controversial is the fact that DAT is a target of stimulant treatment, a finding that has been well demonstrated using PET ligand studies. fMRI studies in ADHD subjects performing attentional tasks (usually go-no go) have also been used to identify key brain regions associated with the disorder, the most frequent finding being decreased striatal activation (Vaidya et al., 1998).

Although the results of neuroimaging studies strongly suggest that characteristic brain regions are implicated in ADHD, no specific abnormality in brain structure or function has been consistently demonstrated. Thus, despite the fact that neuroimaging findings are correctly cited in support of a biologic etiology for ADHD, no single imaging method can be considered as a diagnostic tool.

A variety of studies have examined the potential role of neurotoxins in the pathogenesis of ADHD. Lead toxicity is the most widely discussed, with recent studies focusing on subclinical lead exposure rather than frank toxicity (Gittelman and Eskenazi, 1983; Thomson et al., 1989; He et al., 2000). Lead exposure has been linked not only to inattention and hyperactivity, but also aggressive and antisocial behaviors (Bellinger, 2004). There has also been interest in serum zinc levels in ADHD (Sandyk, 1990), with findings suggesting low levels in hyperactive children. In contrast, high levels of hair zinc may be predictive of stimulant response (Arnold et al., 1990, 2000).

One of the most well publicized and controversial proposed etiologies for ADHD has been a dietary intolerance or food allergy. The most popular, the Feingold diet, eliminated artificial food additives including sugar. Several large-scale studies followed, the findings of which refuted the basic hypothesis (Adams, 1981; Wender 1986; Krummel et al., 1996). Yet selected individual subjects within these studies showed robust responses to the diets, suggesting possible efficacy for some children. Some researchers continue to suggest some efficacy for dietary manipulation in children with ADHD, and especially among children with allergies (Carter et al., 1993; Boris and Mandel, 1994; Kidd, 2000).

Long-term outcome

Traditional conceptualizations of ADHD stated that symptoms remit by adolescence. This perspective was consistent with the notion that stimulant medication has a paradoxical effect in children that reverses by puberty. However, numerous prospective controlled reports have shown that symptoms persist into adolescence and adulthood. These follow-up studies indicate that between one-third and one half of all children with ADHD continue to have the disorder in adolescence, and a larger number have at least some symptoms (Mannuzza and Klein, 2000). Two important caveats emerge from these studies. First, comorbid conduct disorder (CD) predicts a worse outcome and seems largely responsible for the increased rate of antisocial behavior in patients with continued ADHD (Pliszka, 2000; MacDonald and Achenbach, 1999). Additionally, the greater prevalence of substance abuse in adolescents with ADHD is of concern. This finding is consistent with the expected comorbidity between CD and substance-related disorders. Recent studies suggest that ADHD+CD interaction presents a higher risk for substance abuse than either disorder alone (Molina and Pelham, 2003; Flory and Lynam, 2003). Additionally, comorbid internalizing disorders may also be associated with increased rates of substance abuse (Whitmore et al., 1997).

One perplexing finding in studies of long-term outcome of ADHD children has been that long-term treatment does not appear to positively impact functional outcome. Nevertheless, stimulant-treated adolescents and adults likely fare much better than their untreated counterparts by experiencing fewer car accidents, viewing their childhood more positively, stealing less in elementary school, and achieving better social skills and self-esteem. Stimulant treatment has not been found to have deleterious physical effects, although there is persistent concern regarding the impact of stimulants on growth. Stimulant treatment also is associated with decreased social ostracism, thereby promoting a more positive outlook and self-image (Biederman et al., 2004).

Prognosis

- One-third to one half of individuals who have ADHD continue to have the disorder in adolescence and adulthood. An even larger number experience some symptoms but do not meet full criteria for the disorder.
- Comorbid CD predicts a worse outcome and contributes to an increased rate of antisocial behavior in patients with persistent ADHD.
- The presence of comorbid internalizing disorders, such as anxiety and depression, is associated with increased rates of substance abuse later in life.
- In clinical samples, substance abuse comorbidity appears to be decreased by treatment.

PEARLS & PERILS

Explanations for the apparent contradictions between the findings of acute vs. long-term studies (Vitiello, 2001) have focused on adequacy of stimulant dosing, age at initiation of treatment, and consistency of medication administration (e.g. whether the medication was administered two or three times per day, five or seven days per week, or 10 or 12 months of the year). For positive drug effects to generalize, it may be necessary to administer medication on a more continuous basis. This procedure has increasingly become the standard of care, and is reflected in the widespread use of a new generation of extended release stimulants, some of which can be administered once daily, and a new long-acting non-stimulant, atomoxetine.

Differential diagnosis

The diagnosis of ADHD is easier to make when parents recognize the disturbed behaviors early and bring their child for evaluation, and when teachers or daycare workers corroborate the signs of the disorder. However, as noted in DSM-IV-TR one must be cautious in making the diagnosis when children are from disorganized or chaotic home environments, which may lead to difficulty with goal-directed behavior, owing to environmental factors and not ADHD. No research has demonstrated that ADHD is a direct consequence of poorly organized family environments. However, there is some evidence that young people who have suffered abuse or neglect may present with increased activity and/or attentional dysfunction.

ADHD is often grouped with oppositional defiant disorder (ODD) and conduct disorder (CD) to form what are referred to as disruptive behavior disorders. Both ADHD and CD frequently co-occur with ODD. CD is also a common comorbid condition, but less frequently than ODD (Lahey et al., 2002; Jensen et al., 2001). In addition to the high rate of comorbidity among the disruptive disorders, these disorders must also be distinguished from one another as part of the differential diagnosis. Parent and teacher ratings of ADHD, ODD, and CD symptoms show high inter-correlations. In particular, young people with disruptive behavior are frequently rated as inattentive as well. Nevertheless, the essence of each condition is distinct. ODD is a recurring pattern of negativistic, hostile, and defiant behavior. CD consists of a persistent behavior pattern in which a child violates the basic rights of others, as well as major age-appropriate societal norms or rules. In contrast, ADHD is an early-onset disorder of cognitive or neuro-regulatory function, and is not due exclusively to temperamental factors, and family and social adversities. Thus, if ADHD occurs in the presence of severe psychosocial stress, there is increased risk for having comorbid ODD and CD, at the time of presentation or over time.

ADHD must also be distinguished from mood and anxiety disorders, each of which can present with inattention, and in young people, behavioral dysregulation. The situation is made more complex by the fact that both mood and anxiety disorders can co-occur with ADHD as secondary disorders (e.g. a child with ADHD is despondent about academic failure, or approaches new performance situations with anxiety and fear of failure). Here, the key to differential diagnosis is the temporal sequencing of the conditions (Manassis and Monga, 2001). If apparent ADHD symptoms occur in the context of long-standing problems of mood and anxiety, it would make sense to consider a primary mood or anxiety disorder. However, if the history of persistent ADHD precedes the development of mood or anxiety symptoms, one might consider that the internalizing pathology is secondary to ADHD. Discrimination of ADHD and bipolar disorder can be more complex, owing to the often atypical presentation of the latter condition in children and adolescents. How to distinguish between rapid "cycling" of mood and behavior disturbance, as is typically seen in bipolar disorder, and severe hyperactivity, emotional lability, and possible dysphoria related to ADHD treatment, can be most challenging (Masi et al., 2003).

Finally, many children with pervasive developmental disorders (PDDs), including autistic disorder, show behaviors such as hyperactivity, impulsivity, and inattention, and it is often difficult to determine when to diagnose ADHD (Ghaziuddin et al., 1992). Guidance from DSM-IV is not to diagnose ADHD in the presence of a PDD, based on the notion that the ADHD symptoms must not be attributable to another disorder. A diagnosis of ADHD is allowed in the presence of mental retardation. However, in both cases, appreciation that there are ADHD symptoms, and targeting these in treatment, can be beneficial to patients and their families.

Assessment

ADHD is often described as an externalizing disorder, meaning that others experience the behavior as more problematic than the individual himself or herself. Thus, the diagnosis generally requires gathering information from caretakers and other informants (see Key clinical questions). There are no laboratory measures or tests that are pathognomonic for ADHD. A careful history from the parent is usually sufficient to judge whether the presenting behavior meets the DSM-IV criteria. However, this method alone is prone to result in over-diagnosis, as it does not provide any objective standards for "developmentally inappropriate" degrees of hyperactive, distractible, or impulsive behavior. In addition, it does not define functional impairment. Several additional criteria have been suggested as clinically useful for identifying a core group of children with ADHD. These criteria are shown in Table 7.2.

A thorough developmental history adds information to support the longitudinal presentation of symptoms. Parents

DIAGNOSIS

Table 7.2 Suggested additional criteria for ADHD

1. Scores 1.5 standard deviations above the mean on standardized behavior rating scales, such as the Connors Rating Scale, completed by both parents and teachers.
2. Symptom duration of 6 months.
3. Pervasiveness of behavior across multiple settings and across multiple activities in these settings.

KEY CLINICAL QUESTIONS

Screening for core symptoms, pervasiveness of symptoms, and level of impairment as well as family history and knowledge regarding the disorder and therapy is helpful.

- *How much do you know about ADHD? Its treatment?*
- *Is your child more hyperactive, inattentive, and impulsive at school/home/in the playground compared to other children of same age?*
- *Does your child experience difficulties finding items needed for homework/school assignments; does he/she frequently misplace personal items?*
- *Does school frequently call to inform you that your child is disruptive in class and unable to complete schoolwork?*
- *Do you experience difficulties controlling your child?*
- *Does supervising/controlling your child consume a considerable amount of your time? How does this affect you personally?*
- *Do you or any one else in your family have problems with restlessness, time management, or staying focused?*

Diagnosis of ADHD

- The symptoms of ADHD are required to be pervasive and therefore must be present in at least two or more settings (e.g. home and school/workplace) in order to diagnose the disorder.
- Symptoms must be present for at least 6 months with onset before age 7. Sometimes this criteria requires retrospective assessment of symptomatology.
- Later onset may occur in a subset of young people, particularly those with the predominantly inattentive type of ADHD.
- Very young children may be more hyperactive and impulsive than inattentive. The latter symptoms may not appear until beginning school.
- Boys with ADHD are often more overtly disruptive, which results in more frequent referrals. Girls with ADHD may more often exhibit predominantly inattentive symptoms which tend to be under-identified, leading to possible under-diagnosis in girls relative to boys.

PEARLS & PERILS

may report that their children learned to run before they walked. As toddlers, they may have been unable to sit still for any period of time, or to remain seated when expected. An early presentation of aggression is often common in young children with hyperactive/impulsive symptoms. Even when aggression is not present, invading others' space may compromise peer relations. Information about the child's behavior with babysitters, with relatives, and in preschool can be invaluable in documenting this early history.

School-age children with ADHD are more likely to present with symptoms of inattention to salient stimuli, problems with vigilance or sustained attention, distractibility, disorganization, inability to complete tasks, and other stigmata of inattention symptoms. By adolescence, hyperactive impulsive symptoms may be less apparent to others, although the individual himself/herself may experience a persistent sense of restlessness. In contrast to hyperactivity/impulsivity symptoms, inattention symptoms tend to remain high, and may even come more clearly into focus as demands for independent function increase.

There is no single laboratory test that can predict ADHD. Factor analytic studies on the Wechsler Intelligence Scale for Children-Revised (WISC-R) have described a freedom-from-distractibility factor consisting of the Arithmetic, Digit Span, and Coding subtests. A similar factor consisting of the Arithmetic and Digit Span subtests has been described for the more recent WISC-IV (Wechsler, 1974, 2004). However, although there is widespread belief that low scores on the freedom-from-distractibility factor are suggestive of ADHD, findings have not been consistent in discrimination from learning disabilities.

Another test often used for diagnostic purposes is the continuous-performance test (CPT) (Riccio et al., 2002). This task typically requires a patient to scan a series of target and non-target stimuli, and either respond or inhibit response to a specific signal. Measured variables include errors of omission, errors of commission, and response time. However, while the CPT can be a useful assessment task, its diagnostic utility is far from clear (Nichols and Waschbusch, 2004), as there is no absolute standard for interpretation, and several key variables can affect performance. The CPT can be useful in providing adjunctive information on vigilance and impulsivity, and can also be used to monitor treatment response.

A variety of standardized behavioral rating scales have been used in the assessment of children with ADHD, including the Conners Rating Scales, the ADHD Rating Scale and specific subscales of the Child Behavior Checklist. The Conners Rating Scales are symptom checklists that use a four-point rating format for symptom severity. There are two common versions: 93- and 48-item parent rating

Assessment of ADHD

- Caution is needed when making the diagnosis of ADHD in children who have suffered neglect/abuse, since such patients may present with increased acting out and/or inattention.
- Although different neuropsychologic tests may be suggestive of ADHD, no single test can confirm the clinical diagnosis of ADHD.
- Rating scales, including the Conners Rating Scale, the ADHD Rating Scale and Child Behavioral Checklist, may be used as objective measures in the initial and follow-up assessment of children with ADHD.
- Medical conditions associated with ADHD-like behaviors include increased serum lead level, thyroid hormone resistance, and seizure disorder. Routine serum and EEG tests are not cost effective, and are not recommended unless indicated by clinical history or physical exam.

scales (PQ-93 and PQ-48), and 39- and 28-item teacher rating scales (TQ-39 and TQ-28). Several factors may be derived from the scales, but the Hyperactivity Index (HI) is most commonly used to assess and monitor hyperactive behavior. The HI score is derived by adding up and averaging the Likert ratings for all of the variables that address hyperactivity and then comparing this number with age-appropriate norms. The TQ-39 has shown high discriminant validity in differentiating children who are hyperactive from their peers. The Conners Rating Scales have also effectively discriminated between children with ADHD, specific learning disorders, and matched normal controls (Schechter and Timmons, 1985). See Chapter 2 for additional scales.

A criticism of rating scales is their tendency towards unidirectionality with regard to change, measuring only undesirable symptoms. However, movement too far in the other direction is not always appreciated. As an example, the fact that some children seem to become "over-focused" with stimulant treatment is not easily detected on standardized symptom ratings, possibly owing to floor effects. Another problem with unidirectional rating scales is that they only assess pathology, and not the full range of normality, or even exceptional function. With some notable exceptions, most currently available rating scales describe impaired function only, but not individual strengths with regard to the various domains of interest.

There are no medical tests which indicate the presence of ADHD. Two tests that may occasionally provide data regarding a medical basis for hyperactive and inattentive behaviors are the serum lead level and thyroid-stimulating hormone assays. It is fairly well established that lead ingestion can result in hyperactivity and inattention. However,

clinical populations of children with ADHD show little if any elevations in lead levels, and it is unlikely that lead is a significant cause of the disorder. Symptoms suggestive of ADHD have also been reported in patients with generalized resistance to thyroid hormone. Earlier studies have found the prevalence of thyroid abnormalities to be higher in children with ADHD (Weiss et al., 1993), and that ADHD was strongly associated with generalized resistance to thyroid hormone (Hauser et al., 1993). Subsequent research failed to find evidence of generalized resistance to thyroid hormone (Spencer et al., 1995) or any strong correlation between thyroid hormone concentrations and symptoms of hyperactivity and inattention (Stein and Weiss, 2003). Clinically, routine measurements of thyroid functions are not warranted in individuals with ADHD (Elia et al., 1994; Valentine et al., 1997).

Some recent naturalistic studies have found that children with ADHD have an increased prevalence rate of comorbid seizure disorder compared to children without ADHD (3% vs. 0.4%, respectively). Conversely, epilepsy patients are known to have a greater prevalence of other neurologic disorders including ADHD (Dunn et al., 2003). This association poses questions regarding the possibility of a common underlying neuropathophysiologic condition. Nevertheless, normalization of EEG alone does not produce improvement in ADHD symptomatology in the vast majority of cases.

Treatment

Evidence-based treatments for ADHD include behavioral interventions such as parent behavior management training, contingency management, and cognitive-behavioral therapies, administered individually or in group settings, or pharmacologic treatment, with a variety of stimulant formulations and the non-stimulant atomoxetine approved for this indication. For many patients, the optimal treatment is multimodal, meaning the combination of medication and psychosocial treatments, although uni-modal approaches may be sufficient or preferable for many (MTA Cooperative Group, 1999). Multimodal treatment requires the systematic evaluation of subjects from a multidimensional viewpoint, the formulation of a treatment plan to meet the individual needs of each child and family, and the delivery of services targeting symptoms and/or impairment in multiple domains. The primary rationale for multimodal intervention is that ADHD is a disorder with far-reaching consequences in all areas of a child's life, and any single intervention is unlikely to address all of the impaired areas of functioning. Although the term "multimodal" is generally reserved for the combination of medication and psychosocial treatments, it should be noted that psychosocial treatment is itself often multimodal, incorporating different interventions targeting the child, family system, and school setting.

Treatment of ADHD

- Psychosocial treatment modalities for ADHD include parent behavior management training, cognitive behavioral therapy, and educational interventions.
- Food and Drug Administration (FDA) approved pharmacologic agents for the treatment of ADHD include stimulants and atomoxetine.
- Both ADHD and non-ADHD children may show behavioral response to stimulants; therefore, a response to stimulants does not confirm the diagnosis of ADHD.
- A variety of noradrenergic agents such as bupropion, venlafaxine, alpha-2 adrenergic agonists, and tricyclic antidepressants have been used "off label" for ADHD, and may be used after both classes of FDA approved medications have been tried.
- Side-effects or poor response to one stimulant should not preclude a switch and trial of another stimulant or atomoxetine.

Psychosocial treatments

Although medication treatment can lead to improvements in behavior for many children with ADHD, 10–30% of those treated may not show a favorable response, or may have intolerable adverse effects. In addition, some families have a preference not to use medication. Thus, alternative treatment approaches take on added significance. Also, it could be argued that all children with ADHD require psychosocial intervention to improve self-observation or coping skills, and to enhance skills, which are often compromised by their ADHD (Barkley, 2002; Wells et al., 2000).

Parent behavior management training

Among psychosocial treatments, parent behavior management training has been the most widely researched treatment option for school-age children with ADHD, and also those with comorbid CD or ODD (Bor et al., 2002). Parent behavior management training involves training parents to implement behavior therapy programs in the home, to target both home and school behavior, generally using contingency management approaches (Anastopoulos et al., 1993). A basic premise is that positive reinforcement is a powerful agent of change. Parents are taught the principles of positive reinforcement, and how to ignore negative behaviors. A functional behavioral analysis is applied to the negative behaviors, and specific behaviors are pinpointed and their frequencies tracked. Parents learn to establish reward systems, often using tokens or points to track pre-identified positive or negative behaviors. Time out is utilized as a basic method of consequence for negative behaviors that

require immediate intervention. Parent behavior management training has been shown to substantially impact child behavior and compliance. It can also increase motivation to complete tasks. However, it is less likely to directly enhance attentional capacity.

Parent behavior management training can be implemented in either a group or individual format. However, regardless of how it is administered, it requires frequent manipulation of behavioral targets and reinforcers. The fact that specific target behaviors can be the focus of treatment is one of the strengths of parent behavior management training. It also means that this approach is well suited to augment medication treatments, providing an opportunity to focus on specific behaviors and settings. Because this treatment relies on parents as the agent of change for child behavior, and focuses less on direct work with the child, it is best suited to preschool and school-age children. Although some aspects of the intervention are likely to be successful in older children and adolescents (McCleary and Ridley, 1999), behavioral work with this age group almost always requires direct intervention with the ADHD patient himself/herself.

Cognitive behavioral therapy

Even when compliance with parental requests improves, children with ADHD still suffer from myriad difficulties involving social skills, as well as self-esteem. Poor peer relations, aggression and inadequate self-regulation have all been recognized as predictors of poor prognosis. Cognitive behavioral therapy emphasizes problem solving, as well as anticipation and consequences of action. This treatment can be administered individually or in groups. Cognitive behavioral therapy is well suited for use in adolescents and adults with ADHD, who have a need to develop increased self-monitoring capacities, and who have the verbal and self-observational skills that are required for treatment implementation. One type of cognitive behavioral intervention targets social skills directly, and is referred to as social skills training (Fehlings et al., 1991; Antshel and Reimer, 2003). In this treatment, children learn how to inhibit unwanted behaviors, recognize social cues, and determine an appropriate social course of action in the context of certain situations. Although social skills training has considerable face validity, treatment effects have not been robust (Antshel and Remer, 2003). A persistent problem has been its failure to generalize across settings. Nevertheless, some studies have shown that cognitive behavioral therapy and social skills training are able to supplement the effects of medication.

Educational interventions

In 1991 the US Department of Education recognized children with ADHD as eligible for special education services on the basis of Public Law 94–142, Individuals with Disabilities Act, Part B ("other health impaired status"), and

Section 504 of the 1973 Rehabilitation Act. Under Section 504, a person with disabilities is defined as any person who has a physical or mental impairment that substantially limits a major life activity (such as learning). The severity of ADHD will determine whether a particular child fits the definition. Understanding this policy, and accessing services and/or establishing accommodations as necessary, is critical to providing a comprehensive treatment for young people ADHD in school settings (Swanson et al., 1999). Examples of available services include special education, skill development programs, and supervision by a paraprofessional aide, administered either in a mainstream classroom or in a classroom dedicated to young people with specific disabilities. Accommodations may include untimed testing, special seating arrangements, assistance with note taking, and other services which are aimed to permit students to function at their highest possible level.

In addition to providing the requisite educational support, a variety of behavioral approaches can be introduced in classroom settings. Teacher-administered contingency management constitutes the most commonly used classroom intervention. This strategy may take the form of positive teacher attention or token rewards. Negative consequences range from ignoring behavior and verbal reprimands to the use of time out. Concerns in the classroom are two-fold. There are needs for behavioral control as well as for academic achievement. A comprehensive review found that overall, behavioral interventions are superior to medication in specifically enhancing academic performance. However, combined effects are particularly powerful in modifying classroom behavior. Additionally, behavioral interventions can decrease the dose of stimulant medication required to improve classroom behavior and short-term academic performance.

Pharmacologic treatment

Pharmacotherapy (Table 7.3) of ADHD dates to 1937 when Bradley first reported the effects of benzedrine on children's behavior. Since then, the behavioral effects of stimulants, and their role in treating ADHD behaviors, has been well documented. Unfortunately, the use of medications for this condition has been fraught with controversy. The most frequent concerns relate to risk for unwanted long-term side-effects, including growth delay, and the risk for substance use and abuse as ADHD children move into adolescence. Other concerns relate to the perception that stimulants result in affective blunting, or that use of medication will reinforce a child's belief that only external events affect their behavior. However, studies that have examined child attributions re-

TABLE 7.3   **Psychopharmacology of ADHD**

Medication	Total daily dose	Comments
FDA approved		
MPH		
Ritalin (methylphenidate)	10–60 mg bid or tid	Multiple doses
Focalin (d-methylphenidate)	5–30mg bid	May require tid dosing
MPH-extended release		
Concerta	18–72mg qd	May need immediate release supplement
Metadate CD	10–60mg qd or bid	May need immediate release supplement
Ritalin LA	20–60mg qd or bid	May need immediate release supplement
DEX		
Dexedrine/dexamphetamine	10–40mg bid or tid	Multiple doses required
Adderall	10–40mg bid or tid	Multiple doses required
DEX-extended release		
Dexedrine Spansule	10–40mg bid or tid	May need immediate release supplement
Adderall XR	10–30mg qd	May need immediate release supplement
Pemoline	37.5–112.5mg qd	Rare, serious hepatotoxicity
Atomoxetine		
Strattera	1–1.4 mg/kg qd	Non-stimulant
Non-FDA approved		
Imipramine	Up to 5mg/kg	Caution when increased QTc on EKG
Bupropion	3–6mg/kg bid	Caution with seizure history
Venlafaxine	37.5–225mg bid	Risk of pulmonary HTN
Clonidine	0.1–0.4mg tid or qid	Risk of rebound HTN

lated to medication and ADHD symptoms indicate that generally children credit themselves for the gains they make.

Stimulants

Until recently, stimulants were the only approved medication treatments for ADHD, and they remain the most commonly prescribed class of medication for this disorder. Stimulants have well documented efficacy in treating motor overactivity, impulsivity, and inattention, with effects that are among the most robust in all of medicine. Stimulants produce significant improvement in attention, hyperactivity, impulse control, and aggressiveness, leading to better organization of behavior, task completion, and self-regulation. There is fairly robust improvement in social skills, as evidenced by peer ratings (Whalen et al., 1990), and parent and teacher ratings of social function (Smith et al., 1998; Winsberg et al., 1982). There is also improvement in academic productivity, although change in actual academic performance has been more difficult to demonstrate. Although most data with stimulants have been obtained in samples of school-age children with ADHD, there is increasing recognition that stimulants can be used successfully across the lifespan. There are now controlled studies of stimulants in adults with ADHD.

Methylphenidate (MPH) and dexamphetamine (DEX) are the most commonly used stimulants; they are schedule II controlled substances. Pemoline, a schedule IV (i.e. less heavily regulated) controlled substance, had also been frequently used until the mid 1990s when a black box warning regarding potentially severe liver toxicity was issued. Although the different stimulants are often grouped together, the different classes of stimulants have somewhat different mechanisms of action. Data are not convincing that any one stimulant preparation is more effective than any other (Arnold, 2000). However, up to 25% of individuals respond preferentially to one or the other formulation. Thus, multiple stimulant medications should be tried before it is determined that response is not adequate.

Until recently, stimulant prescribing was almost exclusively with immediate release formulations. However, these formulations required multiple daily dosing, reflecting their short behavioral half-life. However, since ADHD is a pervasive phenomenon, and its manifestations may be present in the evenings, at weekends, and during the summer, it stands to reason that treatment needs to target these different times. Very often, children do homework in the evening and may require medication to stay on task. Evening is also an important time for family interactions, and when disruptive behavior can lead to negative family relationships. At weekends and during the summer vacation, ADHD behaviors may affect important peer as well as family relationships and activities. Therefore, many young people with ADHD require medication during these periods to achieve satisfactory social function, even if academic tasks are not

paramount. A variety of factors determine whether medication should be administered throughout the day, or over the summer, including the nature and severity of ADHD symptoms, whether there are other management or coping strategies that can be used, the specific tasks and situations which the child can be expected to face, and the extent to which medication is tolerated.

Since 2000, there has been an explosion in the number of sustained release stimulant treatment options for individuals with ADHD. These formulations eliminate the need to take medication several times over the course of the day, and provide a more consistent profile of delivery. These medications have the added benefit of decreasing the need for in-school dosing, and the associated potential for stigmatization of children with ADHD and diversion of medication. Both MPH (Keating et al., 2001) and mixed amphetamine salts (MAS) (Grcevich, 2001) are now available in preparations formulated to last 12 hours. MPH is also available in two new delivery forms that are each intended to last 8 hours. A new immediate release stimulant treatment, d-MPH (the active stereoisomer of MPH), has also recently come on the market.

Increasingly, stimulants are given in their long-acting forms as a first-line approach. The usual starting dose for Concerta MPH (12-hour formulation) is 18 mg, which is equivalent to 5 mg immediate release (IR) MPH administered three times daily (Pelham et al., 2001; Wolraich et al., 2001). Doses can be increased by 18 mg at a time. There is now also the option to give a 27 mg dose. Metadate CD (8-hour formulation) is available in 10, 20, and 30 mg formulations (i.e. equivalent to 5, 10, and 15 mg IR bid); Ritalin LA (8-hour formulation) is available in 10 mg, 20 mg, 30 mg, and 40 mg formulations. An older sustained release preparation (i.e., MPH – SR) is also still available in both branded and generic forms. Immediate release (IR) MPH can also be used as a primary therapeutic agent, given in either bid or tid dosing schedules. However, its niche increasingly is to supplement the longer-acting preparations, either to achieve more rapid onset of effect or to extend duration of action. When IR MPH is used as a primary option, the usual starting dose is 5 mg. The dose is then increased in 5 mg increments. When a tid dosing schedule is used, the third dose is sometimes sculpted to half the morning or noon dose to prevent insomnia. Three times daily dosing is particularly helpful for providing coverage during homework time, and providing an opportunity for children to interact with parents and peers while experiencing the beneficial effects of medication (Stein et al., 1996). Doses are usually given at 4-hour intervals, since the half-life is 2–2½ hours, and peak activity is seen by 1½–2½ hours. The upper recommended dose for MPH is 60 mg, although use of higher doses may be required in certain cases, and has achieved a certain degree of recognition among experts in the field (Yusin, 2001; Greenhill et al., 2002).

MAS and DEX can often be administered in a similar manner to MPH, and also come in a variety of IR and extended release formulations. Adderall XR (MAS) is the only amphetamine preparation formulated to act for 12 hours (Grcevich, 2001). Brand Adderall or generic MAS is also available in a shorter-acting form, lasting approximately 5–6 hours (Swanson et al., 1998). Dexamphetamine (DEX) is available in both a spansule, with duration of activity comparable to the shorter-acting MAS, and an IR preparation, which lasts approximately 4 hours. A recent study found that DEX spansule and MAS have comparable efficacy and duration (James et al., 2001). DEX and MAS are more potent than MPH, so the initial starting dose and upper dose limit are lower. The recommended dosage range for DEX is 2.5–40 mg. Although DEX has a somewhat longer half-life than MPH, a tid schedule is still often required.

Adverse effects (AEs) of stimulants are generally mild, but can become problematic. The most common AEs are headache, abdominal pain, decreased appetite (with or without weight loss), and initial insomnia. There are slight increases in pulse and blood pressure (BP), which are not very meaningful at the group level (Findling et al., 2001), but can take on greater significance for particular individuals. Affective changes, including blunted affect, irritability, and mood lability can also be seen, either at peak dose or when the dose wears off. Use of longer-acting psychostimulants tends to minimize mood lability and other AEs that are often considered to be a reflection of on-off effects. Motor or vocal tics can develop or, more often, can be exacerbated (Borcherding et al., 1990). However, there has been a convergence of evidence that stimulant treatment does not necessarily exacerbate tics (Castellanos et al., 1997; Gadow et al., 1999; Law and Schachar, 1999), and even some suggestions that these conditions are relatively independent (Coffey et al., 2000; Spencer et al., 2001). There has been concern that stimulants can precipitate psychotic symptoms such as hallucinations (Cherland and Fitzpatrick, 1999), although this problem is very rare and almost always a reflection of excessive dosing or use in individuals with disorders other than ADHD.

A long-term side-effect that has worried many physicians is the possible suppression of growth. Weight loss tends to be short-lived in most individuals, reflecting the transient appetite suppression that is often experienced. The extent to which stimulants affect height attainment is less clear. Some studies suggested that stimulant treated children experienced a decrease in their rate of growth (Poulton and Cowell, 2003), although they tended to catch up in adolescence, when stimulant treatment was often withdrawn. Recent data support the association between maintenance treatment with stimulants and mild growth retardation (MTA Cooperative Group, 2004). For the overwhelming majority of treated young people, height velocity is not a problem with either stimulant (Biederman et al., 2003). However, for selected individuals, there may be concerns. Consequently, monitoring of height is strongly recommended.

Other parameters to monitor in stimulant-treated young people include pulse and blood pressure, and for pemoline, liver function parameters. Although there are generally very few cardiovascular side-effects, tachycardia or elevated diastolic blood pressures are occasionally seen. Youngsters treated with pemoline should have liver enzyme levels monitored upon beginning treatment and regularly thereafter. Although the incidence of severe liver toxicity with pemoline is quite rare, it is strongly recommended to use one of the other stimulant classes first, and to only use pemoline if several other stimulant and non-stimulant treatments fail.

Atomoxetine

Atomoxetine (Strattera) is a new medication with highly potent and selective activity to block the noradrenergic transporter. It is structurally distinct from both the stimulants and the tricyclic antidepressants. Atomoxetine is the first non-stimulant medication approved for the treatment of ADHD, and is the only medication approved for the treatment of ADHD in adults. Atomoxetine has been studied extensively in both children and adults, and initial efficacy data have begun to appear in the literature. Atomoxetine was shown to be effective in reducing both inattentive and hyperactive/impulsive symptoms over a 9-week period in a sample of children and adolescents (Michelson et al., 2001). Doses of 0.5 mg/kg, 1.2 mg/kg and 1.8 mg/kg were studied. All doses were different from placebo, with treatment effects seen at the first post-medication treatment visit, but the highest degree of improvement was found in the 1.2 mg/kg and the 1.8 mg/kg groups and after several weeks of treatment. The medication also produced change in functional measures as well as ADHD symptoms, with the greatest degree of change in the 1.8 mg/kg group. Effect sizes for treatment response vs. placebo have consistently been in the moderate to high range. In a small pilot study, efficacy was relatively comparable to MPH, although that study was not powered to detect differences across treatments (Kratochvil et al., 2001).

Atomoxetine can be administered on either a twice daily or once daily schedule, despite the fact that its half-life in the overwhelming majority of individuals is 4–5 hours. Despite this fact, therapeutic benefit seems to be maintained over the full day, suggesting a dissociation of pharmacokinetic and pharmacodynamic effects. Dosing follows a weight-based schedule, with 0.5 mg/kg representing the most frequently used starting dose. After 1 week, dose escalation to 1.2 mg/kg is recommended. The FDA upper dose range is 1.4 mg/kg, although safety data up to 1.8 mg/kg were collected in pre-marketing trials. Because atomoxetine is metabolized via the cytochrome P450 2D6 pathway, medications that alter this pathway, such as fluoxetine or paroxetine, can affect atomoxetine metabolism, increasing its blood level and half-life.

Adverse effects with atomoxetine have been relatively mild, with sedation and a variety of gastrointestinal side-effects, including decreased appetite, nausea, vomiting, being the most frequently encountered. A small increase in pulse and BP, similar to what is seen with stimulants, is also often seen. Because it is not a stimulant, and because its effects are highly selective for noradrenaline and not dopamine, atomoxetine is thought to not have abuse potential. Also, because it does not cause insomnia it is particularly well suited for use with children who experience sleep irregularities, either due to ADHD or stimulant treatment.

Non-FDA approved treatments

A variety of medications have been used "off-label" to treat ADHD. Although the medications are distinct, they share, as a basic mechanism, the ability to increase norepinephrine neurotransmission. They should be used after both classes of FDA approved medications have been tried, and reserved for cases which do not respond to or do not tolerate FDA approved treatments. Since they are not FDA approved for use in ADHD, informed consent should clearly indicate that this is an "off-label" treatment.

The noradrenergic tricyclic antidepressants, principally imipramine and desipramine, have been the most extensively studied and, until the middle 1990s, were the most often prescribed non-stimulant medication for individuals with ADHD. For desipramine, doses between 2.5 and 5 mg/kg/day have been recommended (Biederman et al., 1989). In the case of both of these medications, cardiac side-effects are of concern and pre-medication work-up must include at least an EKG. Tachycardia and postural hypotension are commonly seen, but are not often problematic. Prolongation of the PR and QT intervals may be a greater source of concern and should be reviewed with a pediatric cardiologist. The decision to prescribe tricyclics for ADHD children must be made with the knowledge that several sudden deaths were recently reported in children taking desipramine (Riddle et al., 1991). Although it has been argued that data do not support the conclusion that tricyclics have a high degree of cardiovascular toxicity in children (Biederman, 1992), proper informed consent should be obtained. It should also be noted that neither imipramine nor desipramine are FDA approved for the treatment of ADHD children.

Bupropion and venlafaxine are chemically unrelated to other known antidepressants. Both have been studied for their potential utility in ADHD. Bupropion has demonstrated efficacy compared with placebo (Conners et al., 1996; Simeon et al., 1986), but it is probably not as effective as stimulants (Casat et al., 1987, 1989) or atomoxetine. There are similar but more preliminary data indicating that venlafaxine might be useful for ADHD (Popper, 1997). Open label studies of adults with ADHD found venlafaxine to be an effective treatment for the disorder. The most common side-effects reported were nausea and sedation (Adler et al., 1995; Findling et al., 1996; Hedges et al., 1995). An open label study in 8- to 17-year-old subjects found significant reductions in impulsivity and hyperactivity as rated by parents (Olvera et al., 1996). However, double-blind placebo controlled trials have not yet been conducted.

Since the mid 1980s, there has been considerable interest in the use of alpha-2 adrenergic agonists in the treatment of ADHD and aggression (Hunt et al., 1985). These agents, originally marketed for hypertension, work by producing increases in central noradrenaline. Initial studies were conducted with clonidine, but the more specific alpha-2 agent guanfacine has recently been the focus of investigation. The alpha-agonists are reportedly most effective in treating symptoms of hyperactivity, impulsivity, and aggression for children with ADHD. Effects on attentional symptoms have been less clear, although a recent study found that guanfacine treatment was associated with improved ratings and CPT measures of attention (Scahill et al., 2001). Because of their role in treating overarousal and aggression, the alpha-2 agonists seem ideally suited for use in children with comorbid ODD/CD/aggression. They have been effective in treating ADHD patients who either have diagnosed tic disorders (Steingard et al., 1993), or are at increased risk to develop them, such as those children with a positive family history of tics. This benefit is particularly important, since as many as 40–60% of patients with Tourette syndrome seen in psychiatric settings have ADHD (Biederman et al., 1991), and many of these individuals have significant behavior problems. Although the alpha-2 agonists seem to be less effective than stimulants in the treatment of ADHD, they may be particularly useful in individuals whose tics worsen on a stimulant medication. The alpha-2s have also been used in combination with a stimulant. However, there have been safety considerations involving this combination, primarily regarding cardiovascular adverse events. However, recent data indicate that combination treatment can be used effectively and safely.

Clonidine has been the most often studied of the alpha-2s. The usual dose ranges from 0.05–0.3 mg total per day, often divided in a three times a day dosing schedule. One of the advantages of clonidine is that it can be used to treat the initial insomnia which sometimes results from late afternoon stimulant use (Rubinstein et al., 1994). Clonidine is available in both tablet form and as a depot skin patch preparation. The latter provides sustained coverage for 1 week, and may be particularly useful for treating children with ADHD whose behavior is characterized by a variable pattern of extreme lability, especially in the early morning, before stimulants and oral clonidine take effect. Guanfacine comes only in an oral preparation. Guanfacine tablets are of 1.0 mg strength, so care must be taken to not confuse the two different doses. Since guanfacine has a somewhat longer half-life than clonidine, it can often be given in a two or three times a day dosing schedule.

The most common side-effect of the alpha-2 medications is sedation, although this tends to decrease after several weeks (Hunt et al., 1985). Dry mouth, nausea, and photophobia are among the other adverse effects reported. At high doses, hypotension and dizziness are also possible. The skin patch often causes local pruritic dermatitis. Glucose tolerance may decrease, especially in those at risk for diabetes. It is important to carefully evaluate cardiovascular function when using the alpha-2 agonists, especially when used in combination with stimulants treatment, since there were reports of sudden death in three cases treated with the combination of clonidine and methylphenidate. Although a review of this situation by the FDA concluded these unfortunate events were not attributable to the combination (Fenichel, 1995), careful monitoring is recommended.

Non-traditional treatment

The presence of EEG abnormalities in children with ADHD has led to a specific treatment in which biofeedback of the EEG rhythm is used to modify and reduce specific abnormalities. The treatment is based on the hypothesis that children who have ADHD are both less able to produce beta activity and more prone to show excessive slow theta activity during periods of excitement compared to unaffected children. Although there has been anecdotal information regarding successful treatment, many subjects receive multimodal interventions along with biofeedback. Despite a burgeoning practice, there have been no publications of controlled treatment or comparison with medication interventions. Similarly, despite the large amount of data that fail to support the utility of most dietary treatments of ADHD, there is still considerable attention given to this form of intervention. These interventions should be considered experimental until more evidence supporting their utility comes forward.

Summary

The abundant interest in ADHD has led researchers to carefully evaluate basic assumptions regarding pathophysiology and treatment. There has been increasing emphasis on syndrome validation and the definition of more homogeneous subtypes, either through better understanding of pathophysiology or clinical presentation. Anatomically, the symptoms of attention disorders may arise from deficits in the anterior and posterior frontal lobes, usually in the right hemisphere, basal ganglia, cerebellum or the reticular activating system. The disorder is highly heritable, with candidate genes for catecholamine function being the most often implicated. Still, despite considerable progress over the past two decades, much is to be learned regarding the neurophysiologic basis and genetics of ADHD. Other data

CONSIDER CONSULTATION WHEN ...

- Symptoms do not improve significantly after adequate trials with one or two stimulants or atomoxetine.
- There are unmanageable side-effects on stimulants or atomoxetine.
- Use of more than one medication is being considered.
- The child and family require more than basic education and parent training.
- There is significant psychiatric comorbidity.
- There is diagnostic uncertainty.
- Parents have major psychiatric illnesses.

point to the importance of environmental influences, or a combination of biologic and environmental factors. Variations in temperament often are described in terms of activity level, vigilance, and potential for distractibility. Whether an infant's behavior represents an early precursor or genetic predisposition for the disorder must be determined. In addition, psychosocial disadvantage seems to have a role in pathogenesis. Children who experience early life trauma, and who are raised in chaotic home environments, seem to be at increased risk. Indeed, it can be difficult to distinguish the behavior of a child in a chaotic home environment from that of a child with ADHD. Although instructive, neuropsychologic investigations have not yet been wholly successful in distinguishing these clinical presentations, recent advances in neuroimaging provide hope that a biological marker will be available in the future. However, this is far from being a reality at present.

There have been considerable advances in psychosocial, psychopharmacologic and multimodal treatment of ADHD. A variety of home and school-based interventions have demonstrated efficacy, and new long-acting stimulant and non-stimulant medications make it possible to target the entire day without having to administer medications in school. It is hoped that the development and dissemination of these evidence-based approaches will produce important benefits in terms of long-term outcome of the condition.

Annotated bibliography

Biederman J, Faraone SV (2002) Current concepts on the neurobiology of attention-deficit/hyperactivity disorder. *J Atten Disord*, 6 (Suppl 1):S7–16.
A comprehensive overview of contemporary models of the neurobiologic basis of ADHD. The authors present data for ADHD heritability, prenatal exposure to substances, psychosocial adversity, structural and functional imaging findings in ADHD patients, and neurochemical mechanisms of ADHD pathophysiology and treatment.
Biederman J, Newcorn J, Sprich S (1991) Comorbidity of attention deficit hyperactivity disorder with conduct, depressive, anxiety, and other disorders. *Am J Psychiatry*, 148(5):564–77.

The authors present the results of a systematic search of the psychiatric and psychological literature for empirical studies addressing the issue of ADHD comorbidity. The results support considerable comorbidity of ADHD with conduct disorder, oppositional defiant disorder, mood disorders, anxiety disorders, learning disabilities, and other disorders, such as mental retardation, Tourette syndrome, and borderline personality disorder.

Greenhill LL, Pliszka S, Dulcan MK, Bernet W, Arnold V, Beitchman J, Benson RS, Bukstein O, Kinlan J, McClellen J, Rue D, Shaw JA, Stock S (2002) American Academy of Child and Adolescent Psychiatry. Practice parameters for the use of stimulant medications in the treatment of children, adolescents, and adults. *J Am Acad Child Adolesc Psychiatry*, 41(Suppl 2):26S-49S.

This practice parameter uses an evidence-based medicine approach derived from a detailed literature review and expert consultation to describe stimulant treatment strategies for ADHD. Although this practice parameter is the latest available version from AACAP, it was developed before the approval of atomoxetine, and does not fully include atomoxetine in the algorithm for ADHD treatment.

Mannuzza S, Klein RG (2000) Long-term prognosis in attention-deficit/hyperactivity disorder. *Child Adolesc Psychiatr Clin N Am*, 9(3):711–26.

The authors present the results of their studies which have traced the developmental course of ADHD from childhood to adulthood, showing that the presence of ADHD symptoms in late adolescence may be considered the greatest risk factor for the development of antisocial behavior and substance abuse and may contribute to persistent poor self-esteem and social skills deficits. This research is one of the most widely cited longitudinal studies of ADHD, but there are several others. Some findings of the different studies seem to vary as a function of the initial sample and assessment methods used.

MTA Cooperative Group (1999) Multimodal Treatment Study of Children with ADHD. A 14-month randomized clinical trial of treatment strategies for attention-deficit/hyperactivity disorder. *Arch Gen Psychiatry*, 56(12):1073–86.

This paper presents the results of a study examining the long-term efficacy (14 months) of pharmacotherapy and behavior therapy for ADHD, given alone and in combination. Results indicate that combined treatment did not yield significantly greater benefits than study-delivered medication management alone for core ADHD symptoms, but may have provided modest advantages for non-ADHD symptom and positive functioning outcomes. Response to medication given in the study was greater than in the community, where doses were lower and the schedule of administration was less frequent. A subgroup of young people treated with behavior therapy only was able to normalize behavior without medication.

CHAPTER 8

Disruptive Disorders and Aggressive Behavior

Niranjan S. Karnik, MD, PhD and Hans Steiner, Dr med univ, FAPA, FAACAP, FAPM

Case presentation

> **CASE 8.1**
>
> Steve is a 12-year-old white boy who arrives at your office in the company of his 36-year-old mother. His mother works full-time and has been estranged from the child's father for over 6 years, and the boy has infrequent contact with his father. A maternal aunt cares for the boy after he returns from school each afternoon.
>
> For the past 6 months his behavior has become increasingly difficult to control at home and school. He has developed a circle of friends who are often reprimanded by school officials for misbehavior and mild to moderate mischief. School officials have called Steve's mother and raised concerns that he may be jeopardizing his academic career – which to this point has been characterized by good grades – by spending time with these new friends.
>
> Steve is brought to your office for an evaluation following a series of incidents where he has begun to harm small animals, and to vandalize property in the company of his new friends.

Steve's case highlights the challenges of providing care to children with disruptive spectrum disorders. While many children have acting out or aggressive behaviors as a normative part of being a child, disruptive behavior disorders distinguish themselves with a predominance of oppositional, defiant, or anti-social behaviors. This area of practice requires clinicians to take seriously the biopsychosocial model and its associated complexity. These behaviors usually are present in multiple spheres, and with a variety of social, psychologic and interpersonal influences. There is a dynamic interaction between the biologic risk and resiliency of the individual's genetic and developmental history.

Aggression and disruptive spectrum disorders represent a cluster of behaviors that are among the most common pre-senting complaints in the practice of child and adolescent psychiatry as well as pediatrics. For the clinician, the aim of an evaluation is to differentiate normal disruptive behaviors from those that represent true psychopathology. Thus, all problematic behaviors do not necessitate either clinical attention or treatment, despite pressure that schools, parents or other practitioners may bring to bear during these evaluations.

Disruptive behaviors and aggression are by definition violations against the rights of others or the intentional breaking of social norms. Thus, a child with autism who engages in physical harm but does so without understanding social rules should not be diagnosed with a primary conduct disorder. In this scenario, the conduct symptoms should be classified as a component of the developmental disorder due to an inability to internalize social patterns, which leads to disruptive patterns.

Since social norms form the definitional basis of disruptive disorders and aggression, the clinician must be prepared to gather social information and realize that social norms are not fixed. These norms differ over time, by location and culture, and often have highly localized patterns. Nevertheless, legal systems enshrine common understandings of basic accepted social patterns, and children who consistently display disruptive patterns are likely to come in contact with the judicial or child protective systems if their behavior is left unchecked.

Etiology

Since these behaviors are so common, and there are so many different pathways that can lead to aggressive and disruptive behavior, a theory which employs multivariate models and is concerned with interactions between multiple variables is better suited to the task of understanding problems which result from complex environment-person transactions. Univariate and main effects models have not been successful in predicting adverse progressions and outcomes.

Disruptive behavior ranges widely in its manifestations, especially when age is taken into account. It is unlikely that there is any one set of specific etiologic factors that can fully explain aggressive and disruptive behavior. Current data best fit a cumulative risk factor model, where the likelihood of disruptive behavior increases as risk accumulates. This model can be expanded to include environmental protective factors and the individual's resilience to improve prediction as to which children develop more significant psychopathology and which do not (Tinklenberg et al., 1996; Steiner and Cauffman, 1998; Steiner et al., 1999; Steiner and Stone, 1999; Edens et al., 2001).

The model predicts that the greater the number of risk factors and the earlier they appear, the higher the probability that the individual will engage in aggressive acts and have serious psychopathology. The mechanism by which this occurs seems to be via multiple interactive loops: factors in the family environment interact with characteristics of the child to produce, at an early age, aggressiveness, impulsiveness, and a disregard for the rights of others. Peers and teachers then reject such children and a new cycle of negative interactions develop.

Biologic factors

In the last 10 years there has been a steady accumulation of data implicating, but not definitively proving, biologic risks for aggressive behavior. These factors include, among other things, genetic factors, central nervous system (CNS) insults, underarousal of the nervous system, neurotransmitter aberrations, and difficult temperament (Raine, 1997; Raine et al., 1997; Raine, 2002; Raine et al., 2002). The effect of these factors is seen most clearly in the context of environmental disadvantage and in the presence of other social risk factors.

Support from some twin studies indicates that aggression and in extreme cases criminality have some degree of genetic contribution. These findings are controversial because other family resemblance studies have failed to replicate genetic linkages.

Other evidence suggests that CNS insults of various types can result in higher rates of disruptive behaviors. These data would seem to be consistent with a continuum of experience linking minor CNS trauma to pervasive developmental problems that have more significant CNS injury. Nevertheless, the degree of injury is not directly correlated with degree of disruption. The location of CNS injury and differential functions of the various portions of the brain play a role as well.

Further support for the role of CNS factors in disruptive behavior in adults comes from neuroimaging. Two hypotheses have received some support: frontal dysfunction associated with aggressive crime and temporal lobe dysfunction associated with sexual offending. There is growing evidence

from a developmental perspective that lends credence to theories about frontal and prefrontal dysfunction in children and adolescents with aggressive characteristics (Blair et al., forthcoming).

Deficiencies in various channels of the autonomic system may be a risk factor for disruptive behavior. The evidence strongly supports low resting pulse as a predictor of future criminality. Evidence from other channels, such as skin conductance (GSR) and EEG is not totally consistent. Overall, the data suggest that there may be a subgroup of antisocial children who are underaroused and not likely to learn readily from and be easily socialized by people in their environment. As a result, these underaroused youths, seek high levels of stimulation to raise their low levels of arousal, and they do so by engaging in risk taking and aggression. Recent research has found reductions in the P300 electroencephalographic waveform further highlighting the prefrontal cortex as a site for underarousal. This theory suggests that these children may be more impulsive and unable to keep themselves from reacting to stimuli. Much of this research has yet to uncover the pathways through which low arousal may work at a psychologic and physiologic level. Other theories in the arena of autonomic dysfunction relate to increased fearlessness, reduced vagal tone, and reduced noradrenergic functioning. Ultimately, these disparate findings may correlate more strongly with one type of aggression or anti-social behavior over others, making the clinical categorization all the more salient to the future of research in this field.

Psychologic factors

A host of psychologic correlates of aggression and disruptive behavior have been found. These include neuropsychologic factors, ease of learning and conditioning, intelligence and personality factors, to name but a few. Whether these are causal factors is not known, nor is it always known how they precisely might operate if they are.

Multiple neuropsychologic deficits, including learning disabilities, prefrontal and frontal lobe dysfunction, left hemisphere dysfunction, and reduced lateralization for linguistic functions have been found in juveniles committing anti-social acts. On the behavioral level, learning and conditioning deficits have been found under a variety of conditions. Aggressive youths also show some characteristic personality traits. They are lower in all of the following: self-restraint, impulse control, responsibility, and suppression of aggression. The characteristics are magnified by posttraumatic stress disorder, which is common among antisocial youths.

Social factors

Among the many social factors that influence disruptive spectrum disorders, three are particularly important – family, peers, and extended environment. The literature clearly supports the theory that adult criminality in families leads to juvenile aggression and disruption. Such families often have concomitant social phenomena such as abuse, neglect, sexual molestation, and other patterns that certainly lead to increased levels of conduct disorders in childhood. Clinicians need to make certain to screen for these patterns when conducting a complete evaluation of an aggressive or disruptive child.

Parenting styles and approach can also lead to poor outcomes for children. A substantial body of research has been amassed which shows that parental absence, lack of supervision, and ineffective parenting can all result in increased levels of aggression and conduct disorder.

Family influences on children's anti-social behavior are not just limited to parent-child relations. Divorce, separation, and unhappy and conflicted marital relationship are also predictive, but less so than the parenting variables. There is recent evidence that familial variables recede in importance as the child goes through puberty. Instead, internal regulators such as restraint and distress, and the quality of peer relationships, which themselves may reflect the effect of earlier parenting, become more important.

Peer influences have been found to be critical to late-onset disruptive disorders and anti-social behavior. These relationships occur at a time when adolescents are seeking to conform to groups, and will often behave in ways to define their identities away from their family and communities of origin, and instead seek to establish new and potentially volatile connections with more non-conformist groups. Peers often provide support for those children who fail to achieve good social relations at earlier ages, and can find rapid acceptance via aggressive or disruptive acts.

Finally, the neighborhood or ecologic environment in which the child has been raised has repeatedly and convincingly been shown to be part of the core risk factors for disruptive spectrum disorders. High rates of unemployment in the neighborhood, low parental social class, poor urban neighborhoods with high crime rates, and poor schools all contribute to risk. High levels of community violence often characterize these environments with well documented injurious effects on children from witnessing such violence.

Protective factors

There are also protective factors that attenuate risk, but much less is known about them (Seligman and Csikszentmihalyi, 2000). "Protective factors" refers to more than the simple absence of risk and to more than the polar opposite of risk factors. Normal or above normal intelligence, an easy temperament, an ability to relate to others, good work habits at school, areas of competence outside school, and a good relationship with at least one parent or another important adult all offer protection against anti-social behavior and delinquency in the presence of significant risk. Prosocial peers as well as a good school, which fosters experiences of success, responsibility and self-discipline, can serve as protective factors. They exert their effect by strengthening core aspects of individual functioning.

Disruptive disorders

The current nosology for disruptive spectrum disorders is problematic on several levels. Chief among these is that fact that they do not reflect well the understanding that has emerged from research on aggression and disruptive disorders. Much of the current nomenclature presumes that normative and non-normative patterns can be distinguished based purely on phenomenology. Increasingly, the social context that surrounds the child has become critical to our understanding of aggression and violence (Karnik and Steiner, 2002; Karnik, 2004; Steiner, 2004). Stealing and robbery with physical harm to others may be considered pathologic in a peaceful middle-class suburb of Pennsylvania, while these same behaviors exhibited by a child in Somalia in the context of an ongoing civil war would be considered appropriate survival techniques. The social environment around the child therefore needs to be taken into account in order to fully understand disruptive behaviors. Despite these limitations, DSM-IV TR has two primary domains for the classification of child and adolescent disruptive disorders: oppositional defiant disorder and conduct disorder. Both of these disorders are on axis I. There is also an important diagnosis in adults which should be considered in the differential of disruptive disorders, anti-social personality disorder. None of these diagnoses includes contextual or environmental variables (APA, 2000).

Disruptive spectrum disorders are best considered as a continuum of impairment or behavioral difficulty. Oppositional defiant disorder represents the least severe form of pathology in this spectrum, followed by conduct disorder, and then finally anti-social personality disorder in adulthood. While there need not be a linear progression from one diagnosis to the next, many children will move through patterns of behavior in escalation and if followed developmentally progress from one to the next. However, many do not.

Oppositional defiant disorder (ODD)

Oppositional defiant disorder (Table 8.1) is characterized by childhood misbehavior toward adults, loss of temper, irritability, anger, and excessive defiance of authority. The usual age of onset is between the ages of 6 and 10, rarely occurring under the age of 3, and with unlikely incidence past the age of adolescence.

It differs from conduct disorder by its emphasis on minor behavioral challenges mostly to parents and other involved adults and maintenance of these behaviors generally within

Table 8.1 Oppositional defiant disorder

Discriminating features

1. Has difficulty complying with adults' rules.
2. Deliberately annoys people.
3. Argumentative.
4. Not caused by psychosis or mood disorder.
5. Behavior more than expected for developmental age.

Consistent features

1. Loss of temper.
2. Blames others.
3. Irritable.
4. Angry.
5. Resentful.
6. Spiteful.
7. Vindictive.

Variable features

1. Behaviors present over at least a 6-month period.
2. Impairment across multiple domains (social, academic, or occupational).
3. Age of onset.
4. Severity.

Table 8.2 Conduct disorder

Discriminating features

1. Escalating pattern of aggression toward animals, people, or property.
2. Theft or property destruction.

Consistent features

1. Violations of parental rules prior to age 13.
2. Behaviors necessitating or resulting in police activity or notice.
3. Truancy.
4. Running away from home.
5. Physical cruelty to people or animals.
6. Lying.
7. Deceitful.

Variable features

1. Time course over 6 months to 1 year.
2. Initiates fights.
3. Bullies people or peers.

the scope of the family unit. Functionally, it is a diagnosis for children that present to the clinician with a pattern of behavior that is troubling, but that usually does not rise to the level where aggressive or intense treatment would be required.

Conduct disorder (CD)

Conduct disorder (Table 8.2) is a further progression of disruptive behavior to the point where there is aggression toward people or animals, destruction of property, deceitfulness or theft, and serious violation of parental or authority rules. The disorder will likely have representation of behaviors across more than one of these domains. It can be specified as mild, moderate or severe, and also by age of onset, with childhood onset occurring before the age of 10. A child cannot be diagnosed with both ODD and CD, since the features of ODD are included in the CD criteria (APA, 2000).

Parents are likely to report the involvement of police as well as school officials, since these behaviors are likely to manifest in multiple contexts. Clinicians should make use of the information and resources that schools and police authorities may have about the child's behavior, but should make diagnostic evaluations independently and always in the interests of the child.

Children under the age of 8 are unlikely to exhibit full symptoms of this behavior, and clinicians should be wary of making this diagnosis in the very young. Boys usually present

at earlier ages than girls, and may present with more violent or aggressive traits than developmentally matched girls.

Phenomenologically, CD usually builds slowly over time. A child or adolescent is unlikely to wake up on a single day and begin burning homes, hitting individuals, and stealing things. The presentation is likely to be slower and more progressive, with small behavioral changes heralding larger ones.

Anti-social personality disorder (ASPD)

Anti-social personality disorder is a diagnosis of adult populations that deserves brief mention due to its unique connection to CD. ASPD is a personality disorder that shares many of the characteristics of CD, but does so in a more severe and protracted form and includes the criteria of a lack of remorse. Many researchers have documented high rates of ASPD within incarcerated populations, and ASPD is considered a very poor predictor of rehabilitative potential.

In DSM-IV TR, ASPD alone among DSM diagnoses requires that a prior diagnosis of CD be made in childhood in order to meet the criteria for ASPD. An individual must meet the criteria for conduct disorder before the age of 15 years (APA, 2000). In terms of taxonomy, this requirement presents a small problem in that CD is an axis I disorder, and ASPD resides on axis II. The implication of this shift has not been fully explained in the current literature on ASPD or CD. Given this connection, a diagnosis of moderate or severe CD should therefore be considered a significant risk factor for future adult psychopathology. Prompt and rapid intervention and aggressive treatment is therefore indicated.

The connection between diagnostic domains is an interesting and important attempt to extend the structure of diagnostic categories across the developmental spectrum. Nevertheless, doing this by crossing axes, and within a domain where the diagnosis of ASPD is even more problematic than CD presents a serious problem in the current DSM nomenclature. Future research needs to explore the developmental course of disruptive spectrum disorders in order to understand the trajectories that these disorders follow.

Assessment

Children with these disorders exhibit problematic behavior that is not considered to be within the normal range (either due to frequency or severity) or due to another psychiatric disorder (see Pearls & perils). Information from multiple sources is essential given the pervasiveness of these behaviors and the natural tendency of many children to not disclose voluntarily information about behaviors that can be criticized by others. And, given the comorbidity of disruptive disorders with other psychiatric disorders, a thorough assessment for other conditions is mandatory. In addition, focusing the evaluation on three aspects of the behavior: pattern, percipients, and degree of disruption can produce valuable information in terms of conceptualizing the problem and treatment options (see Key clinical questions).

Patterns of behavior

When examining children for conduct spectrum disorders, it is vital that the clinician ascertain the pattern through which the behavior manifests. Children who have stable patterns of disruptive behaviors may be more personality driven and apt to be resistant to medication interventions. Conversely, children with fluctuating behavior patterns and varied responses to stimuli might benefit from mood stabilizers and

<table>
<tr><td>

KEY CLINICAL QUESTIONS

- *What type of violent or aggressive patterns does the child engage in?*
  Violence that is episodic, short-term and reactive in nature is more responsive to current treatment strategies of medication and psychotherapy. Conversely, a small minority of children will exhibit patterns that show premeditation, planning, and a true lack of morality. This pattern is more disturbing and less responsive to current forms of treatment, and should prompt referral to experts (Steiner et al., 2003).
- *Is the child rapidly escalating his or her behaviors?*
  In the event that the child is escalating behavior from one level to the next (i.e. goes from vandalism to harming animals or people), then it is essential to ascertain the degree to which changes in the child's life may have precipitated this situation. Escalating behaviors should also prompt rapid referral and treatment, or if indicated hospitalization in order to stabilize the child.

</td></tr>
</table>

antidepressants (see below). The most troubling pattern that clinicians may find is that where children are escalating their behaviors. Shifts from vandalism to harming small animals or interpersonal violence should be a cause for concern and prompt rapid evaluation and possible hospitalization for stabilization if there is credible evidence or threat of self-harm or harm to others (Steiner, 1997; Steiner and Dunne, 1997; Steiner and Stone, 1999; Steiner and Karnik, 2004).

Precipitants: change in friends, environment, family structure, abuse

When evaluating children for disruptive behaviors, it is essential that the clinician try to establish the precipitants or mitigators of behaviors. Information about the social environment needs to be obtained in depth. Taking a simple, traditional history is not sufficient to understand the dynamics of disruptive behaviors. The clinician may need to delve into details of who the child spends time with, where the child spends his or her days, what the child does for recreation, who constitutes the child's peer group, how the child provides for his or her basic needs, and many other facets of life. Collateral information from parents, welfare authorities, juvenile court personnel, teachers and relatives may be required to gain a better picture of the social environment around the child.

Clinicians should be especially attentive to changes in the spheres of influences and the environment around the child. When children suddenly change peer groups, begin to exhibit markedly different patterns of behavior, clinicians need to investigate the nature of these changes (Esbensen and Deschenes, 1998; Maxson et al., 1998; Cureton, 1999; Winfree et al., 2001; Brownfield and Thompson, 2002; Sirpal, 2002). It

<table>
<tr><td>

- Aggressive or disruptive behaviors, in and of themselves, are not exclusive to primary conduct disorders. Other diagnoses must be eliminated including mood, psychotic, substance use and developmental disorders.
- Failure to take a detailed history and utilize multiple sources of information can often lead to premature conclusions and misdiagnosis. In these cases, the outcomes can potentially be devastating for the child who then becomes labeled with a disruptive disorder, which is difficult to undo.
- Despite the significant implications of making a diagnosis of conduct or oppositional defiant disorder, clinicians should do so when the indication is present so that proper attention and treatment can be obtained for the child.

</td><td>

PEARLS & PERILS

</td></tr>
</table>

is vital to ascertain the degree to which these changes may be due to normal developmental changes in the child, and their growth in terms of personality and experience, and to what extent these behaviors may be related to more counterproductive or problematic patterns. In assessing this portion of behavior, the clinician may use as a guide the degree to which the child experiences difficulty in functioning. Some children will find themselves in opposition to their parents or school authorities as they try to assert new identities. Gay and lesbian youth, for example, may display oppositional and disruptive behaviors in the face of strong parental opposition to these emerging identities (Lock and Steiner, 1999). Clinicians need to act as mediators in these situations and work on behalf of their patients to help them come to terms with their identities in healthy ways, while also recognizing that these children may have internalized many destructive patterns such as excessive drug and alcohol use which can be comorbid with disruptive disorders.

One common precipitant that should be screened for is a history of abuse (Garbarino and Garbarino, 1993; Garbarino et al., 1997; Steiner, 1997; Steiner and Dunne, 1997). Abuse can take many forms, from the everyday physical abuse of the schoolyard bully to the profound devastation of sexual molestation. Despite the range of possible abuse, children are apt to experience these violations in very individual ways, and disruptive behaviors or aggression may be the first sign of ongoing or new-onset abuse.

Degree of disruption

Another approach that helps define the nature of disruptive disorders is to attempt to ascertain the degree of disruption. This variable is clearly an interactive process whereby the child exhibits some type of behavior, for instance a very loud temper tantrum on being told he or she has to go to bed. The parents then have their own acceptance level for this type of behavior. This tolerance may fluctuate depending on the number and type of stressors that the parents are facing in their daily activities.

This interaction should not prevent clinicians from having a reasonably and accepted set of standards against which to judge the behaviors described. It is important to realize that a well-meaning parent may present to your office hysterical that her 6-year-old child tore the fichus plant to bits, and she is adamant that something be done. The clinician should recognize that the act deserves some attention, and that it does go against social norms for people to tear apart fichus plants. Nevertheless, it may not be the total disaster that the mother believes has occurred because her tolerance levels appear to be lower at present.

The clinician might wish to use rating scales for this portion of the assessment. Having multiple members of the family as well as siblings and school representatives independently assess the child's behavior can lead to a clearer understanding of the individual child's behavior and the degree of disruption that this behavior causes as well as vital information regarding periodicity and frequency.

Differential diagnosis

It is vital to consider the many comorbid psychiatric disorders that can accompany disruptive disorders. It is rare to see a disruptive spectrum disorder independent of other behavioral features or diagnoses. Additionally, virtually every major diagnostic domain in child and adolescent psychiatry can have disruptive features, which are better conceptualized as expressions of the primary psychiatric disorders.

Mood disorders

Major depression as well as bipolar disorder in their various subtypes can present with disruptive features. Traditional models of depression posit that individuals become slower, less responsive, and sleep more. Conversely, those with atypical depression can eat more and sleep less. In children, depression is often accompanied by somatic complaints. Disruptive behaviors can result from irritability associated with depression and sleep disturbance. The manic or hypomanic phase of bipolar disorder can certainly present with disruptive or aggressive behaviors. See Chapter 10 for more details on mood disorders in childhood.

Anxiety disorders

Posttraumatic stress disorder (PTSD), generalized anxiety disorder, panic attack, or acute stress disorder in children (Chapters 9 and 20) can often present with disruptive patterns. Children, unaccustomed to assessing their internal somatic and sensory system, may be unable to verbalize feelings associated with stress disorders and will often simply "act out" in disruptive ways as a way to present their distress. In these cases, stress disorders like PTSD may have specific triggers, and clinicians should try to ascertain any temporal connection between trigger and disruptive or aggressive behaviors.

Psychotic disorders

As will be evident to most clinicians, psychosis can be evidenced by disruption and aggression. As noted above, children are often unable to reflect their experience in verbal forms, and therefore present their experiences in behavioral patterns. A child who is actively delusional or hallucinating may appear to be responding to internal stimuli and may engage in self-harm or actively attempt to harm others. Such behaviors are often confused with manic aspects of bipolar illness or substance abuse, but can often be differentiated from other domains of psychiatric illness by magnitude and quality of behavior. Please see Chapter 12 for more details.

Substance use disorders

Children who use substances will present with disruptive patterns or aggression in multiple contexts. The active phase of substance use as well as withdrawal can present with disruptive spectrum disorders. Substance use disorders are more completely discussed in Chapter 14.

Pervasive developmental disorders

Children with developmental disorders (Chapter 5) can easily present with disruptive patterns, especially when they are placed in situations where they are forced to break with routine. Asperger syndrome, autism, mental retardation, and other developmental disorders can be associated with aggression, especially since these children have difficulty interacting with children in their peer group.

Treatment

Oppositional defiant disorder

Most available research data suggests that ODD is best treated with individual and family therapy. Under this rubric many different modalities can be used, but the common theme should be to educate the parents on good behavioral management techniques and parenting approaches. Developing consistent structure, expectations, and consequences across all of the child's environments is essential. Children and particularly adolescents can benefit significantly from interpersonal and cognitive-behavioral psychotherapy. These approaches can lead children to understand their own behaviors and their responses to situations from a new vantage point, and the effects of their behaviors on others. The length of therapy cannot easily be predicted and will vary by the specific psychotherapeutic modality and the approach of the clinician. Another new arena for interventions that is re-emerging is an area best termed "sociotherapy." In some ways it harkens back to a previous era of community-based psychiatry and centers on the use of social and community interventions to help facilitate behavioral changes. In the case of ODD, structured after-school programs and weekend activities can significantly help children learn social behaviors and boundaries. If, despite these interventions, behaviors escalate or fail to improve, consideration needs to be given to re-examining the original diagnosis and considering again other comorbid conditions.

Conduct disorder

Conduct disorder is among the most difficult of child psychiatric conditions to treat. All of the approaches outlined for ODD are applicable. There has been interest in developing and examining programs that target all of the dimensions and environments of the child's life to identify problems and appropriate ongoing resources. Several programs offer multi-pronged, simultaneous interventions to improve the child's and family's functioning.

In the context of an acute episode, time may not permit psychotherapeutic or sociotherapeutic modalities to reach their full potential. At these times, it may be appropriate to consider medication in an attempt to modulate the child's aggression. However, it is important to remember that no class of medications has demonstrated consistent efficacy for aggression. In general, medications are more likely to be beneficial for aggressive behavior that is impulsive and environmentally reactive. The first line of therapy for CD would be mood stabilizers or anti-convulsants. The range and choice of mood stabilizers is quite large. Among the best studied medications are valproic acid and its derivatives, as well as lithium. Recent extended release formulations of these medications have made dosing much easier. Clinicians should take a careful medical history before starting these medications and regularly monitor relevant laboratory studies. Possible non-adherence should be addressed while initiating and maintaining treatment. Should mood stabilizers fail to produce an adequate effect, clinicians could consider adding or using an atypical anti-psychotic. This class of medications is being widely used for multiple off-label uses, and can be beneficial when used with mood stabilizers or alone when used in low doses. Attention needs to be paid to possible extrapyramidal and akithitic side-effects, and careful monitoring should be done when prescribing any anti-psychotic.

Should outpatient interventions fail, hospitalization can be used as an intervention of last resort or in the context of acute behavioral de-compensation where the safety of the child or individuals around the child is at risk. Hospitalization should focus on rapid interventions to de-escalate the child, build a safety network around the child, and change the direction of care. Careful follow-up and consideration

---

CONSIDER CONSULTATION WHEN …

- The child potentially has multiple domains of pathology (mood, substance, psychotic or developmental disorder) and presents with disruptive patterns.
- The sources of information (parents, school, friends, activities directors, clergy, etc.) disagree on the basic patterns that are being reported.
- Basic psychoeducational interventions are ineffective.
- Multiple medication trials or psychotherapeutic modalities have failed.
- The child is rapidly escalating in behavior.
- Aggressive or disruptive behaviors may cause harm to the child or others.

of a partial hospitalization, residential placement, or other specialized treatment programs need to be part of discharge planning.

Summary

Disruptive spectrum disorders are among the most challenging clinical problems in the child and adolescent psychiatric field. Both due to their high incidence and the complexity of their etiologies, disruptive spectrum disorders require clinicians to spend time gathering detailed histories and collateral information, explore for potential comorbidities, and then develop creative interventions using the range of options available within therapeutic, environmental, and pharmacologic models of care.

Annotated bibliography

Connor D (2002) *Aggression and Antisocial Behavior in Children and Adolescents: Research and Treatment*. New York, Guilford Press.
This is a comprehensive examination of disruptive disorders in a thoughtful and productive manner from a developmental perspective. Dr Connor
has surveyed the literature on aggression and anti-sociality in childhood and synthesized it into a useful volume that is both a guide for the treating clinician and a reference tool for the researcher or non-clinician.

Furstenberg FF (1999) *Managing to Make It: Urban Families and Adolescent Success*. Chicago, University of Chicago Press.
This book presents recent research from a large study on the factors that led to success in urban populations, which have traditionally been seen as at-risk for disruptive disorders due to high rates of substance abuse and violence.

Raine A (1997) *Biosocial Basis of Violence*. New York, Plenum Press.
This book serves as an excellent review of the field with challenging insights into the ways that biology frames our social experience of aggression and violence. It paints a nuanced portrait of the social and biologic realms in constant flux.

Steiner H (ed.) (2004) *Handbook of Mental Health Interventions in Children & Adolescents: A Developmental Perspective*. New York, Jossey-Bass.
This book is a comprehensive review of the field of child and adolescent mental health. It not only reviews the research of the relevant basic science field, but also presents overviews of the major domains of child psychiatry and current interventions, including comprehensive sections on aggression and disruptive disorders.

CHAPTER 9

Anxiety Disorders

Osvaldo Gaytan, MD, Andro Giorgadze, MD, and Shannon Croft, MD

Introduction

Anxiety disorders are among the most prevalent disorders in psychiatry and are frequently seen in children. In community samples, anxiety disorders have been shown to occur in 5–18% of children. Anxiety is a complex emotional state with psychic, somatic and behavioral components, characterized by apprehension and anticipation of future danger. The perceived danger may be external or internal (for example, a threat to self-esteem or psychologic well-being). It is important to note that children are prone to experience anxiety in a variety of contexts, and that this anxiety response has adaptive and developmental value. However, anxiety disorders are marked by the presence of pathologic anxiety; e.g. anxiety when no real physical or psychologic danger exists, or when the emotional reaction is disproportionate in intensity to the actual danger (Kohn and Keller, 2003). DSM-IV delineates between normal and pathologic behavior, requiring the presence of significant distress and functional impairment before the diagnostic threshold of these disorders can be reached (APA, 1994).

Having an anxiety disorder in childhood denotes an increased risk for the persistence of the disorder into adulthood as well as the emergence of other forms of psychopathology later in life. The association of anxiety disorders with poor self-esteem, limited social skills, and overall impairment of academic performance supports the importance of early assessment and referrals in providing patients with treatment during their childhood and adolescence, thereby, minimizing the long-term sequelae of these disorders. Assessment of children with anxiety disorders is quite complex and requires screening for comorbid conditions such as other anxiety and psychiatric disorders or potential medical causes.

Children are often unable to conceptualize and verbalize their complex emotional states. They may lack insight into their feelings of anxiety, and may instead manifest it through somatic symptoms (racing heart, sweating, difficulty breathing, headache and other pains, gastrointestinal [GI] upset) and behavioral symptoms (freezing, crying, clinging or having a tantrum). Inattentiveness and hyperactivity are common manifestations of anxiety. Avoidance of frightening situations is often present and can be very disabling, affecting social and academic life. Treatment of anxiety disorders, therefore, is generally multimodal, encompassing individual, group, and family therapeutic interventions along with pharmacotherapy as warranted.

This chapter will cover the description and etiology of anxiety disorders, followed by assessment, differential diagnosis and treatment. We have included the section on tic disorders and Tourette syndrome (TS) considering the close phenotypical, clinical and etiologic association of tics with obsessive-compulsive disorder (OCD) and the significant comorbidity of tics with other anxiety, mood disorders, and behavioral problems.

PEARLS & PERILS

- Subclinical levels of anxiety disorders are very common.
- Comorbidity is closer to the rule than the exception.
- In general, earlier age of onset is associated with a more chronic and treatment resistant course.
- A high level of anxiety is a risk factor for acute risk of suicide.
- When asking screening questions, remember that most kids don't usually understand the word "anxiety," ask about things that "irritate" or make a child "angry," "nervous," or "scared" instead.
- Anxiety disorders require higher doses of medication and a longer duration for a full medication trial.
- There is a high rate of remission, even without treatment, for most anxiety disorders.

derman [...] d Morris, 1995). Retrospective [...] al phobia reported that up to 77% [...] or to age 20 (Schneier et al., 1992). [...] genetic susceptibility, family dynam- [...] deling and temperament all have been [...] ole in the development of both specific [...] as. The observation that specific phobias, especia[...] al phobia, aggregate around families lends support to u[...] e role of genetic susceptibilities and of environmental factors such as family dynamics and modeling in the development of phobias. The association of a fear response to a specific traumatic event in a child's life, or a spontaneous panic attack, has been observed in children. Nevertheless, childhood phobic responses do occur spontaneously in settings where parental modeling or social learning cannot account for the presentation. These spontaneous phobias usually occur before age 7 and may be associated with instinctual fears of insects, animals, blood, or bodily injury (Albano et al., 1996).

Recently, the role of temperament in the development and propagation of social phobia has received much attention. It was reported that up to 33% of children identified as being behaviorally inhibited met criteria for social phobia in adolescence (Kagan and Snidman, 1999). The increased risk of developing social phobia in children with behavioral inhibition, as well as the similarities in personality structure between behaviorally inhibited children and those with social phobia, offer a possible focus for future etiologic research.

Selective mutism

The diagnosis of selective mutism hinges on a child's persistent failure to speak in specific social situations where speech is expected (Table 9.5, modified from DSM-IV criteria). Most commonly, children with this diagnosis are reported to speak freely at home, may speak less to family and friends in social situations, and are most often mute when speaking to adults at school and to strangers in public (Dummit et al., 1997). The onset of the illness is reported to be in the preschool years, but may not present as a problem until a child begins kindergarten (Krysanski, 2003). To meet DSM-IV criteria, a child must have symptoms for at least a month (excluding the first month of school when children may be normally shy) and these symptoms must cause significant impairment. Selective mutism should not be diagnosed if the child's reluctance to speak is secondary to unfamiliarity with the language (recent immigrants), embarrassment over speech problems, or if the child is diagnosed with a pervasive developmental disorder, schizophrenia, or any other psychotic disorder (APA, 1994). The ICD-10 uses the term elective mutism, the term used in previous editions of the DSM. In this very similar diagnosis, a child demonstrates an emotionally determined selectivity in speech, though he or she is competent at speaking in some social situations.

DIAGNOSIS

Table 9.5 Selective mutism

Discriminating features

1. Inability or refusal to speak in social situations when speech is expected.

Consistent features

1. Lack of physical etiology for mutism.
2. Functional impairment.
3. Normal fund of knowledge for spoken language.

Variable features

1. Early onset prior to age 6.
2. Difficulties with speech and articulation.
3. Shy temperament.
4. Occurs more often in girls than boys.

Children who are diagnosed with selective mutism may have experienced problems with separation anxiety, sleeping and eating as infants (Steinhausen and Juzi, 1996). Selectively mute children are almost always described as shy or even timid. Social phobia has been seen as a very frequent comorbid diagnosis (Dummit et al., 1997). Other common comorbidities include language delays and enuresis (Steinhausen and Juzi, 1996; Kristensen, 2000). Comorbid diagnoses of depression and externalizing problems are rare (Dummit et al., 1997).

Prevalence estimates have ranged from 0.18–1.9%, but some of this variance may be due to different populations being studied as well as the use of different diagnostic criteria. A recent study based on teacher report on over 2000 children in kindergarten, first, and second grades found a prevalence rate of 0.71% (Bergman et al., 2002). Studies often report a slightly higher ratio of girls to boys with selective mutism (Dow et al., 1995).

As with other anxiety disorders, there have been multiple explanations for selective mutism which include unresolved conflicts, family neurosis, and reactions to trauma (Dow et al., 1995). However, it now seems clear that the majority of children with selective mutism have not been sexually or physically abused (Dummit et al., 1997) as occasional case reports have suggested. Recently, the literature has em-

Selective mutism

- Usually begins in preschool years, but noticed upon entering school.
- Children may communicate nonverbally, in written form or simply whisper.
- Primary disorders of language and hearing must be ruled out.
- Duration of at least 1 month is required.

PEARLS & PERILS

phasized the social phobia and anxiety components of this illness, with some authors proposing selective mutism is simply a variant of social phobia (Black and Uhde, 1995).

Obsessive-compulsive disorder

Obsessive-compulsive disorder (OCD) is a chronic, relatively common condition characterized by the presence of obsessions and/or compulsions (usually both are present), which are time-consuming (take more than 1 hour a day), cause marked distress, or significantly interfere with a child's functioning (Table 9.6, modified from DSM-IV criteria). Obsessions are intrusive, recurrent thoughts, fears, images or other mental events that the person recognizes as the product of his or her mind. Obsessions are experienced as involuntary, distressing, unnecessary, and excessive. The child usually attempts to ignore or suppress obsessions or neutralize them with some other thought or action (APA, 2000). The most common obsessions include fear of contamination and germs, need for symmetry and precision, obsessional fear for safety of self or loved ones, fear of hurting other people or being hurt, obsessive doubting, and somatic obsessions (Swedo et al., 1989). Religious scrupulousness is common in adolescence, while aggressive and sexual intrusive images or thoughts are more common in adults. Obsessions can be triggered by external cue, for example, being near a certain person or object may activate contamination fears (AACAP, 1997).

Compulsions are repetitive behaviors or mental acts that a person feels driven to perform in a certain rigid way (APA, 2000). Compulsions are carried out to reduce distress, prevent some dreaded outcome or performed in response to obsessions. While children may not be aware of any specific

Table 9.6 Obsessive-compulsive disorder

Discriminating features

1. Presence of either obsessions or compulsions.
2. Marked distress or functional impairment must be present.
3. Absence of a physiologic abnormality that would explain symptoms.

Consistent features

1. Obsessions and compulsions take more than 1 hour a day.
2. Children attempt to ignore or suppress their symptoms.

Variable features

1. Most patients have both obsessions and compulsions.
2. Onset of symptoms usually gradual.
3. Partial control of symptoms is common.
4. Academic and behavioral problems are common.
5. Boys tend to develop OCD earlier than girls.

Obsessive-compulsive disorder
- Subclinical obsession and compulsions are quite common in school children.
- Insight and ego-dystonic aspect may be quite variable.
- OCD is a chronic condition with waxing and waning symptoms aggravated by stress.
- Symptoms may change in content and context with time.
- Many children are secretive about their symptoms; may use denial or minimization.
- Comorbidity is the rule with OCD: screen for other anxiety disorders, depression, and tic disorders.
- An adequate trial of medication is 3 months with maximally allowed doses.

dreaded outcome that compulsions are executed to ward off, they may have a general feeling that something bad is going to happen if they do not perform compulsive activities. The most frequently seen compulsions include cleaning rituals, repeating actions until it just "feels right," compulsive touching, arranging things in certain order, compulsive reading or writing, checking behaviors (e.g. doors, locks, stove, brakes), counting, doing things in a certain way or a certain number of times, praying, silent word repetition, and a hoarding (AACAP, 1997). The insight into excessiveness and unrealistic nature of obsessions and compulsions can fluctuate with time even in adults and is not a requirement to make the diagnosis in children.

OCD has a prevalence in children of 1–3%, but subclinical obsessions and compulsions are several times more common (Towbin and Riddle, 2002). OCD has a bimodal peak of onset. In children the mean age of onset is 10 years with a male predominance, while in adults the mean age of onset is 21 years and gender distribution is equal. More than 80% of individuals have the onset of their symptoms before age 18 (Riddle, 1998) and some children have onset as early as 5 years of age (AACAP, 1997).

Historically, psychodynamic factors were implicated in the etiology of OCD with a special emphasis on defense mechanisms (undoing, isolation, magical thinking, and reaction formation) and disturbance during the anal phase of psychosexual development (Freud, 1966). Later theories emphasize the role of conditioned stimuli and avoidance strategies in the pathogenesis of OCD. Currently, several lines of evidence indicate the involvement of the cortico-striato-thalamo-cortical circuit in the pathogenesis of OCD. PET studies show the involvement of the orbital frontal cortex and caudate (Baxter, 1999). Clinical data derived from the studies of psychopharmacologic agents indicate 5-HT and dopamine neurotransmitter systems involvement.

There are a host of different neurologic and medical conditions that can lead to secondary OCD, including postviral

Prolonged exposure, or flooding techniques, makes the child confront the feared stimulus immediately and remain in its presence until anxiety subsides. Obviously this approach requires the child to be able to tolerate high levels of anxiety and should be used only in appropriate situations.

Modeling involves having the frightened child observe anther person interacting adaptively with the feared stimulus. It can be especially useful since it teaches new learning skills. Consider, for example, using modeling for a child in the hospital setting preparing for some procedure. Thought stopping helps with intrusive, negative thoughts. The technique requires the child to interrupt the distressing thought and count backward from 10 to one. Behavioral techniques and CBT have an advantage of long-lasting outcome even after treatment is discontinued. Psychodynamic therapy is difficult to study in research protocols, however, clinical experience suggests that it may be particularly helpful addressing a variety of issues in the child's life including self-esteem, personal relationships, and character styles (Ritvo and Ritvo, 2002; Jacobs, 2003). CBT and other therapies have an advantage of potentially causing long-lasting improvement and no liability in terms of side-effects, however, more severe anxiety (or when therapy is not available) requires medications. In complicated cases, both a pharmacologic approach and therapy can be combined for a better or long-lasting outcome, or therapy can be given to prevent relapse when medication is discontinued.

Several agents have gained increased acceptance as the pharmacologic treatment of anxiety disorders. SSRIs (selective serotonin reuptake inhibitors) are the first-line agents for all anxiety disorders. Benzodiazepines can be effective in the acute management of anxiety. Sometimes they may be helpful as an adjunctive medication when starting SSRIs, since it usually takes several weeks before anxiety symptoms noticeably improve during a SSRI trial. However, they have been shown to be ineffective when used alone in children and adolescents with anxiety disorders (Simeon et al., 1992; Graae and Milner, 1994). If utilized, benzodiazepines should be used sparingly and for short duration, especially because of the chance for behavioral disinhibition (Graae and Milner, 1994), sedation, and dependence/withdrawal issues.

Tricyclic antidepressants (TCAs; imipramine, clomipramine) have been shown to be effective in children with anxiety disorders, but their side-effects and risk of overdose make them less appropriate compared to SSRIs. If SSRIs are implemented as a component of the treatment, it is important to remember that anxiety disorders generally require higher doses than depressive disorders and a longer duration of treatment (3 months) for a full medication trial to be completed. Also, individuals with anxiety disorders may have an initial increase of anxiety with SSRIs. Starting with a low dose and increasing the dose slowly may avoid possible side-effects such as behavioral dyscontrol, agitation, insomnia, and fretfulness. Recently, paroxetine and venlafaxine have been reported to be associated with increased suicidal ideation in youth. Until this issue is further clarified, periodic monitoring for suicidal ideation is warranted in children on SSRIs.

Generalized anxiety disorder

CBT has been shown to be effective in treatment of GAD and is the first-line option for treatment of mild to moderate GAD. Relaxation training, modeling, exposure, role playing, and training in recognizing anxious feelings and somatic reactions can also be helpful. There have been few controlled trials with any medication for the treatment of GAD in children. However, based on adult studies and one large controlled trial in children, SSRIs have become the most popular first-line agent (Freeman, 2002). There are trials for the use of fluvoxamine, fluoxetine, and sertraline showing both effectiveness and safety (Birmaher et al., 1994; Rynn et al., 2001; Walkup et al., 2001). Fluvoxamine was shown in a double-blind trial to be effective in treating GAD, separation anxiety disorder, and social phobia (Walkup et al., 2001).

Panic disorder

It is important to educate patients, family, and even teachers about the nature of the disorder and how they can best support the patients by encouraging and helping them with the use of behavioral and cognitive techniques. The primary goal of education is to reduce the parents' anxiety over their child's panic attack, thereby minimizing any affective modeling and improving the child's own coping skills. Cognitive behavioral therapy for panic disorder concentrates on relaxation techniques such as progressive muscle relaxation, deep breathing, coping self-statements, positive visualization, and self-instruction to control the progressive escalation of physical symptoms. Cognitive approaches that minimize catastrophic thinking are also of great use during an attack. Finally, exposure techniques such as hierarchical-based exposure and systemic desensitization may be especially useful in treatment of agoraphobia in panic disorder, or for panic attacks which are associated with situational triggers. Recently, a multimodal CBT treatment plan that improves a patient's coping skills was shown to significantly diminish agoraphobic avoidance and eliminate panic attacks in adolescents. The treatment gains were maintained over a 6-month follow-up.

Currently, there are no controlled studies for the use of any medication in children or adolescents with panic disorder. The approval of SSRIs in the treatment of panic disorder in adults have led to the use of these medications as first-line agents for children and adolescents when other therapeutic interventions have proven ineffective. There is one report in an open-label study of an 83% response rate to paroxetine in children and adolescents with panic disorder (Masi et al., 2001). Benzodiazepines can be used in some cases to aid children with intolerable panic attacks (Kutcher and Mackensie, 1988). In general, most clinicians reserve benzodiazepines for short-term emergency use in children.

Separation anxiety disorder

Cognitive behavioral therapy, whether individual, family or group based, has become the first treatment of choice for SAD and centers on returning the child to school as quickly as possible. Early in the disorder, especially if the amount of school missed has been minimal, simple behavioral techniques may be all that are needed. Parents should display empathy to a child's anxiety, but should also set firm limits and utilize rewards and praise to encourage the appropriate behavior in the child (i.e. return to school). With more chronic and severe cases, a comprehensive treatment plan needs to be established with the recruitment of parents and school officials if necessary. The mainstay of treatment is the use of systemic desensitization and relaxation techniques, along with positive reinforcement in children and cognitive strategies (positive self-talk, recognizing cognitive distortions, problem solving) to improve coping skills in older children and adolescents (Francis and Beidel, 1995; Labellarte et al., 1999).

Individual, family and group therapy have also been shown to be of benefit, especially if they utilize education and modeling of appropriate behavior, and if they address the issues of separation and autonomy in individual sessions, leading to improved self-esteem and mastery of the patient's conflicts. Partial hospitalization may be warranted if symptoms are severe enough and may aid in the prompt transition back to the school setting after stabilization. In these severe cases, school counselors may be recruited to provide emotional support throughout the day and ease the transition period. If a patient also has panic disorder or a mood disorder, these disorders must be treated first. Although there are studies that show the effectiveness of imipramine, especially in conjunction with cognitive-behavioral therapy (Bernstein et al., 2000), SSRIs have replaced TCAs because of their improved side-effect profile and tolerability. Recently, studies have found that children with anxiety disorders have shown significant improvement on fluoxetine in both an open-label, and a randomly controlled, study (Birmaher et al., 1994, 2003). Imiprimine may still be utilized in treatment resistant cases. Fluvoxamine has also been shown to be effective for SAD (Walkup et al., 2001).

Specific and social phobia

The first line of treatment for simple phobias are the behavioral techniques, such as *in vivo* exposure with contingency management and exposure-based self-control strategies (Morris and Kratochwill, 1998; Silverman et al., 1999a, 1999b). For social phobia, studies have shown support for CBT, whether it is individual, group or family based (Beidel and Morris, 1995; Beidel et al., 2000). In general, systematic desensitization and exposure works better for younger children than does imagined exposure to the phobic object or social situation because of the difficulties children have in visualization and in utilizing and mastering relaxation techniques to cope with elicited anxiety. In social phobia and in some specific phobias, the restructuring of cognitive distortions, as well as improvement of social skills, problem solving and assertiveness training are all integral parts of CBT treatment. Emotive therapy utilizes the creation of stories by the therapist where the child is assigned a strong, hero-like companion to aid the child in confronting the phobic object/situation, and has recently been utilized successfully by more clinicians, but lacks any controlled studies to support its use. Finally, there have not been any controlled studies in the use of medication for treatment of specific and social phobias. Based on treatment of adults with social phobia, most clinicians consider SSRIs as their first-line agents. As with GAD and SAD, fluvoxamine and fluoxetine have been shown to be of benefit in children with social phobia (Birmaher et al., 1994; Walkup et al., 2001).

Selective mutism

A number of treatment strategies for children with selective mutism have been described, but no studies have been adequately controlled, so there is no one clear treatment for selective mutism. Most authors espouse multimodal therapy (Wright et al., 1995), combining different therapies depending on the needs of each particular child and family. Psychodynamic play therapies target underlying conflicts (Krysanski, 2003). Family therapy addresses family patterns that may impact the child's symptoms (Dow et al., 1995). Behavioral interventions have become the most frequently used treatment for children with selective mutism, and address mutism as a learned behavior that may be treated by typical behavior therapy techniques aimed at reinforcing speaking, while decreasing the reinforcement of the absence of speech (Dow et al., 1995). An open trial of fluoxetine (Dummit et al., 1996) showed that 76% of children with selective mutism improved after a 9-week trial with a mean daily dose of 28mg. SSRIs may be a useful adjunctive therapy to refractory cases with significant anxiety symptoms (Dow et al., 1995). Speech and language therapy is indicated when language difficulties have been found during the assessment.

Obsessive-compulsive disorder

Cognitive behavioral therapy (CBT) is considered a first-line therapy for mild to moderate OCD (March, 1995). The behavioral part of CBT includes the exposure of a child to a dependent research groups is that prepubertal bipolar children typically have multiple daily mood swings and that irritability is much more common than euphoria (Wozniak and Biederman, 1997; Geller et al., 2000b).

There are several excellent reviews of the neurobiology of bipolar disorders, but the majority of this information is from adult studies, as there have been relatively few investigations of the neurobiology of childhood and adolescent mood disorders (Post et al., 2003; Manji and Zarate, 2002).

There have been limited molecular genetic studies of children with bipolar disorders. Family risk studies have suggested that early-onset major depression may be a more familial form of the illness than adult-onset major depression (Todd et al., 1993). Two molecular genetic studies in children with bipolar disorders by Geller and colleagues have been reported (Geller and Cook, 1999). It is still very early in our knowledge about the molecular genetics of psychiatric disorders and it is very likely that multiple genes are involved that interact with each other, and are expressed differentially during development (Kelsoe et al., 1993). It is unlikely that a single genetic locus will be identified that causes either depressive or bipolar disorders in children or adolescents.

Structural magnetic resonance imaging (MRI) studies of adults with bipolar disorder have revealed a variety of abnormalities including decreased prefrontal cortex volumes (Sax et al., 1999; Drevets et al., 1997), increases in the volume of the amygdala and putamen (Altshuler et al., 1998; Strakowski et al., 1999; Strakowski et al., 2002), atrophy of the V3 vermal area (DelBello et al., 1999) and larger lateral ventricles (Strakowski et al., 2002). Another common structural MRI finding in adults with bipolar disorder is the presence of white matter hyperintensities whose significance is unknown (Strakowski et al., 1993; Altshuler et al., 1995; Soares and Mann, 1997). Structural MRI studies of children and adolescents with bipolar disorder have also reported a variety of neuroanatomic abnormalities, including an increased incidence of subcortical white matter hyperintensities (Botteron et al., 1995; Pillai et al., 2002; Woods et al., 1995), reduced intracranial volume and increased frontal and temporal sulcal size (Friedman et al., 1999), and reductions in thalamic area (Dasari et al., 1999).

Strakowski et al. reviewed all of the older positron emission technology (PET) and single photon emission computed tomography (SPECT) studies, in bipolar disorders (Strakowski et al., 2000). In many of these studies, the investigators did not report how subjects were diagnosed, how the normality of their comparison group was determined, and how important confounds like concomitant central nervous system (CNS) medication use were controlled for. Despite these limitations, there are suggestions of regional cerebral blood flow (rCBF) abnormalities in both the frontal cortex and temporal cortex, with a general trend being for increased rCBF in these areas during mania and decreased rCBF during a depressive episode.

Functional magnetic resonance imaging (fMRI) is an imaging technique that does not involve exposure to ionizing radiation and has the advantage of better temporal resolution than PET or SPECT. Functional MRI also has the capability of acquiring many more scans in a single scanning session, which allows for signal averaging with block designs with a subsequent increase in the signal-to-noise ratio. The ability to recognize unique identities and various forms of affect in human faces is an essential component of human social behavior (Ekman and Oster, 1979) and the use of neurobehavioral probes like human faces with fMRI allows greater sensitivity and specificity in identifying the neural systems involved in psychiatric disorders (Gur et al., 1992; Breiter et al., 1996; Morris et al., 1996). Yergelun-Todd and colleagues at Mclean Hospital studied 14 adult patients with DSM-IV bipolar disorder and 10 normal controls with a 1.5T system using the Ekman fearful and happy faces as visual stimuli (Yurgelun-Todd et al., 2000). They reported a significant increase in signal intensity in the left amygdala and a reduction of signal intensity in the right dorsolateral prefrontal cortex in response to recognition of fearful facial expressions. While all of their normal controls were able to accurately label 100% of the fearful faces, only 10 of 14 (71%) bipolar patients were able to correctly identify the fearful Ekman faces. Yergelun-Todd et al. interpreted these findings to suggest that there were abnormalities in fronto-limbic circuitry of the bipolar subjects as compared to the normal control subjects.

There have been several studies of bipolar patients using magnetic resonance spectroscopy (MRS), and Soares et al. have recently reviewed the literature concerning MRS in the pathophysiology of adult mood disorders (unipolar and bipolar studies) and summarized the findings from seven ¹H studies in the adult literature to date (Soares et al., 1996). These MRS ¹H studies reported significant choline/Cr abnormalities in the parietal lobes and basal ganglia of adult bipolar patients (Renshaw et al., 1995). Soares et al. (1996) concluded that MRS offers a non-invasive tool for *in vivo* evaluation which can add to the understanding of the neurochemical aspects of the neurobiology of mood disorders.

There are very limited data on the outcome of children and adolescents with BPD. One prospective study which followed 86 prepubertal and early adolescent patients with bipolar disorder type I over a 4-year period of treatment showed that they spent approximately 57% of this time in hypomania, approximately 39% of the time in mania, and approximately 47% of the time with depressive features, confidence intervals of approximately +/- 30% for each value (Geller et al., 2004). At 4-year follow-up, 86 of the patients were assessed and rate of recovery was 87%. However, rate of relapse after recovery was 64%. In these studies, recovery was defined as no mania or hypomania for at least 2 weeks and relapse was defined as having full DSM-IV criteria for mania or hypomania and a Childhood Global Assessment Scale score of less than or equal to 60 for at least 2 weeks.

Bipolar II disorder

Bipolar II disorder (Table 10.9), during which an episode of hypomania occurs, is two to three times more common in children and adolescents than bipolar I disorder. A hypomanic episode is characterized in DSM-IV as an abnormally and persistently elevated, expansive, or irritable mood that lasts at least 4 days. In contrast to a bipolar I disorder, the illness caused by bipolar II disorder is not severe enough to cause marked impairment in occupational functioning (school functioning in children and adolescents), to interfere with social activities or relationships with others, or to necessitate hospitalization, and there are no psychotic features.

Cyclothymic disorder

Cyclothymic disorder (Table 10.10) is characterized by hypomanic episodes without a history of major depressive episodes. In cyclothymia, the child or adolescent is not without symptoms for more than 2 months at a time. Retrospective studies of adults with cyclothymia have shown that adolescence is the most common age of onset for cyclothymia. A significant proportion of adolescents with cyclothymia also are at risk of progressing to bipolar disorder. In a study by Akiskal et al. (1985) of the offspring of adults with bipolar disorder, seven out of 10 adolescents with cyclothymia progressed to mania or hypomania within 3 years of diagnosis.

Assessment

Children and adolescents suspected of having an affective or mood disorder require a thorough assessment (see Chap-

Table 10.9 Bipolar II disorder

Discriminating features

1. Hypomanic episode.
2. Major depressive episode.
3. Never been a manic episode.

Consistent features

1. Severity (mild, moderate, severe).

Variable features

1. Psychotic or catatonic features.
2. Postpartum onset.
3. Partial or full remission.

Table 10.10 Cyclothymic disorder

Discriminating features

1. Multiple episodes of hypomania and depressive symptoms for at least a year.
2. Change from usual functioning.
3. Not related to substances or medical conditions.

Consistent features

1. There is no freedom from symptoms for over a 2-month period.
2. Absence of physiologic condition that may explain symptoms.
3. Impaired academic or social functioning.
4. Absence of a psychotic illness.
5. Hypomanic episodes are present at least 4 days.

Variable features

1. Irritable mood
2. Change in mood is observable by others.
3. Appearance of mania within 3 years of symptom onset.
4. Family history of bipolar disorder.

ters 1–4 for additional information). During an interview, questions that relate to mood symptoms should be asked in a way that allows the interviewer to explore significant areas related to those symptoms. Both children and their parents must be interviewed, since a parent's report alone is not sufficient. Children should be seen individually and suicidal ideation/behavior should always be assessed. Whereas parents are important sources of information regarding the behavioral manifestations of psychiatric symptoms and the temporal course of an illness, children are more able to report subjective symptoms (i.e. sadness, anxiety, grandiosity, elation) and some vegetative symptoms, such as sleep disturbance. Information should be obtained from any other involved, relevant individuals such as teachers and peers (Emslie et al., 1990a; Emslie and Mayes, 1999; Harrington, 2003).

It is important for the physician to systematically assess the child's family psychiatric history. No evaluation of children and adolescents with affective disorders is complete without a detailed biologic history of the family that includes first-, second-, and third-degree relatives. The offspring of adults with an affective illness show high rates of depression and bipolar disorder (Akiskal et al., 1985). When compiling a family history, it is preferable to interview both parents of the patient, even if one parent appears to know the family history of the other. A family assessment should be conducted to evaluate the pre-morbid level of family functioning, the parents' marital relationship (if applicable), and the impact of the illness on the family, as well as the research supporting the efficacy and safety of the newer selective serotonin reuptake inhibitors (SSRIs), SSRIs are considered the first-line treatment for early-onset depression. A recent algorithm for child and adolescent depression has been published and recommends using SSRIs not only as the first-line treatment, but also as a second-line treatment. Other antidepressants and combination treatments are suggested only in later stages of treatment (Hughes et al., 1999). This algorithm was developed based on available research data. Several controlled trials have shown SSRIs to be effective in children and adolescents, including two trials with fluoxetine and one each with paroxetine, sertraline, and citalopram. Recently, there has been concern about increased suicidality in children and adolescents being treated with SSRIs for depression. A review of the published and unpublished trials revealed that young people on SSRIs had a 4% incidence of suicidal ideation and/or behavior (no completions) compared to 2% of those on placebos. The increased incidence was during the early part of treatment. Based on this information, in October 2004, the FDA required drug companies to add a "black box" with this information and what disorders each drug has been approved for to the health professional labeling for the SSRIs, and to modify the information given to patients and their families (FDA, 2004). The American Academy of Child and Adolescent Psychiatry emphasized the need for close monitoring by physicians when children and adolescents are placed on these medications, especially during the initiation of treatment (AACAP, 2004).

The first study to demonstrate an antidepressant medication treatment to be superior to placebo in treating early-onset depression was by Emslie et al. (1997a). In this study of 96 children and adolescents (ages 8–18) with MDD, 56% of those randomized to fluoxetine versus 33% of those randomized to placebo were considered much or very much improved following 8 weeks of treatment. In a study replicating the findings by Emslie et al. (2002), 219 children and adolescents (ages 8–17) with MDD were randomized to 9 weeks of treatment in a multi-site study of fluoxetine versus placebo. Similar to the initial study, 52% versus 37%, respectively, were considered much or very much improved.

In another large, multi-site industry-funded study, 275 adolescents (ages 12–18) with MDD were randomized to paroxetine, imipramine, or placebo for an 8-week acute trial. Based on the primary outcome measure for response (HAM-D) ≤8 and/or ≥50% reduction on the HAM-D, there was no significant difference between the active medications and placebo (66.7% paroxetine, 58.5% imipramine, and 55.2% placebo). However, on a secondary outcome of CGI improvement of "much" or "very much" improved, paroxetine was superior in efficacy to placebo (66% vs. 48%), but imipramine (52%) was not (Keller et al., 2001). This study is important in two ways. It provides additional evidence for some positive effect of SSRIs in the treatment of

adolescent MDD, and reinforces the suggestions that TCAs are not effective in depressed children and adolescents as a group, but may have a role in specific individuals.

A multi-site study of sertraline versus placebo was conducted with 376 children and adolescents (ages 6–17) with MDD. Sixty-three per cent of subjects randomized to sertraline were considered much or very much improved, compared to 53% on placebo (Wagner et al., 2003). Finally, Wagner et al. reported on a multi-site, double-blind placebo controlled study of citalopram in 174 children and adolescents (ages 7–17) with MDD. In this study, a significant difference was seen between the active treatment group and the placebo group beginning after 1 week of treatment. Based on the primary outcome measure (CDRS-R ≤28), citalopram was more effective than placebo (36% vs. 24%; p=0.05). However, based on global improvement (clinical global impression [CGI] improvement of "much" or "very much" improved, citalopram was no better than placebo (47% vs. 45%) (Wagner 2004).

Thus, the SSRIs are generally considered safe and effective treatments for this age group, although clinicians should monitor patients closely for worsening of depression or suicidality, particularly early in treatment. To date, only fluoxetine has received approval from the FDA for the treatment of pediatric depression. Unpublished trials of other newer antidepressants, such as venlafaxine and mirtazapine have not shown a difference between active medication and placebo in the pediatric population.

Dosage for antidepressants in children and adolescents is similar to adult dosing. Dosage for antidepressants has to take into account two factors. First, children are given proportionally more antidepressants for their size because of their faster metabolic rate, which leads to a shorter serum high-life. Secondly, there is substantial individual variation in blood levels (six to 10 times) in similar children of similar sizes receiving the same dose. Approximately 10% of the population metabolizes slowly and can obtain high serum levels on low dosage, whereas others may require very high dosages to achieve a therapeutic level. Children and adolescents should be started at low doses, with dosages being increased slowly as side-effects are tolerated and as clinical condition indicates. As with adults, it may take 4 weeks at therapeutic levels before there is a clinically significant improvement in the level of depression. Plasma levels of the antidepressant are used in research settings to determine metabolism rates and compliance parameters, but practical guidelines for clinical usage is not well established at this time, but may be clinically relevant in the future.

Little has been written about the use of monoamine-oxidase inhibitors (MAOIs) with depressed children and adolescents. There are single case reports of the successful use of an MAOI in children and adolescents who have not responded to TCAs. It is imperative that individuals maintain a tyramine restricted diet while they are taking MAOIs, to avoid the possibility of a hypertensive crisis (Emslie et al., 1999).

When patients do not respond to antidepressants, the physician should consider the addition of lithium. Studies of adolescents (who did not have bipolar disorders) not responding to TCAs alone reveal a good response when lithium was added. Lithium may be particularly useful for children and adolescents who are considered at high risk for bipolarity. This includes patients with family histories of manic-depressive illness, patients with hypersomnia and hyperphagia during an episode of depression, and patients who are psychotic and depressed.

For children and adolescents who have psychotic disorders with their depression (that is, they have hallucinations and delusions corresponding with the onset of the mood disorder), it may be necessary to use an antipsychotic agent with the antidepressant medication. Considering the possible cumulative side-effects from both agents, the physician should select the antipsychotic agent that will be the least bothersome with the smallest dose possible. As the depression remits, so should the psychotic symptoms.

Because of the limited number of studies on the use of antidepressants in children and adolescents, little is known regarding the length of time needed for treatment. Generally, physicians follow adult guidelines, maintaining the antidepressant at the acute phase dose for 6 months after remission and then slowly tapering the medication until it is discontinued.

Although substantial work is needed to identify patients who will respond to medication, antidepressants remain an important therapeutic tool in this age group for the relief of MDD.

Integrating psychotherapy and medication

Only one study has been reported to date on combination treatment in adolescents with MDD. The Treatment for Adolescents with Depression Study (TADS) compared medication (fluoxetine), CBT, combination treatment (fluoxetine and CBT), and placebo in 439 adolescents (ages 12–18) with MDD. Subjects were randomized to one of the four treatment groups for 12 weeks. Based on global improvement (CGI improvement), 71% of those on combination were considered responders, compared with 61% on fluoxetine alone, 43% receiving CBT, and 35% receiving placebo. Combination treatment and fluoxetine alone were more effective than placebo, but CBT alone was not. In this study, combination treatment was associated with the greatest reduction in suicidal thinking, suggesting that fluoxetine plus CBT may offer the most favorable risk-benefit ratio in teens with MDD (TADS Team, 2004).

Bipolar disorders

Most of the research on treatment for bipolar children and adolescents has focused on psychopharmacologic interventions. However, these children and adolescents require a comprehensive treatment plan that includes interventions focusing on helping the individual achieve the highest possible level of function as well as helping the family cope and support their child. All of the non-pharmacologic interventions described above for children with depressive disorders can be helpful for those with bipolar disorders.

Psychotherapies

Child and family-focused cognitive behavioral therapy (CFF-CBT) has been studied as an adjunct to treatment with medication. The focus of this therapy is on assisting the family in coping with the child's excessive reactivity and reducing the role of environmental stressors. One open-labeled study of 34 children with pediatric bipolar disorder showed statistically significant improvement relative to pretherapy functioning (Pavuluri et al., 2004).

Peer relations for these patients can be very difficult for these patients due to their frequent mood swings, poor social skills, and impulsive behaviors. This problem is a major issue that can be worked with in therapy to develop more appropriate social skills. Sometimes referral to social skills group is also helpful. These patients should be encouraged to participate in as many outside groups and activities as appropriate without causing further stressors that may exacerbate their BPD.

Psychopharmacology

Despite the increasing use of traditional mood stabilizing agents and atypical antipsychotics in bipolar children and adolescents there are few published, placebo controlled double-blind studies of the efficacy of any psychotropics in children and adolescents with BPD. Current clinical practice is to treat manic episodes in children and adolescents with BPD as adults with bipolar disorder are treated, using mood stabilizers and antipsychotic agents (Kowatch and DelBello, 2003). The treatment of bipolar children and adolescents is further complicated because these patients often present with a mixed or "dysphoric" picture characterized by frequent short periods of intense mood lability and irritability rather than classic euphoric mania (Findling et al., 2001). Geller and colleagues found in 26 bipolar children and adolescents that "complex" cycling patterns, characterized by brief manic periods lasting 4 or more hours, occurred in 81% of their patients (Geller et al., 1995). This observation has lead to the terms "ultrarapid" cycling, denoting cycles occurring four to 364 times per year and "ultraradian" cycling, denoting those occurring daily throughout the year (Geller et al., 2004).

The traditional mood stabilizers, lithium, sodium divalproex, and carbamazepine have been the standard of care for treatment and maintenance of bipolar disorder in adults (Post et al., 1996). However, recently several other classes of psychotropic agents have been discovered to have mood stabilizing properties, including the atypical antipsychotics, clozapine, olanzapine, quetiapine, and newer antiepileptic drugs, such as lamotrigine and oxcarbazepine. To date, there have been only two double-blind placebo controlled studies of the treatment for acute mania in children and adolescents with bipolar disorder (Geller et al., 1998; DelBello et al., 2002) and one uncontrolled maintenance treatment study (Strober et al., 1990), all of which are described below under the specific medications studied.

A practical treatment strategy based on the extant literature is to first consider whether psychotic symptoms are present or not. The risks of medication noncompliance should be discussed with the patient and their family. Patients and their families should be educated about the common and potential adverse effects of the psychotropic medications that they are prescribed and any concerns addressed before the medication is started. An excellent resource for patients and parents about the adverse effects of psychotropic medication is the book *Helping Parents, Youth, and Teachers Understand Medications for Behavioral and Emotional Problems: A Resource Book of Medication Information Handouts* by Dulcan and Lizarralde (2003). Long-acting medications and medications that are better tolerated should be used whenever possible to enhance compliance.

Treatment of pediatric bipolar disorder

- **Without psychosis**
  - If on medication, taper medications
  - Re-evaluate mood and behavior
  - Still with mood symptoms?
    - Euphoric → lithium
    - Mixed → Divalproex or atypical
  - Non/partial response → mood stabilizer + atypical
  - Once stable - re-evaluate ADHD
  - Still with ADHD symptoms?
  - Low-dose, long-acting stimulants
- **With psychosis**
  - First line
    - Mixed picture → divalproex + atypical
    - Euphoric → lithium + atypical
    - Mixed/manic/depressed → atypical
  - Second line (nonresponders)
    - Divalproex + atypical + lithium
    - Lithium + oxcarbazepine

PEARLS & PERILS

Lithium

Lithium is the most studied medication for children and adolescents with bipolar disorder and is the only medication approved by the Food and Drug Administration (FDA) for the treatment of acute mania and bipolar disorder in adolescents, ages 12–18 years (Kowatch and Bucci, 1998). In a prospective, placebo controlled, investigation of lithium in children and adolescents with bipolar disorders (n=25), Geller et al. found that after 6 weeks of treatment, subjects treated with lithium showed a statistically significant decrease in positive urine toxicology screens and a significant improvement in global assessment of functioning, 46% in the lithium treated group vs. 8% in the placebo group (Geller et al., 1998). This study demonstrated the efficacy of lithium carbonate for the treatment of bipolar adolescents with co-morbid substance use disorders, but did not measure the effect of lithium on mood in these adolescents.

A recent, open-label lithium study showed 63 out of 100 adolescents aged 12–18 responded to lithium treatment after 4 weeks, with 26 achieving full remission (Kafantaris et al., 2003). Risk factors for poor lithium response in children and adolescents with bipolar disorder include prepubertal onset and the presence of co-occurring ADHD (Strober, 1998). In general, lithium should be titrated to a dose of 30 mg/kg/day in two to three divided doses, which typically results in a therapeutic serum level of 0.8–1.2 mEq/L. Common side-effects of lithium in children and adolescents include hypothyroidism, nausea, polyuria, polydypsia, generalized essential tremor, acne, and weight gain. Lithium levels and thyroid function tests should be monitored as in adults.

In one follow-up study of pediatric bipolar disorder, Strober et al. prospectively evaluated 37 adolescents whose bipolar disorder had been stabilized with lithium while hospitalized (Strober et al., 1990). After 18 months of follow-up, 35% of these patients discontinued lithium, and 92% of those who discontinued subsequently relapsed as compared to 38% of those who were lithium compliant, supporting the potential utility of lithium for maintenance treatment for bipolar disorder in adolescents. It is reasonable to maintain a child or adolescent who has had a single manic episode, on a mood stabilizing agent for 12–18 months, and then if they are euthymic and asymptomatic to slowly taper the mood stabilizing agent over several months. If mood symptoms recur, the mood stabilizing agent(s) should be reintroduced. If the child is not responding or partially responding to a mood stabilizer, the addition of a second mood stabilizer or an atypical antipsychotic might be required.

Anti-convulsants

The antiepileptic agents sodium divalproex and carbamazepine frequently are prescribed to treat mania in children and adolescents with BPD. Open-label studies of divalproex in manic adolescents have reported response rates ranging from 53–82% (Kowatch et al., 2000; Wagner et al., 2002; West et al., 1994; Papatheodorou et al., 1995). One open-label study of 90 patients under the age of 18 with a combination of lithium and divalproex showed improvement in all outcome measures by week 8, with 42 patients achieving full remission (Findling et al., 2003). There have also been several case reports and series describing the successful use of carbamazepine as monotherapy and adjunctive treatment in children and adolescents with bipolar disorder (Evans et al., 1987; Puente, 1975). There has been only one study to directly compare lithium, divalproex, and carbamazepine for the treatment of 42 acutely manic or hypomanic children and adolescents during a 6-week random assignment, open prospective investigation (Kowatch et al., 2000). In this study, all three mood stabilizers had large effect sizes with divalproex (1.63), followed by lithium (1.06) and carbamazepine (1.00).

Sodium divalproex can be initiated at a dose of 20 mg/kg/day and this loading dose will typically produce a serum level of 80–110 µg/mL. Common side-effects of divalproex in children and adolescents include weight gain, nausea, sedation, and tremor. There has been much debate regarding the possible association between divalproex and polycystic ovarian syndrome (PCOS). The initial reports of PCOS were in women with epilepsy who were treated with divalproex (Isojarvi et al., 1993). The hypothesized mechanism for divalproex induced PCOS is that obesity secondary to divalproex results in elevated insulin levels, which leads to increased androgen levels, menstrual irregularities, and ultimately PCOS. However, there is continuing debate whether this condition is related to weight gain with divalproex, a direct effect of the drug on steroid metabolism, or an incidental finding. Recently, Rasgon et al. reported that epilepsy, and not the anti-convulsants may be associated with increased risk for PCOS (Rasgon et al., 2000). In contrast, O'Donovan et al. recently reported that rates of menstrual irregularities and PCOS were higher in women with bipolar disorder who were taking divalproex than in those who were not taking divalproex and a comparison group of healthy volunteers (O'Donovan et al., 2002). Further investigations of the risk of developing PCOS for female bipolar adolescents are necessary, and clinicians should monitor female patients treated with divalproex for any signs of PCOS that include weight, menstrual abnormalities, hirsutism, and acne.

Carbamazepine is usually started at a dose of 15 mg/kg/day to produce a serum level of 7–10 µg/mL. Carbamazepine is used widely for seizure management but less commonly than divalproex for bipolar disorder in children and adolescents. This anti-convulsant must be titrated slowly and requires frequent monitoring of blood levels, which can be problematic in children with needle phobia. Its most common side-effects are sedation, rash, nausea, and hyponatremia. One retrospective study of 44 bipolar pre-adolescents showed a statistically significant greater improvement in the group treated with carbamazepine, relative to groups treated with divalproex or lithium as early as the second week (Davanzo et al., 2003). Oxcarbazepine is a chemical analogue of carbamazepine with less PY450 drug interactions and side-effects. There are limited studies in adults with BPD that suggest that it may be helpful as a mood stabilizer (Hummel et al., 2001; Nassir Ghaemi et al., 2002).

Atypical antipsychotics

The atypical antipsychotics have recently become first-line treatments for adults with BPD (Strakowski et al., 2003; Keck, 2003), and this strategy will probably also occur for the treatment of children and adolescents with BPD as data from several ongoing, controlled trials emerge. Several recent case series and open-label reports suggesting that atypical antipsychotics such as clozapine (Kowatch et al., 1995), risperidone (Frazier et al., 1999), olanzapine (Soutullo et al., 1999; Khouzam and El-Gabalawi, 2000; Chang and Ketter, 2000) and quetiapine (DelBello et al., 2002) are effective in the treatment of pediatric BPD. One open-label study of 28 children under the age of 18 showed improvement in aggressive and manic features in 82% of patients treated with risperidone (Frazier, et al. 1999).

There are emerging data from adult and child studies that combination treatment with an atypical antipsychotic and a traditional mood stabilizer may decrease BPD symptoms and improve overall response rates. Tohen and colleagues recently compared the efficacy of combined therapy with olanzapine and either divalproex or lithium to divalproex or lithium monotherapy for the treatment of acute mania in adults and found that the response rate was significantly higher in the combination group (68% versus 45%) (Tohen et al., 2002). DelBello et al. have recently published the results of a controlled trial that examined the efficacy, safety, and tolerability of quetiapine as an adjunct to divalproex for 30 manic or mixed bipolar I adolescent inpatients, ages 12–18 years, who received an initial divalproex dose of 20 mg/kg and were randomized in a double-blind to 6 weeks of quetiapine, which was titrated to 450 mg/day (n=15), or placebo (n=15). The divalproex + quetiapine group demonstrated a statistically significant greater reduction in Y-MRS scores from baseline to endpoint than the divalproex + placebo group. Moreover, Y-MRS response rate was significantly greater in the divalproex + quetiapine group than in the divalproex + placebo group (87% vs 53%). The findings of this study indicate that quetiapine in combination with divalproex was more effective for the treatment of adolescent bipolar mania than divalproex alone. These results also suggest that quetiapine is safe and well-tolerated when used in combination with divalproex for the treatment of mania.

Kafantaris et al. evaluated acutely manic adolescents with psychotic features after treatment with lithium and an adjunctive antipsychotic medication. If their psychosis resolved, the antipsychotic medication dose was gradually tapered and discontinued after 4 weeks of therapeutic lithium levels. The patients were then given a trial of maintenance lithium monotherapy for up to 4 weeks. Significant improvement was seen in 64% of the sample with psychotic features after 4 weeks of combination treatment. However, 43% did not maintain their response after discontinuation of the antipsychotic medication, suggesting that more than 4 weeks of antipsychotic treatment is required for some adolescents with psychotic mania. Successful discontinuation of antipsychotic medication in this sample was associated with first episode, shorter duration of psychosis, and the presence of thought disorder at baseline, suggesting that the more florid and acutely impairing manic episodes are time limited and the antipsychotics can be carefully discontinued (Kafantaris et al., 2001).

Many agents used to treat children and adolescents with bipolar disorder are associated with weight gain. A series of general medical, metabolic problems may occur as a result of increases in weight including type II (non-insulin dependent) diabetes mellitus, and changes in lipid levels, and transaminase elevation (Clark and Burge, 2003; Lebovitz, 2003). Children who experience significant weight gain should be monitored especially closely for these possibilities. Recently, the American Diabetes Association in collaboration with the American Psychiatric Association published a monitoring protocol for all patients prior to initiating treatment with atypical antipsychotic (American Diabetes Association and Association, 2004). This protocol includes: a personal and family history of obesity, diabetes, dyslipidemia, hypertension, or cardiovascular disease; weight and height (so that body mass index can be calculated); measurement of waist circumference (at the level of the umbilicus); blood pressure; fasting plasma glucose and a fasting lipid profile. This group recommended that the patient's weight should be reassessed at 4, 8, and 12 weeks after initiating or

changing therapy with an atypical antipsychotic, and quarterly thereafter at the time of routine visits. If a patient gains more than 5% of his or her initial weight at any time during therapy, the patient should be switched to an alternative agent. These guidelines should be followed in all children and adolescents treated with atypical antipsychotics.

Ziprasidone may increase QTc prolongation and safety data in children and adolescents are limited (Pfizer, 2000). Therefore, ziprasidone should be used with caution in children and adolescents with BPD and a family history of cardiac disease. EKGs should be monitored at baseline and when significant dose increases occur, generally when the dose of ziprasidone exceeds 3 mg/kg.

Stimulants

Most children with BPD will have comorbid ADHD and mood stabilization with mood stabilizers or atypical antipsychotics is a necessary prerequisite prior to initiating stimulant medications (Biederman et al., 1999). A recent randomized controlled trial of 40 bipolar children and adolescents with ADHD demonstrated that low-dose dexedrine can be safely and effectively used for treatment of comorbid ADHD symptoms after the child's BPD symptoms are stabilized with divalproex (Scheffer et al., 2005). Sustained release psychostimulants may be more effective at reducing rebound symptoms in bipolar children and adolescents. A typical dose of such stimulants for a child with BPD and ADHD would be 36 mg/day of Concerta or Adderall XR, 10–20 mg/day.

Other treatments

Electroconvulsive therapy can be an effective treatment for depressive and bipolar disorders. It generally is used for older adolescents when other interventions have failed. There are no controlled studies on its efficacy in children and adolescents, though its effects appear to be similar to those seen in adults (AACAP, 2002). See Chapter 4 for additional information.

Summary

The recognition and treatment of depressive and bipolar disorders in children and adolescents remain major concerns and challenges for physicians, educators, and parents. These disorders are often difficult to manage and referral to a child/adolescent psychiatrist with experience in pediatric mood disorders is often helpful to manage these patients. The morbidity and mortality associated with these disorders among children and adolescents can be decreased by increasing the public's awareness of the seriousness of these disorders. In the future, we will hopefully see research studies that guide physicians in the effective

CONSIDER CONSULTATION WHEN ...

- The child is actively suicidal.
- The child has psychotic symptoms with the mood disorder.
- The child's depression does not improve despite adequate treatment with an antidepressant over a sufficient period.
- The child's symptoms worsen, particularly if mania is suspected, when traditional medical and behavioral interventions are attempted.
- The child develops intolerable side-effects caused by medication.
- The child has comorbid disorders that require treatment.

identification and treatment of both acute and recurrent episodes of both depressive and bipolar disorders.

Annotated bibliography

American Academy of Child and Adolescent Psychiatry (1998) Practice parameters for the assessment and treatment of children and adolescents with depressive disorders. *J Am Acad Child Adolesc Psychiatry*, 37 (Suppl):63S–83S.
Overview of assessment and treatment for depressive disorders in children and adolescents.

Coyle JT, Pine DS, Charney DS, Lewis L, Nemeroff CB, Carlson GA, Toorjoshi PT, Reiss D, Todd RD, Hellander M (2003) The Depression and Bipolar Support Alliance Consensus Development Panel. Depression and Bipolar Support Alliance Consensus on the unmet needs in diagnosis and treatment of mood disorders in children and adolescents. *Journal of American Academy of Child and Adolescent Psychiatry*, 42:1494–1503.
Overview of depression and its treatment in children and adolescents.

Craney JL, Geller B (2003) A prepubertal and early adolescent bipolar disorder-I phenotype: review of phenomenology and longitudinal course. *Bipolar Disord*, 5(4):243–56.
This article is a useful summary of the phenomenology and longitudinal course of a sample of young subjects with early onset BPD.

Emslie GJ, Mayes TL, Laptook RS and Batt M (2003) Predictors of response to treatment in children and adolescents with mood disorders. *Psychiatric Clinics of North America*, 26:110–117.
Discussion of treatment issues in depression.

Fristad MA, Arnold JSG (2004) *Raising a Moody Child: How to Cope with Depression and Bipolar Disorder*. New York, Guilford Press, Inc.
This book is an excellent one for parents who have a child with BPD.

Kowatch RA, DelBello MP (2003) The use of mood stabilizers and atypical antipsychotics in children and adolescents with bipolar disorders. *CNS Spectr*, 8(4):273–80.
This article is a good review of this topic.

McElroy S, Keck PJ (2000) Pharmacologic agents for the treatment of acute bipolar mania. *Biological Psychiatry*, 48(Sep 15):539–57.
This is an excellent summary of the pharmacologic treatment of mania in adults.

CHAPTER 11

Eating Disorders

David A. Waller, MD

OUTLINE

Introduction

The term "eating disorder" is a deceptively simple phrase that refers to an extremely complex group of psychiatric disorders with prominent physical, psychologic, and social dimensions. The physician should be familiar with the diagnostic criteria for each of these disorders and comfortable eliciting them. Differential diagnosis is important, to distinguish one eating disorder from another, to assess for other psychiatric comorbidity, and to rule out concomitant medical illnesses. For each patient, a nutritional assessment must be performed. Where is the patient in terms of height and weight percentiles? A decision must be made based on clinical and laboratory data described below as to what level of care is indicated: inpatient, outpatient, or an intermediate level of intensity. Then a treatment program must be planned that addresses each of the following important dimensions: (1) nutritional state, (2) abnormal eating behaviors and attitudes, and (3) the psychologic meaning of the eating disorder for that particular patient. The above process is made more difficult by the fact that patients with these disorders and their families may deny their existence (or at least their severity), and health-care insurance companies (in the current US "managed care" environment) may be overly focused on curtailing cost of care. These issues set the stage for a series of control struggles between the patient, the health-care team, and the insurance company. All too often the patient does not immediately get better, the physician becomes increasingly frustrated, and the understandable conclusion is drawn that these patients are best avoided. The purpose of this chapter is to provide the necessary information to allow the physician to proceed without undue consternation along appropriate diagnostic and therapeutic paths to help these patients.

A useful approach to these patients and their families involves a developmental perspective. This view should be a familiar frame of reference for pediatricians, child and adolescent psychiatrists, and other health professionals who work with children. Eating disorders may be thought of as the outward expression of underlying problems in psychosocial development in genetically susceptible individuals. It is therefore important in the course of evaluating and treating the eating disorder to assess where the child or adolescent is in terms of accomplishing age-appropriate psychosocial developmental tasks. An important part of treatment constitutes helping the child and family move along the appropriate developmental path. Erikson's stages of psychosocial development (Erikson, 1963) may be especially useful guideposts and are referred to in the course of discussing particular eating disorders (Table 11.1).

Another general principle is that the physician should maintain a good alliance with the patient and family, as well as act as a health-care provider. The atmosphere should be one of mutual respect and teamwork, with an unhurried pace befitting the slow-going that sometimes characterizes developmental progress. For example, at the very beginning of contact with the patient and family in the waiting room, it is useful to allow the patient and family to have input into the decision of whom the doctor first interviews. Then at the beginning of the visit, the physician should find out whose idea it was to come for help, and the reasons this person has for wanting help. Subsequently, each person's views can be elicited, and they may be compared and contrasted. Questions about weight and eating habits should be asked in the context of learning about the patient's life (see Key clinical questions). The process of evaluation thereby becomes therapeutic in the sense that individuality is encouraged, all points of view are respected, and control struggles are avoided to the extent that is possible without jeopardizing the patient's well-being.

In DSM-IV (APA, 1994), eating disorders are described in two separate places for the first time. Feeding and eating disorders of infancy and early childhood are discussed with other disorders commonly beginning in childhood, whereas anorexia nervosa and bulimia nervosa appear in a separate section later in the text. Nevertheless, the latter two disorders commonly begin in adolescence or young

TABLE 11.1

Eriksonian stages

Age	Psychosocial developmental challenge	Ideal outcome
Infant	Basic trust vs. mistrust	Hope
Toddler	Autonomy vs. shame/doubt	Will
Preschool age	Initiative vs. guilt	Purpose
School age	Industry vs. inferiority	Competence
Adolescence	Identity vs. role confusion	Fidelity
Young adulthood	Intimacy vs. isolation	Love
Adulthood	Generativity vs. stagnation	Caring
Old age	Integrity vs. despair	Reflection

adulthood. Criteria for a proposed new eating disorder, called binge eating disorder, appear in Appendix B of DSM-IV. In this textbook, infant feeding disorders, which involve developmental difficulties in the area of attachment and early attempts to establish autonomy, are discussed in Chapter 15.

KEY CLINICAL QUESTIONS

- Screening questions for eating disorders:
  - *What concerns do you have about your appearance and weight?*
  - *Is your current weight too high, too low, or about right?*
  - *What is your ideal weight?*
  - *Which are you worried about, losing or gaining weight?*
  - *How would you describe your appearance/weight?*
  - *What do you see when you look in the mirror?*
  - *What do your friends and family say about your appearance/weight?*
  - *What have you eaten today/ yesterday/last week?*
  - *Where do you eat?*
  - *What type of activities precede eating?*
  - *What are your thoughts/feelings while eating?*
  - *What are you doing to lose/maintain/gain weight?*
  - *How much are you dieting/taking laxatives, other medications/purging/binging/exercising?*
  - *What kind of exercise do you do and how much?*
  - *When was your last menses? Have you missed any?*
  - *How often have you felt sad or worried recently? What were the circumstances?*
- Screening questions for interest in treatment:
  - *What concerns do you have about your weight?*
  - *What have you tried to improve your weight problem?*
  - *What worked? Why?*
  - *What did not work? Why not?*
  - *What do you think would help with this problem?*

Anorexia nervosa

Anorexia nervosa occurs in 0.5–1% of adolescent females in middle to upper socioeconomic classes in industrialized countries. About one in 20 cases is male, and the disorder is being increasingly diagnosed in individuals outside the usual population with greatest incidence. It may be that early recognition and treatment reduces the likelihood of a chronic, even life-threatening, course and it is important to be able to recognize early signs and symptoms of the disorder. Physicians should be alert to children and adolescents who are losing weight but who do not seem to have the appropriate concern about undue thinness. Anorexia nervosa is defined by weight loss of at least 15% of the expected weight for a person's height, age, and gender, or by failure to gain weight so as to be within 85% of the expected weight. Together with low weight is the irrational attitude that there is still a danger of being too fat, which is based on an apparent misconception regarding body size (Table 11.2). A child's weight and height should be monitored in primary care settings, including in adolescence. If persistent weight loss in the absence of medical illness is occurring, the child should be asked how he or she feels about her body size (about right? too fat? too thin?) and whether he or she is more afraid of gaining weight or of losing weight. Patients with anorexia nervosa are always more afraid of gaining more weight.

If the patient is a girl and expected to have menstrual periods, an additional criterion for diagnosis is that she has missed at least three consecutive cycles. Boys with the disorder have an analogous suppression of reproductive endocrine function. A decrease in gonadotropins leads to decreased output of testosterone, a lack of sexual interest, and a diminution of sexual functioning. Amenorrhea is obviously related to weight loss, but it is not totally a function of it. In a small number of women it begins before substantial weight has been lost, and it may persist after weight has returned to a normal level, especially if abnormal attitudes toward body size persist (APA, 1994).

a unique family with multiple individuals affected with anorexia nervosa and/or obsessive-compulsive disorder, an area of linkage on chromosome 11 was identified with LOD score = 2 (Waller et al., 2001). In a large, multi-center study that included obsessionality as a behavioral covariate of anorexia nervosa, Devlin et al. (2002) reported higher LOD scores for loci on chromosomes 1, 2, and 13. As noted above, atypical antipsychotic medications (in addition to SSRIs) may have a role to play in instances of enormous anxiety found in this type of eating disorder. However, the best somatic treatment for anorexia nervosa is food.

The prognosis for this disorder remains quite variable (Waller et al., 2003). For patients who come to medical attention, about half seem to do well: weight is recovered, menstrual cycles resume, and there is not undue concern with weight. However, some patients relapse under stress, and some are never able to emerge from a totally consuming preoccupation with food and body concerns. In these patients, weight often hovers around 80 lb, and social relationships are severely limited. A few patients still die from the disease, and of those patients with a chronic course the mortality rate continues to rise through the years, with deaths attributable to suicide or malnutrition. Thus, the mortality rate for anorexia nervosa remains higher than for any other psychiatric illness (Keel et al., 2003).

Bulimia nervosa

Bulimia nervosa is more common than anorexia nervosa. It affects about 3–4% of young women in the middle-to-upper socioeconomic class, but it is also seen in adolescents, in some males, and in women in lower socioeconomic classes. The defining feature is recurring episodes of binge eating followed by compensatory behaviors to offset the effects of the large amount of food that has been consumed, so the net effect is that the patient is usually of normal weight (Table 11.3). There are two subtypes that are differentiated by the type of compensatory behavior employed by the patient. Most research studies of treatment have focused on patients with the purging subtype, in which episodes of binge eating are followed by self-induced vomiting, often together with laxative or diuretic abuse to get rid of some of the calories. The other, nonpurging subtype is characterized by the patient's fasting, possibly in conjunction with exercise, to compensate for the binges. A binge episode is defined by the consumption of a large amount of food in a discrete time, during which the patient feels out of control of her eating behavior. There is also a frequency criterion: the episodes of binge eating and compensatory behaviors must have occurred at least twice a week for at least 3 months. Appendix B of DSM-IV contains criteria for binge eating disorder, which differs from bulimia nervosa in that there are no compensatory behaviors (Table 11.4).This condition, if validated as a disorder, may account for a substantial number of patients

DIAGNOSIS

Table 11.3 Bulimia nervosa

Discriminating features

1. Recurrent episodes of binge eating with compensatory behavior to prevent weight gain.

Consistent features

1. A sense of lack of control over eating.
2. Absence of anorexia nervosa.
3. Food craving.
4. Absence of a physiologic condition that explains symptoms (e.g. Kleine-Levin syndrome).

Variable features

1. Erosion of dental enamel.
2. Electrolyte disturbances.
3. Esophageal or gastric tears.
4. Callous marks on back of hand (Russell's sign).
5. Salivary gland enlargement.

seen in weight control clinics and may respond to some of the same therapeutic interventions which are effective in treating obesity and bulimia nervosa (see below).

It seems helpful clinically to conceptualize bulimia as a kind of "addiction" in which food is the abused substance (Hardy and Waller, 1989). Patients can often recall the exact time that the abnormal behaviors were no longer in their control, but rather had assumed a life of their own. The abnormal behavior is craved, and the patient may in severe

PEARLS & PERILS

Bulimia nervosa

- Patients are usually of normal weight. This disorder is easily missed unless the physician specifically asks about eating habits and body image.
- May be likened to an addiction, with food being the abused substance. Food is craved, the behavior is kept a secret, and the disorder affects the individual's life in multiple areas.
- Russell's sign (callous marks on the back of the hand) is a tell-tale sign.
- The most common physical finding is erosion of the dental enamel.
- In children with insulin-dependent diabetes mellitus, anorexia nervosa, and bulimia nervosa may appear in the form of recurrent and unexplained episodes of diabetic ketoacidosis. In these instances, the patients purge by not giving themselves their insulin.
- As many as 50% of patients respond to antidepressants, even in the absence of signs and symptoms of clinical depression.
- Bupropion has been associated with seizures when given to these patients.

Table 11.4 Binge eating disorder

Discriminating features

1. Recurrent episodes of binge eating without compensatory behaviors to prevent weight gain.
2. Marked distress regarding binge episodes.

Consistent features

1. A sense of lack of control over eating.
2. Food craving.
3. Absence of a physiologic condition that explains symptoms (e.g. Kleine-Levin syndrome).

Variable features

1. Extreme forms of obesity.
2. Medical complications related to obesity.
3. Other psychiatric disorders.

cases spend all day focused on the next indulgence in this activity. The behavior is often followed by a terrible sense of remorse and a firm intention to do better next time, and the patient experiences a sense of total failure when the behavior recurs. Since there may be few outward physical signs, it is incumbent on the primary caregiver to ask about problems in the area of eating, if this disorder is to be diagnosed before it is firmly entrenched. Even then, the patient may be inclined to be secretive about the matter, sometimes foregoing treatment because of concern that it might not be possible to get along without the disorder.

The most common physical finding is erosion of dental enamel. This results from the presence of stomach acid in the mouth and particularly affects upper teeth, since the tongue protects the lower teeth during vomiting. Thousands of dollars of reparative work may be needed. If diuretics or laxatives are used to assist with purgation, electrolyte disturbances may occur, consisting of metabolic alkalosis and hypokalemia (Mehler, 2003b). The latter may predispose to cardiac arrhythmias. A particularly noxious form of purgation is the abuse of ipecac. Emetine toxicity can result in heart failure and death. Occasionally, violent vomiting can result in esophageal or gastric tears. Enlargement of salivary glands, giving a "chipmunk cheek" appearance, probably results from recurrent vomiting and is mainly of cosmetic rather than clinical significance. A tell-tale sign of bulimia is Russell's sign, the presence of callous marks on the back of the hand produced by the upper teeth when the hand is pushed down the mouth to induce vomiting.

Differential diagnosis

Differential diagnosis is more straightforward than with other eating disorders because of the stereotypical behaviors that occur. Binge eating and vomiting in bulimia ner-

vosa are conscious, voluntary activities. Perhaps the most important medical condition to be excluded is a brain tumor that would essentially have different symptoms: vomiting would be in response to nausea, the compulsive eating would not be so episodic, and it might be accompanied by other neurologic or personality changes. Other examples of organic binge eating disorders include the following syndromes: (1) Kleine-Levin syndrome, typically found in adolescent boys, in which episodes of uncontrolled eating and hypersexuality are associated with periodic hypersomnolence, presumably a result of hypothalamic insult (Waller et al., 1984); (2) Prader-Willi syndrome, a genetic condition in which binge eating and obesity apparently result from a deletion (or absence of paternal contribution) of the long arm of chromosome 15 (Mascari et al., 1992); and (3) Kluver-Bucy syndrome, in which binge eating is associated with visual disturbances and sexual behavioral alterations, and which may have diverse causes (some reversible) (Guedalia et al., 1993). Achalasia, in which the esophagogastric sphincter fails to relax with swallowing, has been mistaken for bulimia (Smith and Christie, 1984), and the metabolic alterations in endocrine disorders such as insulin-dependent diabetes mellitus (Rodin et al., 1986–1987) and hyperthyroidism (Harel and Biro, 1994) may predispose an adolescent to contracting bulimia.

Treatment

Although bulimia nervosa was not codified as a distinct psychiatric illness until 1980, considerable insight into treatment has been gained as a result of placebo controlled research studies in young adult women with the disorder. Two types of intervention have been demonstrated to be effective (Agras and Rossiter, 1992; Mitchell et al., 1993). One is cognitive behavioral therapy (CBT). An example that typifies this approach is that of Fairburn et al. (1993). This manualized program of treatment is divided into three stages. The first stage aims to substitute a pattern of regular eating in place of the patient's habitual binge eating, self-induced vomiting, and laxative abuse. After a period of self-monitoring is instituted, the patient is provided with specific behavioral strategies that prevent overeating. The second stage is more cognitively oriented and involves identifying and challenging thoughts, beliefs, and values that are perpetuating the eating problem. The third stage aims to maintain progress and anticipate future difficulties.

A second approach with demonstrated efficacy in young adult women is the use of antidepressants. Original trials were prompted by the observation that patients with bulimia had increased incidences of past personal history of depression and of family history of depression, and that they sometimes met criteria for depression at the time of diagnosis of bulimia. Surprisingly, it was subsequently found that the presence of depression or depressive symptoms

Binge eating disorder

In DSM-IV, proposed criteria are provided for further study of an eating disorder that is often associated with obesity, binge eating disorder. Marcus and Kalarchian (2003) suggest that research criteria for children with this disorder should include: (1) recurrent episodes of binge eating, defined as food seeking in the absence of hunger and a sense of a lack of control over eating; (2) binge episodes associated with food seeking in response to a negative feeling state like sadness or boredom, or associated with food seeking as a reward or with sneaking or hiding food; and (3) symptoms that persist at least 3 months and are *not* associated with the regular use of purging, fasting, or excessive exercise, in contrast to normal-weight bulimia nervosa, hence the common association of binge eating disorder with obesity (Table 11.4). The importance of binge eating disorder is that it can be associated with especially extreme forms of obesity and with extensive distress and dysfunction, more psychiatric comorbidity (e.g. depression) than is usual with being overweight (Wilfley et al., 2003). A recent dramatic finding is that binge eating is a major phenotype characteristic of severely obese subjects with a mutation in the melanocortin 4 receptor gene (MC4R), indicating that this is an important candidate gene for the control of eating behavior (Branson et al., 2003).

Diagnosis of this disorder depends on systematically incorporating questions about binge eating during the routine history and physical exam, analogous to other questions about potentially self-injurious ingestion behaviors like alcohol and substance abuse. Behavioral weight control programs have been found to help patients with binge eating disorder not only to lose weight but also to stop binge eating (Stunkard and Allison, 2003). Effective medication treatment of binge eating disorder in placebo controlled studies of adults includes the SSRIs, sibutramine, and recently topiramate (Carter et al., 2003). However, there are no Food and Drug Administration approved medications for binge eating disorder.

Summary

By now, the reader should have a healthy respect for the complexity of eating disorders and the challenges inherent in treating children and adolescents who are afflicted with them. A treatment team may be especially helpful, both for providing the different kinds of expertise that the treatment of these children requires and for providing support among those giving help. With patience and persistence, progress can often be made. The eventual resolution of abnormal eating behaviors, improved nutrition, and meaningful psychosocial development can be as gratifying as any health-care triumphs.

> **CONSIDER CONSULTATION WHEN ...**
> - The child continues to lose/gain weight despite appropriate behavioral interventions.
> - Clinically concerning problematic eating attitudes and behaviors persist.
> - Family issues appear to be significantly contributing to or worsening the disorder.
> - A comorbid psychopathologic condition, such as a mood disorder, is also present.
> - The child's weight loss is such that tube feeding or parenteral nutrition is required.
> - Significant dental, electrolyte, or cardiovascular abnormalities occur.
> - Hospitalization is required.

Annotated bibliography

Cummings MM et al. (2001) Developing and implementing a comprehensive program for children and adolescents with eating disorders. *J Child Adoles Psychiatric Nursing*, 14:167–178.
This paper outlines in detail a comprehensive continuum of care treatment program for children and adolescents with eating disorders.

Epstein LH, Roemmich JN, Raynor HA (2001) Behavioral therapy in the treatment of pediatric obesity. *Ped Clin North America* 48:981–993.
This paper describes the elements and implementation of behavioral treatment for obesity in children and adolescents.

Fairburn CG, Harrison PJ (2003) Eating disorders. *Lancet*, 36:407–416.
This paper provides a comprehensive review and synthesis of the literature upon which the treatment of anorexia nervosa and other eating disorders is based.

Fairburn CG, Marcus MD, Wilson GT (1993) Cognitive-behavioral therapy for binge eating and bulimia nervosa: a comprehensive treatment manual. In: Fairburn CG, Wilson GT (eds) *Binge Eating*. New York, Guilford Press.
This chapter is a complete, step-by-step cognitive-behavioral treatment manual for bulimia nervosa.

Lock J et al. (2001) *Treatment Manual for Anorexia Nervosa. A Family-based Approach*. New York, Guilford Press.
This book provides a step-by-step family-based anorexia nervosa treatment program that the physician can use to guide parents to successfully treat their adolescent on an outpatient basis.

Mehler PS (2003b) Bulimia nervosa. *New Engl J Med*, 349:875–881.
This is a comprehensive review of diagnostic and treatment issues, including medication, for bulimia nervosa.

effective preventive measures before the condition reaches this level of morbidity and mortality.

CHAPTER 12

Psychotic Disorders

Karen M. Hochman, MD and Elaine F. Walker, PhD

Introduction

Psychosis involves impairment in a person's perception of reality. This problem can be manifested by abnormal sensory perceptions (hallucinations), thought abnormalities (including disorders of thought content or process), and behavioral disturbances (including catatonia and disorganized behavior). The first challenge for the physician is to determine whether the symptoms present are normative, whether they represent a psychiatric condition, or whether they are a manifestation of specific general medical condition or the physiologic effects of a substance. Psychotic symptoms may be part of a psychiatric condition, such as schizophrenia, mood disorders, and substance-induced psychotic disorders. In addition, children and young people may experience psychotic symptoms associated with anxiety, conduct, and evolving personality disorders. The most commonly used diagnosis for children and young people with true psychotic symptoms is "psychotic disorder not otherwise specified." Symptoms often evolve as the child matures, and may not fit into a particular diagnostic category upon initial presentation.

Although estimates of the prevalence of psychotic symptoms and disorders in childhood vary, there is general consensus that they are uncommon (Volkmar, 1996). Psychotic disorders are extremely rare in children under the age of 10. A Swedish study of first admission rates for various psychotic disorders including schizophrenia, schizophreniform disorder, atypical psychosis, affective psychosis, and substance-induced psychosis reported prevalence rates of 1.8 per 10,000 in children under the age of 13 years, and 17.6 per 10,000 at age 18 years (Gilberg et al., 1986, reviewed in Hafner and Nowotny, 1995). It is apparent that as development progresses, there is a steady increase in the risk of developing psychotic symptoms. This developmental trend is especially pronounced for males (Galdos and van Os, 1995).

In this chapter, we review the current state of knowledge of childhood psychotic disorders. Our discussion will focus on childhood manifestations of the key symptoms of psychosis, with an emphasis on developmental changes in presentation. We then turn to a discussion of treatment strategies. Most of the clinical trials of standard treatments for psychotic disorders have been conducted with adult patients. Thus, the data on treatment of psychotic children are limited. Nonetheless, the available findings indicate that multiple treatment modalities are often needed and generally include pharmacotherapy, psychoeducation for the child and family, supportive therapy for the child and family, educational modifications, and rehabilitative programming.

Background

The diagnostic boundaries for childhood psychoses have changed dramatically over the years (Volkmar, 1996). Prior to the publication of DSM-III in 1980, virtually all serious childhood disorders were viewed as a manifestation of schizophrenia. Even autism was included in the schizophrenia spectrum by some theorists. In fact, prior to the early seventies, infantile autism and childhood schizophrenia were referred to as "the childhood psychoses" or "childhood schizophrenia." Kolvin (1971a) was the first to establish that "infantile psychosis" can be distinguished from "late onset psychosis" in children on a statistical basis, based on differences in: age of onset, clinical features, social class, genetics, and evidence of cerebral dysfunction.

Studies by both Kolvin (1971b) and Rutter (1972) also highlighted the similarity between child and adult-onset schizophrenia. As a result of this landmark research, since DSM-III (APA, 1980), infantile psychosis has been classified as autistic disorder, and the diagnosis of schizophrenia in children and adolescents has been made using the same diagnostic criteria as for adults. Further, the DSM-IV clearly

General medical conditions that can cause psychotic symptoms:

- Delirium.
- Acute substance intoxication (e.g. amphetamines, cocaine, phencyclidine, hallucinogens, solvents).
- Adverse effects of prescribed and over-the-counter medication (e.g. stimulants, corticosteriods, medication with strong anticholinergic effects, such as cold remedies).
- Other toxins such as heavy metals (e.g. lead or mercury).
- Substance withdrawal syndromes (alcohol, benzodiazepines, barbiturates).
- Central nervous system (CNS) anatomic defects.
- CNS tumors.
- CNS infections (encephalitis, meningitis, HIV related conditions).
- Autoimmune disorders (systemic lupus erythematosis).
- Endocrine disorders (thyrotoxicosis, Cushing's disease).
- Metabolic disorders.
- Epilepsy (especially originating from the temporal lobe).
- Degenerative diseases (such as Wilson's disease or juvenile Huntington's chorea).

How do psychotic patients differ from delirious patients?

- Chronically psychotic individuals are rarely disoriented.
- Psychotic patients do not tend to complain of feeling confused.
- Manic excitement rarely lapses into somnolence as delirium can, and depressive stupor is more stable than a lapsing level of consciousness.
- Psychotic speech is characterized by a thread of coherence in contrast to the distractibility of delirium.
- Speech abnormalities in psychotic individuals involve neologisms or idiosyncratic use of language, in contrast to the dysarthric speech often evident in delirium.
- Psychotic patients hallucinate rather than misperceive.

(adapted from Kobayashi, JS, 2001)

confusion fluctuate over the course of a day, frequently with increasing confusion in the early evening (this phenomenon is referred to as "sundowning"). Delirium is often accompanied by perceptual disturbances such as illusions, misperceptions, and a predominance of visual hallucinations. The patient may exhibit an extremely labile emotional state (Kobayashi, 2001).

Substance abuse

It is very common for the adolescent presenting with psychotic symptoms to have a substance abuse history. In adolescents presenting with psychosis, a substance-induced psychotic disorder (Table 12.2, modified by DSM-IV criteria) should be considered, although frequently the substance abuse acts as a trigger or exacerbating factor rather than as a primary etiologic agent (Eisner and McClellan, 1998, referenced in AACAP, 2001). For additional information on substance abuse, see Chapter 14.

Co-occurring substance use

Rates of substance use in children with psychiatric disorders, especially adolescents, tend to be significantly higher than the general population. Some studies report the rate of comorbid substance abuse in adolescents with schizophrenia to be as high as 50% (AACAP, 2001). The "epidemiologic catchment area" (ECA) study found that 47% of adult pa-

tients with schizophrenia experience serious problems with drug or alcohol use, compared with only 16% of the general population. (Mueser et al., 1990). Cannabis use disorders are reported in more than 50% of first episode patients (Green et al., 2003). Rates of nicotine use in schizophrenia patients have been reported to range from 58–90% (Hughes et al., 1986).

Table 12.2 Substance-induced psychotic disorder

Discriminating features

1. Prominent hallucinations or delusions.
2. Evidence from the history, physical exam or lab findings that the symptoms developed during or within a month of substance intoxication or withdrawal.

Consistent features

1. The person has no insight that the symptoms are substance-induced.
2. Medication or substance use is thought to be the cause of the disturbance.

Variable features

1. Symptoms onset did not precede the use of the substance(s).
2. No symptoms during extended periods of sobriety.
3. No evidence of another non-substance-induced psychotic disorder.
4. Symptoms not in excess of what one would expect given the type and amount of substance used.
5. Symptoms don't last more than a month after substance use or withdrawal ends.

It is reasonable to assume that co-occurring substance use disorders carry with them an increased risk of negative outcome in adolescents with psychotic disorders. There is evidence in the adult literature that the use of alcohol and street drugs in persons with severe mental illness is associated with all of the following: poorer response to typical antipsychotic medication, greater treatment non-compliance, increased rates of psychiatric hospitalization, greater risk of homelessness, family problems, unemployment, incarceration, and higher rates of infection with HIV, Hepatitis B and C. (Green et al., 2003).

Mood disorders

Both schizophrenia and psychotic mood disorders tend to present with a mixture of mood and psychotic symptoms. A positive family psychiatric history of mood or of schizophrenia spectrum disorders can be of assistance in generating a provisional diagnosis. However, it is worthwhile to keep in mind that some studies have shown an increased risk of depressive disorders in the family members of schizophrenic youth (Werry and McLellan, 1992, cited in AACAP, 2001).

Negative symptoms of schizophrenia can be mistaken for depression and vice versa. Mania in adolescents is frequently accompanied by severe psychotic symptoms including hallucinations, delusions (which may be mood incongruent or bizarre), and disorganized thinking. Historically, over half of adolescents with an eventual diagnosis of bipolar disorder were originally diagnosed with schizophrenia (AACAP, 1997). The recommended best practice is to follow the patient over time, and reconsider the diagnosis if the child does not respond to treatment and/or if the clinical presentation alters over time (see Chapter 10 for mood disorders).

Schizotypal personality disorder (SPD)

Diagnostic criteria for SPD are the same for children as for adults. It is notable that schizotypal personality disorder (together with schizophrenia and other non-affective psychotic disorders) is over-represented in first-degree relatives of EOS patients. In some cases, SPD precedes the onset of acute psychotic symptoms in children and adolescents. Schizotypal personality disorder is marked by a pervasive pattern of social and interpersonal deficits, discomfort with and reduced capacity for close relationships, cognitive and perceptual distortions, and eccentric behavior. There are frequently: odd beliefs and magical thinking, suspiciousness or paranoia, unusual perceptual experiences, odd thinking and speech, unusual behavior, and constricted or inappropriate affect (APA, 2000). Individuals diagnosed with SPD have never experienced a period of persistent psychotic symptoms, unlike the children and adolescents who meet diagnostic criteria for

schizophrenia. The DSM-IV-TR specifies that the disorder must have begun by early adulthood and cautions against making personality disorder diagnoses before the age of 18.

Recently published findings by Westin et al. (2003) suggest that personality pathology in adolescents resembles that in adults and can be reliably diagnosed in adolescents age 14–18 years. However, the authors suggest that adult diagnostic criteria may not be the optimal way to diagnose these disorders in adolescents. It is recommended that data from adolescent studies be used to develop a classification system for personality pathology in adolescents.

Obsessive-compulsive disorder (OCD)

Children with OCD (see Chapter 9) suffer from intrusive thoughts, ideas or images. They frequently perform mental or behavioral rituals in response to their intrusive thoughts, and in accordance with rigidly applied rules. The compulsive mental acts or behaviors are aimed at reducing distress or preventing a dreaded event or situation. OCD can be difficult to differentiate from psychosis when the child or adolescent does not recognize that the obsessions or compulsions are excessive or unreasonable. Intact reality testing is usually present in adult patients with OCD, but is sometimes absent in young children (AACAP, 1998). Fortunately, most young people suffering from OCD can describe their symptoms in a way that helps to differentiate the obsessive thoughts, ideas, and images from true hallucinations, and delusions. Generally, obsessive thinking is recognized as a product of one's own mind and the experience is ego-dystonic (or emotionally uncomfortable). In contrast, reality testing is absent with true hallucinations and the young person believes the experience to be externally generated and real. Sometimes the bizarre, stereotyped behavior of schizophrenia can appear similar to the rituals of OCD. Generally, the schizophrenic individuals themselves do not recognize the delusions and odd behaviors as either excessive or unrealistic. Both diagnoses should be given when the two disorders co-occur.

Pervasive developmental disorder (PDD)/autism

The pervasive developmental disorders (see Chapter 5) are characterized primarily by: abnormal social relatedness, impaired communication/language development, impaired symbolic play, and a narrow range of interests with onset before 3 years of age. There is often no or limited normal developmental period preceding the onset of the disorder (unlike most cases of EOS and VEOS). Individuals with a PDD are given the additional diagnosis of schizophrenia only when pronounced hallucinations or delusions develop (usually in adolescence) and last for at least 1 month.

Psychologic factors involved in disorders

A 14-year-old male is hospitalized after having a seizure during which his mother states that he started jerking, lost consciousness, and fell to the floor. Further history reveals that he has had a number of these episodes, was started on an anti-convulsant by his pediatrician several weeks ago, and has not been attending school.

Somatoform disorders (conversion disorder)

- Medical work-up is negative.
- Observation reveals that the seizures do not fit typical patterns.
- Additional history reveals that the episodes started when the patient was having problems with his peers at school; now they occur only when the family attempts to get the patient back to school, and also the patient's uncle has epilepsy.
- The patient reports considerable distress but does not appear upset.
- Patient has a seizure when told he is going back to school.

Psychologic factors affecting a medical condition

- EEG reveals seizure activity, serum anti-convulsant level is non-therapeutic.
- When confronted, patient admits that he does not take his medication consistently.
- Further history reveals that patient believes that medication is not helpful and that all individuals with seizures end up being very ill and non-functional adults regardless of interventions.

Factitious disorder (by proxy)

- Medical work-up is negative.
- Patient's mother expresses considerable concern, seems very knowledgeable about medical issues, maintains that patient is very ill, is insistent on extensive medical testing and procedures but does not seem as distressed as would be expected.
- Seizures are witnessed only by patient's mother; when mother absent, patient has no seizures and has no significant complaints.
- Upon video observation of the patient's room, mother is noted to tell nursing staff that patient had a seizure and needs medication when patient had not had any abnormal behaviour.

Malingering

- Medical work-up is negative.
- Observation reveals that the seizures do not fit typical patterns.
- When patient thinks he is not being observed, he is bright and interactive with visitors.
- Further history reveals that patient has been arrested and charged in connection with a stolen car. The seizures started when the patient was informed of his court date, and that if convicted he might be imprisoned.
- When told that he still had to attend court and reminded of the potential serious side-effects of medication, patient admitted that he was pretending to have seizures so that he would not have to go to jail.

disorders represent one end of a spectrum of symptoms and behaviors that, depending on the developmental level of the child or the situation, may be considered normal variants of the behaviors of children and adolescents. Children frequently complain of somatic symptoms, often clearly related to emotional or psychologic stresses or misinterpretation of normal bodily phenomena. Part of normal development is learning to identify emotional responses and issues and express them verbally rather than physically. Additionally, frequently children and adolescents deliberately feign (sometimes overtly produce) symptoms to falsify the sick role or obtain some benefit such as not going to school. However, these behaviors usually are not persistent, significant, and do not involve the medical system (APA, 1994; AAP, 1996; Fritz et al., 1997; Fritz and Campo, 2002).

- Medical assessments should be thorough but reasonable, with care taken to provide ongoing monitoring to provide reassurance and ensure medical problems are not missed.
- These patients are in considerable distress and have "real" disorders which can be diagnosed and treated.
- Distinguishing between these disorders can be challenging and may involve serial assessments and information from multiple informants.
- Providers should monitor and deal with their negative reactions to minimize impact on patient care.
- Psychiatric involvement is beneficial but needs to be carefully approached and implemented in collaboration with ongoing medical assessment.
- Treatment planning should include immediate, short and long-range goals.
- Collaboration and integration of care among disciplines, providers, and institutions is essential.

conversion disorders being most common. Only one case met the criteria for hypochondriasis. A number of these individuals had other psychiatric disorders (Taylor and Garralda, 2003). A study by Campo et al. (1999) of somatizers in a pediatric practice found that these young people were at risk for psychiatric disorders, family dysfunction, functional impairment, and frequent use of health services.

For all of these disorders, the affected individual must meet criteria of severity and distress or impairment. These

Somatoform disorders

Somatoform disorders share the characteristic of having physical symptoms and a degree of impairment, which cannot be explained by a medical condition (Table 13.1). The diagnostic criteria have been established based on adult data, and are used for children and adolescents due to the lack of a child-based research or a developmentally oriented assessment classification. Much of the research has been designed around the presenting, physical symptoms rather than the specific somatoform disorders. Clinician training and experience have been shown to influence the diagnosis, with more experienced practitioners being more accurate. Studies have not been done on the reliability or validity of these diagnoses. Complicating the issue further is the considerable debate about whether certain conditions (i.e. chronic fatigue syndrome, fibromyalgia) are medical conditions or somatoform disorders. Some theorists believe that some of these somatic disorders are better conceptualized as personality disorders. However, many child and adolescent practitioners consider character traits as developing and tend not to identify these behaviors as persistent and fixed. The data suggest that unexplained physical symptoms in childhood predict emotional disorders in adults, though definitive longitudinal studies have not been done. Most of the studies have examined the presence or absence of a physical symptom rather than functional or psychiatric status (APA, 1994; AAP, 1996; Fritz et al., 1997; Fritz and Campo, 2002).

DIAGNOSIS

Table 13.1 Somatoform disorders

Discriminating features

1. Symptom or deficit is not intentionally produced or feigned (malingering or factitious disorder).

Consistent features

1. Significant physical symptoms causing clinically significant impairment or distress in social, occupational, or other important areas of functioning.
2. Symptom or deficit cannot be explained by a known medical condition, direct effects of a substance or is excessive for what is expected from the history, physical examination, or laboratory findings.

Variable features

1. Psychologic factors considered to have an important role in the onset, severity, exacerbation, or maintenance of symptoms.
2. Duration of symptoms (length of time present).
3. Types of symptoms (body system involvement).
4. Requirement that medical treatment be sought out or obtained.
5. Various disorders with own specific criteria.

Conversion disorder

Individuals with conversion disorder have unexplainable deficits or symptoms affecting sensory or voluntary motor function, suggesting a neurologic or other medical condition, which appears to be significantly associated with a psychologic stressor (Box 13.2). There are four subtypes based on whether the symptoms are primarily motor, sensory, non-epileptic seizures, or mixed. Presenting symptoms follow the stressor and may cause more distress among the parents and medical personnel than in the patient. However, *la belle indifférence* (lack of concern by patient) often reported in adults is not always seen in children and adolescents. Frequent symptoms in children and adolescents include non-epileptic seizures, apparent paresis, anesthesia, and gait disturbances. They usually are self-limited, but may be associated with iatrogenic injury if symptoms persist and if there is extensive medical interventions (APA, 1994; AAP, 1996; Fritz et al., 1997; Fritz and Campo, 2002).

Conversion disorder appears to be more common in girls, across all age groups. It most commonly presents in school-age children and adolescents. It is unusual in very young children. There has been a variable association reported with prior medically identifiable illness or injury (10–60%). Psychiatric comorbidity has been inadequately studied. Studies of adults have found high rates of other psychiatric disorders. Case studies of children and adults suggest that often their symptoms mimic those of involved family or a friend with a medical illness. The course is thought to be brief and most resolve within 3 months of diagnosis. The time to diagnosis can be lengthy. Reoccurrence is thought to be unlikely. Family factors seem to have a major role in the expression and maintenance of illness. These families have been identified as having one of two patterns: anxious and preoccupied with disease, and disorganized and chaotic (APA, 1994; AAP, 1996; Fritz et al., 1997; Fritz and Campo, 2002).

BOX 13.2

Conversion disorder

1 One or more symptoms affecting sensory or voluntary motor function that suggests a neurologic or other medical disorder.
2 Psychologic factors are associated with initiation or exacerbation of symptoms because conflict or stressors precede symptoms.
3 Symptoms not limited to pain or sexual dysfunction.
4 Does not occur during the course of somatization disorder.
5 Not better accounted for by another mental disorder.
6 Subtypes of motor, sensory, seizures, mixed.

Somatization disorder

The diagnostic criteria for this disorder are more appropriate for adults and involve having symptoms related to a number of bodily systems over a number of years (Box 13.3). Generally, children and adolescents do not have the duration or variability of symptoms to have somatization disorder, though they may meet the criteria for undifferentiated somatoform disorder (one or more symptoms, duration at least 6 months). Adults with somatization disorder often have the onset of their symptoms in adolescence. However, recurrent somatic complaints are common in pediatric practice, and there may be a higher prevalence rate if a more appropriate set of diagnostic criteria were developed. Several population studies have found a high rate of somatic complaints in children and adolescents. Prepubertal children report recurrent abdominal pain and headaches the most. With age, complaints of limb pain, aching muscles, fatigue, and neurologic symptoms increase. Polysymptomatic presentations may increase with age. Girls report neurologic symptoms most often at all ages. Recurrent pain complaints are equal in boys and girls until after puberty when girls predominate. Family members tend to share the same complaints as the children. Families of somatizing children tended to have more psychiatric symptoms in the parents, family histories of anxiety, depression, and personality disorders, members with chronic physical illnesses, more use of illness as stress reduction, more substance abuse, and more dysfunction than controls. Children and adolescents who have been sexually abused tend to be more somatic. Adults with this disorder have childhood histories of illness with a lack of parental care (APA, 1994; AAP, 1996; Fritz et al., 1997; Fritz and Campo, 2002).

Hypochondriasis

Individuals with hypochondrias misinterpret usual bodily symptoms and develop a persistent, preoccupying fear of having a serious disease despite appropriate medical intervention (Box 13.4). This disorder has not been systemati-

> **BOX 13.4**
>
> ## Hypochondriasis
>
> 1 Misinterpretation of bodily symptoms, causing fears or the idea that one has a serious disease.
> 2 Preoccupation persists despite appropriate medical evaluation.
> 3 Belief not delusional or confined to circumscribed concern about appearance.
> 4 Duration at least 6 months.
> 5 Not better accounted for by generalized anxiety disorder, obsessive compulsive disorder, panic disorder, major depressive episode, separation anxiety, or another somatoform disorder.
> 6 May specify if with poor insight.

cally studied in children and adolescents, and there are no epidemiological data. Unless parents of hypochondriacal children and adolescents are concerned about their child's illnesses, they tend not to abuse medical care. A proxy form has been described where caretakers excessively worry over their children with normal phenomena or minor symptoms. In adults, there has been overlap with obsessive-compulsive disorder and depression. Adults with this disorder are dissatisfied with their medical care and risk harm from unnecessary or excessive medical interventions (APA, 1994; AAP, 1996; Fritz et al., 1997; Fritz and Campo, 2002).

Pain disorder

Pain disorder also has not been systematically studied in children and adolescents. Affected individuals have pain in one or more sites with a significant association of psychologic factors (Box 13.5). An initial physical disorder, such as a sports-related injury may evolve into a pain disorder (Wells, 1996). Given the subjective nature of pain assessment and the limited ability of many children and adolescents to accurately report their pain, these syndromes may be difficult to diagnose and thus under-recognized. Family influences have not been well studied, though there are some

> **BOX 13.3**
>
> ## Somatization disorder
>
> 1 History of physical complaints beginning before age 30.
> 2 Occurs over a period of years with variable physical symptoms.
> 3 Must have history of pain related to at least four different sites or functions.
> 4 Two gastrointestinal symptoms other than pain.
> 5 One sexual or reproductive symptom other than pain.
> 6 One pseudoneurological symptom not limited to pain.

> **BOX 13.5**
>
> ## Pain disorder
>
> 1 Pain in one or more anatomic sites is the predominant focus and warrants clinical attention.
> 2 Psychologic factors have important role in onset, severity, exacerbation, or maintenance.
> 3 Not better accounted for by a mood, anxiety, or psychotic disorder.
> 4 Does not meet criteria for dyspareunia.
> 5 Subtypes:
>   - Associated with psychologic factors.
>   - Associated with both psychologic and a general medical condition.
>   - Acute or chronic.

data that suggests that children with unexplained pain had more family members with problems with pain than those with identified organic causes of their pain. Children who miss school due to pain syndromes may have more maternal reinforcement (APA, 1994; AAP, 1996; Fritz et al., 1997; Fritz and Campo, 2002). Campo et al. (1999) found that recurrent pain complaints by children in a primary care setting were associated with increased risk of psychopathology, functional impairment, family difficulties, and higher health and mental health service use.

Body dysmorphic disorder

There has been no systemic study of body dysmorphic disorder (BDD) in children and adolescents, though there are some data that indicate that the onset for many individuals occurs in adolescence. The literature describes a number of case reports. Some have suggested that BDD may be related to obsessive-compulsive disorder. People with this disorder have a preoccupation with a non-existent or slight defect in appearance that causes clinically significant distress or functional impairment. Normal adolescence involves concern about appearance, but not this level of impairment or distress. Affected individuals are shamed and secretive, so they may not volunteer symptoms. The face is the most commonly involved area of the body. Adults often seek treatment through plastic surgery. The non-delusional form (insight is present) is classified as a somatoform disorder and a delusional form is classified as a psychotic disorder. There is some evidence that both forms are the same disorder, with the delusional variant being more severe. Insight can be difficult to assess in children and adolescents (APA, 1994; AAP, 1996; Albertini and Phillips, 1999; Phillips, 2000; Fritz and Campo, 2002). Symptoms in young people appear to be similar to those of adults. Albertini and Phillips (1999) found in their review that bodily preoccupations most frequently centered on skin and hair, and all subjects reported associated obsessive behavior including camouflaging with clothing, comparing with others, and mirror checking. Most reported impaired social and academic or job functioning and significant distress. A number had dropped out of school, been hospitalized, or made suicide attempts.

Psychologic factors affecting a medical condition

The underlying premise of this disorder is that the severity or exacerbation of the physical symptoms is related to psychologic rather than organic factors in individuals with general medical conditions. There is limited systematic information on these disorders. Most of the literature on this disorder has been focused on describing problems experienced by individuals with a particular medical condition (i.e. diabetes mellitus, asthma). In the past, it was thought that specific psychologic conflicts or personality styles were expressed through particular physical symptoms. Currently, it is believed that psychologic and organic factors can interact to influence the manifestations of a medical condition. Several possible mechanisms have been described. Physically ill young people may engage in behaviors which predispose them to worsening symptoms. Behaviors that may be relevant include activities that may make the individual more vulnerable to disease episodes such as smoking by asthmatics, over or undereating by diabetics. Psychologic factors also may precipitate illness or increase recurrence. For example, stress has been associated with poor short-term and long-term measures of glucose control as well as asthma attacks and dermatitis flare-ups. Psychologic factors may sustain illness by decreasing adherence resulting in significant symptoms and increased morbidity. It also is possible that when psychologic and physical factors have common biologic mechanisms they may act synergistically. For example, cholinergic pathways have been identified as important in both asthma and affective disorders (Rubinstein, 1988; Brown et al., 2003).

Factitious disorder/factitious disorder by proxy

Factitious disorder, also termed Munchausen syndrome, has been described in the pediatric literature, though more attention has been devoted to the proxy form. In this disorder, the individual is deliberately feigning or producing symptoms for the emotional benefits associated with being ill (Table 13.2). In factitious disorder, the motivating factors tend to be more complex and less conscious than secondary material gains. The principal goal is satisfaction of emotional needs through being in the sick role. Generally, there has to be a persistent pattern of fabrication for these diagnoses to be considered (APA, 1994; Forsyth, 2002).

DIAGNOSIS

Table 13.2 Factitious disorder (Munchausen syndrome)

Discriminating features

1. Motivation for the behavior is to assume the sick role (indirectly if by proxy).
2. External incentives for the behavior are absent.

Consistent features

1. Intentional production or feigning of signs or symptoms (physical or psychologic).

Variable features

1. May involve a caretaker producing symptoms in another individual responsible for factitious disorder by proxy (factitious disorder not otherwise specified).

There is little research and information on factitious disorders in children and adolescents. A recent literature review on factitious disorders in youth over the past 30 years identified 42 cases with patients ranging from 8 to 18 years old. The majority of children were female, especially those above 15 years of age. The medical conditions most frequently reported were fevers, ketoacidosis, purpura, and infections. The deceptions ranged from claiming false symptoms to active injections, bruising, and ingestions. The mean duration of falsifications was almost 16 months (range of single incidents to 5 years) before discovery. For those with available data, all of the younger children (14 years old and younger) admitted or did not deny their behavior when confronted, whereas only 55% of the older patients did. The involved youths were described as bland, flat, and indifferent. They also were identified as being depressed, socially isolated, and often obese. Additional diagnoses included dysthymia, oppositional defiant disorder, adjustment disorder, anorexia nervosa, passive dependent personality, and hysterical personality. Many of them appeared to have begun fabricating illness after an experience with the medical establishment through illness. Several expressed an interest in medical careers and one worked part-time in a medical office. A number of patients were described as having enmeshed relationships with their parents or significant family psychiatric histories. Some had parents in medical fields or who were caring for disabled children. Generally, the deceptions of the younger children were more blatant, more readily acknowledged when confronted, and were more likely to resolve. The older adolescents had more complex activities, were more likely to deny even in the context of concrete evidence, and many fled the involved institutions with their families. While these cases were ones with no identified parental involvement, the extent of parental collusion or potential for earlier behavior consistent with factitious disorder by proxy was unclear. The patients and families tended to be lost to follow-up and to reject recommendations for psychiatric interventions (Libow, 2000), though a limited study by Stutts and Hickson (1999) of six cases found that four followed through with a psychiatric referral, including two who had denied fabricating their disease symptoms.

In the proxy form, a caretaker of an individual is producing or falsely reporting symptoms in that individual. It is considered a medically focused type of child abuse. Recently, the American Professional Society on the Abuse of Children published guidelines for dealing with definitional issues in proxy situations. Two separate elements would be distinguished: the child abuse and the psychiatric disorder affecting the perpetrator. The illness of the child would be described as pediatric condition falsification. The caretaker motivation for producing the child's condition would then be assessed, looking for the dynamics of factitious disorder. Factitious disorder by proxy would be a psychiatric description of the caregiver that attributes certain psychologic mo-

tives for this kind of child abuse. The caretaker's emotional gratification can be through assuming the vicarious sick role, enhancing self-identity by acting as a selfless caregiver, or maintaining a relationship with a professional, usually a physician where the caretaker controls the doctor's attention, admiration, and involvement. Additional evaluation would include examining the role of the child, whether he or she was passively or actively involved in the deception. Caretakers who had other motivations for their behavior (i.e. misinterpretation of symptoms, excessive anxiety, psychosis) would not be considered to have factitious disorder by proxy (Ayoub et al., 2002). Rosenberg (2003) additionally has proposed criteria for definitive and possible diagnosis of factitious disorders by proxy by either exclusion or inclusion.

Common presentations in factitious disorder by proxy include gastrointestinal, neurologic, infectious, dermatologic, and cardiopulmonary symptoms. Younger children are more likely to be victims. Pediatrics has developed algorithms to help with some of these presentations; for example, distinguishing apnea from suffocation. There is considerable need to develop additional clinical algorithms to help differentiate actual illness from simulated ones. Due to the difficulty of obtaining information on families involved with factitious disorder by proxy, little systematic data are available. The perpetrator appears concerned and caring. Often, there is a history of prior exposure to the health system from previous care, training, or employment. They initially are considered model parents and have close, friendly relationships with the medical providers. The caretakers frequently are described as not appearing adequately upset or distressed when discussing the child's health problems and suffering. There is significant comorbidity, with a number of children having histories of failure to thrive, accidental injuries, or neglect. There is some information that indicates that they may share some characteristics of families with victims of other types of abuse. Some of the families have been described as having diffuse boundaries among members, overly rigid boundaries with the outside world, parental entitlement, and intergenerational histories of domination or abuse of children by adults. They also demonstrate significant family histories of somatoform disorders and preoccupation with illness. The majority of perpetrators are mothers, though in many cases the father also is in the home. Fathers often are viewed as absent or passive in terms of their parenting. When the fathers are the perpetrators, they generally are described as difficult, demanding, and overbearing by hospital staff. The perpetrators often fabricate about other areas of their lives. The psychopathology of the mother may be related to the experience of abuse or rejection in childhood, a pathologic relationship with her child, and rewards through the health system. Assessments of the mothers have revealed significant histories of self-harm, drug abuse, factitious disorders, and personality disorders. However, a number of the mothers have appeared to have no notable psychiatric problems. The recidivism rate of mothers with factitious disorder by proxy is very high. Literature describing the children is scant (Forsyth, 2002; Sheridan, 2003).

Sheridan (2003) described a recent literature review of factitious disorder by proxy, with children as the victims. She identified 451 cases in 154 journal articles published between 1972 and 1999. Of the cases described, approximately equal number of boys and girls were affected. A minority of the cases had their race identified and the majority was Caucasian. Three-quarters of the cases were diagnosed before age 6. The duration from initiation of symptoms to discovery averaged almost 2 years. For approximately 60% of the cases, the symptoms appeared to be actively produced, with almost 50% of the cases having episodes while the child was hospitalized. The most frequent methods were suffocation, drug administration, and poisoning. The most frequent problems were apnea, anorexia/feeding problems, diarrhea, seizures, cyanosis, behavior, asthma, allergy, fever, and pain. All victims appeared to suffer short-term harm, with approximately 7% with long-term or permanent disability, and 6% were dead, with an average age of death of 18.83 months (range 1.5–96 months). The most common cause of death was apnea. The child was placed out of the perpetrator's care in about one-third of the cases. There were 210 siblings, of whom 25% were dead and approximately 60% had similar or suspicious symptoms to those of the identified victim. The perpetrators were much more likely to be mothers, with almost equal numbers of boy and girl victims. In the instances in which the father was the perpetrator, the victim was three times more likely to be a boy. Employment or training in a health-related profession was described in almost 30%, with a similar percentage having features characteristic of factitious disorder. Twenty-three per cent had a psychiatric diagnosis, most commonly depression or some type of personality disorder. Almost 22% reported a history of abuse (childhood or domestic). Confirmation of the diagnosis included symptom resolution with separation from the caretaker, video confirmation, and admission by the perpetrators (11%).

Consequences of factitious disorder and factitious disorder by proxy can include multiple medical providers, unnecessary medical interventions, probable short- and long-term morbidity and potential mortality, psychologic symptoms, psychiatric disorders, social impairment, and educational deficits. Older children and adolescents may collude actively with their caretakers. Morbidity and mortality can occur through the caretaker's actions or the physician's interventions (Forsyth, 2002). In many of these cases, the involved medical providers and health systems had a significant role in perpetuating the problem. Often, these children and their families had numerous providers in different medical systems that had limited or no communication with each other. These children received mul-

tiple work-ups and interventions, even though there were a number of signs that should have raised suspicion such as symptoms inconsistent with generally accepted medical disorders, symptoms consistent with extremely rare or unusual diseases, no improvement despite usually successful treatments, and parents who gave false histories. Some of the involved professionals, physicians, and others refused to believe that the caretakers had factitious disorder by proxy and actively attempted to protect them. Additionally, concerns about legal system involvement often complicated making the diagnosis and intervening, as did the reactions of the health-care professionals (von Hahn et al., 2001; Forsyth, 2002; Sheridan, 2003).

The outcome of factitious disorder by proxy has been described as variable depending on severity of the symptoms and the treatment provided. A significant minority of the children died or had permanent disability. Several studies describe some of the children as continuing to fabricate medical illness. A number had ongoing psychologic problems such as somatic complaints, emotional disorders, conduct problems, and school problems. Over half of the children followed in one study were still with their biologic mothers. The outcome was better for children and families who participated in an intensive, inpatient program. However, these cases were selected based on the possibility of treatment responsiveness and may not be representative of most individuals with this disorder (McGuire and Feldman, 1989; Forsyth, 2002; Sheridan, 2003).

Given the rarity of these disorders and the probable multiple factors involved in their etiology and presentations, Eminson and Jureidini (2003) have suggested that research and possible interventions should be targeted at earlier stages in an attempt to prevent development of these problems. They identify potential targets such as vulnerable populations (i.e. parents with somatization histories, many unexplained symptoms during pregnancy, frequent or inconsistent utilization of medical centers with the identified or other child, or distorted perceptions about children's health). Another focus is the medical system (i.e. improvement of medical history taking, care coordination, and focus on psychosocial issues).

Malingering

Despite being a common consideration in the differential diagnosis of children and adolescents presenting with medically unexplainable symptoms, there is little literature or few data on malingering in youth in medical situations. Most studies examining children's ability to deceive have not been done in clinical settings. To meet the criteria for malingering, the child or adolescent must be deliberately lying about or producing the symptoms with the knowledge that they are not ill and with the objective of obtaining some benefit or avoiding some aversive situation (Table 13.3). The inducement is not related to the perceived benefits of being sick. Generally, malingers tend to feign symptoms rather than produce disease or injury (Williams and Hirsch, 1988; Oldershaw and Bagby, 1997).

A major consideration in considering this diagnosis is determining the child's abilities and intent to deceive. The children first must recognize that false statements can mislead others, and that they must convince others that the false statements are true. Also, to malinger, the child must understand the connection between the feigning of physical symptoms and obtaining the external incentive. Additionally, children and adolescents vary on their ability to identify and accurately label their physical and emotional states and may be misleading without deliberately lying. Malingering is a type of intentional deception, and as such does not include unintentional forms such as self-deception or psychologic defenses such as repression. Young people also are vulnerable to misunderstanding clinical questions due to their cognitive abilities and emotional states and often will not disclose their lack of understanding. Typically, youth improve in their ability to deceive and to accurately identify their psychologic and physical states as they mature. Such developmental factors mean that malingering probably is most likely in older school-aged children and adolescents. However, as with all clinical issues with children and adolescents, it is important to consider their environmental context and influences, particularly the knowledge and involvement of their caretakers (Wells, 1996; Oldershaw and Bagby, 1997). There are case reports in the literature involving parents instructing their children to malinger (malingering by proxy) for financial and other reasons (Cassar et al., 1996; Roberts, 1997; Stutts et al., 2003).

Table 13.3 Malingering

Discriminating features

1. Motivated by external incentives such as avoiding school or work, obtaining financial compensation, evading criminal prosecution, or obtaining drugs.

Consistent features

1. Intentional production or feigning of signs or symptoms (physical or psychologic).
2. Marked discrepancy between claimed distress or disability and objective findings.

Variable features

1. Involved in the legal system.
2. Lack of cooperation during diagnostic evaluation and in complying with treatment.
3. Conduct disorder or anti-social behavior.

Not much is known about the consequences of malingering or malingering by proxy. Before discovery, the risks include unwarranted medical procedures and treatments, which may be problematic, either short or long term, causing unnecessary morbidity or mortality. Psychologic complications may include the incorporation of the sick role into the young person's self-identity, the use of multiple medical providers as well as the prevention of developing more adaptive skills to obtain rewards or cope with stresses. Additional negative consequences may include the critical and disapproving reactions of the treating professionals, which may impact clinical care.

Assessment

All of these disorders have persistent or medical symptoms that cannot be adequately explained by accepted medical illnesses. As part of the assessment, it is essential to carefully review the child's history, including information from previous providers whenever possible. Attempts should be made to distinguish between symptoms that appear to relate to organic disease and those that seem to be connected to psychologic issues or to be fabricated. Often, there are sustained discrepancies between the history, the physical exam, laboratory results, and the general appearance of the child. Support for the connection of psychologic or environmental factors can include: onset of symptoms after specific trauma or stress; disability or handicap out of proportion to reported symptoms; clear secondary gain; and exacerbations linked to stressful events. It is essential to obtain information on how all of the involved individuals (child, caretakers, involved family, school personnel, and others) understand the child's illness and treatment in terms of etiology, responsiveness, prognosis, and impact on functional abilities. These families often have become isolated and overly focused on the child's symptoms and illness. Generally, it is not helpful to convey any doubts that the medical team has about the nonorganic nature of the child's symptoms. If these individuals and families had the ability to identify their emotional needs and utilize appropriate coping strategies to manage them, they would not be complaining of physical symptoms and seeking medical interventions (Wells, 1996; Forsyth, 2002; Fritz and Campo, 2002).

Having a psychiatrist as part of the treatment team and involved early in the process can be helpful. Having the caretaker, child, and family evaluated by the psychiatrist may aid in the diagnostic process, especially in terms of trying to understand family relationships, psychologic attributions about the illness, contributing psychologic and environmental issues, and relevant psychosocial information. The psychiatric evaluation should be presented to the family as an integral aspect of the medical evaluation, since stress and chronic illness often are comorbid. It should focus on the physical problems and their impact with questions about psychologic and psychiatric functioning included in that framework. A psychiatric evaluation of the caretakers can be helpful in elucidating their attributions about the illness, relationships to the child, and special aspects of their connections to the health system as well as information about their backgrounds, emotional functioning, and additional possible medical and other fabrications. The psychiatrist also can assess the child and family to provide information on their functioning, level of distress, and potential sources of support. Children of school age and older should be seen individually with an emphasis on exploring their understanding of their illness and psychologic functioning. Clinical interviewers should emphasize open-ended questions, but evaluations particularly with the children also may require multiple narrower questions, which cover all likely possibilities. Observations of the child's and family's behavior and interactions in medical settings should be considered as well as information from other involved agencies or institutions such as schools, child protective services, or the juvenile justice system. Attempting to maintain a therapeutic alliance with the child and caretaker is optimal so that adequate care can be provided and to minimize the patient and family going to new health providers (Forsyth, 2002; Fritz and Campo, 2002).

These disorders are diagnosed using a psychiatric classification system, either the DSM-IV or ICD-10. Somatoform disorders and factitious disorders are considered clinical disorders and are placed on axis I in the DSM multi-axial classification. Psychologic factors affecting a medical condition and malingering are defined as other conditions that may be a focus of clinical attention. They also are on axis I. Medical conditions are coded on axis III (APA, 1994). To help primary practitioners with diagnosing psychiatric disorders, there is a DSM version designed for pediatrics (DSM-PC). The DSM-PC organizes symptoms into developmental variations, problems, and disorders. There are examples given in each division for various age groups, describing possible presentations based on developmental considerations. The disorders section describes the DSM-IV criteria for the relevant psychiatric disorders. One section describes pain and somatic complaints, with the disorder section on somatoform disorders. Factitious disorders and malingering are included in the possible diagnoses to be considered. Another section discusses psychologic factors affecting medical conditions (AAP, 1996).

Somatoform disorders

Children and adolescents with disorders in this classification are not conscious that their physical symptoms are a manifestation of emotional conflict or issues. While the available literature suggests that missed medical conditions are unlikely, it is important to review the medical

---

KEY CLINICAL QUESTIONS

Somatoform disorders
Identification of possible psychologic or environmental factors:
- *What are your ideas about how you got this problem?*
- *Who else do you know with this type of problem?*
- *How has this problem interfered with your life? What aspects?*
- *How is your life different since you got ill? What can/can't you do?*
- *What happened right before you became ill?*

Body dysmorphic disorder
- *Is there some aspect/part of your appearance that you are very unhappy about?*

Psychologic factors affecting a medical condition
Possible reasons for treatment non-adherence:
- *What is your understanding of your disease and treatment?*
- *What happens to individuals with your disease?*
Identification of possible psychologic or environmental factors:
- *How has this problem interfered with your life? What aspects?*

Factitious disorder (by proxy) – questions for caretaker
Possible positive aspects about health care relationships:
- *What is good/bad about being in the hospital/your doctor/being ill?*
Possible previous exposure:
- *Who has been ill/connected to health-care professions?*
Data on whether understanding matches affect:
- *What is your understanding of this disease and treatment?*
- *What happens to individuals with this disease?*
Ability to be reassured, continued need for additional interventions:
- *What would you think if the team told you that this problem is not life-threatening and does not need any further medical interventions?*

Malingering
Possible external incentives:
- *How has this problem interfered with your life? What aspects?*
- *How is your life different since you got ill? What can/can't you do?*
- *What happened right before you became ill?*
- *How is school going? Are you in trouble with the court? I your family?*
- *How long do you think you are going to be ill/in the hospital?*

---

evaluation for adequacy. Involvement of the psychiatrist in the assessment needs to be done carefully. Often, both providers and families are more familiar and comfortable with physical disorders and feel stigmatized by the inclusion of psychiatry. These patients and families often feel misunderstood by their physicians and interpret psychiatric referral as abandonment. Continued participation by the medical team is essential. The diagnosis of these disorders should include the exclusion of organic causes as well as positive signs of psychologic factors. Suggested indicators of somatoform disorders include: temporal continuity of symptoms with significant psychologic stress; prior history of somatization; social or familial reinforcement of symptoms; model for symptoms within the family or environment; co-morbid psychiatric disorder; apparent communicative or symbolic meaning of the symptoms; violation of known anatomic or physiologic patterns by symptoms; and responsiveness of symptoms to placebo, suggestion, or psychologic treatment. Information from the school can be very helpful, since school avoidance due to learning or social problems can be integral components of the psychologic stress. Similarly, family dynamics and issues may be underlying factors, especially if there is a family model for disease or the child has separation fears. Exploring the family's understanding of and response to the child's symptoms is crucial to comprehending the factors maintaining and perpetrating the situation. Questions about concerns about appearance and body image should be asked to screen for body dysmorphic disorder (Phillips, 2000; Fritz and Campo, 2002).

Psychologic factors affecting general medical conditions

This set of disorders is diagnosed when children and adolescents with previously identified medical problems have persistent or recurrent symptoms related to their medical illness for which the underlying organic abnormality is not an adequate explanation for the frequency or severity. The symptoms appear to be temporally associated with psychologic issues or environmental events, to be related to behaviors, which increase the patient's vulnerability to illness, or to be the consequence of non-adherence to treatment recommendations. Non-adherence often has significant psychologic causes. It is essential to ensure that the patient and family have been adequately educated about the medical treatment, can understand the information, and that implementation is possible (i.e. adequate financial resources). Again, the psychiatrist should be presented as a part of the medical team, involved to provide consultation and possible complementary care to ongoing medical care. The assessment should focus on the medical illness and all of its parameters and ramifications with psychosocial information being asked about in that context (Rubinstein, 1988; Brown et al., 2003).

Factitious disorder/factitious disorder by proxy

Individuals with this disorder are aware of their actions and falsifications, but are seeking emotional gratification through their interactions with the health system and professionals. All of their behavior is geared towards engaging and maintaining involvement in the medical care. These disorders are difficult to assess and diagnose. They are not suspected for a long time and then providers often are discomforted by their suspicions, and verification is very challenging. Disbelief and disagreement among the medical providers can complicate the evaluation and management. Indications that this diagnosis should be considered include: the working medical diagnosis is a very rare condition or experienced clinicians have never seen such a case; symptoms only occur in the caretaker's presence; the mother is very involved with hospital staff, is always present and has an unusual affect when discussing her child's health; caretakers are resistant to reassurance about the child's health; usually successful treatments don't work; there have been multiple diagnoses and medical providers; increasingly invasive and unusual procedures; dead or unusually ill siblings; false information in other areas of the child's or family's histories; and caretakers with extensive histories of personal illnesses or past medical professional experience. Observation of the mother's behavior and habits can be helpful, as can laboratory testing (i.e. blood typing, toxic screens for family medicines, household products).

Additional interventions include monitoring symptoms by separating the child and caretaker, video surveillance, and observing through one-way mirrors. Searching the patient's room and caretaker's belonging also has been utilized. A number of these strategies may be difficult to employ due to ethical and legal considerations. It can be helpful to involve the hospital legal team when considering how to proceed. As much as possible, participating providers should attempt to maintain a positive alliance with the child and caretaker (Forsyth, 2002).

Malingering

Concerns about malingering arise when there appears to be some motivation for being ill that involves avoiding adverse situations (i.e. school) or obtaining some benefit (i.e. hospital gifts at Christmas) that the child is aware of and is pretending to be sick to achieve (Wells, 1996). During the assessment, providers should monitor any negative responses that they may have to the possibility of malingering and attempt to maintain a therapeutic relationship with the child and family. The young person is deliberately being deceitful, however, there are underlying psychologic issues and these individuals are troubled and in distress. Usually, it is essential to obtain information from others such as schools, extended family, and community agencies to confirm the potential secondary gains in addition to evaluation of the child and caretakers (Williams and Hirsch, 1988).

Differential diagnosis

Distinguishing between the disorders described above involves making decisions about the presence of an identifiable medical condition, the relationship of psychologic or environmental factors to the symptoms, the intent of the patient or caretaker, and their level of awareness (Fig. 13.1). The medical evaluation and monitoring should be reasonable and ongoing to ensure that organic causes of the symptoms are unlikely. Children and adolescents often have significant somatic symptoms as normal responses to experiences like bereavement. Generally, these symptoms are time limited. Typical presentations of a number of psychiatric disorders in children and adolescents include somatic complaints.

Depressive, anxiety, eating and psychotic disorders all can have significant physical symptoms but have other characteristic symptoms, which are prominent (APA, 1994; Fritz and Campo, 2002).

Treatment

Treatment approaches should be individualized for each unique patient. However, for most of these disorders, designing a treatment plan that includes coordination between medical providers, usually with the primary care physician as the coordinator and integration of a psychiatrist either as a provider or consultant. These patients and families are often reluctant to be in psychiatric care and it may have to

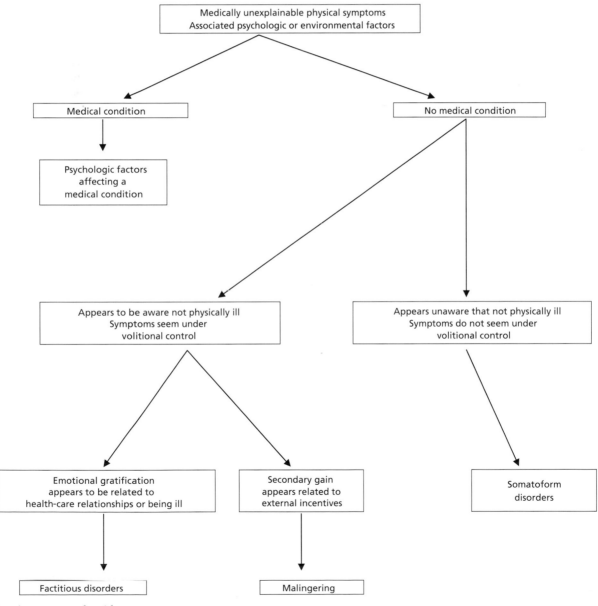

Fig. 13.1 Assessment algorithm.

be a long-term goal. It can be helpful to consider treatment in stages with having immediate, short-term, and long-term goals. Immediate goals can be cessation of inappropriate medical interventions, ensuring the safety of the child, engaging the family in treatment, and arranging ongoing care. Short-term goals can be preventing further unnecessary medical interventions, maintaining reasonable medical monitoring, symptom reduction, and steps to initiate age-appropriate activities. Long-term goals can be appropriate use of medical care, resolution of symptoms, development of appropriate coping skills to deal with psychologic and environmental issues, and resumption of age-appropriate activities. Often, other agencies such as the schools, child protective services, juvenile justice system, and other community institutions need to be involved (Forsyth, 2002; Fritz and Campo, 2002).

These patients and the families elicit multiple responses in medical professionals and hospital staff, often very negative ones. Providers can feel frustrated, angry, and betrayed. By the time the diagnosis is made, there can be beliefs that these patients and families are abusing health-care resources, they are wasting the professionals' time, and no intervention will help. And the health team can feel guilty about the delay in diagnosis and possible iatrogenic harm to the child. The psychiatrist can help in these situations by providing education on the psychology and dynamics of these disorders, the possible beneficial interventions as well as aiding the staff in processing their reactions (Forsyth, 2002; Fritz and Campo, 2002).

Somatoform disorders/psychologic factors affecting general medical condition

Given that these patients and families conceptualize their problems as physical, treatment approaches are more likely to be successful if they are presented as being primarily medically oriented. The rehabilitation approach should be utilized with a focus on resuming normal activities even with the persistence of symptoms. A primary physician should be identified and should remain involved with regular contact with the patient and the family to monitor the medical condition and provide consistent reassurance that additional medical interventions are not necessary and counterproductive. Important components of treatment include de-emphasizing a final diagnosis and concentrating on increasing function; ensuring a thorough and adequate medical work-up; minimizing number of treating physicians and use of hospitalization; making use of benign, face saving interventions such as physical therapy, heating pads, lotions, vitamins, exercises; and regular physician contact that does not require illness exacerbation. Pain should be adequately managed with medication. A number of behavioral techniques have been identified as beneficial for pain management and can be helpful as adjuncts to medication. Behavioral management also is

essential to reinforce appropriate coping behavior, increase adherence to the treatment plan, and decrease secondary gain related to being sick. Education on the treatment approach and its rationale, symptoms to be concerned about, systems of communication with medical providers, and possible problem solving strategies are important (Rubinstein, 1988; Fritz and Campo, 2002; Brown et al., 2003).

Often, convincing these individuals that psychiatric care is appropriate is a lengthy process. Formally labeling patients as having a psychiatric disorder can impede treatment. It is beneficial to emphasize the difficulties of having physical problems and the tendency of multiple factors to exacerbate symptoms. Emphasizing the role of stress in the exacerbation of symptoms may be helpful in convincing these families of the utility of psychiatric care. It may be helpful to treat significant anxious or depressive symptoms with psychotherapy and medication. For patients willing to obtain psychiatric care, supportive, individual, and group psychotherapies have been demonstrated to be helpful for adults, though there are no data on children and adolescents. Family cognitive behavioral therapy for recurrent abdominal pain has shown greater reduction of pain, fewer relapses, and more function than controls with usual pediatric care (Fritz and Campo, 2002). There are some data that individuals with body dysmorphic disorder respond to selective serotonin reuptake inhibitor (SSRI) antidepressants as well as to cognitive behavioral therapy techniques such as cognitive restructuring, exposure (e.g. social situations), and response prevention (avoiding compulsive behaviors). Antipsychotics alone appear to be unlikely to be effective though may be helpful as augmentation to an SSRI when the patient is delusional or has poor insight (Phillips, 2000).

Factitious disorders

Ideally, the providers who have developed the best therapeutic alliance with the caretakers confront the patient's family with the team's impressions. Minimizing the number of individuals involved is best. Having the psychiatrist present can help with support and with clarification of the psychiatric aspects. The aim of the confrontation is to inform the child's caretakers of the potential harm to the child and possible consequences. Occasionally, mothers will confess, though most will continue to deny their activity. Engaging in extensive attempts to convince the mother to agree with the diagnosis is not productive. Prior to the confrontation, there should be a plan for the child's supervision and safety as well as additional care that the mother may need (i.e. psychiatric hospitalization). Child protective services should be notified, with recommendations for the child's ongoing care. Children often are resistant to being removed from their families. They may need psychotherapy to help with separation from their caretakers, developing an identity not defined by being sick, and resuming age-appropriate activities. Many of these children may be returned to live with the perpetrator. Thus, if possible, trying to maintain an ongoing relationship with the child and family so that appropriate medical and psychiatric care can be provided is optimal. This situation is extremely difficult for all involved and the hospital staff and other providers may need to discuss their concerns and reactions during the process (Forsyth, 2002).

Malingering

When developing the treatment plan, it is important for the health providers to recognize and appropriately deal with their reactions to these patients and families. Malingering tends to produce negative responses in providers, who often feel manipulated, betrayed, and taken advantage of (Williams and Hirsch, 1988). Often, the initial reaction is that these patients do not need ongoing care and that they require punishment. However, children and adolescents rarely are incorrigible criminals or slackers who cannot be rehabilitated. These young people have psychologic and environmental variables, which explain their malingering and can respond to interventions. In addition to coordination between medical and psychiatric providers, it is essential to include school personnel and other involved agencies. Often, it is necessary to involve child protective services or the juvenile justice system to provide additional structure and resources. Overall, the treatment should focus on ameliorating any contributing factors (e.g. appropriate school placement for school avoidance due to academic failure). The goals and resources for treatment should be identified before confronting the patient and family. A few key members of the team should present the team's conclusions and recommendations without accusations and criticisms. A helpful framework can be that the patient clearly is having difficulties; the team wants to help but that medical care is not the appropriate intervention.

Summary

Identifying and managing these disorders is challenging due to the complicated and poorly understood interactions between physical and psychologic factors which produce

CONSIDER CONSULTATION WHEN ...

- There is concern about excessive utilization of medical care.
- Medical symptom presentations are unusual.
- Typically effective medical treatments are ineffective.
- Impairment of function exceeds the level expected.
- Psychologic issues or environmental stressors appear associated.
- Psychiatric symptoms in child or caretaker are significant.

and influence disease in children and adolescents. Additionally, young people suffering from disorders in this spectrum require ongoing care coordinated among several providers and systems. Considerable research needs to be conducted to develop diagnostic criteria more appropriate for children and adolescents, to describe the courses and outcomes, as well as to identify effective interventions.

Annotated bibliography

American Academy of Pediatrics (1996) *The Classification of Child and Adolescent Mental Diagnosis in Primary Care: Diagnostic and Statistical Manual for Primary Care (DSM-PC)*. Elk Grove Village, IL, American Academy of Pediatrics.
Manual based on the DSM-IV, written for pediatric practitioners. It is organized into two sections: situations (issues related to the child's environment) and child manifestations (behaviors demonstrated by the child). Symptoms are grouped into developmental variations, problems, and disorders. There are examples given in each division for various age groups, describing possible presentations based on developmental considerations. The disorders section describes the DSM-IV criteria for the relevant psychiatric disorders.

Brown LK, Bruning K, Fritz GK, Herzog DB (2003) Somatoform disorders. In: Weiner JM and Dulcan MK (eds) *Textbook of Child and Adolescent Psychiatry*, 3rd edn. Washington DC, American Psychiatric Press, pp. 751–763.
Overview of somatoform disorders and psychologic factors affecting medical conditions.

Campo JV, Jansen-McWilliams Comer DM, Kelleher KJ (1999) Somatization in pediatric primary care: association with psychopathology, functional impairment, and use of services. *Journal of American Academy of Child and Adolescent Psychiatry*, 38:1093–1101.
Survey of somatic symptoms presenting in pediatric primary care practice.

Forsyth BWC (2002) Munchausen syndrome by proxy. In: Lewis M (ed.) *Child and Adolescent Psychiatry: A Comprehensive Textbook*, 3rd edn. Philadelphia, Lippincott Williams & Wilkins, pp. 1223–1230.
Overview of factitious disorder by proxy.

Libow JA (2000) Child and adolescent illness falsification. *Pediatrics* 105:336–342.
Review of literature describing cases of factitious disorders in children and adolescents in the past 30 years.

Phillips KA (2000) Body dysmorphic disorder: diagnostic controversies and treatment challenges. *Bulletin of the Menninger Clinic*, 64:18–35.
Overview of body dysmorphic disorder.

Sheridan MS (2003) The deceit continues: an updated literature review of Munchausen syndrome by proxy. *Child Abuse and Neglect*, 27:431–451.
Review of literature describing cases of factitious disorder by proxy from 1972 to 1999.

CHAPTER 14

Substance Use Disorders

Steven L. Jaffe, MD

Introduction

There was a downward trend of alcohol and drug abuse in teenagers during the late 1980s and early 1990s which was followed by a sharp increase in 1993. This increase, which was primarily related to marijuana use, continued until 2001. Thirty-day prevalence for 12th graders for marijuana use peaked at 23.7% in 1997. Since 2001, there has been a significant decrease, with the 12th grade 30-day prevalence decreasing to 21.2%. In spite of this, daily marijuana use has remained at 6% (Johnston et al., 2004). Perceived harmfulness of marijuana has significantly decreased despite its increased potency (Schwartz, 2002).

Alcohol continues to be the illegal substance that is most abused by teenagers, with a 30-day 12th-grade prevalence of 47.5% for use in 2003 and 30.9% for binge drinking. Of major concern is that a third of high school seniors admit to having been in a car where the driver has been drinking. LSD use, which peaked in 1997, has shown a sharp decrease in the past few years, decreasing to an annual prevalence of 1.9%. MDMA ("ecstasy"), which also peaked in the late 1990s, has also shown a sharp decrease with teenagers realizing its high risk. Inhalants ("huffing") have a peak use in early adolescence (8th grade.) Inhalant use slowly decreased in the 1990s but has slightly increased by 2002–2003, with an annual prevalence in 2003 of 8.72% for 8th graders. Types of inhalants include gasoline, fluorocarbons (Freon) used in air conditioners, butane, Scotchgard, and even household bleach. Cigarette smoking has recently decreased, but the past month use of 24.4% for high school seniors in 2003 continues to be much too high. An increased use of the prescription narcotic OxyContin in the past 2 years may be the beginning of a very dangerous new trend.

Adolescents tend to use alcohol and drugs in an inverse relationship to their recognition and understanding of the risk of harm. Thus, this recent increase in general use corresponds to a decreased perceived risk of harm. Many factors, such as lack of education about the risks of drugs and the glamorization of alcohol and drugs on television and in the music industry, appear to have contributed to the increase of use. Although teenagers are highly educated in the use of computers, they are poorly informed about the realistic and actual risks of alcohol and drugs. Since early use correlates directly with a later degree of use and with the use of more than one drug, the increase in use by 8th graders is an alarming trend.

In recent years, increasing the age of legal alcohol consumption has been considered as a primary method of decreasing alcohol and drug use in the teenage population. However, the trends discussed in this chapter have devastated the possibility of increased age as a significant influential factor. Suicides, homicides, and accidents account for 80% of teenage deaths, and alcohol and drugs are involved in one half of these cases. The extensive use and abuse of alcohol and drugs during the preadolescent and adolescent years, as well as the strong contribution of drugs and alcohol to emotional problems, indicate that whenever there are problems in the teenage years, the physician should consider that alcohol and drugs may be a contributing factor.

There are a number of risk factors that have been described as correlates to serious substance abuse in adolescents (Box 14.1). When the physician sees a teenager and family with these types of problems, alcohol and drugs need to be considered as part of the clinical picture. The most influential factor

> **BOX 14.1**
>
> **Risk factors for serious substance abuse in adolescents**
> - Parent or other relative with substance abuse or dependency problems.
> - Low achievement, especially in school.
> - Poor self-esteem.
> - Aggressive or impulsive personality.
> - Family instability.
> - History of sexual or physical abuse.
> - Psychiatric disorder, especially depression.

for a teenager having problems with alcohol and drugs is a relative, such as a parent, grandparent, aunt, or uncle, who has a history of alcohol or drug addiction. The physician should specifically ask whether a relative had problems with drugs and alcohol. Specific attitudes and a lack of achievement by the teenager also correlate with alcohol and substance abuse. Such attitudes include the teenager thinking poorly of him or herself, not liking school, not achieving or dropping out of school, and smoking cigarettes, as well as rebellious and delinquent behavior. The aggressive or impulsive teenager is at high risk for substance abuse.

Additionally, if the teenager's friends have the same characteristics (i.e. they are aggressive or delinquent) or if the teenager's friends use drugs or alcohol, the adolescent in question is at high risk for drug or alcohol use. In terms of family problems, disruption and dysfunction within the family correlate with alcohol and drug abuse in teenagers. Thus, parental separation, divorce, lack of clear discipline, and especially the lack of positive relationships within the family all increase the likelihood that a teenager will use or abuse alcohol and drugs. Teenagers who have been sexually or physically abused, who have had a depressive episode, or who have had problems in school because of behavior, attention-deficit/hyperactivity disorder (ADHD), or learning disabilities are at increased risk for alcohol and substance abuse.

Research indicates that teenagers become involved in alcohol and drugs through a pattern of progression, which begins with abstention and moves to the use of beer or wine and cigarettes, hard liquor, marijuana, problem drinking and then other drugs (Kandel, 1975). Thus, it is extremely unusual for a teenager who is using cocaine to never have tried marijuana. In contrast with adults, teenagers often do not give up the drug of the previous stage but continue to use it along with the new drugs. Therefore, teenagers tend to be multiple drug users. For example, many abuse alcohol, marijuana, and LSD during the same period. Cigarette use is a method of learning to smoke and thereby is a gateway to the use of marijuana. An exception to this pattern of staged progression is inhalants, where 8th graders have the highest rate of use.

While most teenagers use alcohol and drugs occasionally and without negative consequences (71% of high school seniors drank alcohol during 2001), half of those have had a binge episode in the past month. These youths become the high risk behavior groups who become involved with driving after drinking, unprotected sex, and aggressive acts. Teenagers need to understand that it takes only one time to kill yourself and/or your car passenger. Any use of more than alcohol and marijuana is worrisome and of course, regular use of alcohol and/or marijuana is extremely problematic.

Diagnosis

As with much diagnostic work, the history of the patient holds much of the diagnostic information. The physician quickly develops hypotheses when listening to and observing the patient and tests them with further inquiry. The evaluation of an adolescent who may be abusing drugs or alcohol, but is not about to admit to it, calls on a physician's greatest skills in relationship building, empathic confrontation, and knowledge of popular substances and patterns of abuse. Since it is usually a family member who brings the young person for an evaluation, a more complete picture can be obtained from an additional source. The formal DSM-IV diagnosis is relatively easy to generate once the psychosocial data are forthcoming (APA, 1994). The criteria are straightforward and serve the physician well because of their checklist nature (Tables 14.1 and 14.2). There are a number of types of substance use disorders which are classified by the substance being used. Generally, young people can meet the criteria for substance abuse or dependence. Substance intoxication or withdrawal tends to be diagnosed in emergency rooms and young people often do not have significant withdrawal symptoms.

PEARLS & PERILS

Drug and alcohol abuse

- If there is a problem in the teenage years, alcohol and drugs may be involved.
- If there are any problems in feelings, actions or thinking, drugs and alcohol may be causing the problems.
- The greater the problem with alcohol and drugs, the more the teenager will lie about his or her drug and alcohol use. Therefore, information from family, peers, and school is important.
- Teenagers tend to be multiple drug users.
- If a teenager is not asked about drugs and alcohol, he or she will usually not volunteer this information.

DIAGNOSIS

Table 14.1 Substance abuse

Discriminating features

1. Recurrent use with significant negative consequences.
2. Never met the criteria for substance dependence for the substance.

Consistent features

1. Failure to fulfill major role obligations at work, school, home.
2. Recurrent substance use in physically hazardous situations.
3. Recurrent substance-related legal problems.
4. Continued substance use despite having persistent or recurrent social or interpersonal problems.

Variable features

1. Types of substances.

DIAGNOSIS

Table 14.2 Substance dependence

Discriminating features

1. Recurrent use with inability to moderate or control use.
2. Severe impairment in function.
3. Corresponds to addiction.

Consistent features

1. Tolerance.
2. Withdrawal.
3. Larger amounts or longer period than intended.
4. Persistent desire to quit/cut down.
5. Unsuccessful attempts to quit/cut down.
6. Considerable time spent in activities necessary to obtain, use, or recover from effects of the substance.
7. Important social, occupational, or recreational activities given up/reduced.
8. Use is continued despite knowledge that the substance has caused or exacerbated a persistent or recurrent psychologic or physiologic problem.

Variable features

1. Types of substances.
2. With/without physiologic dependence.
3. Course.

BOX 14.2

Substance-related disorders

Types of disorders:

- Substance abuse
- Substance dependence
- Substance intoxication
- Substance withdrawal
- Substance-induced delirium
- Substance-induced persisting dementia
- Substance-induced persisting amnestic disorder
- Substance-induced psychotic disorder
- Substance-induced mood disorder
- Substance-induced anxiety disorder
- Substance-induced sexual dysfunction
- Substance-induced sleep disorder
- Substance-related disorder NOS
- Polysubstance dependence
- Other (or unknown) substance-related disorders

Substances:

- Alcohol
- Amphetamine
- Caffeine
- Cannabis
- Cocaine
- Hallucinogen
- Inhalant
- Opioid
- Phencyclidine
- Sedative – hypnotic or anxiolytic

Additionally, young people with symptoms consistent with another psychiatric diagnosis thought to be due to substances can be diagnosed with a substance-induced disorder, such as substance-induced mood disorder (Box 14.1). The physician needs to be aware that 40–90% of adolescents with substance abuse or dependence have a comorbid psychiatric disorder. Common diagnoses include ADHD, conduct disorder, mood disorders, and anxiety disorders (Jaffe, 1996).

Assessment

Because of the widespread use and possible severe detrimental consequences, the primary care physician should screen all adolescents for substance abuse. Early detection and treatment saves lives. When talking to the teenager and his or her family about alcohol and drug use, the physician must be knowledgeable and comfortable approaching these issues. The teenager who is abusing alcohol and drugs will quickly notice if the physician knows little about the ways drugs and alcohol are abused, their effects, and the problems associated with their use. However, if the physician has personal experience with drugs or alcohol, this fact should not be mentioned.

Additionally, the physician should not become too chummy, since the teenager will then treat the physician as another teenager. An attitude of interest, concern, and seriousness mixed with a little humor in the context of the physician's usual style is often the best approach. Any change in feelings, mood, behavior, or cognitive functioning may be related to problems with alcohol and drugs. The physician should ask specific details of a teenager's activities and experiences, since these reveal the details of life. For example, asking "How's school?" yields little. Asking about the details of the day, what a teacher is like, the nature of the teenager's relationship to the teacher, and grades in a specific course often reveal many important data. Be aware that the parents often do not know the extent of their child's alcohol and drug use. Tarter (1990) presents the importance of exploring problems in all domains of the adolescent's life. These include physical health status, aggressive behavior problems, psychiatric disorders, social skills, family relationships, school adjustment, peer relationships, work adjustment, and recreation.

Physicians may learn a great deal about what alcohol/drugs are being used in their community by asking the adolescent what their peers are using. Anglin (1987) describes a schema for interviewing teenagers about their alcohol and drug use. This commonly used framework includes a psychosocial assessment, whereby home and family relationships are explored in detail and functioning at school is covered. Peer relationships, leisure activities and employment, and self-perceptions are carefully reviewed. Of course, these issues must also be explored with the family. Teenagers tend to deny and hide their drug use. Therefore, changes in feelings, actions, and thinking must be carefully explored in an open non-accusatory way with the family. The physician must at all times act as an ally of the parents and as a knowledgeable and concerned professional who is there to help the teenager. To explore alcohol and substance use with a teenager, Anglin suggests an ordered discussion of the substances the teenager ingests. Thus, questions move from dietary patterns to prescribed medications, over-the-counter medications, and the use of other substances. The discussion of actual substance abuse may move from tobacco to alcohol, marijuana, and other drugs. If a teenager is reluctant to discuss his or her own actions, asking what his or her peers do and do not do may give insight to what he or she does or does not do. It is often helpful to ask questions such as "How many times a month do you smoke pot?" rather than "Do you smoke pot?" This approach may help the teenager to lower his defenses and prevent him from immediately answering "No" to every question.

The well-known CAGE (screen for alcohol abuse) screening questions were developed for adults and are not very useful for adolescents. During the past several years, a number of screening and evaluation instruments have been developed that specifically assess adolescent substance abuse. The CRAFFT, a screening instrument developed in a medical setting is extremely useful and has been validated (Box 14.3). Two or more "yes" answers suggest serious problems with substance use and indicate that further evaluation is needed (Knight et al., 1999). Teenagers should also be questioned about the following important issues: taking risks, such as driving or being in a car when using alcohol or drugs, breaking the law, somatic effects, such as memory difficulties resulting from marijuana use, and changes in school achievement. With a heavy alcohol/drug user, a time line for each drug (Table 14.3) including onset, peak use, and use in past 60–90 days should be explored.

Confidentiality

Issues of confidentiality are difficult in their clinical application and vary with the style and judgment of the physician. Although promising the teenager absolute confidentiality may yield more information, this approach can be extremely problematic. Much of the information may be of a life-threatening nature (for example, the teenager may reveal that he or she drives while tripping on LSD), and these behaviors need to be brought to the attention of the parents. If the teenager is clearly endangering him or herself or others, it is an indication for confidentiality to be broken. The risks of drugs and alcohol are often life-threatening but may not be immediate and clear. This condition calls for the consideration of relationships and the involvement of judgment in the decision-making process. One method of handling the situation is to interview in the presence of the parents. Thus, the teenager reveals the specifics of the high-risk behavior directly to his or her parents.

KEY CLINICAL QUESTIONS

Screening for substance use

Adolescents who use substances tend to have friends or family who do and usually are not functioning as well as they could. Assuming that the patient is using drugs and asking specific questions about use is more likely to get accurate data.

- *What school do you go to?/what grade?/how are your grades?*
- *What extracurricular activities are you involved in?*
- *Who lives at home? What do you do together? How do you get along?*
- *Have you been involved with the police or juvenile court?*
- *Do any of your family members use drugs?*
- *Who are your friends?*
- *What kind of activities do you do with them?*
- *Which of your friends use tobacco/alcohol/drugs (list several types)?*
- *Where and when do they use?*
- *How much do you use tobacco/alcohol/drugs?*
- *Where and when?*
- *With whom?*
- *What do drugs do to/for you?*
- *How do you get and pay for the drugs?*
- *Do your parents know?*

For each drug:
- *When started – age, circumstances*
- *When became regular use (2–3 times/week)*
- *When became daily use*

Last use:
- *What do you like/not like about drugs?*

Screening for interest in treatment:
- *Are there any reasons that drugs are bad?*
- *Does using drugs cause any problems for you?*
- *Have you tried to cut down/quit? What happened?*
- *What do you think about getting treatment?*

BOX 14.3 The CRAFFT

C – Have you ever ridden in a car driven by someone (including yourself) who was high or had been using alcohol or drugs?

R – Do you ever use alcohol/drugs to relax, feel better about yourself, or fit in?

A – Do you ever use alcohol/drugs while you are by yourself or alone?

F – Do you ever forget things you did while using alcohol/drugs?

F – Do your family or friends ever tell you that you should cut down on your drinking or drug use?

T – Have you ever gotten into trouble while you were using alcohol or drugs?

TABLE 14.3

Drugs and their effects

Drugs	Street name	Effects
Cannabinoids		
• Marijuana	Dope, ganja, grass, herb, blunts, joints, Mary Jane, pot, reefer, weed, chronic, hemp	Euphoria, slow thinking, confusion, selective attention deficits, short-term memory loss, anxiety, panic, respiratory infections, tolerance, addiction
• Hashish		
Hallucinogens		
• LSD	• Acid, cubes, microdot, yellow sunshine	• Altered state of perception and feelings
• Mescaline	• Buttons, cactus, peyote	• Increased temperature, heart rate (HR), blood pressure (BP)
• Psilocybin	• Magic mushrooms, purple passion, shrooms	• Decreased appetite, numbness, paranoia, flashback, persistent mental disorders
Stimulants		
• Nicotine	• Cigarettes, cigars, snuff, bidis, chew	• Chronic lung and cardiovascular disorders, strokes, cancer, tolerance, addiction
• MDMA	• Ecstasy, Adam Eve, peace, Stp, X, XTC	• Mild hallucinogenic effects, increases tactile sensitivity, empathetic feelings, hypothermia, cardiac and renal failure, liver toxicity
• Amphetamine	• Dex, beenies, black beauties, LA, speed, truck drivers, uppers	• Increased alertness, energy, BP, HR, tremor, loss of co-ordination, irritability, delirium, weight loss, insomnia
• Methamphetamine	• Crank, crystal, glass, ice, meth	• Aggression, violence, psychosis, paranoia
• Methylphenidate	• MPH, R-ball, vitamin R	• Memory loss, tolerance, addiction
Depressants		
• Barbiturates	• Barbs, reds, tooies, yellows	• Decreased anxiety, pulse, respiration, sedation, drowsiness, fatigue, confusion, tolerance, addiction, withdrawal can be life-threatening
• Benzodiazepines	• Ativan, Valium, Xanax, Klonopin	• Sedation, drowsiness, excitement, slurred speech, withdrawal after physical dependency can be life-threatening
• Flunitrazepam	• Rohypnol, forget-me-pill, mexican Valium, roffies, rope	• Visual and gastrointestinal disturbance, urinary retention, memory loss on drug
• GHB	• G, Georgia home boy, grievous, bodily harm, liquid ectasy	
• Methaqualone	• Quaalude, ludes, quad	• Sedation, drowsiness, nausea, vomiting, headache, poor reflex, slowed speed, seizures, coma, death
Dissociative anesthetics		
• Ketamine	• Cat Valium, special K, vitamin K	• Increased HR, BP, memory loss, delirium
• PCP	• Phencyclidine, angel dust, love boat, peach pill	• Panic, aggression, violence
Opiates		
• Codeine	• Captain Cody	
• Fentanyl	• Apache, China girl, dance fever, goodfella, TNT, Tango & Cash	
• Heroin	• Dope, H, horse, junk, skag, skunk, smack, white horse	Pain relief, euphoria, sedation, respiratory depression, tolerance, addiction, coma, death
• Morphine	• Miss Emma, monkey, white stuff	
• Opium	• Laudanum, paregoric, big O, black stuff, block, hop	
• Oxycodone	• Oxycontin, oxy, OC, killer	
• Hydrocodone	• Vicodin, vilar, watson, 387	
Inhalants		
• Solvents	• Paint thinners, gasoline, butane	• Muscle numbness, depression, memory loss, sudden death
• Nitrous oxide	• Laughing gas, boppers, snappers, whippets	
Anabolic steroids	• Anabol, oxandrolone, durabolix, roids, juice	• No intoxication, increased BP, liver cysts, hostility, shrinks testicles, aggression, premature growth cessation

* Modified from NIDA (National Institute of Drug Abuse) website, www.drugabuse.gov

Urine drug screening

Issues of judgment and risk taking also involve judgments about urine drug screening. The physician should be familiar with the local laboratory, the types of urine drug screening that can be done, and the cutoff points for positive tests. A urine drug screen is only valid if it is unadulterated and if it is actually the teenager's urine. Therefore, urine for drug screens needs to be obtained under observed conditions. Resistance to giving a urine specimen for a drug screen correlates with chance of being positive. Teenagers who ask "Don't you trust me?" should be answered with "No. Show me you are not using drugs." Adults should not be put off by the numerous ploys of shifting the issue from the teenager's possible drug use to issues concerning relationships or others. Urine drug screens (Box 14.4) should not be done on a routine basis, but only when there is reasonable suspicion of drug use.

Adolescent urine drug screening mainly shows evidence of marijuana use, because cannabinoids last for 3–4 weeks

after they are smoked on a regular basis. Most other drugs are only present for 1–2 days. Alcohol levels are determined from breath or blood testing.

Treatment

When determining how to deal with alcohol and drug abuse in teenagers, understanding the stage of involvement is often extremely helpful. For the teenager who is only involved in experimental or social use, education and counseling is needed. If the teenager has progressed to more regular use, then the addition of individual, group, and family therapy, as well as an abstinence contract, is needed. The abstinence contract involves the teenager who is using drugs more than occasionally, but maintains that he or she will have no problem stopping. The teenager agrees to regular urine testing and counseling and promises not to use drugs or alcohol.

In this treatment strategy, the teenager's progress determines whether more intensive treatment modalities are needed. For example, a teenager who has been doing poorly in school and has had hostile confrontations with his or her family may agree to counseling and an abstinence contract. If this teenager stops smoking marijuana, his or her urine drug screens will be negative after the 2 or 3 weeks it takes for the tetrahydrocannodinol (THC) to be eliminated from the body, and his or her behavior, relationships, and school achievement will return to their pre-drug levels. More intensive treatment will not be needed. However, if the teenager is unable to abstain from drugs and alcohol, further rules will be broken, family relationships will be disrupted, failures will increase at school, at work, and elsewhere, and deteriorating behavior will help the physician determine that a more intensive treatment program is needed (Table 14.4). Additional treatment methods include a partial hospital program, 12-step program, and residential treatment (Box 14.5). Box 14.6 shows the names and addresses of self-help and advocacy groups that may be helpful resources for recovering teenagers and their families.

It is important to note that teenagers who are serious abusers of alcohol and drugs may have numerous co-existing disorders, especially ADHD, conduct disorder, learning dis-

---

BOX 14.4

Urine drug screen

Period (days) that substances may be detected after last use:

- Cannabiniods
  2–8 days after acute use
  14–42 days after chronic use
- Amphetamines
  1–2 days
- Barbiturates
  3–14 days
- Benzodiazapines
  2–9 days
- Cocaine
  1–4 days
- Opiates
  1–2 days
- PCP
  2–8 days

LSD, psilocybin, and ecstasy (MDMA) are usually not tested on routine drug screens.

TABLE 14.4

Substance use treatment

Level of use	Experimental use	Regular use	Preoccupation with use	Chemical dependence
Level of care and treatment facilities	A 1–2	B 1–2+	C 1–6+	D 1–9+
	Education Counseling	Individual and group therapy Family therapy Abstinence contract Motivational interviewing	12-step program AA/NA meetings Cognitive-behavioral theraoy Intensive outpatient & partial hospital program	Hospital, residential programs Therapeutic community

BOX 14.5 Treatment methods for teenagers who use drugs and alcohol

Experimental (recreational use)
- Education helps adolescents and parents learn about alcohol and drugs and their detrimental effects.
- Excellent information and pamphlets for distribution may be obtained at no charge from the National Clearinghouse for Alcohol and Drug Information Publications Catalog (1–800–729–6686).
- Counseling, talking with the adolescent about his or her life and drug use.

Regular use
- Individual, group and family therapy, done by a mental health professional.
- Abstinence contract, written agreement not to use drugs, to have regular urine drug screens, and to abide by home rules (privileges and consequences) as developed by the parents and the adolescent.
- Motivational interviewing, empathic non-confrontational technique allowing teen to explore negative consequences.

Preoccupation with use
- 12-step program, attending regular meetings of Alcoholics Anonymous or Narcotics Anonymous; establishing a sponsor and completing the steps.
- Partial hospital program, attending a program during the day or evening that includes therapy groups, family programs, individual therapy, creative activities, and school.

Chemical dependency
- Hospital program, acute and intermediate level of care.
- Residential program, long-term intermediate level of 24-hour care and therapeutic program.

BOX 14.6 Self-help and advocacy groups
- Adult Children of Alcoholics (ACOA); P.O. Box 880517; San Francisco, CA 94188; (415) 931–2262. Addresses the trauma of growing up in an alcoholic family.
- Alcoholic Anonymous/Narcotics Anonymous; 16155 Wyandotte Street; Van Nuys, CA 91406; (818)780–3951. Narcotics Anonymous (NA) is a national network of more than 2000 regional groups. They are closely patterned after Alcoholics Anonymous (AA). NA groups are conducted by recovered drug addicts, who follow the AA program to aid in rehabilitation. NA publishes a variety of helpful materials for its members, including a directory of group meetings.
- Families Anonymous (FA); P.O. Box 528; Van Nuys, CA 91408; (818)989–7841. Self-help group patterned after AA.
- Mothers Against Drunk Driving (MADD); 669 Airport Freeway, Suite #310; Hurst, TX 76053; (817)268-MADD. Membership is open to all parents, including fathers. Promotion of public policy against drunk driving.
- National Clearinghouse for Alcohol and Drug Information (NCADD); P.O. Box 2345; Rockville, MD 20852; (301)468–2600
- National Federation of Parents for Drug-Free Youth (NFP); 8730 Georgia Avenue, #200; Silver Spring, MD 20910; (301)585–5437. Activities include Project Graduation and Safe Homes.
- NIDA (National Institute of Drug Abuse) website, www.drugabuse.gov
- National Parent-Teachers' Association (PTA); 700 North Rush Street; Chicago, IL 60611; (312)787–0977. The nation's largest child advocacy association.
- Parent Resources and Information for Drug Education (PRIDE); Robert Woodruff Building, Volunteer Services Center, Suite #1012; 100 Edgewood Avenue NE, Atlanta, GA 30303; (800)241–9746. Information and referral resources for parents and others.
- Students Against Driving Drunk (SADD); P.O. Box 800; Marlboro, MA 01752; (617)481–3568. Chapters in high school and colleges; weekend hot-line service to provide safe rides.

(adapted from American Academy of Pediatrics: Evaluation by interview. In: Schonber SK (ed) *Substance Abuse: A Guide for Health Professionals*. Elk Grove Village, Ill., 1988 author.)

orders, depression, or histories of physical or sexual abuse. Full evaluation and treatment of co-existing psychiatric disorders is needed. Because of the extensive use, abuse, and high risk of drugs and alcohol in the teenage population, it is essential for all physicians working with teenagers to become knowledgeable and effective in dealing with this aspect of a teenager's life.

Jaffe's (2001) *Adolescent Substance Abuse Intervention Workbook* instructs the adolescent to concretely explore how 12 areas of his or her life have been negatively affected by substances in an effort to move them to recognize a need to stop using. Intervention with the parents is needed to help them set limits, stop any enabling behavior and allow the teenager to experience the consequences of their alcohol/drug use.

Primary care physicians need to become knowledgeable of the child/adolescent psychiatrists, psychologists, substance abuse counselors in their geographical area who like

working with adolescents and understand substance abuse. Teenagers who are depressed, suicidal, aggressive, flunking school, breaking family values, and continue to use alcohol/drugs warrant referral. If the teenager tells a physician about

- Full psychiatric evaluation is needed because substance abuse often co-exists with one or more psychiatric disorders (especially mood disorders, behavior disorders such as ADHD and CD, and anxiety disorders).
- Failure of treatment usually indicates that a more advanced stage of use was actually present. Treatment modalities of this more advanced stage are indicated.
- Detoxification is not usually needed for adolescents because of the following:
  - adolescents tend to be in better physical condition than adults
  - adolescents tend to use multiple drugs
  - marijuana, LSD, and cocaine, which are commonly used by adolescents, do not require detoxification
  - heavy alcohol abuse is often episodic without the development of physical addiction.
- Although it is rare in adolescents, physical addiction to alcohol, sedatives, or minor tranquilizers can have life-threatening withdrawal symptoms and necessitates detoxification. Recently, there has been an increased use of minor tranquilizers, especially alprazolam (Xanax) and clonazepam (Klonopin).
- Treatment of comorbid ADHD or depression may help the associated symptoms but does not make the teenager stop using alcohol/drugs. Teenagers use alcohol/drugs because of curiosity and the euphoric/positive/fun feelings produced. Later, they learn that alcohol/drugs temporarily help them escape negative feelings. Thus, specific substance abuse interventions with the teenager and all the family are needed to begin to develop abstinence.

CONSIDER CONSULTATION WHEN ...

- There is life-threatening behaviour.
- The young person is unable to abide by abstinence contract.
- There is significant psychiatric comorbidity.

The website for NIDA (National Institute of Drug Abuse) www.drugabuse.gov is an excellent source of information on the drugs, diagnosis, treatment, and prevention.

Summary

Exploration and evaluation of substance abuse is one of the most difficult and challenging areas for the primary care physician. Interventions result in the saving of numerous adolescent lives. Outcome studies indicate that after intensive treatment and after-care participation, 50–70% of substance dependent adolescents have positive results. These results are as positive as other treatments for chronic diseases (AACAP, 1997).

Annotated bibliography

Anglin TM (1987) Interviewing guidelines for the clinical evaluation of adolescent substance abuse. *Pediatr Clin North Am*, 34:381–398. *This article provides a wonderful detailed description of an interview method.*

Jaffe SL (2001) *Adolescent Substance Abuse Intervention Workbook: Taking a First Step.* Washington, DC, American Psychiatric Press. *A structured, sequential treatment approach.*

Knight JR, Shrier LA, Bravender TD et al. (1999) A new brief screen for adolescent substance abuse. *Arch Pediatr Adolesc Med*, 153:591–596. *Description of substance abuse screen for clinical practice.*

Tarter RE (1990) Evaluation and treatment of adolescent substance abuse: a decision tree method. *Am J Drug Alcohol Abuse*, 16:1–46. *Overview of triage for treatment of adolescent substance users.*

alcohol and drug problems, it is imperative for the physician to explore these issues, educate the teenager and his or her family, determine the extent and stage of usage, and help the teenager obtain treatment.

Clinical Conditions and Situations

Sandra B. Sexson, MD

CHAPTER 15

Issues in Infant Psychiatry

Ayelet Talmi, PhD and Robert J. Harmon, MD

Introduction

Psychiatrists, pediatricians, and family practitioners see infants* from birth to 36 months in their practices and in academic and research settings. In recent years, the field of infancy and early childhood, and more specifically, infant mental health, has provided a wealth of information about emotional, intellectual, motor, and sensory patterns in infancy. Contributions to the science of infancy have included a substantial body of evidence regarding the types of challenges that can interfere with optimal development. Consequently, we are becoming better able to create, maintain, or improve conditions for healthy development. Prevention and intervention efforts may begin before babies are born or conceived, as in the case of interventions that target spacing subsequent children. However, gaining a comprehensive understanding of a child and family's circumstances in order to formulate an effective, preventatively oriented treatment approach is challenging.

Understanding the difficulties and developing a treatment plan with young children is harder to accomplish than with older children and adults for several reasons. First, despite enormous variation in children, their families, and the particular challenges being considered, infant distress

---

* This chapter describes issues relevant to infants and young children from birth to 3 years of age. According to common convention in the field of infant mental health, the terms "infant" and "young child" are used interchangeably in this article to describe very young children. Similarly, we recognize that many different people take care of children from birth to 3. For the sake of flow, the terms "parents," "mother," "father," "caregivers" will also be used interchangeably to denote relationships with important attachment figures.

signals often appear very similar. Second, since development occurs so rapidly over the first 3 years of life and multiple lines of development are highly interrelated, several observations over time are necessary to distinguish typical variations in development from patterns that may indicate a chronic problem. Most importantly, infants and young children need to be understood in context. The relevant contexts range from their relationships with their primary caregivers and families, to their cultural backgrounds, to the impact of events in their communities. Each of these contexts and the interrelationships among them impact infant development on an ongoing basis.

Infant mental health

In the last century, research and clinical work with infants and young children has provided a wealth of information about the origins of both typical and atypical development. Early experiences of deprivation, abuse and neglect, organic and medical complications, and relationship problems often appear in the histories of children and adults with difficulties (Fraiberg and Fraiberg, 1980). Even in the face of tremendous neural, emotional, and relational plasticity, scientific evidence suggests that development in the first few years of life sets the foundation for later capacities, achievements, and challenges (Shonkoff and Phillips, 2002)

A brief history

For the field of psychoanalysis, the mysteries of adult personality development lay in infancy. While Sigmund Freud based his theoretical framework on the early relationship between infants and their parents, it is Anna Freud who is credited with launching the field of child analysis. As early as the 1920s, Anna Freud was practicing psychoanalysis with children. Her pioneering clinical and theoretical work emphasized the techniques of child analysis, infant behavior and development, childhood stress and relationships, and play. Colleagues and contemporaries included René Spitz, a leading figure in psychoanalysis, infant observation, and child deprivation. Spitz's films and writings about infancy, *Hospitalism* and *Anaclitic Depression* (Spitz and Wolf, 1946; Spitz, 1946), chronicled infants' early emotional development in the context of separation from parents. Margaret Mahler and D.W. Winnicott both based much of their theory on the very early relationship between the mother and the infant. Winnicott described the "good enough" mother who provided a relationship in which her baby could survive and thrive, and also wrote about the "goodness of fit" as the match between the parent and the baby. Winnicott did not separate the baby from its context arguing that "there is no such thing as a baby" (Winnicott, 1960, p. 586).

John Bowlby and James Robertson studied hospitalized infants. They identified three stages in the response to maternal separation: protest, despair, and denial/detachment (Bowlby et al., 1952). Bowlby's development of attachment theory emphasized the evolutionary importance of maintaining contact with a caregiver with respect to the safety and emotional development of the infant. Exploring the mechanisms of Bowlby's theories through systematic observations of infant-mother interactions, Mary Ainsworth and her colleagues identified four patterns of relationships between infants and their caregivers – secure, avoidant, resistant, and disorganized – each with its own distinct patterns of both infant and caregiver behaviors (Ainsworth, 1967; Ainsworth et al., 1978; Main and Solomon, 1986). By the early 1960s, a wealth of research about the infant-mother relationship existed.

In the 1960s Selma Fraiberg presented her work on congenitally blind infants. Fraiberg and her colleagues described parent-infant psychotherapy and detailed approaches for clinicians from various disciplines who were working with infants and their families. In her work, Fraiberg used parental responses and reactions toward the child to inform treatment. The goal was to help the infant-parent relationship emerge in a space free of the distortions and displaced affects that engulfed their contexts. She helped professionals understand the importance of identifying the language of infancy and helping caregivers key into what the baby was saying. "Ghosts in the nursery" (Fraiberg et al., 1975) was the first paper on clinical infant mental health and remains an essential reading for infant specialists.

In the 1970s, as the clinical work in infant mental health continued to evolve, researchers continued to explore infant development and the influencing factors (Sameroff and Chandler, 1975). The Clinical Infant Development Program (CIDP), a comprehensive assessment and intervention program with at-risk infants, was created at the National Institute of Mental Health (Greenspan and Wieder, 2003). In 1977, ZERO TO THREE: National Center for Infants, Toddlers, and Families emerged from CIDP. Today, ZERO TO THREE is one of the leading organizations in promoting and advancing the field of infant mental health. ZERO TO THREE conducts training programs (e.g. diagnostic classification, reflective practice), sponsors leadership initiatives, publishes texts and videos on infancy and early childhood, advocates on behalf of infants and toddlers on local, national, and international levels, interfaces with media and professionals regarding infant mental health, and houses resource centers for parents and professionals.

Defining infant mental health

Infant mental health is synonymous with health, social, and emotional development. Zeanah and colleagues describe infant mental health as a "state of emotional and social competence in young children who are developing appropriately within the interrelated contexts of biology, relationships and culture" (Zeanah et al., 2000b, p. 14). Similarly, ZERO TO THREE: National Center for Infants, Toddlers, and Families considers infant mental health in the context of the developing capacity of infants and children from birth to 3 years to "experience, regulate and express emotion; form close and secure interpersonal relationships; and explore the environment and learn" (ZERO TO THREE, 2003). The first years of life reflect a period of rapid growth and change, including dramatic increases in the differentiation and complexity of a young child's social and emotional development.

Infant mental health and infant development more generally occur within the context of the family, community, and cultural expectations for young children. While the infant-caregiver relationship is the focal context in which infant mental health emerges, this relationship is embedded in other contexts that interact and influence human development (Bronfenbrenner, 1979) and in this case, infant mental health.

Cultural considerations regarding infant mental health include how infant mental health is understood within the particular culture. Additionally, adult goals and expectations for infants and for child development shape interactions and experiences in which infants grow. Cultures also vary with respect to childrearing practices used to promote, protect, and restore infants' and young children's mental health.

Infant development

No discussion of infant difficulties or the practice of infant mental health can begin without a solid understanding of typical development in the first 3 years of life. For practitioners working with infants and young children, developmental theories offer useful guidelines for predicting future development and evaluating whether an infant is on a healthy trajectory. Developmental perspectives attempt to explain a child's progression and maturation (Metcalf and Rowe, 2000). Infancy and early childhood is a time of rapid change linked to behavioral, cognitive and social-emotional advances. Typically, future development or current developmental level is predicated upon what already exists or has emerged. Importantly, developmental discontinuities are also evident, often marking key transition periods. The central role of experience in development must also be underscored. Experiences impact development differently depending on when they occur.

Key developmental theorists

While no single theory can adequately capture the complexity of human development, a number of key theorists emerged during the 20th century. Combining clinical experience, systematic observation, and experimental designs, Jean Piaget, Sigmund Freud, Erik Erikson, Anna Freud, John Bowlby, and their students and collaborators contributed a wealth of information about the progression from infancy to adulthood. These individuals, among the many other developmentalists exploring the earliest years of life, were perhaps most influential in informing the fields of infant psychiatry and infant mental health.

Especially relevant to infants and young children, Piaget emphasized the infant's active role in exploring the world and attempting to master it. His explicit account of cognitive advances during the first few years of life (i.e. sensorimotor and preoperational stages) provide an avenue for understanding how young children learn about and understand their worlds.

Sigmund Freud's theory of personality development and the stages he proposed sparked both psychoanalytic and developmental avenues for understanding and working with issues in infancy and early childhood. The Id, Ego, and Superego and the psychosexual stages (e.g. oral, anal, phallic) emerged from Freud's work. Erik Erikson elaborated upon Freudian theory to encompass social and cultural dimensions. Erikson's work identified the importance of interpersonal relationships above and beyond intrapsychic conflicts in shaping development. He articulated drives that moved people toward life and those that move people away with tension between these goals, creating typical crises in the life cycle. In Erikson's eight-stage model of normal development, each stage presents both intrapsychic and interpersonal balances that must be achieved. Future development depends on previous accomplishments.

Anna Freud expanded her father's theoretical framework and therapeutic approach to the realm of childhood. Credited with founding the field of child analysis, Anna Freud's theories of ego defense and development emerged from her clinical work and extensive observations of young children in nurseries during the 1930s and 1940s. Together with her collaborators, Anna Freud provided foster care to many young children and attempted to help them form attachment relationships by providing continuity of caregivers and encouraging their mothers to visit frequently.

Credited with developing the field of attachment, John Bowlby's work has had profound implications for the science of relationships. Trained as a psychoanalyst, Bowlby departed from drive theories and conceptualized infants' relationships with their caregivers based on ethologic (the study of animal behavior), modern evolutionary theory, and control systems theories. Bowlby described attachment behaviors as those that maintain a child's proximity to a caregiver in order to avoid harm. Over time and with consistent interactions with a familiar caregiver, the infant learns to tolerate the anxiety associated with brief separations and is able to move away from the caregiver in order to explore the environment. Bowlby's work highlighted the social origins of relationships between infants and their caregivers.

Importantly, developmental theories have been challenged because many of them rely on infant characteristics and abilities, often at the expense of familial and environmental influences. As discussed previously, infant development cannot be understood without understanding the context in which the infant exists.

Transactional model

The Transactional Model, developed by Sameroff and his colleagues (Sameroff and Chandler, 1975; Sameroff and Fiese, 2000), proposes that developmental outcomes are the products of interactions over time of a child's life and his or her experiences and environment. Continuous dynamic interactions between the child and his or her family and social contexts shape infant outcomes and the infant-caregiver relationship. Social relationships will amplify certain child characteristics and minimize others so that an infant born with certain characteristics will develop differently depending on the relationships and environment to which he or she is exposed.

Importantly, the earliest research on the transactional model suggested that the mechanism by which early risk influences development is often through negative effects of child characteristics on caregivers and the caregiving relationships (Sameroff and MacKenzie, 2003). Consider, for example, the situation when an infant is born prematurely. Premature infants are often medically fragile, developmentally immature and exhibit greater physiologic, motor, and state disorganization and fewer self-regulation capacities (Als, 1982). Because they have medical complications, are less responsive and available for social interaction, and provide diffuse and less predictable cues (Goldberg, 1979), their parents or caregivers may experience difficulties in taking care of them. Caregivers are likely to interpret infant unavailability according to their own frameworks. Such frameworks may include things like guilt about having a baby early, memories of a traumatic birth, postpartum depression, worries about financial issues related to hospitalization, and lack of social support. Caregiver responses, therefore, will be based not only on what the infant brings into the situation, but also on their experiences and interpretations of infant behavior. Parents who are having difficulties coping with the Neonatal Intensive Care Unit (NICU) environment, who are experiencing life stressors, or who are trying to manage their own mental health difficulties are likely to respond to a premature infant very differently than parents who are coping well, have access to resources, and are psychologically healthy. In the former case, preterm infants' characteristics may increase parents' difficulties in determining appropriate responses, decrease infants' experiences of sensitive and appropriate caregiving, and ultimately create a cycle in which parents feel less efficacious and infants experience fewer contingent interactions. More challenging interactions may also detract from some of the joy and pleasure inherent to parenting. In the latter, parents may be psychologically and physically available to the infant, enhancing their awareness of the infant's cues and their ability to provide continuity of caregiving. The infant, in turn, will experience this responsiveness across repeated interactions, experience greater behavioral organization, and ultimately develop adequate self-regulation strategies.

As illustrated in this example, the Transactional Model requires an understanding of the complex interactions among child characteristics (prematurity), caregiver characteristics (mental health, availability), and environmental factors (NICU, stressors). Such information is a prerequisite for drawing conclusions in evaluations, making appropriate treatment recommendations and, more globally, understanding child development.

Developmental accomplishments

The following section will detail some developmental accomplishments routinely observed during the first 3 years of life. We will provide an overview of development in the motor, cognitive, and social and emotional domains. Early development can be segmented in countless ways. Age groupings in the present chapter were selected to reflect some coherency across domains, emergence of new skills, and transitions that commonly signify developmental shifts.

As with any discussion of development, readers must be cautioned to use the information provided only as a guideline. Achieving or not having achieved particular milestones during a specific time period indicates neither giftedness nor delay. Typically, a comprehensive professional assessment is necessary to determine the extent and implications of developmental delays.

Prenatal development

The rapid advances in fetal development from a single cell to a complex organism makes prenatal development a time of particular interest to practitioners working with infants. Scientific and technological advances have afforded us a literal window into the world of the developing fetus. From three-dimensional photographic records of the fetus at each stage of development (Nilsson and Hamberger, 2003) to studies documenting the impact of prenatal exposure to teratogens (Lester et al., 2000), maternal stress, and chemical agents (e.g. pesticides), the role of the environment in shaping development is evident.

Typically, the protected uterine environment provides everything that the baby needs to develop appropriately. The mother's body supplies nutrition, hormonal cycling, physiologic regulation, motoric input, modulated sensory stimulation and more. However, because development occurs so rapidly during pregnancy, perturbations to the fetus may have dramatic consequences with respect to infant outcomes. Maternal substance abuse (i.e. drugs, alcohol, and tobacco) may directly damage the developing nervous system and other organs or result in preterm delivery, which is associated with numerous developmental risks. Physical damage to the fetus may occur as the result of physical injury of the mother, inadequate blood/nutritional resources, and disease. Other risk factors during pregnancy include maternal viral infections and malnutrition.

Prematurity and obstetric complications necessitate special consideration with respect to infant development. Many premature infants experience ongoing medical complications that alter their development. Compounding these effects are the psychosocial aspects of beginning life in the NICU and experiencing an altered relationships with caregivers. In cases of congenital anomalies, genetic abnormalities alter developmental trajectories from the start. Importantly, this does not suggest that environment impacts development less. An infant diagnosed *in utero* with Down syndrome would be at risk for even greater developmental difficulties if he or she did not receive adequate nutrition during the prenatal period.

To optimize prenatal development, prevention efforts typically target providing prenatal care to mothers (e.g. folic acid, routine obstetric appointments, and access to nutritional resources). Other efforts aim to reduce exposure to teratogens by treating substance abuse. Mental health-oriented prevention programs typically consider psychosocial factors, including maternal psychologic health, family environment, and social support networks in addition to the above.

The neonatal period (0–2 months)

While little empirical evidence exists to suggest that the experience of being born has lasting psychologic impact on emotional development, the circumstances surrounding a birth certainly have the potential to impact later well-being. Among many elements, the physical environment of the labor and delivery room (e.g. a comfortable, home-like appearance versus the sterile operating room), the similarity between parents' expectations of bringing a child into the world and the reality of the unfolding event, and the history that families bring with them to the hospital (e.g. having experienced previous perinatal losses) may all impact the emerging relationship between and infant and his or her family. Consider the marked differences between a routine vaginal delivery, a planned Cesarean section, and an emergency delivery resulting from a placental abruption; or whether the first moments of life begin in a mother's arms as opposed to starting life in a transport incubator on the way to the Neonatal Intensive Care Unit. For some infants, the neonatal period lasts a couple of months, while for others it may last for 6 months, as in the case of an infant born at 24 weeks. Supporting the emerging relationship regardless of the circumstances under which it begins is critical to promoting development and is a central aspect of early work with infants and their parents.

Importantly, the infant-parent relationship begins long before the baby is born and oftentimes, before the baby is conceived. Expectations about what an infant will be like and the psychologic relationship between parents and the baby develop throughout pregnancy (Cohen and Slade, 2000). They become especially salient during the third trimester, as delivery approaches and the corresponding physical changes clearly indicate that another person is there. Fertility history and previous birth experiences are among the many factors that impact expectations of childbirth and parenting. The birth of an infant may differ markedly for parents who have struggled for years to conceive a child in contrast to parents with a history of perinatal loss. For the family with fertility problems, the birth may be a time of joyous celebration. In contrast, the family with a history of perinatal loss may experience tremendous fear and anxiety about this baby's survival coupled with trauma and grief stemming from past events. Clearly, history and prenatal relationship building blocks shape the way parents interact with newborns and, therefore, impact infant development.

Once outside of the protective uterine environment, a newborn is suddenly faced with the challenge of breathing, ingesting and eliminating nutrients, regulating body temperature, and directly processing environmental stimuli, among other things. Initially, newborns depend on adult caregivers to provide a substantial amount of regulation (e.g. changing a wet diaper, selecting appropriate clothing, providing food) for basic systems. During the first months of life, responses of others to distress and social initiations impacts infants' understanding of what is expected of them and what they can expect of others. Repeated interactions with nurturing, protective, stable and consistent caregivers are essential to healthy development and form the foundation of attachment relationships.

Newborns have an array of behaviors that they use to communicate physiologically driven needs. Most commonly, adults identify distress in the form of crying or fussing as a primary mode of communication. However, newborns exhibit subtle and overt cues that signal organization or disorganization. Physiologic (e.g. breathing, heart rate, skin color changes), motor (e.g. extensions and flexions, tremors, fanning of fingers and toes), and state (e.g. transitions between states, types of available states) changes all indicate whether an infant is able to approach a situation or is in need of withdrawing to regroup (Als, 1982). For example, an infant who turns pale, pauses breathing and then resumes at a rapid rate and starts looking away or falling asleep while someone is trying to play with him is communicating that the social interaction is too challenging at that moment in time. Responding to these subtle cues might include pausing and allowing the infant to recover and resume the interaction by initiating a gaze.

The temperament literature (Chess and Thomas, 1991) suggests that infants are born with characteristic styles of behavior that evolve into consistent patterns. Caregivers respond to this style and their responses shape future behaviors. The "goodness of fit" between an infant's behaviors and a caregiver's style impact the manner in which development unfolds. For example, the combination of a baby displaying high levels of negative emotionality and the baby's parent having a low frustration tolerance may create a pattern of negative and hostile interactions.

With respect to the attachment system, precursors of attachment are based upon both infant and caregiver behaviors. The infant must have a sufficient repertoire of behaviors to communicate with the caregiver. At the same time, the caregiver should demonstrate awareness and responsiveness to infants' cues, flexibility in responding (Browne et al., 1996), and well-timed responses to infant signals (Kelly and Barnard, 2000). At birth, newborns show a preference for their mother's voice and smell. Visual input is best when it is the distance of a caregiver's face from the baby when the baby is being held (i.e. 6–12 inches away). In fact, the human face is one of the most interesting things for a newborn to see because it is designed with distinct focal points (the eyes), contrasting colors (darks and neutrals), and moves from time to time.

Over the course of the first months, newborns become better able to track objects and orient to sounds. Newborns appear to respond well to soft, high-pitched voices and soothing, cooing sounds. While often interpreted as social and responded to with delight, smiles during sleep or waking in the first 4–6 weeks of life are reflexive in nature. The social smile typically emerges between 4 and 8 weeks. "Cooing" also emerges during the second month of life and vocal conversations between infants and caregivers can take place. While movement is typically limited to less controlled extremity and head movements with some tucking of the trunk, an infant's jittery and jerky movements become increasingly smoother during this period and startles begin to disappear.

Early infancy (2–9 months)

The rapid physical and developmental advances continue during the next few months of life. During this period, patterns of behavior emerge and families generally develop rhythms and routines based upon the infant's signals and factors in the environment. Caregivers can generally recognize and respond to the infant's efforts at communicating in addition to anticipating circumstances under which the infant will require support or intervention. Sleep-wake cycles become more regulated, shifting from shorter periods of sleep interspersed with feedings and alert times to several hours of undisturbed sleep followed by longer awake periods and regular naps. Motor and social advances drive cognitive development and the capacity to explore the environment.

Motor accomplishments are the products of improved coordination of movements and increased physical strength and control. The jerky and uncoordinated newborn movements tend to disappear. Initially, improved control of the head and body enables infants to track and follow objects, reach for them and ultimately transfer them between hands and to others. Exploration of the infant's own body increases. Early body movements and wiggling lead to rolling over and eventually scooting, crawling, or moving around. Most infants can bear weight on their legs and enjoy jumping up and down while being supported by a caregiver. Postural control also enables infants to sit up and explore the world differently because of their upright position and free hands. Some infants may also be standing with assistance, pulling up on objects, or even standing on their own and taking some steps. Refined hand control enables infants to be more purposeful in their efforts to pick up and manipulate small objects. New skills lead to exploration of the environment and development of play routines.

This period evidences remarkable changes in communication abilities and social exchanges. With longer periods of alertness and a growing capacity to attend and process the environment, young infants are able to engage in social interactions that form the basis of conversational skills. Verbalizations increase in response to seeing something stimulating in the environment, experiencing a need, or engaging in a social interaction. Cooing and gurgling become babbling of vowel and consonant combinations, from which emerge first words. Infants often acquire and use signs to communicate (e.g. waving, pointing) their intent during this period.

Increased capacities in attention and memory are markers of cognitive development at this time. Because of the developmental shift in representational capacity, infants exhibit changes in their engagement with objects. The trajectory evolves from infants losing interest in an object the moment it is out of sight, to looking for missing objects, to recognizing a partially hidden object, to searching for missing objects after they are hidden. These representational capacities impact the social and emotional domain as well, and infants become keenly aware of their primary caregivers and evidence distress when the caregivers are absent.

Repeated interactions with familiar and nurturing caregivers reinforce infant recognition of important attachment figures. Differential responses to parents are evidenced during this period with bigger smiles, body movements, and movement toward these close and important figures. Once these attachment bonds have been formed and maintained, the likelihood of forming additional attachment relationships decreases, barring unforeseen circumstances. Separation anxiety, or distress and discomfort at actually being separated from the caregiver or at the perceived threat of separation, emerges. Distress at seeing strangers, aptly named "stranger anxiety," also manifests itself at this point in development. As attachment relationships become more firmly established, infants notice and mind the absence of their attachment figure. By the same token, infants recognize unfamiliar people (and situations) as such and make efforts to move away from then and toward the safety of their attachment figures.

Later infancy (9–12 months)

Toward the end of the first year, locomotion advances and coordinated motor systems facilitate very active exploration and manipulation of the environment. Most infants can sit up, crawl toward or away from people and objects, and walk a few steps without support. Manipulation of objects as tools (e.g. a spoon) emerges as fine motor skills improve. Early signs of self-care behaviors and strides toward independence may appear. For example, older infants may pull clothing off, feed themselves, and carry desired objects to and from places.

Communication abilities continue to improve with consonant vowel combinations becoming first words (e.g. "ball," "mama," "bye-bye"). Infants begin to make meaningful distinctions between sights and sounds in their environment. They are able to use routines and predictability as signals for what happens next or what is expected of them in addition to facilitating transitions between events. Intentional communication is apparent and older infants may become frustrated when they are not understood.

Socially, older infants actively interact with others (e.g. peek-a-boo, building and knocking over blocks, singing songs), watch and imitate what others do, and delight in repetitions of favorite activities. They continue to express a preference for people and may even possess favorite objects. Social interactions continue to function in a regulatory capacity, helping infants manage their own affective experiences while simultaneously providing an enriching context for learning about the environment around them. Caregivers can elaborate experiences, narrate situations, communicate information (e.g. naming objects and activities), and demonstrate new skills all within the context of these interactions.

Cognition and caregiving also interact in that infants develop the capacity to jointly attend to and share the viewpoint of the caregiver as well as request that caregivers attend to what they see. In a series of famous experiments using a "visual cliff," researchers demonstrated that 1-year-olds used "social referencing" to visually check with their mothers before embarking on an ambiguous task (Klinnert et al., 1986). If the mothers' facial expressions communicated joy or interest, most infants proceeded with the task, while expressions of anger or fear tended to prevent infants from completing the task.

Attachment relationships are typically solidified by the time infants reach 12 months of age. In securely attached dyads, a separation from the attachment figure results in distress, while reunions result in seeking comfort from and proximity to the caregiver, which alleviates distress (Ainsworth et al., 1978). Having a secure base typically enables the young child to actively explore the environment and supports optimal cognitive, social, and emotional development.

Early toddlerhood (12–18 months)

With the accomplishment of walking (then running and jumping) comes physical exploration and manipulation of a toddler's surroundings. Over these few months, toddlers figure out how to build tall towers and knock them down, lift and carry objects, push and pull things, turn and open and close toys, climb on the playground or on furniture, dance, hop and jump, throw balls, pound objects, and make more refined movements with utensils and writing implements.

This active exploration provides the foundation for cognitive leaps and increases in knowledge about how things in the world work. Toddlers learn about means-ends relationships, physical and spatial characteristics of objects, and relationships among objects (e.g. in/out, up/down). Repetition and practice helps toddlers refine their skills. Because toddlers have the ability to access much of the environment, conflicts with parents often arise about what is appropriate

or accessible. Thus, parents of toddlers find themselves having to set more limits, create more boundaries, and say "no" or redirect their children's behavior.

While communication skills continue to improve, the young toddler still has difficulty communicating clearly when relying exclusively on words. The young toddler may string together two or three words (e.g. "more milk") to communicate a desire or thought. Vocabulary increases over this period and toddlers are very interested in naming objects and having others name things for them.

Daily routines of playing, eating, self-care, and sleeping become increasingly important in helping the young toddler organize his or her world and prepare for events in the future. While still too young to comprehend these issues, rituals and routines also help toddlers learn the "rules," including such things as appropriate behavior at the table, cleaning up, and sharing with others. Continuity and predictability in structured environments provide a sense of safety and comfort for the toddler; he or she knows what to do and what will happen when he or she does it. This continuity and predictability extends to relationships with caregivers. Toddlers are very sensitive to separations from their caregivers. In addition to separation anxiety, young children may experience other fears. Sudden noises, large or unfamiliar objects, or strangers might evoke distress. Relationships with caregivers also provide important information about how to behave. Toddlers are keen observers of parent behavior and are likely to imitate things they see their parents doing, regardless of whether they understand the nature of the behavior. Aside from modeling behaviors, parents also reinforce or punish toddler behaviors, thereby informing toddlers of what they consider right and wrong.

Toddlerhood (18–36 months)

Perhaps the most salient developmental accomplishment of toddlerhood is the capacity for symbolic representation. Toddlers learn to use words and symbols to communicate their internal and external experiences. Pretend play affords toddlers with a mechanism to control both the outside world and express and work out their inner thoughts and feelings. While language development varies tremendously, many toddlers experience a language explosion between 18 and 24 months of age. By the time children are 2, their expressive vocabulary includes between 100–200 words and they can understand several hundred more. By age 3, young children are able to communicate using sentences.

Independence and self-assertion are central characteristics of toddler development. Toddlers may assert their wish to do things on their own while not having the requisite skills to complete the activity. Definite opinions and preferences emerge and are communicated, often at inopportune moments. These assertions and moves toward independence may increase the level of conflict between the toddler and his or her parents. Obtaining cooperation from a toddler involves setting clear guidelines for choices, which usually means letting the toddler choose between one of two options that the parent is willing to support. Temper tantrums and low frustration tolerance necessitate anticipation of circumstances that will be challenging and the application of a consistent and clear intervention.

Relationships with parents remain central throughout toddlerhood. Although independence and the ability to do things on their own increase, toddlers elicit parental involvement in play and caregiving. Because they are avid explorers but cannot accurately assess situations, toddlers require close supervision and structure in order to ensure their safety. Some toddlers obtain additional security and comfort from particular special objects (e.g. a blanket) and may turn to these objects in times of distress or transition. The use of these "transitional objects" is particularly appropriate in situations where parents are not available.

With peers, toddlers move from parallel play, where toddlers play next to each other and may or may not be engaged in similar activities, to associative play where cooperation and joint involvement are observed. Toddlers are able to recreate routines and engage in elaborate pretend games (e.g. cooking dinner) that reflect their own experiences and understanding about how the world works.

Other considerations in toddlerhood include the arrival of a new sibling. For firstborn children, having to share what was once the undivided attention of parents may be quite challenging. Again, parental response to the situation is critical in terms of supporting the toddler through the transition. Some toddlers may begin daycare or preschool, necessitating assistance with that transition. Changes in the environment are likely to impact the toddler, and consequently, the toddler's behavior and should be documented and considered during assessments.

Evaluating infants

General guidelines

Evaluating infants is challenging. Clinicians attempt to capture the dynamic unfolding of biologic potential within a specific, ever evolving environmental context. Transactions between multiple determinants influence the developmental process and broaden the arena for assessment. Infants, young children, and their environments appear to be in constant flux. Seen on one day, a baby may appear a certain way, while the next time the baby may seem very different.

The many changes in early childhood necessitate that clinicians accurately diagnose infants according to uniform standards using valid and reliable assessment tools and classification systems. Such diagnostic precision enables professionals and families to speak the same language and ensure that individuals who use the same term mean the same thing.

Moreover, when appropriately diagnosed, infants may meet certain eligibility criteria that afford them and their families access to necessary therapeutic and supportive services. In current and emerging systems of health-care, provision of services is linked to diagnoses. Standard diagnostic criteria are important not only for reimbursement for services, but also in designing and developing programs. Negative consequences of diagnostic classification systems include labeling and stigmatizing of individuals. Concerns about the "self-fulfilling prophecy" also emerge in thinking about diagnoses, particularly when they have been associated with poor prognosis. However, when used with proper training, a comprehensive, systematic assessment of interaction patterns, individual differences, and regulatory patterns should lead to identification of both strengths and vulnerabilities in major developmental areas, relationships, and the environment of the child (Harmon and Murrow, 1995).

Additional research and outcome studies on diagnostic assessment and classification in infancy are vital to advancing the field of infant mental health. Emerging research suggests that the Diagnostic Classification: 0–3 system (ZERO TO THREE, 1994) can help clinicians identify diagnostic issues and establish treatment guidelines for infants and young childhood through comprehensive assessment (Weston et al., 2003). Additional studies suggest that the DC: 0–3 may capture certain disorders better than the DSM-IV (Frankel and Harmon, 1996). Without an empirically validated classification system for infants and young children, professionals run the risk of labeling infants according to adult mental health criteria that do not capture the richness or complexity of these children's situations. Using adult diagnostic labels is harmful in that it connotes a host of difficulties that are not manifested similarly in infancy.

A thorough evaluation should include:
- Developmental history including prenatal and perinatal events.
- Social history and current environment, including cultural factors.
- Physical examination.
- Psychosocial screening.
- Multiple observations of infant-caregiver interaction.

Incomplete evaluations:
- Focus on the presenting concerns without understanding the context in which they emerge.
- Depend on reports from one source without confirmation through observation or from another source.
- Offer the perspective of a single discipline rather than integrating information from various disciplines with information about the child.
- Do not assess whether the infant's performance was representative of typical functioning and capacities.
- Are not relationship-based.

PEARLS & PERILS

Numerous issues complicate the early identification of infant mental health issues (Eppright et al., 1998). First, without specific diagnostic criteria, established developmental norms and standardized assessment tools, it is difficult to determine what is typical and atypical. Downward extension of adult diagnostic systems does not adequately capture mental health issues in the infant population. Moreover, assessment is difficult because of rapid changes in development, new levels of organization, and the changing meaning of specific behaviors or "developmental appropriateness." Second, lack of verbal communication by infants and young children limits our ability to ask questions about mental health issues in traditional, adult-centered interviews or self-report forms. Instead, mental health evaluators must rely upon behaviors and relational dynamics to determine mental health status. Recognition that infant mental health diagnoses exist primarily in the context of relationships is essential for accurate diagnosis. As with adults, environmental and organic factors confound mental health issues.

Assessment of infants and young children is a dynamic process that involves multiple evaluations over a period of time (three to five sessions at a minimum) and input from a variety of sources (caregivers, childcare providers, professionals from different disciplines). Sources of information typically include parent or caregiver reports of history, direct observation and interaction with the infant, observation of parent-infant interactions, parental reports of infant behaviors, and if available, another report of infant behaviors in a different setting (e.g. daycare). The diagnostic process in and of itself is considered to be an opportunity for relationship building, intervention, and treatment planning. Consequently, parents and caregivers are encouraged to ask questions and offer contributions throughout the evaluation. Additionally, feedback in the form of clarification of behaviors observed, parental questions, and goals for the evaluation may be provided after each assessment session.

The following sections provide information about methods of assessing infants and young children. While much of the information can be generalized, unique circumstances may dictate additional procedures or alternate methods. For example, legal involvement may necessitate individuals with specialized skills or advanced degrees conducting assessments (e.g. forensic evaluations, child custody evaluations). Working with young children in foster care may also be complicated. In this case, flexibility and adaptability in combination with familiarity with legal requirements aids in establishing who has guardianship of the child, communicating with various service agencies, and obtaining histories from several individuals.

Clinical interview

The clinical interview provides an opportunity to begin an ongoing conversation about the reason for referral, while at the same time serving as the starting point for building relationships with families and providing support and clarification about their unique circumstances. Because the focus is on the process as much as the content, information gathering and relationship building generally spans a number of sessions. The purpose of the interview is both to obtain a thorough understanding of historical and environmental factors that may contribute to the etiology or manifestation of the presenting problem and to form a working relationship with families. Empathic, reciprocal and supportive communication styles foster alliance and trust. Engaging in such a process ultimately enables the clinician and the family to "see the same child" (Seligman, 2000). The clinical interview also affords the clinician an opportunity to observe the infant-parent relationship.

In order to develop appropriate recommendations for intervention, it is helpful to obtain information about relevant areas of child functioning, child and family history, and the present context in which the child lives. Identifying information (name, age, race, ethnicity, address) is typically obtained during intakes to schedule initial appointments and should be verified early in the process. Throughout the clinical interview, the clinician observes the parent-infant relationship, the infant's individual functioning and developmental status, the parent's presentation, and the family system. The clinician also attends to the developing relationship between him or her and the family and to information regarding the family's capacity to utilize interventions and support (Seligman, 2000).

With respect to information about the infant, it is important to address in detail the presenting symptoms and behavior, the developmental history, and past and current functioning across a number of domains (affective, cognitive, motor, sensory, interactive). Obtaining specific information about the duration, frequency, and severity of symptoms or behaviors and about any relational or environmental factors that exacerbate or ameliorate the difficulties is important. The clinician should document when difficulties began and assess whether there were any identified precipitants (e.g. the birth of a sibling). In addition to detailing areas of difficulties, consider probing for information about areas of strength and adaptive functioning. Daily functioning may include information about sleeping, eating, relationships with others, elimination patterns, and routines.

When assessing infants, a mental status examination provides useful information about current level of functioning. Document individual infant characteristics such as appearance, reaction to situations, self-regulation, motor skills, speech and language, thought processes, affect and mood, play behaviors, and cognitive development (Benham, 2000). Consider exploring relatedness to caregivers, examiners/ providers, and age mates in multiple settings in order to determine how the infant is functioning.

It is also helpful to understand the caregiver's perspective on the reason for referral, the referral source, and how the child's behaviors are affecting the family. If the caregiver was not the referral source, discrepancies in perceptions about the extent to which the infant or young child is exhibiting difficulties may exist. Obtaining permission to speak with other providers or review records may provide additional information about history or perspectives on current difficulties. Involvement of social services or the legal system should alert the clinician to the importance of obtaining a release to speak with representatives from these agencies regarding child and family functioning in the context of systems issues that may be relevant.

Detailed history about pregnancy and delivery and developmental accomplishments helps contextualize current difficulties. In obtaining a history, consider including questions about maternal well-being, maternal substance use, exposure to stressors or traumatic events, and prenatal care during pregnancy. Attempt to understand the nature and course of the pregnancy and delivery, attending to important psychosocial elements (e.g. desire for the pregnancy, past pregnancy history, social support) as well as the medical course. Prugh's "Five Questions" approach (Prugh, 1983) provides a relationship-based way to obtain some of the history. Questions progress from asking how the mother is feeling in general, to concerns about the baby, what the baby's name is and where it came from, exploring "violations of expectation" concerning the pregnancy, delivery, and about the baby, to reflections on the pregnancy and thoughts about the future as well as the support systems and services for the mother and baby.

Careful documentation of newborn characteristics that might compound current presentations, including low birth weight, intracranial hemorrhages, birth asphyxia, central nervous system problems (e.g. seizures or infections), sensory impairments, and congenital anomalies, is also important. After discharge from the hospital, ascertain the nature of eating, sleep-wake, and elimination routines and document any difficulties in these areas. Subsequent hospitalizations and serious illnesses should also be documented. In order to evaluate developmental accomplishments, consider using one of the screening tools described in the next section. Important domains to consider in infancy and early childhood include sensory development, motor milestones, language development, social and emotional capabilities, and relationship factors.

Family history of medical, psychiatric, or psychosocial difficulties should also be documented. The clinician would benefit from understanding past history and current symptoms of parental mental illness, mental retardation, substance use, and impairment in functioning. Developmental and relationship histories of the caregivers and siblings may also be explored. Pay particular attention to history of traumatic events, chronic stressors, and other sociodemographic factors that might compound past or present difficulties. Experiences of violence at the interpersonal or community level should be documented and reported as mandated by law.

Because the environment has tremendous influence on infants, it is critical to understand what the environment is like. Who lives with the infant? What is the nature of their relationship with the infant? What resources do the family have and what resources do the family need? Is the infant exposed to or experiencing violence or neglect? Under what conditions does the infant live? Is the infant getting his basic needs (e.g. food, shelter, care) met? What other agencies are involved with the family and what is the nature of their involvement? Attempt to obtain a picture of each of the environments in which an infant spends a lot of time. These environments may include the home, daycare settings, and the neighborhood or community.

The initial assessment period offers a window into the infant-parent relationship. Careful observation and documentation provides essential information about the extent to which the relationship provides a nurturing context for infant development. The dynamic exchange between caregivers and infants suggests that observing one will provide information about the other and observing the relationship will provide information about both. For example, parents

KEY CLINICAL QUESTIONS

- *Why are you here today?*
  Determine the caregiver's understanding of the reason for referral.
  Identify caregiver concerns and questions.
  Begin by listening and respecting the caregiver, which helps establish rapport.
- *What is a typical day like? (Or, describe a typical day.)*
  Assess patterns of sleep and waking, eating, social time and any difficulties or concerns surrounding tasks of everyday living.
  Examine family routines and environmental consistency, continuity, and predictability.
  Obtain a baseline of adaptive functioning (may want to have the caregiver describe good days and bad days if a discrepancy emerges).
  Identify areas for intervention and support.
- *What things do you love about being (child's name)'s parent?*
  Assess the child's strengths and unique characteristics.
  Help focus the caregiver on positive aspects of the relationship.
  Identify reinforcing elements of the relationship that can be bolstered.
- *How does your experience compare with what you were expecting when you thought about parenting (child's name)?*
  Assess expectations and violations of those expectations or disappointments.
  Identify hopes and wishes that can inform treatment planning and recommendations.
  Provide information that may correct unrealistic demands.

who are emotionally available to their infants are able to help infants regulate their own affective experiences. Similarly, nurturing and responsive parents have infants who are generally secure and have high self-esteem. Other parent and infant characteristics that may merit exploration include: protection/vigilance and safety, comforting/comfort seeking, teaching/learning and mastery, play/play and imagination, discipline and limit setting/self-control and cooperation, and structure and routines/self-regulation and predictability (Zeanah et al., 2000a).

All of the information provided during a clinical interview and in any subsequent observations should be contextualized within the infant and family's culture. Culture has been conceptualized as "a distinct system of meaning or a cognitive schema that is shared by a group of people or an identifiable segment of the population" (Coll and Magnuson, 2000, p. 97). Typically, daily interactions within the family embody beliefs and values that transmit culture across generations. Understanding cultural and personal child-rearing approaches and beliefs provides insight into existing dynamics. For example, behaviors that might be "problematic" in one culture may be acceptable and even desirable in another. Diversity extends far beyond race, ethnicity, and culture to include factors such as generational status, socioeconomic status, gender, age, and sexual orientation. Diversity issues should be openly acknowledged and addressed in interactions with families and in interpretations of behaviors or assessment results. The goal of assessment and intervention is to help reach a mutual understanding about the young child within his or her unique context.

Assessment tools

A variety of assessment instruments is available for use with infants and young children and their families. Ranging from screening instruments that provide snapshots of developmental achievements to parent self-report measures of problem behaviors to comprehensive dimensional assessment procedures, these measures are designed to identify early social, emotional, and developmental difficulties that may be targeted for early intervention or prevention efforts.

Screening instruments

Screening instruments are designed to provide rough approximations of infant functioning in a timely and cost-effective way. Information is often used to identify infants in need of further evaluation and intervention. Large numbers of infants may be screened (e.g. Apgar scores), or screening can be more targeted on the basis of individual or group risk factors or concerns. Collected at a single time point and with broad strokes across domains, screening instruments may over- or underestimate infant functioning or fail to capture individual differences in development. As such, infants may

either be incorrectly denied access to necessary interventions or be targeted as "at risk" by virtue of their performance on global measures.

Parents are often used as sources of information for screening instruments either through self-report measures or interviews. Forms may also be available for completion by daycare providers or teachers. A few screening tools utilize observation of the young child. Table 15.1 provides an overview of several instruments used to assess infants and young children during the first 3 years of life. The table presents the names of the instruments, appropriate age ranges, and approximate administration times.

In selecting the appropriate screening instrument, it is important to consider how the measure was developed, who the target population is, and whether it demonstrates adequate reliability and validity. Reliability refers to whether the same score would be obtained by the same child if tested at other points in time. Validity addresses whether the instrument measures what it is supposed to measure. Predictive validity refers to the measure's relationships to characteristics that appear in the future. Assessment in infancy and early childhood is complicated by the fact that scores on many tools are not highly related to long-term developmental outcomes. Concurrent validity describes the relationship between scores on the screening instrument and scores on other assessments conducted at the same time (e.g. Bayley Scales of Infant Development).

Developmental assessments

Psychologists or other specially trained professionals (e.g. early childhood educators, developmental specialists) may conduct comprehensive developmental assessments of infants and young children using standardized, empirically validated tools. These tools typically require substantial training in administration, scoring, and interpretation prior to their use with infants. For a detailed discussion of developmental assessments and screening instruments please refer to *Infant Assessment* by M. Virginia Wyly.

In the newborn period, several assessment systems provide information about a range of newborn behaviors and capabilities. These assessment systems examine newborn sensory, physiologic, motor, and state functioning and elicit various reflexes. Evaluators consider the interplay among these domains of functioning in the context of the infant's medical risk factors (Brazy et al., 1993) and sociodemographic circumstances.

Brazelton Neonatal Behavioral Assessment Scale

The NBAS assesses a newborn's ability to respond to social and nonsocial stimuli through a series of graded manipulations that promote different states and levels of arousal. Throughout the evaluation the infant is an active participant who makes purposeful efforts at regulating incoming

TABLE 15.1

Assessment tool	Age range	Administration time
Ages and Stages Questionnaires: Social–Emotional (ASQ:SE; Squires, Bricker & Twombly, 2002)	6–60 mths	10–15 mins
Assessment of Preterm Infant Behavior (APIB; Als, 1984)	Preterm Infants	45–90 mins
Bayley Scales of Infant Development-II (BSID-II; Bayley, 1993)	15 days–42 mths	30–90 mins
Brief Infant Toddler Social Emotional Assessment (BITSEA; Briggs-Gowan & Carter, 2002)	12–36 mths	10–15 mins
Child Behavior Checklist for Ages 1½ to 5 (CBCL; Achenbach & Rescorla, 2000)	18 mths to 5 yrs	15–20 mins
Denver Developmental Screening Test II (Frankenberg et al., 1990)	0–6 yrs	30 mins
Devereux Early Childhood Assessment (DECA; LeBuffe & Naglieri, 1998)	2–5 yrs	5–10 mins
Mullen Scales of Early Learning (MSEL; Mullen, 1991)	0–68 mths	15–60 mins
Neonatal Behavioral Assessment Scale (NBAS; Brazelton, 1973)	0–6 wks	30–60 mins
Parents' Evaluation of Developmental Status (PEDS; Glascoe 1997)	0–9 yrs	> 5 mins
Parenting Stress Index (PSI; Abidin, 1995)	< 12 yrs	20–25 mins

environmental stimuli. The infant's capacity to habituate to stimuli, self-organize, and maintain robust states are also examined. Considerable skill is required in order to elicit the infant's best performance and score the instrument reliably. More recent adaptations of the NBAS include using the assessment as a demonstration to provide parents with information about their infants' responses to environmental stimuli (Brazelton, 1990; Fowles, 1999).

Assessment of Preterm Infant Behavior (APIB)

Using the NBAS as a template, Als developed the APIB for use with preterm and fragile infants (Als, 1984). The five subsystems in the synactive theory (physiologic, motor, state, attentional-interactional, and self-regulation) are assessed before, during, and after the environmental manipulations. The examiner evaluates the infant's ability to adapt to manipulations and tolerate stimulation in addition to detailing disorganized and organized behaviors throughout the examination.

Beyond the newborn period, numerous developmental assessments exist. These instruments assess cognitive development, information processing, parent-infant interaction, emotion and temperament, and play, among other things. Reviewing each of these domains and the accompanying instruments and methods is beyond the scope of this chapter. Instead, we will discuss a few key instruments that are commonly used in infancy and early childhood.

Bayley Scales of Infant Development-II

The BSID-II (Bayley, 1993) includes a mental scale, a motor scale, and an infant behavior record for infants aged 15 days–42 months. Items are arranged in developmental order and many items can be scored through incidental ob-

servation. The mental scale includes 147 items measuring language, object permanence, problem-solving, imitation, perceptual-motor integration, and visual and auditory attention. The motor scale has 111 items tapping gross and fine motor skills. The Infant Behavior Record describes infant behavioral traits observed over the course of the examination. The examiner completes it after the exam is finished. Domains evaluated include sensitivity to stimuli, interest, energy, affective arousal, and social responsiveness. The caregiver also responds regarding whether performance on the exam reflected the infant's typical affect, activity level, and ability. While the scales provide important information about current developmental status, the scores are limited in their ability to predict later intellectual performance.

Mullen Scales of Early Learning

Based on a neurodevelopmental model, the MSEL (Mullen, 1991) ranges from birth to 68 months. The instrument uses five scales to assess: gross motor base, visual receptive organization, visual expressive organization, language receptive organization, and language expressive organization. Scores reflect infant strengths and areas of concern.

Diagnostic classification

Before 1994, the *Diagnostic and Statistical Manual of Mental Disorders* (DSM; American Psychiatric Association, 1994) was the only available system for classifying disorders in infants and young children. For infants and young children, few diagnostic classifications in the DSM-IV and other adult classification systems are appropriate. These systems, developed, validated and used with older children and adults, do not consider many of the developmental issues and char-

KEY CLINICAL QUESTIONS

- *What concerns might indicate a need for further developmental evaluation?*

  For newborns, neurobehavioral difficulties (e.g. tremors, seizures), state issues, feeding problems, high levels of chronic irritability, sensory deficits, history of major medical conditions or complications.

  Significant delays in milestones (e.g. motor, communication, interactional).

  Behavioral issues including outbursts, rages, withdrawal, anhedonia, impulsivity, lack of inhibition, self-injurious.

  Regulatory difficulties including problems with sleeping, eating, elimination, daily routines, sensory processing, and interacting.

  Cognitive abilities and adaptive functioning.

  Developmental regressions where previously acquired skills are lost or new skills are not being acquired.

- *What is the reason for referral? In other words, what is the clinician hoping the evaluation will reveal?*

  Clarify the nature of concerns and how the information will be used.

  Provide an opportunity to collaborate with the caregiver in understanding concerns and current circumstances.

  Provide diagnostic clarification when the presenting symptoms can be the manifestation of different underlying difficulties.

- *What information can comprehensive evaluations provide?*

  Diagnostic impressions and integration of presenting symptoms in the context of a thorough history and of the psychosocial environment.

  Treatment planning including specific behavioral and systemic targets for intervention, modalities of intervention, frequency and duration and expected results.

  Clarification regarding the current level of functioning and prognosis for the future.

BOX 15.1

DSM-IV disorders diagnosable in infancy and early childhood

- Mental retardation
- Motor skills disorder
- Developmental coordination disorder
- Pervasive developmental disorders
- Autistic disorder
- Rett syndrome
- Childhood disintegrative disorder
- Asperger syndrome
- Pervasive developmental disorder NOS
- Attention-deficit and disruptive behavior disorders
- Attention-deficit/hyperactivity disorder
- Feeding and eating disorders of infancy or early childhood
- Pica
- Rumination disorder
- Feeding disorder of infancy or early childhood
- Other disorders of infancy, childhood, or adolescence
- Separation anxiety disorder, early onset
- Reactive attachment disorder of infancy or early childhood
- Stereotypic movement disorder
- Disorder of infancy NOS

---

acteristics of disorders relevant for the under-3 population. As detailed in Box 15.1, the DSM-IV criteria for certain disorders may be used to classify disorders seen in infancy and early childhood. However, these diagnostic categories do not adequately capture the complexity of infant difficulties. In contrast to the DSM-IV, the Diagnostic Classification: 0–3 (DC: 0–3) is unique in that it was developed to assess vulnerabilities, difficulties, and adaptations of infants and young children across major developmental areas. The system is described in detail in the next section.

History of Diagnostic Classification: 0–3

The *Diagnostic Classification of Mental Health and Developmental Disorders of Infancy and Early Childhood (DC: 0–3)* is the product of an 8-year effort by a multidisciplinary Diagnostic Classification Task Force comprised of clinicians

and researchers. DC: 0–3 is designed to focus attention on all key aspects of young children's experiences including relationships with important adults; individual differences in motor, sensory, language, cognitive, and emotional development; the child's capacity to organize experience; family patterns; and psychosocial factors in the environment that affect the young child. Using this framework, an individual or team is able to collect and integrate information regarding the child's vulnerabilities, strengths, adaptive capacity, and level of functioning across major developmental areas.

In the course of evaluating infants and young children and formulating diagnostic possibilities, the DC: 0–3 assesses the contribution of constitutional/maturational factors, interactional capacities, emotional functioning, relationship quality and characteristics, and family and environmental factors. Each of these domains alone or in combination with others may impact diagnostic and treatment decisions. Issues that arise during the course of an evaluation should be integrated into a comprehensive treatment plan or preventative intervention that addresses them.

Axis I, primary diagnosis

The primary diagnosis generally reflects the core elements and features of the disorder as expressed through the maladaptive behavior of the child. As can be seen in Table 15.2, diagnoses range from traumatic stress disorder to disorders of affect, to adjustment disorders and regulatory disorders.

TABLE 15.2

The multiaxial system

Axis I: Primary Diagnosis
  100. Traumatic Stress Disorder
  200. Disorders of Affect
  300. Adjustment Disorder
  400. Regulatory Disorders
    • Type 1: Hypersensitive Type
    • Type II: Under-Reactive Type
    • Type III: Motorically Disorganized, Impulsive
    • Type IV: Other
  500. Sleep Behavior Disorder
  600. Eating Behavior Disorder
  700. Pervasive Developmental Disorders or
      Disorders of Relating and Communicating
Axis II: Relationship Classification (based on the PIR-GAS)
  901. Overinvolved relationship
  902. Underinvolved relationship
  903. Anxious/tense relationship
  904. Angry/hostile relationship
  905. Mixed relationship – specify
  906. Abusive relationship
    • Verbally abusive relationship
    • Physically abusive relationship
    • Sexually abusive relationship
Axis III: Medical and Developmental Disorders
Axis IV: Psychosocial Stressors
Axis V: Functional Emotional Developmental Level

(reprinted with permission from the Zero to Three Press).

Axis II, relationship classification

Three aspects of a relationship are evaluated and categorized on axis II. During the evaluation, observers attend to the behavioral quality of the interaction, its affective tone, and the psychological involvement of each of the participants. The Parent-Infant Relationship Global Assessment Scale (PIR-GAS) is used to assess the quality of infant-parent relationship. Relationship problems may or may not occur with symptomatic behaviors. Ability to rate relationships using the scale is not predicated upon knowing the reason for the relationship problem. Scores on the PIR-GAS range from 90 (well adapted) to 10 (grossly impaired). PIR-GAS subscales cluster scores into three levels: no disorder (80–99), tendency to disorder (40–79), and disorder (10–39). See the diagnostic decision tree presented in Figure 15.1 for more detailed information about axis II.

Axis III, medical and developmental disorders and conditions

Axis III details any co-existing physical (including medical and neurologic), mental health, and/or developmental disorders. For example, a congenital anomaly (e.g. cleft lip) would be recorded on this axis. A chronic medical condition such as asthma would also be recorded on axis III.

Axis IV, psychosocial stressors

Axis IV details the forms and severity of psychosocial stress that are influencing factors in various disorders. Considerations include severity of stressor (intensity and duration at that intensity level), suddenness of initial stress, frequency, and unpredictability of its recurrence. The same stressor may impact a child very differently depending on the developmental level, chronological age, endowment, and ego strength of the child. Axis IV also documents the availability and capacity of caring adults to serve as protective buffers and help children understand and cope with the stressor. The Stress Index identifies sources of stress (e.g. abduction, adoption, loss of parent, natural disaster, parent illness), their duration (acute to enduring), and the overall impact of each event (none, mild, moderate, severe).

Axis V, functional emotional and developmental level

Axis V documents essential processes or capacities including attentional factors, interactive displays, and communicative functions appropriate for different developmental levels. For example, infants at all ages are assessed with respect to their ability to engage in mutual attention with a caregiver while representational skills and affective communication are not assessed until infants are 18 months or older. Assessment is based on observations of infants interacting with parent(s) or another significant caretaker. The Functional Developmental Level Rating Scale rates quality of child's play with each significant caretaker and summarizes a child's overall functional level. Infants and young children are classified along a continuum ranging from "has fully reached expected level" to "not mastered any prior level" with points in between.

Guidelines for using the DC: 0–3 system

One of the more valuable features of DC: 0–3 is the guidelines, or "diagnostic decision tree," an example of which is included in Figure 15.1. As can be seen in Figure 15.1, the clinician is asked to consider various aspects of the relationship and the intensity, frequency, and duration of difficulties in determining the appropriate diagnostic classification. It is important to note that while a relationship may not meet diagnostic criteria, it may still be characterized by certain features or tendencies that should be detailed on axis II. The decision tree approach to diagnosis is based on the evaluator paying attention to disorders often overlooked and "ruling out" environmental, constitutional, or interactional problems which may need immediate attention or a specific treatment approach (such as infant-parent psychotherapy).

The guidelines presented below assist the clinician in systematically evaluating the infant and making appropriate

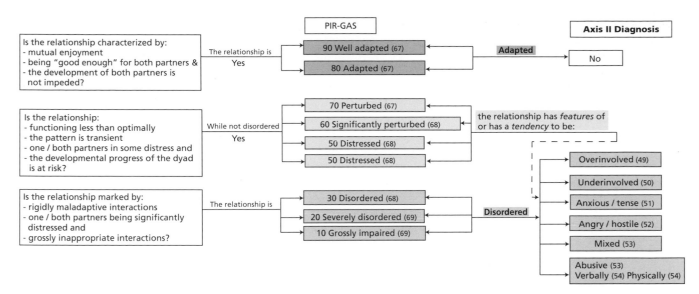

Fig. 15.1 Diagnostic Classification 0-3: decision tree – axis II (relationship disorder classification). Assess the relationship for each parent-child dyad, whenever possible. If there are difficulties in the relationship, then assess for the intensity, frequency and duration of the disturbance. A "tendency" is not given a diagnosis, but a note is made on axis II that the relationship has features of or a tendency to be overinvolved, underinvolved, anxious/tense, angry/hostile, mixed or abusive. Adapted from ZERO TO THREE /National Center for Clinical Infant Programs. Diagnostic Classification: 0-3; Diagnostic Classification of Mental Health and Developmental Disorders of Infancy and Early Childhood. 1994. [Northcutt & Wright (2002) ©Funding for Dr Northcutt provided by First Five Sacramento Commission].

diagnostic decisions. They have been adapted with permission from ZERO TO THREE.

1 If there is a clear severe or significant stressor or trauma to account for the disordered behavior or emotions, then traumatic stress disorder should be considered initially. This would be the appropriate progression if, for example, the young child had recently been in a serious automobile accident.

2 If there is a clear constitutionally or maturational-based sensory, motor, processing, organizational, or integration difficulty related to the observed maladaptive behavioral and/or emotional patterns, then a regulatory disorder should be considered initially. Children born prematurely frequently display regulatory difficulties resulting from a combination of being born early, having an immature nervous system, and beginning life in the critical care environment of an NICU rather than being at home with their families.

3 If the presenting problems are mild, < 4 months duration, and related to a clear environmental event, then an adjustment disorder should be considered initially. A family that recently relocated or a toddler who started daycare within a few months of the evaluation may fall into this category.

4 If there is neither a clear constitution- or maturational-based vulnerability, nor a severe or significant stress/ trauma and the problem is not mild, of short duration, and not related to a clear event, then the categories of mood and affect disorders should be considered initially.

5 Disorders of multiple delays, including communication and social relatedness, are distinct and usually involve chronic patterns of maladaptation (e.g. pervasive developmental disorders) and an ongoing pattern of deprivation (e.g. reactive attachment disorder). Even when underlying constitutional or maturational vulnerabilities or clear stressors are present, these disorders usually take precedence over other categories and are exceptions to the above general rules. This guideline would apply in cases where parents present a history including elements such as not achieving typical milestones, unusual or extreme behaviors (e.g. self-injurious behaviors), and serious communication delays. Alternatively, a history may include pathogenic care in addition to infant behavioral or constitutional factors.

6 If the problem is specific to a certain situation or a relationship to a particular person, an adjustment disorder and a relationship disorder should be considered. Difficulties with one parent or in a particular context (e.g. daycare) that result in behavioral changes and symptoms that extend beyond the relationship would fall into this category.

7 If the problem only involves a relationship without other symptoms, use axis II instead of axis I. That is, if difficul-

ties emerge exclusively in the context of a specific relationship, for example, with one parent, criteria would not be met for an axis I diagnosis.

8 Reactive attachment disorder is appropriate when there is inadequate basic physical, psychologic and emotional care. Concerns about the relationship or attachment are to be considered in the relationship axis or other diagnoses related to the present symptoms.

9 Assess the underlying basis for common symptoms such as feeding and sleep disorders, which may be separate problems, part of various diagnostic categories, an ongoing relationship pattern, or regulatory and pervasive developmental disorders. Thus, a child with a sleep disorder as a result of posttraumatic stress disorder or a mood disorder or a child who is very anxious in daycare and refuses food and vomits only in that setting, do not meet criteria for feeding and sleep disorders. This differs from a child who has a primary eating problem with food refusal in all situations or a child with sleep onset difficulties without other symptoms. Careful history taking, observation, and assessment of various contextual factors will enable the clinician to obtain diagnostic clarification.

Selected diagnostic categories and case studies

Regulatory disorders

Regulatory disorders emerge in infancy and early childhood. They are characterized by an infant's difficulties in modulating both internal organization and incoming environmental stimuli. Symptoms of regulatory disorders often get communicated during history taking that reveals difficulties doing the routine things infants and young children "should" be doing (e.g. eating, sleeping, playing with others, learning in their environments).

Internally, infants with regulatory disorders may exhibit less physiologic stability (e.g. maintaining a steady heart rate, regular respirations, and good oxygenation) and less organized state behaviors, including a more limited repertoire of available states (e.g. full range of states from deep sleep to quiet alertness to a robust cry), more rapid transitions between states (e.g. abrupt shifts from asleep to extremely fussy) instead of smooth transitions, and the shorter durations of a state. The capacity of a young child to attend is dependent on state organization and, therefore, difficulties in attending and in sleeping are also characteristic of regulatory disorders. Eating and elimination patterns require a combination of internal and external modulation and may be problematic. Gross and fine motor difficulties may also be evident. A poorly regulated infant is likely to demonstrate affective disorganization as a limited range of affect, the inability to modulate affective expression, or constricted or expansive affective tone. Chronic disregulation may ultimately result in language and cognitive difficulties.

In order to be diagnosed with a regulatory disorder, an infant must display at least one sensory, sensory-motor, or processing difficulty in addition to evidencing behavioral symptoms: over- or under-reactivity to sensory stimulation includes noises, visual input, tactile stimulation and pain, odors, and temperature. Sensory-motor difficulties may be seen in oral-motor difficulties or incoordination resulting from poor muscle tone or hyper/hyposensitivity, balance problems, hyper/hypotonicity of muscles, and deficits in motor planning skills, modulation of motor activities, or fine motor skills. Deficits in processing capacities may be presented as limitations in auditory-verbal processing, articulation, visual-spatial processing, or attentional difficulties.

Young children diagnosed with regulatory disorders are categorized into one of four types. Type I, Hypersensitive Type, describes children who are fearful and cautious or negative and defiant. These children may become easily overwhelmed by their environment and retreat with very little input or they may over-react to environmental input with behavioral outbursts and refusals. Type II, Under-Reactive Type, characterizes children who are withdrawn or difficult to engage or self-absorbed. These infants may require a great deal of input to notice what is happening in the world around them and may be less responsive to typical social overtures, making it more challenging to interact with them. Young children meeting criteria for Type III, Motorically Disorganized/Impulsive, Regulatory Disorders, may appear erratic, inattentive, uncoordinated, and chaotic. They often demonstrate poor planning and processing capacities and have difficulties completing routine, developmentally appropriate tasks. These children may later meet criteria for attention-deficit/hyperactivity disorder. If one of the first three types does not characterize the infant, Type IV, Other, is used.

Mood disorders

Mood disorders are related to a young child's affective experience and behavioral expressiveness. Symptoms arise as part of the child's functioning rather than as the result of a particular situation or in the context of a specific relationship. In contrast to children with regulatory or developmental disorders, children with mood disorders do not exhibit major constitutional or maturational difficulties or severe developmental delays. While mood symptoms are frequently expressed within a particular relationship or seen in caregiver-child interactive patterns, the interactive difficulties are related to the child's general affective and behavioral difficulties and are not unique to the relationship or situation. Thus, a critical aspect of diagnosing mood disorder in infancy and early childhood involves determining whether symptoms are a

Alina's story

Alina, a 5-month-old hospitalized infant, and her mother were referred by a nurse working with them. Nurses, physicians, and therapists reported having a difficulty communicating with Alina's family. These professionals reported that they were unable to effectively engage in treatment with Alina because her mother would not allow them access to the child, would undo what they did, and did not appear to be listening to and incorporating their suggestions. Professional after professional indicated that Alina's mother did not seem to be able to read the baby's cues and that she frequently overwhelmed the baby.

Alina was born at term and diagnosed with a number of congenital anomalies, including a heart condition, for which she was awaiting transplant. Additionally, she was microcephalic and was extremely sensitive to sound and touch. Medical professionals were concerned about her ability to see and more generally, about Alina's prognosis. The neonatalogists, specialists, and nurses had all met with the family a few times to discuss potential paths and choice points. After one such conference, the mother stated that she just wanted to let nature take its course and did not want to provide extreme levels of intervention. The very next day she told the nurse caring for the baby that the baby was on the heart transplant list and was likely to receive a new heart very soon.

During the assessment period, a number of issues emerged. First, a neurobehavioral examination confirmed Alina's frailty and sensitivity to environmental input. Alina was easily overwhelmed by even distal environmental input presented during sleep and did not demonstrate an ability to habituate after repeated presentation. She showed her distress through rapid breathing, color changes, decreased oxygen saturation, and prolonged motor instability. She had fleeting alert states during which she was available for social interaction and had difficulty maintaining a deep sleep because of her sensitivity to the environment and the demands of the hospital environment. An assessment by an expert revealed a profound visual impairment: Alina could sense light and dark but had little acuity. A second and critical issue involved Alina's mother's own mental health issues. Her mother presented with unusual interpersonal communication skills, including avoidant behaviors and extreme mistrust of new people, disorganized behaviors (e.g. losing things and seeming quite scattered), memory and attentional difficulties, and alternating sad or very angry affect. Despite repeated conversations with professionals who were telling her the same things about her baby, Alina's mother continued to ask the same questions and interact with Alina in ways that directly contradicted what she had been told. Diagnostically, a Regulatory Disorder, Hypersensitive Type, was considered because of Alina's extreme sensitivity and over-reactivity to environmental stimulation and her visual impairment. Because of the intrusive nature of her mother's interactions, difficulties in the infant-parent relationship suggested that the relationship could be characterized as disturbed (PIR-GAS = 40, tendency to be overinvolved).

Treatment involved several different elements. Initially, Alina's mother had difficulty talking with or even making eye contact with the specialist. During one early meeting when the specialist offered the mother papers that she had requested, the mother grabbed the papers, said "thanks but I have so many papers I'm not sure I can read these," and returned immediately to reading her magazine. After spending several days developing a working alliance with the mother and answering her many questions, the specialist gently began offering information about Alina in the context of her mother's interactions with her. Information about Alina's signs of stress and about her attempts to regulate environmental input were discussed and demonstrated. For example, during a bath the specialist pointed out how Alina's breathing became more regular when her mother turned off the radio, dimmed the lights, moved slowly, and talked to her in a very soft voice. The specialist also arranged for an examination by an expert in visual assessment and offered to be present during both the evaluation and feedback. Intervention also involved informing hospital professionals about Alina's sensitivities and working with them to develop appropriate plans of care that would not overwhelm Alina. Unfortunately, the circumstances did not permit the specialist to provide the amount of support necessary to directly address Alina's mother's mental health issues. Instead, these were addressed as they pertained to the infant-parent relationship.

Over the course of several weeks, Alina's condition stabilized to the point of being ready for discharge. Because others in her environment changed the nature of their interactions with her and provided more external regulation to support her emerging abilities to self-regulate, Alina's reactivity decreased. However, she still required extensive support and structure in order to help her maintain her balance and not become overwhelmed. Importantly, Alina's interactions with her mother also improved to the point where her mother could anticipate Alina's response to a situation and take measures to prevent her from becoming overwhelmed. This case illustrates the various types of interventions provided by infant mental health specialists in a consultation and liaison model in hospital settings.

---

general feature of the child's functioning or whether they are relationship or situation-specific. As mentioned previously, if the symptoms appear primarily in the context of a relationship, a relationship disorder (axis II) would be considered.

Mixed disorder of emotional expressiveness

Infants and young children beginning to internalize difficulties regulating affect may suggest a diagnosis of mixed

Sam's story

Sam was a 3-year-old referred by his pediatrician because of head banging. Sam and his mother had both remained hospitalized for 1 week following his birth due to a maternal infection that he also contracted. His early development was characterized by difficulties in motor and language development. He also had an esotropia and was clumsy. At the age of 15 months, Sam's mother had a second son. At that time, Sam began to head bang when he did not get his way. Over time, he developed a hematoma on the front of his head from chronic head banging. His language continued to be a problem. Sam's mother seemed overwhelmed and unsure what to do. Her younger son was developing normally and seemed to be ahead of her older son, whom she could not manage nor communicate with.

During the assessment phase, several things became evident. First, Sam's mother was very depressed and her marriage was stressed by her son's behavioral difficulties. Second, the "identified patient" clearly had difficulty regulating affects and when frustrated, banged his head, often threatening his parents and the evaluator that he would do so. Diagnostically, a Regulatory Disorder was considered given his problems (from birth) with motor and language development and his visual problems. We were also concerned about the effects of his chronically banging his head and wondered whether he might have symptoms consistent with head trauma. However, from a diagnostic perspective, a mixed disorder of emotional expressiveness was also considered, because Sam had difficulty identifying and expressing emotions and often seemed confused about feeling states. It became clear that there were also problems in the parent-child relationship, although the quality of the relationship was not considered disordered (PIR-GAS=50, features of a disorder).

Treatment of this family involved several components including: 1) focusing quickly on the mother's depression, including psychotherapy and medication; 2) mother-child therapy sessions to help mother develop better strategies for dealing with her son's anger and head banging; 3) physical, occupational, and speech-language therapy for Sam's motor and language problems; and 4) some conjoint sessions with the parents to focus on marital issues. Most of the interventions were of short duration and the family successfully regained their equilibrium. The therapy with Sam focused on helping him identify his emotions, particularly angry and sad feelings, and giving him alternative ways to express his feelings. Foot stamping, rather than head banging, was encouraged when he could not tell adults that he was angry or upset and negotiate a more adaptive solution.

Over time, Sam was able to express his frustrations, needs and wants, and the foot stamping was no longer needed. So, although Sam had clear constitutional vulnerabilities, a several year history of his inability to express his emotions and his mother's inability, primarily because of her own depression, to help him regulate those emotions, lead to the development of a mixed disorder of emotional expressiveness. What was particularly striking about this dyad was that the PIR-GAS score at the end of treatment (with the mother) had increased to 78, clearly of much less clinical concern.

disorder of emotional expressiveness. This disorder is characterized by: 1) problems expressing developmentally appropriate emotions, 2) absence of one or more specific affects that are expected based on developmental level, 3) constricted range of emotional expression compared to developmentally appropriate expectations, 4) disturbed intensity of emotional expression that is inappropriate for developmental level, and 5) affect that appears reversed or inappropriate to situations (e.g. expressing happiness when being reprimanded).

Infants at risk

Infants born preterm

When a baby is born prematurely, serious, ongoing medical and physical complications may require hospitalization in the NICU for days and sometimes months. Regardless of the reason for the early birth or the hospital course, disruption of the typical relationship between parents and their newborn may adversely affect the emerging parent-child relationship. As a consequence, the baby's mental health and overall development may be impacted.

Alfonso's story

Alfonso's family came to take care of him every afternoon during the 6 months he spent in the NICU. His mother had to wait for her husband to come home from work before coming to the hospital because the family had only one car. Alfonso's siblings, both under 4 years of age, came with their parents and wanted to play with their very sick brother. It was hard for them to understand why they could not touch or hold him and why they had to come to the hospital instead of taking Alfonso home. His parents often had to focus on the siblings or divide their attention, which led to turn-taking with Alfonso. While staff wanted the family to be with Alfonso, some people got frustrated at the level of activity at his bedside when the children were there. However, the family did not have alternative childcare resources, nor did they want to be apart from their children. Additionally, Alfonso's father only spoke Spanish, making communication with hospital staff challenging. He was often forced to wait for his wife to translate the exchange for him.

For preterm infants and their parents, many relationship disruptions can emerge during pregnancy, delivery, and hospitalization. These disruptions can affect the emerging infant-parent relationship. Prenatal and postnatal disruptions include events such as diagnosis of a congenital anomaly during pregnancy, medical complications, preterm delivery, and long-term hospitalization. Parental factors such as maternal depression, grief, traumatic experiences, family violence, and language barriers may also disrupt the parent-infant relationship. Infant factors that might disrupt relationships include exhibiting disorganized behaviors and behaviors that are hard to read, having difficulty calming and quieting, and being sleepy or unable to socially engage. Finally, with respect to the hospital and NICU environments, numerous elements including hospital policies, relationships with professional caregivers, and access to resources (e.g. money, transportation, privacy, comfortable chairs) may impact the infant-parent relationship.

A preterm birth violates parental expectations about pregnancy, childbirth, parenting, and development (Macey et al., 1987). Because pregnancy ends early and sometimes abruptly, parents of preterm infants experience disruptions in the normative biologic, physical, and psychologic changes associated with pregnancy. They also miss out on traditional rituals, such as baby showers, naming ceremonies, and the baby's first bath that mark the transition to parenthood.

Despite efforts to provide family-centered care and developmentally supportive practices that promote parental involvement with their preterm babies (Davis et al., 2003), parents of preemies often experience guilt, anxiety, and depression (Gennaro, 1988; Maloni et al., 2002); elevated symptoms of posttraumatic stress disorder (DeMier et al., 2000); and anger, helplessness, hopelessness, terror, and ambivalence about the baby's survival (Easterbrooks, 1988; Tracey, 2000). While research suggests that mothers' anxiety and depression decrease during the months after their babies are discharged from the NICU (Brooten et al., 1988), mothers of high-risk, very low birth weight children report high levels of emotional distress even 2 years after the child's birth (Singer et al., 1999). Supportive relationships within and beyond the family bolster parents' well-being during the crisis of a preterm birth, facilitate infant-parent interactions, and promote infant development (Miceli et al., 2000).

Many contextual factors affect the relationship between parents and their preterm baby. These include: the financial burden on parents; the ease or difficulty of travel to the NICU; the needs of siblings; the quality of the marital relationship; and family history. Typically, a number of these contextual factors interact, creating an even more complex picture of family functioning.

The preterm baby's condition powerfully affects what he or she can bring to the parent-infant relationship. Neurologic immaturity and medical complications make preterm babies capable of less physiologic, motor, and behavioral organization and modulation (Als, 1982) than infants born full-term. Thus, a preterm infant may be fussy and irritable, but cannot be soothed by a feeding because it may hurt when he or she eats. The baby whose underdeveloped lungs require high-frequency ventilation may not be able to be held. The infant who does not have the energy to wake up and look at his or her parents even for brief periods misses the most basic early relationship-building opportunities.

The infant factors discussed above may affect relationships well after the baby's discharge from the NICU. Preterm infants may experience ongoing health, academic, and emotional difficulties that create chronic stress for their families (Blackburn, 1995). Even when difficulties are not "diagnosable," they may present challenges. Sensory overload, difficulties with transitions, and laborious efforts to complete schoolwork emerge repeatedly in parents' descriptions of life with prematurely born children.

Disruptions in the relationship between preterm infants and their parents occur for many reasons and may be associated with infant outcomes across a broad range of developmental domains. From 20–50% of infants born preterm meet criteria for a physical, emotional, or cognitive disability (Lorenz et al., 1998). Family stress places children born prematurely at high risk for maltreatment. The risk of maltreatment among children with disabilities is more than three times greater than among typically developing children (Sullivan and Knutson, 2000).

Nurturing and cultivating the infant-parent relationship during the perinatal period is critical. It is the infant-parent relationship that can protect the preterm baby from risk and foster healthy long-term development. Clinicians can promote the mental health of preterm babies and their families by using psychoeducational interventions to teach parents and caregivers about preterm infant development, including similarities to and differences from typical development. Clinicians working with preterm infants and their families should take into consideration the above-mentioned relationship disruptions and assess for their potential impact on the current relationship and on presenting problems. Understanding the family's experience in the NICU is also a critical element to working effectively with them. The case below illustrates some of the complex dynamics that families face. These factors operate above and beyond the fact that their baby is medically fragile and hospitalized.

Prenatal exposure to substances

According to the National Institute on Drug Abuse (NIDA), approximately 5.5% of pregnant women use an illicit drug during pregnancy (National Institute on Drug Abuse, 1996). Drug use estimates vary by sociodemographic characteristics including race and family income. Specifically, drug use during pregnancy is higher for African American women and for women living below the poverty level and in inner-city neighborhoods. Methodologically, it is difficult to study exposure to a single substance, since drug use is frequently poly-substance use, co-occurring with alcohol, tobacco, and other substances. Moreover, drug use also has high comorbidity with mental illness and involvement with the legal system (Lester et al., 2000), both of which have tremendous implications for infant development. With any prenatal substance exposure, it is also important to consider the postnatal effects resulting from growing up in an environment where substances are being used.

In the mid-1980s, awareness of cocaine use during pregnancy spread to the national level. Sensationalized by the media, "crack babies" were expected to have severe developmental consequences resulting from prenatal exposure. NIDA figures suggest that about 45,000 infants exposed to cocaine are born each year (National Institute on Drug Abuse, 1996). More recent literature, based on longitudinal developmental studies of children exposed to cocaine *in utero*, suggests that the effects of prenatal exposure to cocaine are subtler than initially predicted (Lester et al., 2002) but certainly not benign. Findings suggest that prenatal exposure to cocaine affects neurobehavioral development, attention, affect and temperament, and arousal regulation (Lester et al., 2000). Subtle differences in IQ scores and on measures of receptive and expressive language translate to millions of dollars annually in special education services necessary when children with specific deficits require services (Lester et al., 1998).

Fetal alcohol syndrome (FAS) was identified in the late 1960s. FAS is characterized by deficits in growth, physical structures, and in central nervous system functioning and is a leading cause of mental retardation (Fitzgerald et al., 2000). Subsequent to its identification, studies examining the effects of prenatal exposure to alcohol began emerging. While alcohol is considered a teratogen (i.e. an agent that crosses the placenta and circulates in the fetus during gestation and later causes birth defects in the baby), its effects on developmental outcomes vary depending on the timing of exposure and the dose (Streissguth, 1997), with the central nervous system most affected by exposure to alcohol. Infants exposed prenatally to alcohol show the most enduring changes in neurobehavioral functioning relative to their non-exposed counterparts.

Clinicians working with infants and young children would benefit from understanding what substances an infant might have been exposed to prenatally and whether there is ongoing exposure. Other substances to consider include illicit drugs, nicotine exposure *in utero* resulting from maternal tobacco use, exposure to second-hand smoke after birth, and exposure to maternal medications, including mood stabilizers and antidepressants.

Child abuse and neglect

Although a chapter of this volume is devoted to child abuse and neglect, writing about infants and young children necessitates a discussion of the issue. The field of infant mental health was influenced and actually grew out of early observations of parental neglect, maternal separation, and the impact of being raised in institutions on young children's development (Bowlby et al., 1952). Although cruelty to children has been documented throughout history and around the globe, it was not until 1962, when Dr Henry Kempe and his colleagues (Kempe et al., 1962) at the University of Colorado School of Medicine, explicitly named child abuse as a major health concern with devastating developmental consequences in a landmark paper entitled "The Battered Child Syndrome." By 1963, all states in the United States had laws protecting children under 18 from non-accidental serious physical injury, sexual exploitation or misuse, neglect, or grave emotional or mental injury resulting from acts of commission or omission by parents, legal guardians, or caretakers.

Maltreatment of infants and young children varies by cultural practices and values and according to biologic predispositions of both children and caregivers (Huberman et al., 2000). Child abuse cuts across all socioeconomic, racial, and ethnic groups. Categories of abuse include physical abuse, sexual abuse, neglect, and emotional abuse. For fragile infants and young children, rates of child abuse and neglect are even higher. Epidemiologic research revealed that the prevalence of maltreatment of children with disabilities was 31% as compared with 9% in children without disabilities (Sullivan and Knutson, 2000).

Child abuse and neglect includes exposure to extreme violence, whether it be domestic violence, community violence, or war conditions. Infants and young children are highly susceptible to their surroundings. Conditions of chronic chaos, fear, danger, and battle, whether experienced by their caregivers, their neighbors, or strangers, influence their capacity to develop secure relationships that form the foundation for later development. Situations of extreme deprivation, poverty, or stress in which caregivers do not have the resources to invest in infants may be considered as extreme neglect and have similar developmental consequences. Examples include infants and young children across the globe who are raised in orphanages and infants in communities and countries where deprivation is so severe and infant mortality rates are so high that parents are forced to stop providing basic care to one child in order to save another.

Children who have been abused, neglected, or exposed to violence may evidence indiscriminate sociability and unpredictable social cues, making it difficult for others to interact

Consider consultation with a multidisciplinary child protection team and report to the police or a local department of human services as mandated by law and ethical guidelines when there is:

- Physical evidence of injury (e.g. skin lesions, bone deformities, anogenital findings of past or recent trauma, multiple episodes of bodily trauma at various stages of healing, "shaken baby syndrome").
- Verbal disclosure of abuse by the child or a trusted person who knows the child.
- Inappropriate sexual play or knowledge.
- Growth deficiency or sudden shift in growth pattern to far below standard growth curve.
- Repeated use of medical system resulting from illnesses whose origins are unknown or unexplained (Munchausen syndrome by proxy).

with them. Pathogenic care clearly deviates from expected interactions between children and their caregivers and has marked consequences for development. In some cases, severely compromised interactions may warrant a diagnosis of Reactive Attachment Disorder.

Other infants at risk

Other groups of infants are at risk for poor developmental outcomes. Among these are infants who are born into conditions of extreme deprivation and infants who are HIV positive. In this section, we will briefly consider each of these groups.

Both globally and in the United States, infants are born into and raised in conditions of extreme deprivation. When basic resources like food and water are not readily and routinely available, physical, cognitive and emotional development are jeopardized. Infants and young children may die of starvation, dehydration, dysentery, or diseases that may be preventable under other circumstances. Deprivation also includes the absence of parents or caregivers, as in the case of infants reared in orphanages, in war zones, or those whose parents have died because of other epidemics. For example, the global human immunodeficiency virus (HIV) epidemic, particularly in sub-Saharan Africa, leaves hundreds of thousands of infants orphaned each year. In some cases, clinicians working with infants and young children in the United States may be asked to consult with families who have adopted infants from other countries. Understanding the impact of extreme deprivation on child development is essential in working with these families.

Concern regarding infants exposed to HIV continues. Although considerable progress has been made in reducing the amount of maternal-fetal transmission of HIV, with clinical trials reporting transmissions rates below 2%, the pragmat-

ics of pharmacologic regimens, cost, and surgical deliveries limit the affordability and feasibility of such interventions (Kourtis, 2002). Importantly, HIV status is often a correlate of multiple difficulties, including conditions of poverty, drug exposure, and chronic illness. HIV status is associated with growth and developmental delays in infants (Pollack et al., 1996). Such delays may be compounded by factors such as having caregivers who are HIV positive and coping with illness and death. Family functioning may be dramatically altered depending on the stage of illness, whether death is imminent, and the cause of infection. For example, an infant living in a family where chronic substance use caused the infection may face repeated separations from his or her caregiver because of the drug use and its social and legal ramifications. In working with families where HIV infection is

Kyra's story

CASE 15.4

Kyra, a 32-year-old, HIV positive, African-American woman was referred by the social worker at the home for pregnant women where she was living. Kyra was in her fourth month of pregnancy and was being treated with antiretroviral therapy to decrease the likelihood of transmitting the virus to her baby. During the clinical interview, a number of salient issues emerged. First, Kyra was in treatment for crack cocaine use. Although she denied current use, she indicated that she had been asked to leave her previous placement because she "went missing for a weekend on a crack binge." Kyra indicated that she was aware of the detrimental effects of cocaine use during pregnancy. A second important issue concerned the placement in out-of-home care of Kyra's 3-year-old son. James lived with Kyra's mother and Kyra sporadically dropped in to see him but was unable to live in her mother's home or consistently follow the treatment plan developed by social services.

Kyra's involvement with the medical, legal, and human welfare systems was extensive and required continual communication and collaboration among treatment providers. Individual psychotherapy involved bi-weekly, in-home therapy that initially centered on grief work with Kyra surrounding her HIV status. Kyra felt tremendous remorse and guilt about her drug use and the possibility that she would transmit a lethal virus to her unborn child. Kyra appeared committed to continuing her medication regimen. However, she was unable to maintain her sobriety or sever ties from a social circle that perpetuated her addiction. About 6 weeks into treatment, Kyra disappeared for a weekend. When she returned, she acknowledged having used drugs and was asked to leave her placement. Unfortunately, because she did not have a place to live, Kyra had to relocate to a different community and was no longer able to access the services she had been receiving.

an issue, clinicians may consider the impact of environmental factors, stage of the illness, social stigma regarding the illness, and the profound isolation and fear these families face knowing that without a cure, they may be permanently separated from their infants by death.

Treatment issues

Treatment settings and modalities

Infants and young children may be seen in a variety of settings. Clinic and office-based evaluation and treatment are available and utilized by some consumers of infant services. Parents may bring their children to offices for developmental and medication evaluations and therapy. Among these, specialty clinics serve the needs of targeted populations. For example, clinics provide follow-up care for infants who were hospitalized in the NICU, evaluations of infants who were adopted internationally, or see infants who are HIV positive. Infants and young children may also be seen in the context of programs providing services to parents, and in particular, to mothers (e.g. substance abuse treatment, postpartum depression groups). In addition to these more traditional settings, assessment and intervention frequently occurs in other contexts where infants and young children are seen.

Not uncommonly, parents and caregivers raise concerns about behavioral and developmental issues at routine pediatric visits. Alternatively, the primary care physician may be alerted to an issue through observation of the child at such a visit. For medically fragile infants and young children, treatment may begin almost immediately after birth and take place in a hospital setting. Evaluations, consultations, and interventions with mental health professionals, physicians, developmental specialists, and others often occur at the infant's bedside. Because it is often difficult for parents and caregivers of young children to leave the house and attend the various appointments they have scheduled, home visitation programs offer treatment in the convenience of the family's home. Daycare and educational environments also provide contexts for evaluating and treating infants and their families. Professionals working with infants and their families benefit from being flexible about the context in which concerns emerge and services are provided. Such flexibility will afford greater opportunity to conduct comprehensive evaluations that take into consideration the various contexts and relationships in which infants function.

We share the recent concern raised by Zito and colleagues (Zito et al., 2000) regarding dramatic increases in the prevalence of medication usage in preschool-aged children. In the face of inadequate research (e.g. randomized, double-blind controlled clinical trials) regarding the effects of medication on young children and in light of recent concerns by the Food and Drug Administration regarding the effects of selective serotonin reuptake inhibitors (SSRIs) (Davis et al.,

2003), we contend that medication should not be used as a first-line intervention in children under 5 years of age. Only after psychologic, behavioral, and family interventions have been implemented and deemed inadequate to alleviate the symptoms should pharmacologic intervention, in the context of a complete psychiatric evaluation, be pursued (Harmon and Riggs, 1996). This recommendation is consistent with the principle of doing no harm that we are bound to uphold as physicians and mental health professionals treating young children.

Infant-parent psychotherapy

Psychotherapy with infants and young children from birth to 3 often involves working with both infants and their parents. Rather than working exclusively with the infant or treating the parent using an individual psychotherapy model, the dyadic relationship is the identified patient in infant-parent psychotherapy. Stemming from a rich psychoanalytic tradition, the goals of infant-parent psychotherapy are to bolster and support social and emotional functioning, and development more generally, through improving the infant-parent relationship. Specifically, treatment centers around "aligning the parents' perceptions and resulting caregiving behaviors more closely with the baby's developmental and individual needs within the cultural, socioeconomic, and interpersonal context of the family" (Lieberman et al., 2000, p. 472).

The relationship between an infant and his parent can be accessed through infant behaviors, the interaction between the parent and the infant, infant representations of the self and the parent, parental representations of the infant and of the self, and the parent-therapist relationship. Each of these "ports of entry" may be of immediate clinical attention, enabling the therapist to enter the system (Lieberman et al., 2000). Clinicians focus on salient clinical issues in order to access mutually constructed meanings subsumed within the relationship.

Fraiberg and Fraiberg (1980) eloquently described the nature of infant-parent psychotherapy:

> "In treatment, we examine with the parents the past and the present in order to free them and their baby from old 'ghosts' who have invaded the nursery, and then we must make meaningful links between the past and the present through interpretations that lead to insight … We move back and forth between present and past, parent and baby, but we always return to the baby (p. 61)."

Infant-parent psychotherapy typically involves joint meetings with the baby and the parents or caregivers present. In some cases, particularly as babies move into toddlerhood, treatment may also include separate sessions with the parents in addition to joint sessions. Similarly, in circumstances where the infant requires additional treatment to address specific developmental issues or vulnerabilities, additional individual treatment with the infant may be indicated. Flexibility and collaboration with other treatment providers is essential. Regardless of the work being done in individual modalities, the infant-parent psychotherapist attempts to maintain a focus on implications for the relationship.

Although the infant-parent relationship may be the focus of evaluation and treatment, we should not neglect the mental health and social support needs of parents, primary caregivers, families, and communities with babies and young children. Parental psychiatric disorders, substance abuse or dependence, and sociodemographic stressors must be addressed and treated in order to promote optimal infant mental health and development. Many infants and young children are affected by the untreated mental health needs of their families, ongoing exposure to violence, and the psychologic consequences of living in depleted and devastated communities (Shonkoff and Phillips, 2000).

Prevention

The malleability of infants and young children and the profound impact of the environment on development make the first 3 years of life especially appropriate as targets for preventive efforts. Goals of prevention efforts have included, among others: improving pregnancy and newborn health outcomes by providing information and access to prenatal care and decreasing exposure to teratogens; lowering incidence of child abuse and neglect through parent education, providing support, and psychotherapy; increasing the time between subsequent births; improving the infant-parent relationship; and enhancing developmental outcomes through the provision of services and enriched environments. Models of prevention range from home visitation by nurses and paraprofessionals during the prenatal and postnatal periods (Olds et al., 2002) to early childhood intervention efforts as exemplified by Early Head Start programs (Robinson and Fitzgerald, 2002). The following is a detailed description of one such preventive intervention, the Chicago Health Connection's Doula Project.

Chicago Doula Project

Chicago Health Connection's (CHC) community-based doula model is rooted in the service community and is a culturally sensitive approach to pregnancy, childbirth, infant development and family support. The Doula Model provides opportunities prior to labor and delivery to enhance the mother's knowledge of proper prenatal care, early brain development and the critical role they play in shaping the emotional, social and cognitive development of their children. CHC's consulting and technical assistance provide a flexible framework for replicating this model based on the priorities of an organization and the unique needs of the service community.

The Doula program is *one* component of an array of support services that are offered to pregnant and birthing women by the partner agency. In many cases, doula participants are also receiving health services, prenatal care and social services. Follow-up services by the partner agencies are provided, such as long-term home visiting, postnatal care and Head Start programs.

Doulas are full- or part-time salaried laywomen recruited from the communities served by the community partners. Doulas come from a variety of sources, local schools, churches, Head Start programs and hospitals, and are generally natural leaders in the community. Successful doulas share certain qualities: a commitment to helping young women "own" their birth; a capacity to form strong trusting relationships, and an ability to meet women where they are and to listen and respond to their needs. A doula's relationship with the mother begins as soon as the agency is notified of the pregnancy. Regular contact throughout the pregnancy includes accompanying the client on at least one prenatal care visit, helping her develop a birth plan, and providing labor and delivery classes. When labor begins, the doula is available to the mother, helping her determine if she is actually in labor, and supporting her through labor, delivery, and the first few hours postpartum. The doula visits the mother at home during the first working day after hospital discharge, up to five times a week during the first week, two or three times the second week and one to two times in weeks three and four. During the second month postpartum, the doula continues to visit the home at least once a week. At the end of 6–12 weeks, the doula steps back from her relationship with the mother, and the agency steps in to provide ongoing postnatal services.

Preliminary findings about doula support show that when doulas provided continuous emotional support to young, low-income mothers, the women had significantly shorter labors, were more likely to be awake after labor, and were more likely to interact and talk to their babies immediately following labor than women who had not received doula support. In a study of 229 births in the Chicago Doula Project, C-section rates were 8% for single births (compared with 14.5% for US teens and 12.8% for Chicago teens), epidural rates were 11.4% (compared with 50% nationwide), and only 10.5% of participants received inadequate prenatal care (compared to 17.6% for Chicago teens). Breastfeeding initiation rates were 80% (compared with 47.3% for US teens, and 42% for all Illinois women). The sites report that their teen moms are holding their babies more, talking to them more, and are more comfortable talking about their births (Abramson et al., 2000).

Summary

Practitioners who work with infants, young children, and their families know all too well that applying adult standards to evaluation and treatment of this population is not in the best interest of either the patient or the clinician. Developmental science and the field of infant mental health have contributed much to our understanding of the first 3 years of life. As discussed throughout this chapter, diagnosis and treatment of infants and young children requires an extensive knowledge base, specialized skills, and approaches that take into consideration both the child and the context in which the child exists. Infants and young children must be understood within their important and close relationships, at multiple points in time, and with a thorough assessment of developmental level.

We close this chapter with some thoughts about infants and young children that we hope will inform those who work with them:

- Infants need close and secure interpersonal relationships.
- Infants must explore the environment to learn and grow cognitively and develop a sense of mastery.
- Infants learn through their interactions with adults how to regulate their emotions, attention, and behavior.
- Family, community, and cultural expectations must always be considered in work with young children and their families.
- Clinical infant mental health is a relational construct that begins with the transition to parenthood.
- The theoretical framework for work with young children is developmental within a systems perspective. Psychodynamic and behavioral approaches can be used to work with infants, young children, and their families.
- The field of infant mental health continues to evolve, but the development of Diagnostic Classification: 0–3 has been an important first step in understanding developmentally sensitive diagnostic issues in young children.

- Clinical work in the first years of life creates an excellent opportunity for research related to basic developmental processes, prevention, intervention, and clinical disorders.

Annotated bibliography

Osofsky JD, Fitzgerald HE (eds) (2000) *WAIMH Handbook of Infant Mental Health*, vols I–IV. John Wiley & Sons, Inc., New York.
A comprehensive review of the field on infant mental health detailing the promise, progress, and future directions of the field with international perspectives. Volume I offers "Perspectives on Infant Mental Health." Volume II addresses "Early Intervention, Evaluation, and Assessment." Volume III examines "Parenting and Child Care." Volume IV reviews "Infant Mental Health in Groups at High Risk."

Shonkoff JP, Phillips DA (eds) (2000) *From Neurons to Neighborhoods: The Science of Early Childhood Development.* National Academy Press, Washington, D.C.
Provides a detailed evaluation and integration of the science of early childhood development. The book reviews contemporary research, answering questions and making policy recommendations for young children and their families.

Wyly MV (1997) *Infant Assessment.* Westview Press, Boulder, CO.
A comprehensive overview of infant assessment in the first 3 years of life. Topics include screening tools, newborn assessments, cognitive assessments, and interactional evaluations.

Zeanah CH Jr. (ed.) (2000) *Handbook of Infant Mental Health*, 2nd edn. The Guilford Press, New York.
An excellent resource for information on various topics in infant mental health. Chapters include information on contextual factors, treatment, and specific disorders and clinical presentations.

ZERO TO THREE (1994) *Diagnostic Classification of Mental Health and Developmental Disorders of Infancy and Early Childhood.* Zero To Three/National Center for Clinical Infant Programs, Arlington, VA.
The definitive diagnostic manual for use in the birth to 3 population. The manual details the multi-axial system and describes diagnostic criteria for a range of disorders relevant to infants and young children.

CHAPTER 16

Common Behavioral Issues in Clinical Practice

Mary Lynn Dell, MD

Introduction

Physicians in clinical practice see many children and families whose primary concerns are not straightforward medical or psychiatric nature, but may have aspects of both physiologic and emotional disorders, or, if not attended to properly and in a reasonable amount of time, may compromise their physical and/or mental health. Examples of problems falling on a continuum with both medical and behavioral aspects include early childhood feeding disorders, sleep disturbances, enuresis, and encopresis. Likewise, because clinicians who treat children are believed to be knowledgable about a broad array of topics and situations that may affect children, pediatricians, family practitioners, child and adolescent psychiatrists and psychologists may be consulted about life events and transitions such as parental separation and divorce, adoption, and the deaths of important people in children's lives. Clinicians treating children may also be viewed as experts about general cultural influences on child-rearing. Needless to say, acquiring and maintaining expertise in these areas, in addition to the continuing educational requirements of practical pediatric practice, is demanding. However, for clinicians who strive to recognize and treat these conditions on the interface between pediatrics and psychiatry, and those who are attuned to the emotional and physical needs of children and families in stress and transitions, the rewards are great – especially for the child, adolescent, and family.

This chapter will look first at disorders with both physical components and psychiatric overlay, including feeding disorders of infants and young children, enuresis, encopresis, and sleep disorders. Next, life transitions and situations with potential implications for physical and emotional health will be explored, including separation and divorce, adoption, and bereavement in childhood. Finally, the role of culture and religion/spirituality in parenting and caring for children and adolescents will be considered.

Feeding disorders in infancy and early childhood

For all children, especially those under 3 years of age, mealtimes and other eating opportunities are necessary not only for growth and nutritional purposes, but also for physical contact with caregivers, social interaction with caregivers, siblings, and others, gross and fine motor and sensory development, the expression of one's needs and personal preferences, and autonomy and mastery of one's body and environment. Mealtimes showcase not only a young child's physiologic drives, but their personalities and relationships with significant others as well. Understandably, great concern for a child's physical and emotional health, as well of those of caregivers, are aroused when the processes of eating, physical growth, and relating to others in an age-appropriate manner during meals are problematic or stunted.

The term "feeding disorders" is preferred overwhelmingly to "eating disorders" to emphasize the interactional or dyadic relationship with caregivers in the process of feeding babies and young children, as well as to help differentiate anorexia and bulimia nervosa and related syndromes that have different developmental, psychodynamic, and medical considerations. Historically, feeding disorders fell under the larger diagnostic umbrellas of failure to thrive, hospitalism, deprivation or psychosocial dwarfism, and environmental, psychosocial, and maternal deprivation (Chatoor, 1997). These designations were descriptive in some but not all instances, and not as helpful as clinicians would desire for diagnosis and treatment of these children and their families over the duration and course of the problem. A large step forward, especially in distinguishing between feeding disorders with or without physical failure to thrive, was the inclusion of this disorder in DSM-IV as "feeding disorder of infancy or early childhood." The DSM-IV diagnostic criteria included failure to eat adequately leading to a failure to gain adequate weight or actual weight loss over a minimum of 1 month, onset before 6 years of age, and the disturbance not due to or better explained by lack of food, a general medical condition, or another psychiatric disorder that interferes with adequate food intake or healthy eating (APA, 1994).

Clinicians seeing infants and toddlers with disordered eating in daily practice may find the work of Chatoor a more complete paradigm than DSM-IV for understanding the developmental and relational aspects contributing to the condition, as well as rationales behind treatment strategies. Chatoor has described three stages of feeding development, during which adaptive and/or maladaptive features may be manifested by the infant and/or primary caregiver. In the homeostasis stage, birth through 2–3 months of age, the baby adapts to life outside the uterus and establishes an individual rhythm of sleep, wakefulness, eating, and elimination. The caregiver learns how to interact with the infant with mutual reciprocity, reading the baby's cues and responding in ways that enable emotional interactions satisfying to both in addition to meeting all physical needs. In the attachment stage, from approximately 2–8 months of age, the interactions of the infant toward the caregiver during the feeding experience become much more animated and deliberate, with verbalizations and behaviors intentionally seeking engagement with one or two primary care providers. The separation phase generally spans from 9–18 months of age. During this stage, the healthy infant and young toddler displays greater autonomy and initiative at meals and is transitioning from being fed to independent eating.

Disruption of the developmental tasks inherent to these three stages may put the infant at risk for a feeding disorder, especially if there is environmental chaos and an impaired relationship with the primary caregiver. Chatoor (2002) has distinguished six subtypes of feeding disorders based on this developmental model. All entail growth deficiencies, manifested as weight loss, failure to gain weight, and/or nutritional deficits. These subtypes include:

1 Feeding disorder of state regulation – newborn-onset; infant unable to achieve a calm, alert state necessary for feeding.
2 Feeding disorder of reciprocity (neglect) – in the absence of an underlying medical etiology or pervasive developmental disorder, the infant lacks social responsivity and developmentally appropriate interaction with primary caregiver (smiling, verbalizations, visual connectivity, etc.).
3 Infantile anorexia – in the absence of an underlying medical disorder or precipitating traumatic event, the child refuses adequate food intake for at least a month, accompanied by apparent lack of hunger and interest in food.
4 Sensory food aversions – the child refuses to eat specific foods due to bothersome textures, appearance, or smells; onset may occur when a new food is introduced; associated with oral motor delay or coordination problems.
5 Feeding disorder associated with concurrent medical condition – in the presence of a documented, related medical problem, the child shows interest in eating but is unable to sustain feeding long enough to meet his or her needs.
6 Posttraumatic feeding disorder – feeding difficulties, even food refusal, follow a single traumatic event (e.g. choking, intubation), or repeated affronts to the oropharyngeal area that distress the child; associated with anxiety before or during a feeding opportunity, and/or generalization of fear of objects related to feeding (bottle, utensil, food).

Evaluation of feeding problems must be grounded in the same multidisciplinary approach required for subsequent treatment. Chewing and swallowing are deceptively complex in coordination, and underlying medical concerns contributing to upper gastrointestinal (GI) tract problems, as well as middle and lower GI tract irregularities, pulmonary, endocrine, infectious, and other conditions affecting oral intake, must be considered and ruled out (Table 16.1). General pediatricians and pediatric subspecialties may need to be consulted. In addition, speech pathologists, nutritionists, psychologists, and social workers are invaluable throughout the assessment and treatment process (Rudolph and Link, 2002).

The vast majority of infant feeding disorders involve impaired relationships between mother/caregiver and child, or severe stresses or illness affecting the mother's ability not only to successfully feed her child, but to nurture and care for her offspring in other facets of life as well. The mother may be suffering from undiagnosed, untreated, or inadequately treated mental illness herself, including depression, substance use, posttraumatic stress disorders, or psychotic disorders. She may have had poor to non-existent parenting herself, and may not be able to read physical, emotional, and behavioral cues from her infant necessary for caring for her child's physical and emotional needs. Social stresses such as homelessness, violent surroundings, inadequate childcare, and poverty affect one's ability and resources to interact with one's infant in healthy ways, especially if the infant has medical problems or any special needs. Psychiatric and social services assessments of individual parents and the entire family system are crucial to understanding and treating the baby's feeding problems. Also, observation of one or more meals or feeding opportunities with the child and mother is extremely helpful for diagnosis and understanding the quality or the emotional interactions between them. Videotaping these sessions permits closer study, comparisons for later stages of treatment, and tools for parent education throughout one's work with the family.

Treatment must address each of the three subsets of the feeding interaction, including the infant alone, the parent

Table 16.1 Medical causes of feeding disorders in infancy and early childhood

Anatomic anomalies

Cleft lip and/or palate
Laryngeal cleft, cyst, or malacia
Subglottic stenosis
Tracheomalacia or tracheal rings
Esophageal atresia, strictures, or vascular rings
Tracheoesophageal fistula
Tonsillar enlargement
Chin, jaw, nasal or dental anomalies
Masses or abscesses
Foreign bodies

Cardiac

Congenital heart disease/anomalies
Cardiac failure
Cardiomyopathy

Endocrine/genetic/metabolic

Thyroid abnormalities
Parathyroidism
Hypercalcemia
Trisomy 18, 21
Velocardiofacial syndrome
Organic acidemias
Glycogen storage diseases
Urea cycle disorders

Gastrointestinal

Gastroesophageal reflux
Dumping syndrome
Poisonings/caustic ingestions
Crohn's disease

Infectious

Candida
HIV
Esophagitis
Epiglottits
Cytomegalovirus
Herpes simplex

Nervous system

Cranial nerve palsies
Brain stem tumors (gliomas)
Sensory deficits (blindness, anosmia)
Cerebral palsy
Mental retardation
Myelomeningocele
Arnold-Chiari malformations

Table 16.1 (*Continued*)

Neuromuscular conditions

Myopathies
Muscular dystrophies
Myasthenia gravis

Pulmonary

Asthma
Bronchopulmonary dysplasia
Tracheal intubation
Tachypnea

be treated by the appropriate specialist or discipline (e.g. occupational or physical therapy, speech pathology). The caregiver's medical and psychiatric conditions also require treatment. This usually entails forming a trusting, therapeutic relationship with a therapist who not only assists with practical needs, such as medication prescriptions and therapy for depression, referral to 12-Step programs and social service agencies, but also a relationship that provides some correctives to significant past relationships that were emotionally hollow or abusive and may be contributing to difficulties nurturing and connecting emotionally with the child. Significant explanation and reinterpretation of the child's behavior and emotional cues is involved, as well as behavioral modification of many of the child's and parent's maladaptive interactional patterns during mealtimes. In cases in which close work with feeding, medical, and psychiatric teams does not result in sufficient improvement in the child's physical, cognitive, and emotional development, temporary or permanent alternative placement of the child may need to be considered. In most situations, however, both professionals and primary caregivers need to recog-

PEARLS & PERILS

- Underlying and predisposing medical conditions must be diagnosed and treated.
- Feeding disorder is usually dyadic – evaluation and treatment must address child factors, parent factors, and the specific interaction and relationship of child and parent.
- Multidisciplinary approach to assessment and treatment is essential.
- Successful treatment may span weeks or months – patience and perseverance by primary caregiver and health-care professionals are also essential.
- Suspect when young child with malnutrition, growth retardation, or weight loss has had multiple placements and/or caregivers with potentially poor emotional attachments.

alone, and the mother/child dyad. The infant's predisposing medical conditions and developmental delays should

CONSIDER CONSULTATION WHEN ...

- Child with medical problems continues to lose weight or does not eat well despite adequate management of underlying disorder.
- Child failing to thrive has poor interactional patterns – eye contact, body conformity to holding or cuddling, persistent irritability, apathy, withdrawal.
- There is a suspicion of psychiatric, social, or other stresses affecting mother's ability to care for a child failing to gain or losing weight.

KEY CLINICAL QUESTIONS

- *How does your baby respond to you when you try to feed him/ her?*
  May give clues to baby's temperament, interpersonal relatedness, fearfulness, defensiveness, and other factors the child brings to the feeding situation.
- *What were mealtimes like for you (mother) when you were a young child? Are there other stresses you are dealing with now that are adding to your worries about your child?*
  May give clues about mother's past and current emotional states and environmental/social factors affecting he ability to care for and nurture her child.

nize that treatment of childhood feeding disorders requires persistence, dedication, and patience from all involved.

Elimination disorders

Enuresis

Enuresis is one of the most common problems encountered in pediatric practice, with 40% of 3-year-olds, 30% of 4-year-olds, 20% of 5-year-olds, 10% of 6-year-olds, and even 1% of 18-year-olds and older adults estimated to experience nighttime wetting. The disorder is highly familial, with three-quarters of enuretic children having a first-degree relative who was also enuretic. On average, males outnumber females greater than two to one. Public education over the past three decades has done much to educate parents about normal ranges of toilet training and bladder control, hopefully decreasing the shame and stigma – even punishment – suffered by enuretic children as they mature and the problem either resolves on its own and/or they learn to deal with persistent wetting. Similarly, the vast majority of enuretic children have neither serious, nor even minor, medical or psychiatric issues contributing to their problem. Additional education, reassurance, and if needed, rather simple, individualized treatment plans address most cases of this common diagnosis.

Most children complete toilet training between the ages of 2½ and 4, though it is quite common for nighttime bedwetting to occur 2–3 times a week, gradually diminishing in frequency, through age 5. In developmentally normal children, enuresis cannot be diagnosed before the age of 5, involves repeated urination into clothes or in bed a few times a week for at least 3 consecutive months, or is significant enough to cause distress or impaired functioning in interpersonal, social, academic, or occupational realms (Table 16.2). This pattern of voiding cannot be explained in entirety due to a medical condition or as a medication effect, such as a diuretic prescribed for cardiac conditions (APA, 1994). In addition, enuresis may be categorized as primary, voluntary bladder control never attained; secondary, bladder control or nighttime dryness attained in the past but now lost; nocturnal, nighttime only; diurnal, during the daytime; and nocturnal and diurnal.

Though few children have medical conditions underlying or contributing to enuresis, clinicians should take a complete medical history and examine the child to verify that is the case for this particular patient (Box 16.1). The history should inquire about frequency, amount, odor, color, time of day or night of urination, pain or difficulties during actual urination, changes in sleep or presence of sleep irregularities, such as nightmares, terrors, sleepwalking, or snoring, content of diet, including types, amounts, and timing of fluid and solid food intake, as well as family history of enuresis. Abnormalities on physical examination consistent

---

DIAGNOSIS

Table 16.2 Enuresis

Discriminating features

1. Voiding of urine into clothes or bed after the age of 5.
2. Not due solely to a general medical condition or medication/substance effect.
3. Symptom duration a concern for at least 3 months or if duration is shorter, must be causing impairment or distress in school, at work, or in relationships.

Consistent features

1. Family history in first-degree relatives.
2. Males affected more often than females.

Variable features

1. May be primary (never toilet-trained) or secondary (bladder control achieved).
2. May be voluntary or involuntary.
3. May occur during the day, night, or both.
4. Often occurs after major life stress or transition (divorce, move, significant death).
5. May be comorbid with encopresis, sleepwalking, and sleep terrors.

BOX 16.1

Medical causes of enuresis

- Urinary tract infection.
- Diabetes mellitus.
- Diabetes insipidus.
- Neurogenic bladder.
- Urethral obstruction.
- Ectopic ureter.
- Spinal cord abnormality.
- Severe constipation causing pressure on the bladder.
- Irritation or reaction to soaps, laundry detergent, bubble bath.
- Excessive caffeine intake.
- Medication side-effect (diuretic prescribed for cardiac insufficiency).

with an underlying medical etiology for enuresis include fever, pain on palpation of kidneys or bladder, abnormal anal wink, palpable fecal and other pelvic masses, hair tufts, dimples, or skin discoloration over the lumbosacral spine, or abnormal lower extremity reflexes, power, strength, motor, or sensory findings (Robson, 2001; Jalkut et al., 2001). Obviously, concerns elicited on history and physical examination may require further diagnostic evaluation and referral to pediatric nephrologists, urologists, radiologists, or others. A screening routine urinalysis may be indicated, especially in cases of secondary enuresis.

Assuming the absence of medical concerns, inquiry into concurrent child and family stressors is indicated. For instance, developmental regression may be expected during transitions such as moves, school changes, births of siblings, divorce, deaths of significant others, and even changes in trusted babysitters. Though enuresis in the presence of these transitions is understandable and nonpathologic, the child and family may still benefit from a referral to a mental health clinician for supportive therapy and help with adjustment during and after those significant life changes.

Treatment strategies include psychologic support, behavioral techniques, and pharmacology. Often the reassurances that there is no underlying serious medical etiology, the enuresis is statistically likely to recede with continued growth and maturation, and coaching on practical management

PEARLS & PERILS

- High spontaneous recidivism rates, i.e. 10% prevalence at age 6 to 1% at age 18.
- Reassurance, education, and simple behavioral management strategies are extremely helpful.
- Best treatment results often achieved through combination of behavioral, conditioning, and pharmacologic treatments.
- Rarely caused or accompanied by serious medical or psychiatric problems.

such as restricting caffeine intake, and redistributing fluids to a predominantly morning and afternoon pattern (different than nighttime fluid restriction, which is generally not helpful!), using plastic mattress covers under sheets, and being mindful not to blame or ridicule the child, are among the most helpful interventions a clinician can provide. Positive reinforcement and rewards for dry nights and clothes are often helpful. A subset of enuretic children with decreased functional bladder capacity may benefit from bladder training, consisting of incremental increases in fluid intake accompanied by increased times urine is held before voiding. Urethral sphincter muscle tone may benefit from intentional interruption, then resumption, of urine stream mid-flow. These strategies may also augment positive results from other forms of treatment.

Arousal systems, also called urine or bladder alarm systems, are the most successful nonmedical interventions, with reported success rates of 40–75% after 12 months in motivated children. Urine drops complete a circuit that set off an audible or vibrating alarm to awake the child, similar to a pager. Early during its use, the child awakens and completes voiding into the toilet. Over time, a conditioned response is created such that the physiologic stimuli that proceed actual urination become the inhibitors of voiding (Jalkut et al., 2001). These devices are relatively inexpensive ($30–75), can be ordered online, and used by the child independently of parents.

Historically, the pharmacologic treatment of choice for enuresis has been the tricyclic imipramine. Given at bedtime, typically 25 mg for children under 10 years, and no more than 50 mg for older children, the medication is generally well tolerated, but its benefit is lost when discontinued. High relapse rates, coupled with concerns about cardiac arrhythmias and ease of accidental or intentional overdose by the identified patient or other family members, has led to a decline in the popularity of tricyclics in the treatment of enuresis. Desmopressin acetate (DDAVP), a synthetic analogue of vasopressin that reduces urine production by increasing water retention and urine concentration, has gained popularity in recent years. Available as a nasal spray (10 micrograms per spray, usual starting dose two sprays) or in tablet form (typical dose 0.6 mg), DDAVP has reduced wet nights in up to 90% of participants in certain clinical trials (Fisher, 2003). Both DDAVP and imipramine can be combined with urine alarms, usually augmenting treatment success rates.

Individual, family, and group psychotherapies are not helpful for enuresis alone. However, these modalities can be quite helpful for life transitions and stressors, such as moves and divorce, which frequently accompany enuresis, especially the secondary type. Depression, low self-esteem, and other psychiatric sequelae of enuresis may also benefit from therapy. The bottom line is that mental health referral is indicated at any time, regardless of whether or not there is an identified precipitant or stressor, that the child's self-esteem,

CONSIDER CONSULTATION WHEN ...

- Child's self-esteem is suffering, he/she is becoming socially withdrawn, depressed.
- Family, home, and/or school interactions focus on or scapegoat the enuretic child.
- Enuresis is accompanied by encopresis.
- Child and/or family is having difficulty coping with an accompanying stress or life transition.
- Enuresis is accompanied by unusual behavioral or mental status changes.

KEY CLINICAL QUESTIONS

- *Has anything changed in the child's life recently?*
  Identifies stressors, major life changes, and transitions.
- *How does the bedwetting make you feel about yourself?*
  Identifies low self-esteem, depressive, anxiety symptoms, and other consequences of the enuresis.
- *How is the enuresis affecting your family?*
  Identifies maladaptive handling of the problem, blaming, scapegoating.

DIAGNOSIS

Table 16.3 Encopresis

Discriminating features

1. Repeated defecation or passage of feces into clothes, floors, or other inappropriate places.
2. Occurs at least monthly for 3 months.
3. Child is 4 years of age or the developmental equivalent.
4. Not explained solely by a medical disorder other than one causing constipation or by medication effects (laxatives).

Consistent features

1. Fecal mass on rectal or abdominal examination.
2. Treatment-resistant constipation with stool seepage.
3. Males outnumber females 2.5-6:1.

Variable features

1. Presence or history of medical condition predisposing to constipation (fever and dehydration, medication side-effect, painful anal fissure, hypothyroidism).
2. Primary or secondary.
3. Daytime only or daytime and nighttime.
4. May present without constipation and overflow incontinence.
5. Accompanying life stress or transition, general anxiety, social phobia about public restrooms/defecation, oppositional defiant or conduct disorders.

relationships with siblings or parents, or developmentally expected activities or interactions are suffering as a result of enuresis, whether the realm of distress is the family and home, school, in the child's social environment, or his or her internal emotional world.

Encopresis

Compared to enuresis, encopresis, or the passing of feces outside a toilet in clothes and other inappropriate places after an age when bowel training should have been achieved, is a much more serious social and psychiatric problem (Table 16.3). According to DSM-IV, soiling may be purposeful or involuntary, occur at least once a month for 3 months after the age of 4 or the equivalent developmental age, and not be due solely to a medical etiology other than one directly causing constipation or to the direct action of a particular substance (e.g. laxatives). The inappropriate passing of fecal material can be subcategorized according to the presence or absence of constipation and overflow incontinence (APA, 1994). Encopresis with constipation and overflow incontinence involves stool seepage, at any time of the day or night, around a rectal fecal mass resulting from constipation detectable on physical examination, radiograph, and/or by history. The leakage of stool stops after the constipation is treated. In contrast, encopresis without constipation and overflow incontinence lacks fecal mass and constipation, fecal material is typical in content and consistency for the individual patient, soiling is irregular in occurrence. This form is more likely to be found in children and teens with oppositional defiant and conduct disorders.

Similar to enuresis, encopresis is more common in males than females by estimated ratios of 2.5:1 to 6:1, and may be found in as much as 3% of patients in general pediatric outpatient clinics and 25% of referrals to pediatric gastroenterologists. Generally accepted prevalence rates are 2.8% at 4 years, 1.9% at 6 years, 1.6% at 10–11 years, with high rates of spontaneous remission making this a rare problem after the 16th birthday. Though DSM-IV does not classify encopresis as primary or secondary, as many as 60% of affected children report having been continent of stool for a period of at least a year before soiling began. Episode frequency usually exceeds the minimum required for DSM-IV diagnosis, often occurring several times daily and most often in the afternoon (Fisher, 2003; Glader and Rappaport, 2001; Walsh and Menvielle, 1997).

Though 90% of all cases of encopresis are due to constipation with leakage around the fecal mass, thorough history taking and physical examination are necessary to determine any underlying or comorbid medical disorders (Box 16.2). A detailed description of bowel movements is essential, including consistency, frequency, smell, duration; whether in clothing or inappropriate places such as floors, closets, or drawers; history of toilet training and current toileting practices and hygiene; accompanying abdominal pain, flat-

ulence, distention, vomiting, bloody stools, painful defecation, growth failure, polyuria, dysuria; numbness, tingling,
pain, or motor weakness extending from the lumbosacral
area to the lower extremities; and dietary history. Many encopretic children have co-existing urinary tract infections
that require appropriate treatment. Sexual abuse must also
be ruled out as part of a thorough psychiatric history. Delayed bowel training and inappropriate bathroom habits are
not uncommon in mentally retarded and developmentally
delayed children, as well as those with psychotic symptoms
of any origin. Anxious children may fear using public rest-
rooms, leading to soiling accidents that usually are limited
to their underwear. Impulsive children, especially those
with attention-deficit/hyperactivity disorder, may not be
capable of anticipating bathroom needs ahead of time when
facilities are available, or they may ignore physiologic urges
to defecate when they do experience them due to their
higher levels of distractibility. They may have difficulty sitting still for a sufficient amount of time to relieve themselves
adequately, and they may not attend to post-defecation hygiene, leading to smearing in their clothes that can confuse
the correct diagnosis (Mikkelsen, 2002; Rockney, 1999).

If an underlying medical problem is suspected by history or from physical examination findings (which must
include visual inspection of the perianal area and a digital
rectal examination!), additional work-up is indicated. Those
studies may include abdominal imaging (usually an x-ray is
sufficient), urinalysis, urine culture, serum electrolytes and
calcium, and thyroid function tests. Anorectal manometry is
reserved for those few children with anal pressure and sensation abnormalities, or highly treatment refractory constipation. Rectal biopsy, with or without anorectal manometry,
is indicated if Hirschsprung disease is suspected. Fortunately, 95% of encopretic patients suffer from "functional"
constipation with secondary fecal leakage, and benefit from

routine, straightforward treatment (Fisher, 2003; Mikkelsen,
2002; Rockney, 1999).

Education about the pathophysiology and self-perpetu-
ating character of encopresis, for parents, youths, teachers
and other significant adults in the child's life, is a most important first treatment step. Blame and scapegoating of the
child and/or the parent is counterproductive and should
be avoided. Many variations of treatment programs are
employed successfully, but all follow the general strategy
of clearing out a fecal mass or impaction when one exists;
establishing a regular toileting practice or protocol that becomes part of the child's daily routine and fosters healthy
bowel and bladder habits; diet modifications if indicated,
including adequate amounts of fluids and fiber; and the regular use of stool softeners, bulking agents, and/or laxatives
as needed for maintenance therapy (Fisher, 2003; Mikkelsen,
2002; Rockney, 1999).

Most encopresis treatment regimens begin with bowel catharsis, usually comprised of a series of enemas for break-up
and flushing out of the fecal impaction. Catharsis may also
include suppositories and balanced electrolyte solutions
for the child to drink to assist in clearing the gastrointestinal tract from above. In severe cases, the insertion of a na-
sogastric tube is indicated for larger volumes of fluids to be
administered for the flushing out process. Even in circumstances in which regular or periodic enemas are required
after the initial phase of bowel cleansing and disimpaction,
parents should not administer the enemas to their child for
psychodynamic and punitive concerns. Stool softeners or
laxatives are prescribed, typically twice a day, to facilitate
soft, regular stools and avoid constipation and a repeat of
the encopresis cycle of constipation-fecal impaction-stool
leakage (Box 16.3). If mineral oil is recommended, the child

BOX 16.2 Medical causes of fecal soiling
- Functional constipation and fecal retention.
- Febrile illness and dehydration.
- Anorectal lesions (fissures, stenosis, atresia, ante-rior position), often leading to painful defecation.
- Neurogenic (Hirschsprung disease, cerebral palsy, spinal cord disorders, pseudo-obstruction, hypoto-nia).
- Endocrine/metabolic (hypothyroidism, hypercal-cemia, diabetes insipidus, renal acidosis).
- Inflammatory bowel disease.
- Irritable bowel syndrome.
- Laxative use.
- Constipation secondary to medication side-effects (nonlaxatives, prescription and over-the-counter).
- Physical (and/or emotional) consequence of sexual abuse.

BOX 16.3 Medications for constipation and encopresis
Stool softeners
- Docusate (Colace)
- Lactulose
- Mineral oil
- Psyllium

Laxatives
- (Bisacodyl) Dulco-lax
- Fletcher's Castoria
- Pericolace
- Phillips' Milk of Magnesia
- Senna (Senekot)

Rectal suppositories
- Glycerin
- Dulco-lax

Enemas
- Mineral oil
- Sodium phosphate (Fleets)

- Look for underlying or predisposing medical condition.
- Inquire about past or ongoing sexual abuse.
- Inquire about recent life stressors or transitions (birth of sibling, move, divorce, starting or changing schools, etc.).
- Inquire about possible accompanying social phobias about public restrooms/defecation, generalized anxiety, oppositional defiant and conduct disorders.
- Treatment results are best with combined behavioral and medical management.
- Child and parents need ongoing encouragement and support for following treatment plan on a daily basis.
- Individual therapy indicated for child with low self-esteem, withdrawal, or other psychologic symptoms secondary to encopresis.
- Family may benefit from family therapy for coping with problem, communication skills, other concomitant stressors.

KEY CLINICAL QUESTIONS

- *Has the child had any recent illnesses or health changes lately?*
  May unlock underlying or contributing medical concerns.
- *Does the child endorse being sexually abused, or do parents suspect he/she has been sexually abused?*
  Unlocks the trauma of sexual abuse so medical, psychiatric, individual, and family treatment can occur.
- *Have there been any major changes recently in the life of your child or family?*
  May unlock psychosocial and other stressors contributing to encopresis.
- *Has your child had any emotional or behavioral problem in the past? Recently?*
  May unlock clues about comorbid anxiety, mood, and behavioral concerns.

should take a multivitamin every day to prevent fat-soluble vitamin deficiencies (Fisher, 2003; Mikkelsen, 2002; Rockney, 1999).

Behavioral components of the treatment plan include having the child sit on the toilet for 10–15 minutes approximately 20 minutes after finishing a meal to capitalize on the naturally occurring urge to defecate due to the gastrocolic, or gastroilial, reflex. Diligent sitting on the toilet and bowel movements in the toilet are rewarded with verbal praise, stickers, or other tangible rewards. Negative reinforcement also has a role, in the form of required bathing after soiling, washing dirty clothes, and cleaning other objects or surfaces contaminated by feces. Parents must remember that clean clothes are not the fail-safe sign of continence and should not be what is rewarded – pants are also clean if the child is withholding or retaining stool. When first introduced, biofeedback was thought to be a quite effective treatment, either alone or in combination with education, behavioral techniques, and medical management. At this time, reviews are mixed, though for some children and clinicians this op-

CONSIDER CONSULTATION WHEN...

- Child shows signs of anxiety, depression, social withdrawal, or is severely ostracized or scapegoated.
- Child has been or is strongly suspected to have been abused sexually or physically.
- Oppositional defiant and conduct disorder symptoms are problematic.
- Family is unable to comply with treatment regimen, be supportive of the child, or deal with precipitating or concomitant stressors.

tion has been quite helpful (Fisher, 2003; Mikkelsen, 2002; Rockney, 1999).

Two psychiatric concerns are foremost when working with an encopretic child and his or her family. The first is to minimize the stigma and blame that usually accompanies the problem, thereby nurturing improved self-esteem in an effort to avoid depression, social withdrawal, poor social skills, and other longer-term emotional sequelae. Secondly, treatment plans should be implemented as soon as possible for comorbid psychiatric conditions, including psychotic disorders, anxiety, depression, oppositional defiant and conduct disorders. Schools and daycare providers must be fully informed of the problems and included in management strategies if the conditions are to improve. Educational, medical, and rehabilitative services need to be re-evaluated for children with mental retardation and lesser forms of developmental delay. Time limited individual and family therapies are helpful if encopresis is part of a maladaptive reaction to stressful life transitions, such as the birth of siblings, moves, or parental divorce. If sexual abuse is suspected, child protective services must be notified, the child's home and environment scrutinized for safety from continuing threats and assaults, and appropriate evaluation and therapy begun as soon as possible. Many children benefit from supportive therapy for self-esteem issues arising from chronic soiling, and family therapy may improve communication and be helpful in bolstering interpersonal relationships at home that have suffered as a result of the dynamics that frequently surround encopresis.

Sleep disorders in childhood and adolescence

Primary care physicians are asked frequently about childhood sleep problems, and even when child psychiatrists are consulted for non-sleep emotional and behavioral concerns, altered sleep is often a sign or symptom of the underlying psychiatric problem or a potential side-effect of treatment. Therefore, because sleep problems prior to adulthood can be either very age-specific and time limited or, especially in later adolescence, quite similar to typical adult sleep disorders, a review of normal developmental sleep patterns may be helpful.

At birth, sleep can be differentiated into an active phase, called rapid eye movement sleep (REM), and a quieter, less active phase, called non-rapid eye movement sleep (NREM). REM consists of muscle tone inhibition, irregular breathing, phasic electromyographic (EMG) activity, low voltage and irregular electroencephalographic (EEG) activity, and increased cerebral blood flow and metabolism compared to NREM sleep. Until 3 months of age, babies go directly from wakefulness to REM sleep, but by 4 to 6 months of age, NREM sleep has differentiated into its four typical stages with REM following stages III and IV of NREM, or slow wave, sleep. During the rest of childhood until adolescence, REM onset follows 60–75 minutes of NREM sleep. Adolescents experience a physiologic delay of sleep onset compared to the earlier childhood pattern (Handford and Vgontzas, 2002; Kotagal, 2003).

Physiologically, sleep-wake cycles are regulated by the suprachiasmatic nucleus in the hypothalamus. The close relationship of sleep to body temperature is not coincidental, for body temperature is also regulated by the hypothalamus. Parents frequently note that if their child exercises vigorously before bedtime, he or she has delayed sleep onset. This is likely to do with increased body temperature secondary to physical activity. Conversely, children are likely to be most difficult to wake up around 4 a.m., when body temperature is usually at its lowest. Melatonin secretion by the pineal gland is greatest in the evening before sleep onset, facilitating falling and staying asleep at night. Other neuroendocrine substances with secretion related to the sleep cycle include prolactin, testosterone, and growth hormone (Kotagal, 2003).

In daily life, these physiologic aspects of sleep are reflected in changes in typical sleep patterns and total hours spent in sleep by healthy children. Infants, until approximately 3 months of age, alternate sleep and wakeful periods approximately every 2 hours, for total sleep times of 16–20 hours per day. Gradually, the infant is awake for longer periods during the day and sleeps for longer periods during the night. "Settling," or sleeping through 5 hours a night for a period of 4 weeks, occurs by 3 months for 70% of term infants, 6 months for an additional 15%, and by 12 months for 90% of babies (Howard, 1999). Contrary to what many parents and professionals have believed in the past, most, and probably all, babies have multiple awakenings during the night, though they do not always stir or cry and awaken parents. By 1 year of age, children sleep 13–16 of every 24 hours, including 2–3 hours during the day.

Compared to prepubertal children, adolescents need more sleep. Two to 5-year-olds decrease their sleep hours from 13–11 hours on average, with daytime naps decreasing in length and frequency until they are usually abandoned. The ability to sleep through the night continues to improve, with approximately only 10% of 5-year-olds having significant nighttime awakenings. Six to 12-year-olds need somewhat less total sleep than preschoolers, and though they are perhaps the best sleepers from a physiologic standpoint, parents experience more complaints of sleep problems (anxiety, fears, nightmares, bedtime resistance) than at earlier ages. Adolescents require anywhere from 8 to 11 hours of sleep per night, more so than prepubescents. Teens experience a well-documented phase delay around the time of puberty leading to delayed sleep onset and morning awakening times. This fact of physiology, coupled with lifestyle factors, leads to sleep disturbances in as many as 30% of adolescents (Glaze, 2004; Howard, 1999).

Careful history taking is crucial to accurate diagnosis of sleep problems. All children, adolescents, and their parents should be asked about the time the child goes to bed, time of actual sleep onset, time and duration of awakenings during the night, time of final morning awakening, and number and duration of daytime naps. The amount, timing, and content of television and media viewing and computer use may affect sleep, especially increasing sleep onset difficulties. Changes in routine across weeknights and weekends and recent psychosocial stressors may either affect sleep temporarily or start a pattern of disrupted sleep that is difficult to correct. The presence of medical conditions and psychiatric conditions and medications that might affect sleep should be discussed (Boxes 16.4 and 16.5). If the child or adolescent has not been diagnosed with a medical problem affecting sleep, the clinician should still inquire about such signs and symptoms as snoring, mouth breathing, perspiration at night, restless sleep, gastroesophageal reflux, and symptoms consistent with a seizure disorder. Parents of infants and preschoolers should be asked about the sleeping environment, including the type of bed, whether the child sleeps alone in his or her own room or shares a room or bed with siblings or parents, the sleeping position (back, stomach, semi-upright), timing of last feeding or meal, use of pacifier, and need for soothing behaviors such as rocking or patting or being held by parents.

Mood and daytime behaviors, especially irritability, motoric hyperactivity, and degree of apparent sleepiness are helpful to know. Older school-age children and adolescents should be queried about amount of homework and the hour it is typically finished, duration and timing of extracurricular activities and part-time jobs, timing of exercise, meals, and heavy snacks, and other behavioral contributors to excessive daytime sleepiness and insufficient sleep (Box 16.6). Questions should be asked about sleep paralysis, hypnagogic hallucinations, and restless legs. Adolescents should also

BOX 16.4

Medical conditions affecting sleep

- Asthma
- Atopic dermatitis
- Auditory impairments
- Cerebral palsy
- Chromosomal disorders (Down, Prader-Willi, Pierre Robin)
- Chronic ototis media
- Colic
- Craniofacial anomalies
- Cystic fibrosis
- Encephalitis
- Enlarged tonsils and adenoids
- Fever
- Gastroesophageal reflux
- Kleine-Levin syndrome (rare)
- Medications (psychostimulants, steroids, theophylline)
- Menstrual-associated periodic hypersomnia (rare)
- Migraine and cluster headaches
- Mononucleosis
- Neuromuscular diseases
- Obesity
- Obstructive sleep apnea
- Pain disorders
- Seizure disorder
- Sickle cell disease
- Structural lesions of brain cortex, cerebellum, brainstem
- Thyroid dysfunction
- Visual impairments

BOX 16.5

Child and adolescent psychiatric disorders with accompanying sleep problems

- Acute stress disorder
- Adjustment disorders
- Attention-deficit/hyperactivity disorder
- Autism
- Bipolar disorder
- Conduct disorder
- Depression
- Developmental learning disorders
- Enuresis
- Generalized anxiety disorder
- Mental retardation
- Pervasive developmental disorders
- Posttraumatic stress disorder
- Psychotic disorders
- Reactive attachment disorder
- Rett syndrome
- Simple phobias
- Substance abuse disorders

BOX 16.6

Nonmedical causes of excessive daytime sleepiness and insufficient sleep

- Early school starting time
- Erratic or too late bedtimes
- Extracurricular activities
- Family and social activities (non-school-related)
- Mood and anxiety disorders
- Parent work schedules
- Part-time jobs
- Night terrors
- Sleep deprivation
- Sleep talking
- Somnambulism
- Stimulation from television, computers, videos, media

be asked about the extent and timing of excessive daytime sleepiness and trouble attending to complex tasks, such as driving, that might result in accidents. Teenagers may also experience cataplexy, or very sudden sleep onset. The presence of mood, behavioral, and substance abuse problems, the intentional use of caffeine and over-the-counter preparations to stay awake or induce sleep, academic performance, and school tardiness or absence are also important pieces of information to gather. The keeping of detailed sleep logs or diaries by children, adolescents, and their parents over a 2-week period can yield much information helpful to the diagnostic process as well. Inquiry should be made about what the child and family has already tried to remedy the sleep problem and whether or not it was helpful (Givan, 2004; Glaze, 2004; Kotagal, 2003; Mason and Thornton, 2002; Meltzer and Mindell, 2004; Shapiro, 1999).

A thorough physical examination should follow the careful sleep history, and include height, weight, head circumference, determination of body mass index, and blood pressure. The head and face should be inspected for abnormal or disproportionate facial features, enlarged tongue, and dental malocclusion. Sleep apnea may accompany nasal septum problems, nasal polyps, swollen nasal turbinates, tonsillar hypertrophy, and mouth breathing. Central and peripheral neurologic examination should be done, for hoarseness, decreased gag reflex, and abnormal cranial and deep tendon nerve responses may indicate neurologic contributors to disordered sleep. Vision and hearing screening updates are also indicated. The chest wall and spinal column should be inspected for disconfiguration leading to restricted breathing, such as pectus excavatum and scoliosis. Thorough cardiac examinations should be done to rule out underlying heart disease with or without pulmonary involvement (Glaze, 2004; Kotagal, 2003; Mason and Thornton, 2002).

After completion of the history and physical examination, specific testing may be appropriate to assess further the presence of disordered sleeping. The gold standard for diagnosing sleep disorders is polysomnography, during which the child or adolescent goes to sleep, usually in a sleep lab, and is monitored via electoencephalography (EEG); eye, chin, and peripheral muscle electromyography (EMG); echocardiography (EKG); pulse, blood pressure, and respiratory rate; pulse oximetry to record oxygen saturation; nasal airflow, chest and abdominal wall movements, and carbon dioxide detection measures. Most labs also audio and videotape the sessions to capture sleep positioning, snoring, or other unusual noises. All data are then analyzed by a pediatric sleep specialist and correlated with sleep history and physical examination. Another diagnostic procedure is the multiple sleep latency test (MSLT), which can document and measure sleepiness in an older child or adolescent. The MSLT monitors EEG, chin and orbital EMG to measure the time between sleep onset and the start of REM. A sleep onset time of 7–10 minutes in children suggests hypersomnolence, and two or more episodes of sleep onset REM sleep in five readings is consistent with narcolepsy in adults and adolescents. Finally, some sleep centers are including actigraphy in pediatric sleep disorder work-ups. The patient wears a microcomputer device that looks like a wrist watch for 1–2 weeks. The device records and stores skeletal muscle activity. The activity measures correlate closely with sleep and awake time, and is especially helpful in cases of circadian rhythm disorders, such as delayed sleep phase syndrome, and narcolepsy (Givan, 2004; Glaze, 2004; Kotagal, 2003; Mason and Thornton, 2002).

In addition to the sleep disorders included in DSM-IV, clinicians should be aware of the International Classification of Sleep Disorders (ICSD). Developed in 1990 through collaboration of several professional organizations worldwide devoted to the study and treatment of sleep disorders, the ICSD distinguishes between primary sleep disorders (dyssomnias and parasomnias) and secondary sleep disorders due to underlying medical and psychiatric conditions (Handford and Vgontzas, 2002; Kotagal, 2003). Both the DSM-IV and ICSD classifications have their own merits, but are in general agreement about sleep disorders commonly seen in childhood and adolescence. Based on age and development, we will now consider the more common specific childhood sleep disorders.

Sleep-onset association disorder

One of the most common complaints physicians hear from parents is that their infant, toddler, or preschooler just does not want to sleep at night – they are hard to get down to sleep in the first place, then wake up in the middle of the night, demanding parental attention for significant periods of time before finally falling back asleep. Parents report having to give their infant or toddler another bottle in the middle of the night, hold, rock, sing to them, cuddle, read, or lie down next to them in bed before the child goes to sleep.

The common denominator in these situations is that the child has come to associate parental contact and interaction with the process of going to sleep, and has not mastered the self-soothing abilities necessary to calm themselves and drift back to sleep on their own (Table 16.4). Though all children wake up several times a night, especially at the end of a sleep cycle, by their first birthday close to 70% are able to return to sleep without signaling their parents. Estimates are that 20–30% of all children qualify for this diagnosis at some point, most commonly between the ages of 6 months and 3 years of age. In the absence of medical problems, treatment is behavioral, and hinges on modification of parental behaviors as much as those of the child.

The first step is assuring parents that nothing is seriously wrong with their child, and that redirection of the child's sleep patterns in the middle of the night begins with modification of the initial bedtime routine. Evening schedules and routines from supper throughout the rest of the evening should be as consistent as possible. General sleep hygiene principles, such as starting the bedtime portion of the evening schedule in the child's room, including putting on pajamas and actual sleeping itself, should be discussed with the parents and followed as strictly as possible. Though the specific plan is tailored to the individual child in the context of his or her family, the general principles and trajectory are basically the same. At the appointed bedtime hour, parents are instructed to place their child in his or her bed, turn the lights out, and step out of the room. For the first few nights the parent may stand next to the bed and touch and verbally comfort the child without picking him or her up. For the next few nights the parent can stand next to the bed, verbally comfort the child, but not touch him or her in any way. When the child cries, the parent should step back into the room where the child can see the parent, but refrain from talking

---

DIAGNOSIS

Table 16.4 Sleep-onset association disorder

Discriminating features

1. In the absence of medical problems, child is unable to fall asleep without parental presence and interaction.

Consistent features

1. Needs parental presence and interaction to return to sleep in the middle of the night.
2. Inconsistent evening routines and bedtime rituals.

Variable features

1. Most common in children 6 months to 3 years of age.
2. Presence of temporary or chronic parental, marital, or family stressors.

- Usually time-limited, even without treatment.
- Treatment is behavioral, requiring modification of parental interaction with child at bedtime and during night awakenings.
- Consistent evening routines and bedtime rituals are essential.

to or picking up the child. When the child calms down, the parent leaves the room again, gradually decreasing the time spent in the child's room when he or she cries and increasing time away when the infant or toddler is quiet. Though the first several nights may be hard emotionally on both child and parent, the child should soon be able to tolerate the parent's absence from the room as he or she is falling asleep, learning how to calm himself or herself early in the evening so he or she can repeat the self-soothing process and fall asleep alone after other awakenings during the night.

Parents should not be discouraged if this process needs to be repeated after an illness, move, birth of a sibling, or other stress. Even without treatment, this problem typically resolves over time after the third year of life (Givan, 2004; Glaze, 2004; Howard, 1999; Mason and Thornton, 2002).

Nightmares

Virtually all children have an occasional frightening dream, and nightmares occur in approximately 50% of individuals between the ages of 3 and 6 years and are part of normal development. These events gradually decrease in frequency over time, though a few adolescents will continue to report frightening dreams unrelated to stress or changing life cir-

CONSIDER CONSULTATION WHEN ...

- Child and/or parental sleep deprivation puts any family member at physical or emotional risk.
- Parents are unable or unwilling to try behavioral interventions but still insist that something needs to be done.

KEY CLINICAL QUESTIONS

- *Describe your family's evening routine and bedtime rituals.*
  May unlock disorganization or chaos contributing to the child's sleep problems.
- *Is there anything worrying you that makes bedtime more difficult than it might be otherwise?*
  May unlock parental, marital, or other stressors needing more specific attention.

cumstances. Nightmare disorder is diagnosed when these dreams recur often enough to affect functioning at school and home, primarily due to anxiety and sleep deprivation. The child awakens from REM sleep during the second half of the night, or later stages of a long nap, is easily oriented and has detailed recall of the disturbing dream imagery. Young children often describe scary animals and monsters, while older children's nightmares more commonly include humans and frightening events such as falling, physical injury, and death. Unlike sleep terrors (see below), the child with nightmares responds positively to adult comfort and reassurance. A child's developmental inability to distinguish reality from fantasy may increase proclivity to nightmares, especially after viewing violence or frightening content on television or via other media (Table 16.5). Nightmares may also occur in association with fevers or with any medication that affects the usual phases of the sleep cycle at night. Parents are advised to try to minimize the likelihood of nightmares by monitoring the content of television and

Table 16.5 Nightmare disorder

Discriminating features

1. Repeated awakenings from nighttime sleep or long naps with vivid memories of frightening dreams.

Consistent features

1. Occurs during the second half of the night.
2. The child is easily oriented and consolable upon awakening.

Variable features

1. Viewing of frightening TV, movies, or other media before going to bed.
2. Presence of acute or chronic family stress.

- Child usually responds well to adult comfort and reassurance.
- Childhood nightmares are usually part of normal childhood development.
- The inability of young children to distinguish fact from fiction predisposes them to adverse effects of frightening stories and images on television and other media.

CONSIDER CONSULTATION WHEN ...

- Acute or chronic family stress is contributing to nightmare occurrence.
- Child or family sleep deprivation jeopardizes physical or emotional health.

KEY CLINICAL QUESTIONS

- *What do you watch on television before going to bed at night?*
  May unlock the fact that the viewing of scary material on the media is contributing to or precipitating nightmares.
- *Is there anything you are really scared or worried about?*
  May unlock a significant fear or anxiety that is contributing to or precipitating the nightmares.

Table 16.6 Sleep terrors

Discriminating features

1. Abrupt awakening from sleep with accompanying autonomic arousal, including perspiration, tachycardia, tachypnea, pupillary dilation.
2. Amnesia for the episode.

Consistent features

1. Usually in first third of the night during transition from stage II-IV NREM to REM sleep.
2. Child is unresponsive to others.
3. Confused or disoriented if awakened.

Variable features

1. Usually only one episode per night; child may cry out or have incoherent vocalizations.
2. May occur during long naps.
3. May occur on consecutive nights or over intervals of days or weeks.
4. May be triggered by abrupt, unexpected loud noises or sudden pain (otitis media, abdominal gas).

media viewing, especially in the evenings, and setting firm limits if indicated. This media screening by parents should also include cartoons, the scary and violent content of which frequently is under-recognized. When nightmares do occur, parents should comfort their child, take his or her fears seriously, reassure him or her that he or she and everyone else in the house is safe, and facilitate the child's expedient return to sleep. Transitional objects, night-lights, and double-checking locks, doors, and windows while the child is still awake may also be helpful. It is permissible and comforting to the child to climb into bed with parents or a sibling after a bad nightmare, but care must be taken to make sure such behavior does not reinforce night awakenings. Both child and parents often find it helpful to discuss the nightmare the next day (in broad daylight!) to help the child learn to deal with his or her anxieties and fears (Anders, 1997; Glaze, 2004; Handford and Vgontzas, 2002; Mason and Thornton, 2002).

Sleep terrors

Sleep terrors (Table 16.6), also called night terrors, are exhibited on at least one occasion by approximately 20% of all children, with 1–6% having two or three per week. Males are affected more than females, and as many as 75% of affected children have first-degree relatives who also have experienced sleep terrors or sleepwalking. Sleep terrors typically occur during the first third of the night during transition stage III-IV NREM sleep to REM sleep. The child awakens abruptly without warning, screams or cries out loudly, has

a glassy-eyed stare, may point to people and objects not present, as if hallucinating, and exhibits autonomic signs of fear, including tachycardia, tachypnea, diaphoresis, and pupillary dilation. The degree of panic and inability to recognize even familiar family members is quite disconcerting for parents, who rush to the child but are unable to console him. If awakened at the time of the episode, he is quite confused and disoriented, and will usually take longer to return to sleep than if left alone. When not awakened, episodes

CONSIDER CONSULTATION WHEN ...

- Child or family restricts activities significantly due to sleep terrors.
- Child or family experiences sleep deprivation that potentially jeopardizes physical or emotional health.

KEY CLINICAL QUESTIONS

- *Have you had schedule changes that have caused increased fatigue or sleep deprivation lately?*
  Unlocks potential triggers or precipitants.
- *Are you taking any medications or using any substances that seem to be affecting your sleep?*
  Unlocks potential triggers or precipitants.
- *Has anyone else in your family had sleep terrors or been a sleepwalker?*
  Unlocks family history consistent with diagnosis of sleep terrors.

- Usually begins between the ages of 4 and 12 years and resolves spontaneously during adolescence.
- Children with sleep terrors do not have a higher incidence of psychiatric or emotional problems.
- Parents should not wake up the child during an episode unless recurrent episodes disturb other family members, in which case the child should be awakened before the time the episodes usually occur.
- Sleep terrors may be exacerbated by sleep deprivation, fatigue, alcohol, sedating medications, sleep-wake cycle disruptions, physical and emotional stress.

typically last 5–20 minutes, and the child returns to sleep relatively soon. A hallmark feature of sleep terrors is that the child is amnestic for the event the next morning. Optimally, parents should not awaken the child from a sleep terror episode, but observe to assure safety. However, if the episodes are keeping others in the household awake on a regular basis and leading to compromised physical and emotional health, parents should try *anticipatory awakening*, in which the child is awakened approximately 15 minutes before the usual time of the episode. In extreme situations, diazepam 2–5 mg or imipramine 10–25 mg may be prescribed to be taken before bedtime to suppress REM sleep. Medication must be monitored closely and should be viewed as a temporary measure only. There is no evidence that childhood-onset sleep terrors are associated with childhood psychopathology, though some children with sleep terrors may develop somnambulism or sleepwalking at a later age. Children and parents should be reassured that sleep terrors usually resolve spontaneously before or during adolescence (AACAP, 1998, 1999; Anders, 1997; Dworkin, 1999; Glaze, 2004; Handford and Vgontzas, 2002; Kotagal, 2003; Mason and Thornton, 2002; Shapiro, 1999).

Somnambulism (sleepwalking)

Somnambulism (Table 16.7), or sleepwalking, like sleep terrors, occurs when the transition from Stage III-IV slow wave sleep to REM is disrupted. Predisposing factors include fever, sleep deprivation, obstructive sleep apnea, other physical illness, alcohol or sedative hypnotic medications, and acute and chronic stress. Estimates are that up to 40% of all children have at least one sleepwalking episode, and that up to 6% of children sleepwalk frequently, 2–3% more than once a month. Sleepwalking is six times more common

- Safety is paramount. Safety-proof the house and lock doors and windows with special safety locks difficult for the sleepwalking child or adolescent to unlock during an episode.
- Sleep deprivation, loud noises, physical illness, fever, obstructive sleep apnea, alcohol and sedative use, psychosocial stressors may exacerbate tendency to sleepwalk.
- Sleepwalking is usually not associated with childhood psychopathology.

in monozygotic than dizygotic twins. Onset usually begins between the ages of 6 and 8 years, may peak at around 12 years, then spontaneously abates during late adolescence. Sleep terrors and sleepwalking may be comorbid and are hypothesized to share genetic and neurophysiologic characteristics. Up to 80% of sleepwalkers have first-degree relatives with either somnambulism or sleep terror disorder. All sleepwalkers should be examined by a physician to rule out the presence of a seizure disorder that may resemble somnambulism.

During the event itself, the child gets up out of bed, and engages in complex motor activity that usually consists of walking but may include eating, going to the bathroom, going up and down stairs, unlocking doors, and even riding a bicycle. They may return to bed before awakening, or wander until falling asleep elsewhere away from their room. It is generally ill-advised to awaken a sleepwalker, but observe them closely for the possibility of injury or accident. If accosted, they may become agitated, though they usually are unresponsive to or even unaware of the presence

DIAGNOSIS

Table 16.7 Somnambulism (sleepwalking)

Discriminating features

1. Repeated occasions of leaving the bed while sleeping and walking or engaging in other complex motor activities.

Consistent features

1. Occurs during first third of sleep time.
2. Child is unresponsive to others and difficult to awaken.
3. Amnesia for the episode but regains clear sensorium shortly after the event.

Variable features

1. Type of activity and amount of danger entailed.
2. May eat and talk during episode.
3. Duration varies from a few to 30 minutes.
4. May or may not awaken before returning to bed.
5. Sleepwalking child may also have sleep terrors.

CONSIDER CONSULTATION WHEN ...

- Sleepwalking puts the child and family at risk of physical harm, either from actions during the episodes themselves or as a result of sleep deprivation.
- Sleepwalking is exacerbated by acute or chronic psychosocial stressors.

KEY CLINICAL QUESTIONS

- *Have you gone through each room of your house to make sure the windows and doors have locks and there is minimal chance of your child being injured during a sleepwalking episode?*
  Unlocks how the family is addressing the risks and dangers of sleepwalking on a practical note at home.
- *Can you think of any new concerns or anything that might be troubling your child now?*
  Unlocks the possible existence of psychosocial stressors exacerbating somnambulism.

of others. They typically have a glassy-eyed stare and blank facial expression. Though the sleepwalker may be engaging in relatively sophisticated activity, physical coordination is impaired, increasing the risk of physical injury during the episode. The event typically lasts less than 30 minutes and the child will have no memory of it the following morning or upon awakening. It is crucial that parents of a sleepwalking child accident-proof their house to the greatest extent possible to minimize the risk of injury to the child and others in the home. Locking doors and windows at night, the installation of special locks or latches difficult for the sleepwalker to undo during an episode, moving furniture out of major walking paths throughout the house, providing the child with a ground level bedroom, and putting gates at the top and bottom of staircases are minimum measures that are indicated. As in sleep terrors and confusional arousals, some families find that anticipatory awakenings before the times the child usually sleepwalks is helpful. Late afternoon naps of an hour or less in duration may benefit some sleepwalkers. On rare occasions for severe cases, very low dose diazepam or imipramine has been reported to mitigate severity and frequency of sleepwalking, but medication use must be cautious and accomplished only with strict monitoring (AACAP, 1998, 1999; Anders, 1997; APA, 1994; Handford and Vgontzas, 2002; Mason and Thornton, 2002; Shapiro, 1999).

Insomnia

Unlike some of the other childhood sleep disorders, insomnia (Table 16.8) is a much more descriptive, subjective, and difficult-to-pin-down diagnosis. For one thing, it can be a symptom that accompanies numerous other sleep, medical, and psychiatric disorders, as well as a prescription medication side-effect. Normal development and developmental variants in pediatric sleep patterns, the effects of psychosocial and environmental influences on children's sleep, the effects of childhood illnesses, the inevitable variations of routine in even the most organized of households, and

the fact that caregivers raise insomnia as a complaint much more often than the identified patient – all these factors potentially complicate accurate definition and remediation of any legitimate clinical concerns. Parental interactions with each other, parenting styles and approaches to the child, and the child's own temperament are also important variables.

Obviously, when insomnia is a symptom of another sleep disorder, such as circadian rhythm disorders, narcolepsy, restless legs syndrome, or sleep-related breathing disorders, treatment measures should target the underlying problem(s). This same strategy applies to sleep problems secondary to general medical conditions, other psychiatric disorders such as anxiety, mood, attention-deficit/hyperactivity, and substance use disorders. If insomnia is due to a prescription medication side-effect, the child, family, and physician should re-examine the need for the medication, the possibility of dose reduction, or alternative agents that may offer comparable benefit but with less detriment to restorative sleep. After these factors have been ruled out or addressed, a child is considered to have primary insomnia if he or she has significant difficulty in terms of frequency, severity, or duration, initiating and/or maintaining sleep, and this difficulty is adversely affecting school performance, mood, behavior, and learning or cognitive development. The complaint is significant and should be taken seriously whether reported by the child, parent, or both.

Primary insomnia, or difficulty sleeping in the absence of contributing medical and psychiatric factors, is also referred to as learned or behavioral insomnia. These terms acknowledge that associations causing physiologic arousal, prevent and interfere with sleep, and diminish daytime functioning are largely conditioned responses or learned patterns of attitudes and behaviors. These maladaptive habits and cognitions about sleep, especially when combined with genetic vulnerabilities and overlying medical or psychiatric conditions of acute or chronic natures, intensify the deleterious physiologic, cognitive, and emotional effects of sleep deprivation.

A common cause of insomnia in infants, toddler, and preschoolers, sleep-onset association disorder, has already been discussed. School-aged children, adolescents, and even adults, may find the following measures helpful for managing insomnia, both primary and, in many cases, secondary:

1 Age-appropriate and consistent bedtime rituals and schedules
2 Age-appropriate sleep environment, quiet, relatively free of bright lights and noise
3 Age-appropriate and consistent morning wakening times, despite amount of sleep and disruptions during the night
4 Restrict time in crib/bed to actual bedtime/sleeptime
5 Cognitive restructuring for parent and child – "I actually did fall asleep last night, and even if I don't fall asleep quickly tonight I know I will eventually"

DIAGNOSIS

Table 16.8 Insomnia

Discriminating features

1. Significant difficulty (severe, chronic, frequent) initiating and/or maintaining sleep.

Consistent features

1. Negatively affects daytime behavior, school performance, mood, development, or ability to learn.

Variable features

1. May be reported by parent, child, or both.

6 Use of relaxation techniques, including deep diaphragmatic breathing, meditation, guided visual imagery, progressive muscle relaxation

7 Avoidance of all caffeine-containing beverages, foods, and medications from mid-afternoon throughout the evening

8 Avoidance of stimulating television programs, videos, video games, movies, and books after supper, and exclude these items from the child's bedroom

9 Avoidance of nicotine, alcohol, and other substances of abuse, especially in the afternoons and evenings

10 Encouragement for homework completion as early in the evening as possible

11 Avoidance of strenuous physical activity at least 1–2 hours before bedtime

12 Developmentally appropriate nap lengths that occur in early to mid-afternoon

Though commonly insisted upon by desperate parents and older children and teens, there are insufficient data and experience to endorse pharmacology as a treatment of choice for childhood insomnia. Physicians are understandably reluctant to prescribe, for long-term use especially, sleep-inducing medications for developing brains that have no randomized, placebo controlled trials substantiating clinical efficacy and short- and long-term safety. Regardless, certain medications are prescribed on a fairly predictable basis for insomnia, including antihistamines, benzodiazepines, chloral hydrate, clonidine, and melatonin. Antihistamines, especially diphenhydramine, are used primarily for their sedating side-effect profile. While this medication may reduce sleep latency and the number of awakenings during the night, it does not improve nightmares, trouble awakening, and may detract from sleep quality, leave the child jittery and excitable, and result in increased daytime sleepiness. Other side-effects are possible, attributed to the drugs effects on other neurotransmitters, especially acetylcholine. While benzodiazepines, especially diazepam, are helpful with severe sleep terrors and somnambulism, routine use for primary insomnia is not advisable. This class of medications may mask sleep problems instead of improve them, cause rebound insomnia, induce tolerance, and cause excessive daytime sleepiness and clouded thinking. Some physicians prescribe choral hydrate as a hypnotic for time limited use in

CONSIDER CONSULTATION WHEN ...

- Sleep deprivation is jeopardizing the physical and/or emotional health of the child and family.
- Insomnia persists despite adherence to strict sleep hygiene guidelines and attempts at behavioral management.
- School performance is suffering.

KEY CLINICAL QUESTIONS

- *What do you eat and drink after supper, and what activities do you engage in before going to bed?*
  May unlock problems with evening routines and inconsistent sleep hygiene practices.
- *What time does your child nap and for how long?*
  May unlock excessive daytime sleeping patterns that reinforce nighttime insomnia.

children (50 mg/kg up to 2 grams at bedtime). Though some young patients benefit in the short run, all children should be monitored for the idiosyncratic reactions of confusion, disorientation, and paranoia, as well as the side-effects of nausea, vomiting, gastrointestinal distress, dizziness, and fatigue. Tolerance may develop in as brief a period as 1–2 weeks, and the medication should be tapered to prevent withdrawal seizures and delirium. Clonidine, a central alpha adrenergic agonist, has been helpful for children with attention-deficit/hyperactivity disorder and a few other neurologic conditions. It should not be used, however, in healthy children, and risks include bradycardia, hypotension, and rebound hypertension. Melatonin, the principal hormone secreted by the pineal gland in the brain, is now available over the counter. Serum melatonin levels are high at night and lower during the day. Taking oral melatonin, considered to be a dietary supplement by the Food and Drug Administration, is believed to have a phase-setting effect on sleep, enhancing sleep onset. In adults, melatonin has been reported to be helpful for circadian rhythm sleep problems, such as jet lag and delayed sleep phase syndrome. In children, sleep problems due to blindness, delayed sleep phase syndrome and other circadian rhythm dysfunctions, as well as individuals with certain midline brain defects, such as agenesis of the corpus callosum, may respond favorably to melatonin. Melatonin may enhance immune function, and should not be used by patients with immune and lymphoproliferative disorders and those who take corticosteroids and immunosuppressant agents. Finally, care should be given when purchasing this and any supplement over the counter. These products contain inconsistent and variable amounts of the active substance and may contain unspecified adulterants (Glaze, 2004; Meltzer and Mindell, 2004; Pelayo et al., 2004).

PEARLS & PERILS

- Observance of good sleep hygiene and behavioral management are the treatments of choice.
- Daytime naps should be limited to no later than early afternoon, if permitted at all.
- Medications have a very, very limited role in the treatment of childhood insomnia.

Obstructive sleep apnea

Obstructive sleep apnea is known to affect 3–5% of all children and adolescents (Table 16.9). However, those figures may be an underestimate of the true incidence, given the education of physicians and the public about signs, symptoms, and long-term sequelae, especially as the incidence of obesity had increased in children, adolescents, and adults.

The affected individual has increased upper airway resistance, due to physiologic and/or anatomic reasons, and is unable to maintain a completely patent airway. This is especially true when sleeping on one's back during the night or extended naps. This leads to hypopneas, partial obstructive events, and apneas, periods of time during which there is no airflow. The resulting hypoxia, hypercapnea, and sleep arousals lead to sleep fragmentation, which in turn produces physiologic, cognitive, and behavioral problems. While the diagnosis in adults refers to complete obstruction, partial obstruction in children and adolescents is enough to produce untoward physiologic effects. Parents and siblings of affected youth report loud snoring, gasping, diaphoresis, restless-

---

DIAGNOSIS

Table 16.9 Sleep-disordered breathing (obstructive sleep apnea)

Discriminating features

1. Inability to maintain patent upper airway due to increased upper airway resistance secondary to anatomic or physiologic reasons.

Consistent features

1. Periods of time during which there is no airflow *(apneas)* and partial obstructive events *(hypopneas)* lead to *sleep fragmentation*.
2. Loud snoring, gasping, diaphoresis, long periods of sleep without breaths.
3. Affected child may be obese.

Variable features

1. Daytime hypersomnolence, irritability, mood swings, inattention, aggression, hyperactivity, poor academic functioning, mouth breathing, nocturnal enuresis.

PEARLS & PERILS

- Primarily caused by hypertrophy of tonsils and adenoids – treatment of choice is tonsillectomy and adenoidectomy.
- Incidence rising with increase in obesity.
- Longer-term complications include failure to thrive and developmental delay in young children and cor pulmonale, hypertension, and death in all age groups.
- Overnight polysomnogram with multiple apneas, hypopneas, and oxygen desaturations is diagnostic.

KEY CLINICAL QUESTIONS

- *Does your child snore loudly most nights?*
  May unlock possible upper airways resistance.
- *Do you find yourself listening to your child at night and wondering how long it will be before he takes his next breath?*
  May unlock apneic periods during sleep.

---

ness, noticeable periods during which no breaths are taken. Sometimes sleeping upright or with several pillows to prop up the head and neck are reported to help. Consequences of apnea observed during the day include hypersomnolence, increased irritability, mood swings, aggression, hyperactivity, inattentiveness, poor academic functioning, nocturnal enuresis, and daytime mouth breathing. Longer-term complications include failure to thrive and developmental delay in younger children, and cor pulmonale, systemic hypertension, and death in all age groups.

Historically, at least before the current obesity epidemic, obstructive sleep apnea of childhood peaked anywhere from 2–6 years of age, primarily caused by hypertrophy of the tonsils and adenoids. For these children, the degree of apnea is not necessarily proportional to the degree of discernible hypertrophy and not all children are cured by tonsillectomy and adenoidectomy, leading to the conclusion that a combination of structural and neuromuscular considerations combine to produce apnea. Other factors that predispose to obstructive sleep apnea include pulmonary disease of any type, craniofacial abnormalities, especially micrognathia and hyperglossia, hypotonia, neuromuscular disease, and a family history of sleep apnea or other sleep disordered breathing problems.

The clinical history may be suggestive and consistent with obstructive sleep apnea, but is not sufficient alone to make the diagnosis. An overnight polysomnogram demonstrating multiple apneas and hypopneas with frequent oxygen desaturations (often <80%) is diagnostic. The most effective treatment, estimated to resolve symptoms in 70% of affected children, has been tonsillectomy and adenoidectomy. Weight loss is becoming increasingly important as more cases of sleep apnea are caused or exacerbated by obesity. Another surgical intervention, more commonly performed in adult apneics but also possible in younger patients, is uvulopalatoplasty. This procedure removes redundant or extra tissue in the oropharynx that may impinge on the airway and impede airflow. Tracheostomy is still an option in extreme cases, but was more commonly performed in past years before uvulopalatoplasty became popular. Some children may also require supplemental oxygen and/or noninvasive ventilatory support, such as a device used during the night to deliver continuous positive airway pressure, either temporarily or indefinitely. Sometimes training the child to sleep on his or her side is helpful. The nonstimulating tricyclic antidepressant protriptyline has benefited some adult patients, but there are no studies using this medication in children with sleep apnea (Givan, 2004; Handford and Vgontzas, 2002; Kotagal, 2003; Mason and Thornton, 2002; Pelayo et al., 2004, Shapiro, 1999).

Other considerations in child and adolescent sleep medicine

Clinicians are well advised to approach each child and family individually and with an open mind when evaluating sleep practices. Few aspects of daily living are as influenced by cultural backgrounds and values as is sleep. For instance, a traditional American emphasis on fostering independence and autonomy in the young child would leave physicians to believe that infants are left to sleep alone in their own beds whenever possible. However, a more realistic scenario is that more children in the United States share beds with parents and siblings than previously believed, a practice that may also reflect the increasing numbers of families from ethnically diverse backgrounds in many areas of the country today. Similarly, nontraditional parental work schedules and childcare arrangements may necessitate bedtimes and schedules that may seem problematic, at least on first glance, but are actually understandable and work well for a particular child and family. Perhaps the best approach for clinicians is to prioritize healthy physical, emotional, cognitive, academic, and interpersonal growth and development, and then assess whether or not the child's sleep habits and patterns within his or her family and household setting are promoting these desired areas of growth and maturity.

Parental separation, divorce, and remarriage

Parental separation, divorce, and remarriage are so commonplace in contemporary society that professionals working with children and families, especially physicians, may not take the time to systematically review and consider the effects on individual children as they are encountered in routine primary care. Indeed, for at least a decade, statistics have verified that approximately 50% of all marriages end in divorce, with half of all first divorces occurring before the seventh anniversary. Approximately 85% of divorced adults remarry, with 40% of those unions also ending in divorce.

Over 1 million children a year experience parental divorce, and a sizable minority of young people live in two, three, or more family and step-family constellations before the age of 18 (Dell, 1995; Wallerstein, 1999; Wallerstein and Corbin, 2002).

One of the premier researchers in this area, Judith Wallerstein, makes a point especially relevant to pediatricians and other health-care professionals who have long-term relationships with children and families. Dr Wallerstein observes that: "Divorce is a process of social and psychological change in the individual and in family relationships that can extend over many years. ... Divorce is not a time-limited event for the adults or the children involved, in part because a complex undulation of changes including remarriages and redivorces and love affairs leads up to and, in turn, is set into motion by the marital rupture. These changes often occupy a significant portion of the adult's postdivorce life. They typically occupy a significant portion of the youngster's childhood and adolescence and, as we are learning, of his or her own young adulthood" (Wallerstein and Corbin, 2002, p. 1276).

Two points merit special emphasis: 1) divorce is a process, its effects may manifest differently at different stages of development, and these should be explored at regular intervals; and, 2) the dynamics in the stages of separation, divorce, and remarriage share many features in common, while some considerations are also unique to each stage.

- The primary care physician may be the only helping professional who has a longitudinal relationship with children and families to follow them and monitor long-term coping and adjustment to these significant changes in their lives.
- Extra effort on the part of the primary care physician may be required to maintain routine well child appointments and continuity of care, especially during stressful times when parents may be distracted by conflicts, legal proceedings, and their own emotions and adjustment to marital changes.
- As much as possible, for the best interests of the child, pediatricians should maintain good working relationships with both parents before, during, and after divorce.
- Regularly check patient registration forms and chart face sheets – these may provide valuable hints at important changes in the family and in the child's life.
- Allow extra time or schedule an extra appointment to permit adequate time with the child and parents, especially during key times of transition (i.e. custody changes, remarriage).
- Be familiar with mental health clinicians of all disciplines in your practice area for referrals of children, adolescents, and families dealing with separation, divorce, and remarriage.

For the convenience of discussion, we will consider these processes in the common chronological order of troubled marriage, separation, divorce, a post-divorce adjustment period, then remarriage and step-family issues.

Though divorce is perceived widely to be stressful and deleterious for children, evidence is accumulating that living in a home replete with high levels of marital strife and conflict is not any healthier. Many of the emotional, behavioral, and academic problems first named after divorce are actually identifiable for as many as 4 years before in households with struggling marriages. Similarly, poor child-parent relationships reported post-divorce are often evident several years before legal action is filed and finalized (Kelly, 1998).

From the child's perspective, one of the most, if not the most traumatic, milestone in the divorce process is the event of separation and actual physical leaving of one parent from the original intact family household. Especially for younger children, the moment of separation may be more distressing than when they are first told of the separation and/or divorce, and even the legal finalization of the divorce. Children of all ages may become confused if significant time lapses between being told of the separation and when one parent actually leaves. Children may feel just as sad, angry, and lonely during parental separation as many adults imagine they will become at the divorce itself. This time also may be harder on children because of the diminished emotional availability of the parents, who are in the throes of dealing with their own emotions. In addition, the emotional vicissitudes of separation are rarely brief, sometimes extending for several years before the divorce is finalized, and then often for years afterwards if key issues relevant to the child remain charged and conflictual (Wallerstein, 1999).

One of the chief stressors for children of parental separation, divorce, and remarriage is the level of conflict between marital partners or the divorced parents. Though studies over the years have contradicted each other on whether children fare better in stressful, intact homes with poor parental marriages or in divorced homes with potentially happier parents, agreement does exist that frequent and intense conflict between parents, whether married and living together, separated, divorced, or divorced and remarried, is the single greatest determinant of children's emotional and physical adjustment and long-term outcome. This is especially true if the conflict is frequent or intense, and renders the children fearful, depressed, anxious, or feeling caught in the middle between the two parents. Not only do the children learn poor and ineffective methods of conflict resolution, but they may model parental aggression, verbal and physical. Perpetual wrangling between parents also drains the adults of the physical and emotional reserves they need to nurture their relationships with their children. Fortunately, in the majority of cases, parental conflict does lessen in the first few years after separation or divorce (Kelly, 1998; Pruett and Pruett, 1998; Wallerstein and Corbin, 2002).

Violence in high-conflict marriages, separation, and divorce may be of the classic battered-wife nature (violence perpetuated by husbands against wives throughout their relationships). However, in order to avoid asking a "near-miss" question that may skirt over important information, such as "Did your father ever hit your mother?", clinicians should be familiar with additional scenarios. Other patterns of violence include those initiated by females, an interactive aggression started by either men or women, then continued primarily by men, or violence related to the divorce trauma itself and controlled by the person being abandoned or left by the other partner. Witnessing violence between parents may affect emotional and moral development adversely, as well as the child's future romantic and marital relationships. It also leads to a greater incidence of adjustment problems and psychopathology. If a physician suspects or knows of violence between parents, he or she must inquire about and be extra attentive to indications that the child may also be involved in or a victim of the domestic abuse as well (Kelly, 1998; Pruett and Hoganbruen, 1998; Wallerstein and Corbin, 1999).

"Doctor, how do we tell our child we are getting a divorce?"

Even divorcing parents who are at odds about nearly everything will agree that this is one of the most difficult, even heartbreaking, tasks they have ever faced. Though the sophistication or the language used and the extent of the explanations will vary according to the developmental age of the child, in optimal situations the following elements should be included when children are informed that a divorce is coming.

1 Though the mother and father are not getting along well and will no longer live together and be married, each parent still loves each child in the family just as much, if not more, than before the decision to divorce.
2 The parents did everything they could to try to work things out and avoid separation and divorce (if true!), but after thinking about what is best for everyone, they have decided to divorce.
3 The child did nothing to cause or hasten the divorce – it is not your fault!
4 The child will continue to see the parent who is leaving regularly. Though the schedules and specifics may be changing and in flux for a period of time, his or her relationships with both parents will continue.
5 The parent who is leaving the family household will be OK – he or she will have a safe place to stay, enough food to eat and clothes to wear. (It is helpful for children to see the parent's new living quarters as soon as possible to help relieve these doubts.)
6 It is OK to feel sad, angry, relieved, or all mixed up about this – the parents sometimes feel the same way. Both par-

ents will try to be available to the child to talk about these feelings and the changes the divorce will bring, and to answer questions as they arise.

7 Though there may be some changes as everyone gets used to the new living arrangements, both parents would like other areas of the child's life to continue as before, including school, friends, extracurricular activities, household chores, and relationships with grandparents and significant others.

8 As time goes on, if there are any additional changes or something the child should know, the parents promise they'll share it with him or her as soon as they can.

Parents should exercise discretion and good judgment about what specific information they give their children. While they do need to be given a straightforward explanation about the reasons for the divorce, explicit details about one spouse's extramarital affairs and sexual exploits are not appropriate to share. It is often helpful to identify one or two adults outside the family whom parents and child respect and trust, perhaps a clergyperson, close family friend or neighbor, as a safe person the child may talk with also. Informing the child's primary teacher at school may also be helpful, especially if reactions to the changes at home are reflected in his or her mood, academics, or peer relationships. Again, remember that divorce is a process that spans years. A child who was 6 years old when the parents separated and 8 years old when the divorce was finalized will be affected in different ways, have new questions, and need more detailed explanations of the divorce and its consequences at 10, 13, 16, 18, and older ages (Wallerstein, 1999).

Children's initial reactions to divorce

For all age groups, it is reassuring to know that the vast majority of children adapt and cope quite well with the changes divorce brings. While emotional and behavioral reactions can be expected, they diminish in intensity over the course of the first year and are responsive to parental understanding and as much consistency as possible. Initial reactions common to all age groups, though expressed in developmentally different ways, include anger, depressive symptoms, crying, aggression, noncompliance with daily rules, some acting out, regression, academic difficulties, isolation, increased dependency and clinginess, fear, anxiety, confusion or difficulty concentrating, somatization, and appetite and sleep disturbances. Factors negatively affecting early post-divorce adjustment include continued conflict between the parents, ongoing legal action regarding visitation and custody, lessened availability or abandonment by one or both parents, parental psychiatric illness, lack of support from outside the immediate family, financial problems, and troubled relationships with new adults taking on stepparent roles (Dell, 1995; Kelly, 1998; Pruett and Pruett, 1998; Wallerstein, 1999; Wallerstein and Corbin, 2002).

BOX 16.7

Responses to divorce by age

Up to 2 years old
- Lethargy
- Withdrawal
- Sleep disturbances
- Feeding/eating disorders
- Spitting up/vomiting
- Fussiness
- Irritability
- Inconsolability
- Excessive crying
- Restlessness
- Clinginess
- Exaggerated fear of unfamiliar people or situations
- Inappropriate lack of anxiety with unfamiliar people or situations

Preschoolers
- Confusion
- Belief that separation is temporary
- Regression
- Denial
- Irritability
- Aggression
- Guilt
- Fear
- Separation anxiety
- Inhibited play
- Fear of being replaced

6- to 8-year-olds
- Understanding that divorce is final
- Egocentricity: "Maybe I did something to cause the divorce"
- Anger at custodial parent
- Suppression of anger
- Attraction to noncustodial parent
- Loyalty conflicts
- Fear
- Grief

9- to 12-year olds
- Denial
- Anger
- Superficial satisfactory coping
- Disrupted sense of personal identity
- Easily caught on one parent's side
- Somatization

Adolescents
- Greater independence, resourcefulness, maturity
- Anger, resentment
- Withdrawal, isolation
- Depression
- Worries about own future sexual and marital relationships
- Concern about finances

(reprinted with permission from Dell ML (1995) "Divorce – are you ready to help?" *Contemporary Pediatrics* 12(5): 57-66)

Even infants are sensitive to the stresses and changes in the family. Physiologic responses to conflict and aggression include increased heart rate and blood pressure, postural defensiveness and freezing, crying, and even attempts to physically distance themselves from the situation. Despite the fact that their caregivers may be distracted by marital strife, infants continue to demand immediate care, especially adequate food, sleep, and physical intimacy. When these needs are not met sufficiently, babies may become irritable, excessively fussy, cry more, experience an increased incidence of vomiting, feeding and elimination problems, sleep irregularities, and signs of autonomic hyperarousal. If deficient or inconsistent caregiving is prolonged, the young one's capacities for basic trust and eventual independence may be compromised. The infant's temperament and goodness of fit with parent temperaments are also factors in the child's longer-term adjustment and ability to form relationships with others (Dell, 1995; Kelly, 1998).

Toddlers experience many of the same emotional and physical signs and symptoms of adjustment as infants. As they gain greater physical mobility and language blossoms, they may be able to express their emotions through play and even verbally to parents and other adults. For children whose parents work outside the home, a consistent childcare provider during the separation and divorce process is very important for maintaining consistency and some measure of stability.

Preschoolers (ages 3–5) are the age group most prone to behavioral regression in response to major life changes. They are becoming individuals, and learning how family and society expect them to behave in certain situations. Divorce is disruptive to these processes, particularly to continued learning about gender roles and moral development. They may understand that their parents no longer live in the same home, but not understand that this and other changes are permanent. A looming, often unspoken fear is that if one parent has left, the other will, too, leaving the child totally abandoned. The egocentricity of this age may lend to the beliefs that he or she is personally responsible for the break-up of the marriage, or that family unity can be restored simply because the child desires or commands it to be so. Parents may also have to deal with resurgent separation anxiety, sleep disturbances, bedwetting, irritability, and aggression at times when their own energy is depleted (Dell, 1995; Wallerstein, 1999; Wallerstein and Corbin, 2002).

School-age children may be categorized into two groups – 6–8-year-olds and 9–12-year-olds. The younger group can better understand the permanence of divorce and some contributing factors, but retain just enough magical thinking to deny the divorce and its consequences are real. They still wonder if anything they did contributed to the events, and feel rejected by both parents, especially the one who leaves to live elsewhere. They may act out against or completely suppress their anger toward the custodial parent, and worry about and want to spend more time with the noncustodial parent. The older group tends to suffer setbacks in peer relationships and academic functioning in the first year after the divorce. They may try to convince others that they are untouched about the changes in their lives, but they may be suffering a great deal silently. Somatic symptoms in the absence of the usual corresponding pathophysiology, including headaches, stomach-aches, and sore, aching limbs, are common in this age group. However, a significant minority of children may express their anger overtly, verbally and in hostile, potentially dangerous ways. Most preteens respond favorably to continued, supportive interactions with both parents, and encouragement and praise for maintaining good efforts in school and the extracurricular activities in which they are involved (Dell, 1995; Roseby and Johnston, 1998; Wallerstein, 1999; Wallerstein and Corbin, 2002).

Adolescents who cope well with their parents' break-up develop earlier and greater independence, maturity, and resourcefulness than they might have otherwise. Other teens struggle with depression, anger and resentment, shame, embarrassment, and feel "caught in the middle" between parents. They have a more realistic picture of the world outside the family, leading to worry more about finances and practical concerns than younger children, especially as the diminished cash flow affects college, clothes, and entertainment. As they are beginning to date and approach adult-like love relationships, they may experience doubt and anxiety about their ability to form and maintain healthy relationships with members of the opposite sex. More adolescents than previously thought are prone to depression, substance abuse, sexual acting out, and even suicidality during the first 12–18 months post-divorce. Adolescents benefit from calm, stable adults outside the family to talk with and encouragement to look forward and invest in academic and extracurricular activities that will bolster their self-esteem and keep them in contact with others outside the home (Dell, 1995; Kelly, 1998; Wallerstein, 1999; Wallerstein and Corbin, 2002).

From a psychodynamic perspective, Wallerstein has identified six tasks that an individual must complete to deal effectively with parental divorce. Though a child may start these tasks at the time of the actual divorce, completely working through them is an ongoing process through adolescence and early adulthood. These tasks are:

1 acknowledging the reality of the marital rupture
2 disengaging from parental conflict and distress and resuming customary pursuits
3 the resolution of losses
4 resolving anger and self-blame
5 accepting the permanence of the divorce
6 achieving realistic hope regarding relationships

The first two tasks are usually worked through in the first year after the divorce, tasks 3–5 are worked through and revisited several times in later childhood and adolescence, and the final task becomes particularly important in older adolescence and young adulthood. Together, these six goals provide not only a description of what an individual must address growing up as a child of divorce, but they also provide a working outline for therapists treating individuals, families, or groups of same-aged children from divorced families (Wallerstein and Corbin, 2002).

Custody considerations

Over the last 20 years, most divorce and family courts have moved away from the automatic assumption that the best needs of the child are always with the mother, or in cases when the divorcing parents do not include an acceptably fit biologic or adoptive mother, the adult who is the child's "psychologic parent." Increasingly, society and the legal system have recognized the importance of the father to the child's continued healthy development, not just by awarding more generous visitation privileges, but by decreeing joint and even primary physical and legal custody to fathers. Indeed, many states now operate under the assumption that families will enter into a joint custody arrangement, at least initially, unless one parent refuses to participate as a custodial parent or there is a significant concern that joint custody is not in the best interests of a particular child in a particular family and divorce situation (Dell, 1995; Pruett and Pruett, 1998; Wallerstein, 1999; Wallerstein and Corbin, 2002).

Many states began enacting joint custody in the 1980s. Joint legal custody means that both parents have the rights and responsibilities to participate in decisions of major importance to the child, such as education, health, and medical care, but it does not necessarily include recommendations for the minor's physical living arrangements. Joint physical custody entails everything included in joint legal custody, plus the sharing of the child's physical living arrangements between the parents, whether near-equal time in geographically proximate residences, alternate seasons or years if parents have relocated to distant communities, or another mutually agreed upon arrangement. Many professionals specializing in the divorce custody process prefer the term "joint parenting" to describe both types of joint custody (Pruett and Pruett, 1998).

In the eyes of many judges and divorce courts, joint custody is the simplest and best way to recognize the importance of invested fathers in their children's lives before divorce, and to encourage continued involvement post-divorce. True joint physical custody, with children living for nearly equal amounts of time in each parent's new household, is estimated to occur in only 10–20% of joint physical custody families. Many families at the time of divorce genuinely may be committed to joint parenting, but over time fall into the common pattern of mother as primary parent, assuming most or all responsibilities for food, clothing, medical appointments, and other routine but necessary needs. On the other hand, joint parenting receives high marks from families, especially from fathers and children, when parents are able to separate their marital conflicts from the parenting tasks, set residual anger aside, and commit to partnering with their ex-spouse to meet and exceed the physical, emotional, and other needs of the child. Wallerstein has identified six factors that contribute to joint custody/joint parenting arrangements that are helpful to children.

1 Both parents make parenting a high priority in their lives and order the rest of their lives and decisions according to their parenting commitments.
2 Both parents are observant and sensitive to their child's needs and desires, especially as these change over time according to the child's growth and development.
3 Each ex-spouse respects the other as a competent parent, and is able to communicate effectively with the other about the child and parenting matters.
4 Both parents can accept some ambiguities and differences in parenting styles around routine or daily aspects of living, such as toilet training, times of meals, television viewing guidelines, etc.
5 Both parents focus on assisting the child to make smooth transitions between parents and households.
6 The living arrangements are structured to facilitate seamless transitions between households, causing minimal to no disruption of the child's educational, social, and extracurricular activities and interests.

(Pruett and Pruett, 1998; Roseby and Johnston, 1998; Wallerstein, 1999; Wallerstein and Corbin, 2002)

Joint custody does not work well when parents retain high levels of conflict after the divorce, cannot work together cooperatively for the best interests of the child, or when shared parenting is the default plan because neither ex-spouse wants the responsibilities of parenting. When joint custody is ordered by the court in highly conflicted families, or when one or both parents are not motivated and invested in the arrangement, the children are at greater risk for psychologic, academic, social, and even physical maladjustment. Even in optimal shared custody situations, flexibility on the part of everyone is essential, and in years subsequent to the divorce, many families go through times when a child will spend more time with one parent than another for a variety of different reasons. Some studies have noted, for instance, that joint physical custody may be easiest during the school-age years, as compared to the preschool and adolescent years when the child has more unique developmental needs and personal pursuits. Ideally, assessments of each individual child, both parents, and the family constellation, either as part of a mediation process, at the suggestion of attorneys, or by the parents' initiative, should be completed before the divorce is finalized. These assessments may provide helpful information to be considered in visitation and custody decisions (Pruett and Hoganbruen, 1998; Pruett and Pruett, 1998; Roseby and Johnston, 1998; Wallerstein, 1999; Wallerstein and Corbin, 2002).

Remarriage and stepfamilies

Most divorced adults remarry, and they, their children, new spouse, and new spouse's children form stepfamilies. If this trend continues at its current rate, it is possible that by 2010 remarried families will outnumber intact first-marriage families. Another way to frame the prominence of this family constellation is to state that one half of all Americans will become stepchildren, stepparents, or step-grandparents during their lifetimes. Indeed, the life of this common family configuration in which so many children are raised is born itself from divorce and loss (Townsend, 2000).

Generally, remarriage contributes to the happiness and well-being of children when parents are happier individuals, feel supported by another adult in their parent roles, are not as lonely, and feel less stressed financially. If stepparents do not try to replace the same-sex biologic parent, but work diligently to develop their own independent and unique relationship with the child, the youth may experience meaningful and satisfying relationships with all adults in the parenting roles, whether original or stepparents. In some cases, child-stepparent relationships may begin on a rocky footing, only to improve gradually over time with familiarity and the passing of months and years during which the stepparent does not usurp the role of the primary same-sexed parent. In yet other situations, initial conflicts and resentments simmer, even boil over, for years and are never resolved. This may be more likely if the child suspects one parent of infidelity with a stepparent when still married to the child's other parent, whether true or not. Also, adolescents from stepfamilies tend to leave home at slightly younger ages than peers from intact original families (Pruett and Pruett, 1998; Wallerstein, 1999).

Based on her research, Wallerstein has identified eight issues for children in stepfamilies (Wallerstein, 1999):

1 complex relationships with new family members
2 changed relationships within the original family, especially in the mother-daughter relationship
3 geographical separation and relocation
4 unrealistic expectations about new family harmony
5 more difficult adjustment for older children and adolescents than for younger children
6 new strains in the stepfamily and accompanying fears of even more instability
7 rivalries and competition between parents and stepparents
8 development of new family rituals, values, and routines while continuing to remember and honor those of the previous family

A ninth challenge not named explicitly by Wallerstein, though it certainly may influence elements of all eight areas, is the matter of discipline. Does the stepparent have the desire to be involved in that part of the child's life? If so, under what circumstances? Do the child's parent and stepparent agree about methods and timing? Which adult has the ultimate determination about what behaviors, attitudes, and language are acceptable in the blended household? Ideally, these are issues that the parent and stepparent considered before the marriage and changes in the family living situation.

Few, if any, families bear any similarity to the projected order and bliss of the Brady Bunch. Familiarity with some of the struggles children from stepfamilies may experience permits pediatricians to be more perceptive and helpful when caring for these children, their parents, and stepparents.

Long-term outcomes

The majority of children raised in divorced and remarried households adjust well and lead reasonably happy, productive lives. The initial reactions in the first year post-divorce, whether good or bad, do not necessarily correlate with long-term outcomes. The high divorce rate in the United States, coupled with the stresses inherent to a change of this magnitude in a child's life, results in children of divorce and remarriage being over-represented in outpatient psychiatric populations, both in the private and public sectors. By the end of adolescence and beginning of adulthood, children of divorce are three to four times as likely as peers from intact, never-divorced families to have received psychotherapy. The proportions of children and adolescents from divorced homes requiring inpatient psychiatric care is even greater, reaching over 75% of total inpatient cases. Children of divorce also tend to present to the educational systems with higher rates of learning and behavioral disorders (Dell, 1995; Wallerstein, 1999).

Much of what is known about long-term outcomes for children from divorced families comes from Judith Wallerstein's California Children of Divorce study. Interestingly, data from this longitudinal research indicate that initial post-divorce responses do not predict long-term psychosocial adjustment for either children who had difficulty adjusting to the divorce at the time it occurred, or for children who seemed to adjust well to the event at the time. And, just as 10-year outcomes in this study did not reflect immediate post-divorce adjustment, neither were the 15-year outcomes consistent with how the study participants were doing at the 10-year mark. Though the research team cannot identify common themes or links predicting successful or poor outcomes at these milestone anniversaries, they do note that many children who were doing well at 10 years post-divorce were very well parented or received significant help from at least one parent or grandparent, though typically not by both parents. Many had taken greater personal responsibility for themselves as they matured, which did not lessen disappointment due to divorce and lack of parental involvement, but fostered pride and confidence in themselves. Many well-adjusted youths and young adults had found other adult mentors or role models in an effort to compensate for what they may have been lacking from one or both parents. Type and frequency of parental visitation was unrelated to the child's adjustment. Instead, a key element of subsequent adjustment was whether or not the child felt rejected by his or her father. In remarried families, the 10-year follow-up demonstrated a reluctance of step-parents to take a significant parental role in the lives of their stepchildren. In general, remarriage was not associated with good or poor adjustment, except for situations in which children were extremely young at the time of the divorce and did appear to benefit from parental remarriage (Wallerstein, 1999; Wallerstein and Corbin, 2002).

Most children of divorce reported ongoing stresses after the event, especially financial. Continuing hostility between their divorced parents was a common stressor, half of the study participants endured a second parental divorce, and 60% felt rejected by one or both parents (Wallerstein, 1999; Wallerstein and Corbin, 2002).

Clinicians working with divorced parents and children also need to be aware of gender differences in these outcome studies. Though sex-role behaviors in preschool girls appears not to be affected by divorce, there is some evidence that preschool boys from divorced families may spend more time playing with girls and younger children and be more socially isolated than same-aged male peers from non-divorced families. In the California Children of Divorce study, at 18 months after the divorce girls had become better adjusted since the time of the actual event, but boys were experiencing increased psychologic adjustment problems. Other studies have found that boys from divorced families perform more poorly on academic testing than matched control groups from intact families. However, girls may experience increased turmoil in adolescence and young adulthood as they enter dating and long-term relationships with the opposite sex. Ten years after parental divorce, Wallerstein's cohort of young adult females reported a higher than expected rate of short-term romantic and sexual relationships than same-aged women from non-divorced families, often with older men. They entered into psychotherapy more often to work on issues of commitment, abandonment by male figures, and separation from their mothers. Data from the 25-year anniversary of the California Children of Divorce study indicate that adult men who experienced parental divorce as a child feel less competent in their relationships with women, less able to influence women's feelings or behavior, and are anxious about losing everything they have worked for – as if they are particularly vulnerable to disaster (Kelly, 1998; Pruett and Hoganbruen, 1998; Roseby and Johnston, 1998; Wallerstein, 1999; Wallerstein and Corbin, 2002).

In summary, immediate, intermediate, and long-term adjustment to parental divorce is influenced by an intricate, complicated mix of variables (Box 16.7), including age of the child at the time of the divorce; gender; amount of violence experienced or witnessed; the amount of continuing parental conflict; the child's individual temperament and resiliency; genetic vulnerabilities to psychiatric and medical illnesses; access to other adults for emotional support and role modeling; the quality of individual relationships with mother, father, stepparents, and grandparents; quality of parenting by all adults in that role; access to activities in which the child can compensate or sublimate for the losses of divorce, such as academics, athletics, music, and other endeavors; economic resources; and professional mental health care when desired and indicated.

The role of the pediatrician in families of divorce

Familiarity with the information presented in this section about the effects of separation and divorce on children of different developmental stages, the effects of marital and divorce-related stresses on parents, current trends in post-divorce custody in the geographical area where physicians practice, the general issues facing stepfamilies, and intermediate and longer-term effects of divorce is central to the pediatrician's recognition of divorce-related concerns as they may present in clinical practice.

The pediatrician working with divorced families may need to be more vigilant about both the routine well child and sick child care. The distraction of the divorce and the accompanying energy drain may put these children at greater risk for missed immunizations, poorer nutrition, and delays in bringing ill children into the office for care. The simple question "Has anything changed at home?" is a simple but effective way to keep up with changes in parental marital status and family composition. A quick check of the child's registration information or the face sheet in the chart at every appointment is a habit that pays off well for the physician trying to keep abreast of these changes. For instance, changes of address, telephone numbers, and third party payers may clue caregivers in to the fact that there have been significant changes in a household.

After learning of a divorce or remarriage, the physician may remind parents of the developmental and individual child temperament differences and how coping and adjustment to separation, divorce, and remarriage are influenced by these factors. Some pediatricians schedule an additional appointment to permit additional time to talk with children and divorcing parents about how family members are coping presently and what to expect in the near future. Extra time is important to allow children and parents to ask as many questions as they desire about the life-changing events they are living through (Box 16.8).

Though the general supportive measures a skilled and caring primary care physician may provide are very helpful to many families, others do need additional attention

BOX 16.8

Questions about divorce

Questions parents ask

- Is it harmful for children to see their parents fighting?
- How can I prevent my child from being "caught in the middle?"
- Is divorce better or worse for my child than our present home situation?
- How do I tell my child about the divorce?
- How do I help my child with his or her feelings about the divorce?
- Should I talk to my child about my feelings? How?
- How will divorce affect my child emotionally, physically, academically, socially?
- How do you think my child is coping with the divorce? Does he or she need counseling?
- What are the best custody and visitation arrangements? Joint custody?
- How do we handle visits with grandparents?
- How will a move and changing schools affect my child?
- I just don't have any energy for my child since the divorce. What should I do?
- My child hasn't been eating or sleeping well. What should I do?
- Our marriage broke up because one of us is homosexual. Do we tell our child? How?
- How can I help my child adjust to living on a tighter budget?
- How long should I wait before dating and remarrying?
- How do I prepare my child for a new parent and stepfamily?
- I fear my ex-spouse is abusing my child emotionally, physically, or sexually. What should I do?

BOX 16.8 (continued)

Questions children ask about divorce

- Why do my parents have to get a divorce?
- Is it my fault?
- Can I get them back together?
- What's going to happen to me and my sisters and brothers?
- What's going to happen to the parent who moved out? Will I see him or her again? Will he or she still love me? Will he or she forget about me?
- Will I have to change schools? Why?
- Why can't we buy and do all the things we used to before the divorce?
- Did my parent fall in love with someone else?
- Why is my parent so sad (angry) all the time?
- Will I see my grandparents and other relatives anymore?
- Where will the pets live? Who will take care of them?
- I don't need parents. Why can't I do what I want and take care of myself?
- Can you help me?
- I hate my parent for what he or she did to us.
- People are treating me differently and making fun of me.
- I'm having trouble in school.

(reprinted with permission from Dell ML (1995) "Divorce – are you ready to help?" *Contemporary Pediatrics* 12(5): 57–66)

these categories and the extent of the effects on children for the rest of their lives, becoming adept at working with these issues is tremendously important.

from mental health professionals. Pediatricians should be familiar with a range of psychiatrists and therapists in his or her community, for adults as well as children and adolescents. Physicians should also be familiar with the services offered by these clinicians for all age groups, including comprehensive assessments, individual and group therapy, family therapy, psychotropic medication evaluations and management, psychologic testing, and educational/academic evaluations and consulting. Primary care physicians should ask that they remain apprised of the work done be other clinicians, and should remind families that they are available in between annual physical examinations and sick child visits to assist them with any questions or concerns. Caring for children and adolescents of separation, divorce, and remarriage in a complete, thorough manner does require extra time and effort on the clinician's part. However, in view of the numbers of families who find themselves in

KEY CLINICAL QUESTIONS

- *Have there been any changes at home or with your family since the last time we saw each other?*
  May unlock the occurrence of parental separation, divorce, or remarriage.

To the child:
- *Do you have any worries about yourself or either one of your parents that you might like to talk about?*
  May unlock key to child's fears, emotions, and concerns about him or herself, and provide key information into the level of functioning of the parents.

To the parent:
- *Do you have any worries about yourself or your child that you might like to talk about?*
  May unlock key to parent's fears, emotions, and concerns about self, and provide key information as to the level of functioning of the child.

CONSIDER CONSULTATION WHEN ...

- Parents and/or children appear depressed, anxious, or are not coping well with issues of separation, divorce, or remarriage.
- A child from a disrupted family is not progressing in a developmentally appropriate manner physically, emotionally, socially, or academically.
- A parent or child misses appointments for routine well child care.

- Make no assumptions about how adopted children and their families should look, feel, behave, or be like – this limits the physician's clinical sensitivities and powers of observation!
- Pay close attention to available medical and biologic family histories, the physical examination, laboratory studies, and dental, vision, and hearing screenings of newly adopted children.
- Adoptive parents may need extra time and anticipatory guidance during office visits and over the telephone – especially if they have no other biologic or adopted children.
- Though adopted children are over-represented statistically in psychiatric and learning disabled populations, the great majority of adopted children do well physically, emotionally, behaviorally, and cognitively.
- Research and be prepared to provide information on all aspects of the adoptive process and subsequent coping, adjustment, and community resources for adoptive children, adolescents, and their family members.

Adoption

The past three decades have seen renewed interest in adoption, as well as significant changes in the characteristics of those involved in the process. In the United States, the number of healthy infants given up for into adoption by young unmarried mothers has steadily declined, a result of the availability of contraception, the wider access to elective pregnancy terminations, and a social trend of single mothers choosing to keep and raise children conceived out of wedlock (Derdeyn and Lamps, 2002; Sherry and Nickman, 1999). This actual decrease in the absolute numbers of infants available for adoption has coincided with many women postponing pregnancy and motherhood until their thirties and forties, only to be unable to conceive their own biologic children and turning to adoption for their best chance to acquire a healthy newborn to raise. At least 2% of children in the United States are adopted. Adoptions can be private, independent, intrafamilial, extrafamilial, international, across racial and ethnic groups, and involve foster care and older children and adolescents with special needs. Though adoptive parents may be traditional heterosexual married couples with or without other children, single adults and gay couples have been approved at increasing rates. Surrogacy has also introduced new legal, psychologic, and practical considerations into the adoption process (Derdeyn and Lamps, 2002; Sherry and Nickman, 1999). Primary care providers are in unique positions to educate adoptive parents about normal growth and development, monitor for physical and emotional problems, and advocate for all involved in the adoption process.

The joy and many positive aspects of adoption may be accompanied by a paradoxical sense of loss, even for adoptive parents who are receiving a child into their family. For many couples, adoption means that they are fully acknowledging emotionally that they cannot conceive a biologic child of their own. The pain of this loss and its shattered dreams may have been compounded by years of frustration, painful medical procedures, considerable financial expenditures, feelings of inadequacy and inferiority as complete adults, and perceived shame and embarrassment in their family and social relationships. Children who are older when adopted lose familiar caretakers, same-age companions, and may have to change schools or move to a different city or state. Even children adopted as infants will need to deal with losses and "what ifs" related to being given up and not raised by their biologic parents (Derdeyn and Graves, 1998; Derdeyn and Lamps, 2002; Sherry and Nickman, 1999; Stevenson-Moessner, 2003).

Types of adoption

Adoptions are facilitated through public agencies or through independent or private organizations or sources. Licensed agencies, whether public or private, share as much medical and other information about the child with the adoptive family as possible, and provide counseling and other resources to the adoption triad of birth parents, child, and adoptive family before, during, and after the child changes custody. Major drawbacks to some *private adoptions* are that supportive services for the adoptive triad, if offered at all, may be very time limited, not all known and relevant information about the child and his or her biologic background is shared, and procedural shortcuts may have legal ramifications later in time. Historically in the United States, adoptions have been *closed*, meaning that after legal papers were signed there was no contact between the biologic and adoptive families. Increasingly, adoptions have become *open*, with varying degrees of contact between the two parties. Ideally, the biologic and adoptive families, with assistance from the adoption agency, determine the parameters for openness prior to the adoption. The shift toward open adoptions was given a boost in 1987 by the National Adoption Task Force of the

Child Welfare League of America, which recommended that after an adopted child reaches the age of majority, agencies should assist them in contacting birth families if those individuals were willing to become involved with the adopted child. In some adoptions of older children, openness permits respect of biologic relationships and other relationships familiar to the child, while permitting the establishment of a new legal and permanent home. Open adoptions work especially well for families with strong religious and spiritual beliefs, and nontraditional adoptive parents such as singles and gay and lesbian couples, perhaps because these groups look to larger community support more than many traditional families. Openness may not be advisable in situations in which the biologic parents have been declared unfit for ongoing problems such as substance abuse or criminal activity, or after adversarial court proceedings (Derdeyn and Graves, 1998; Derdeyn and Lamps, 2002; Lears et al., 1998; Sherry and Nickman, 1999; Silverstein and Roszia, 1999).

A great fear for many adoptive parents is that the adoptive process in an advanced stage or, even a legally finalized adoption, might be reversed and the child removed from the new home. *Adoption disruption* is more likely to occur if the child was adopted previously or is older. In truth, it is often adoptive parents who change their minds. Common factors in those situations include more highly educated adoptive mothers, surprise at the number or severity of the child's problems, unresolved fertility issues, insufficient preadoption counseling, and inadequate information given to them about the child beforehand. When adoption is disrupted, both the child and the family who had anticipated the adoption need emotional support and therapy (Derdeyn and Graves, 1998; Derdeyn and Lamps, 2002).

Infant adoption is the type that comes to mind for most of the general public. The legal arrangements may have been made during pregnancy, and in open adoptions the adoptive parents may even be present at the delivery. Infant adoptions may be intrafamilial, for instance, an aunt adopting her sister's baby, becoming the legal mother and raising the baby as if she had given birth to the child. Many infant adoptions are also international, given the declining number of healthy infants available for adoption in the United States. Attachment research has supported overwhelmingly that infants adopted in the first year of life are as apt to develop healthy attachments and relationships with others as nonadopted babies, especially in the presence of warm, consistent caregiving environments (Carlson, Sampson, and Sroufe, 2003).

Adoption of older children can be quite rewarding for both adoptive families and the child. However, special support is needed for all involved, especially if the child has been abused or neglected, has been in foster care or group homes, has experienced adoption disruption, or has special physical, emotional, or educational needs. Children adopted at older ages do have higher incidences of emotional and be-

havioral problems. They may have been raised up until that point in an environment of a different ethnicity or language. Older children have also been affected by more situations of separation and loss. Prospective parents interested in adopting an older child should take extra care and time to find out as much as possible about the child's background and experiences to facilitate a smoother transition into a new home and family (Carlson, Sampson, and Sroufe, 2003; Derdeyn and Graves, 1998).

Special needs adoptions involve children who are 10 years of age or older, and have significant medical, psychiatric, developmental, or intellectual concerns. Half of special needs children involve those with mental retardation or emotional problems. They may also have lived in foster care for 4 or more years and may have experienced one or more adoption disruptions. Difficulty finding adoptive homes is increased if these young people are from minorities or part of a large sibship. Up to half of all adoptions through public agencies involve special needs children. Despite higher disruption rates than other types of adoption, most are successful with social work support, considerable preparation and training of adoptive parents, and monetary subsidies to help care for the extra requirements and professional care these children may require. Special needs adoptions also go more smoothly when the adoptive father is very involved and invested in the child's emotional and physical care. Careful consideration on a case by case basis as to openness is indicated. Because the children are older, may have siblings living elsewhere, and have had other placements, they have made emotional attachments to other significant individuals and they may benefit from ongoing contact with them. This can be especially true for children who have been adopted across racial and ethnic lines. On the other hand, continued contact with those who may have neglected or abused them may be contraindicated. As physicians see these children more frequently than those without special needs, they are in unique positions to assess their medical and emotional adaptation over time (Derdeyn and Graves, 1998; Hollingsworth, 1998; McRoy and Grape, 1999; Sherry and Nickman, 1999; Silverstein and Roszia, 1999).

International or foreign adoptions have increased in popularity in the last two decades, especially among single adoptive parents and other nontraditional families, coinciding with the decrease in the number of healthy infants to adopt in the United States. The number of international adoptions and the countries from which children are adopted varies with the world political situation. For instance, adoptions from Eastern Europe and China increased dramatically in the mid-1990s secondary to political changes and shifts in countries' adoption policies. Prospective parents typically travel to the child's birth country to meet the child for the first time and complete arrangements, then parent(s) and child return to the United States together. Difficulties may arise if the infant has been abused and neglected severely before adoption, or if medical care has been suboptimal. International adoptions of older children may be complicated by language considerations if the child is speaking. Occasionally, determining an accurate birthdate is difficult when written records are poor or absent. Regardless of these negative factors, this type of adoption is typically quite satisfying to both adoptive children and families (Derdeyn and Graves, 1998; Sherry and Nickman, 1999; Mitchell and Janista, 1997b).

Transracial or interracial adoptions, particularly adoptions of African-American children by Caucasian families, are somewhat controversial among professional social work organizations. Those favoring transracial placements say that there is no professional literature to say that white parents are unable to adequately parent a child of color; that there are not enough minority adoptive parents to absorb the number of same-race children awaiting adoption; that the most important consideration should be the provision of permanent, committed, nurturing homes; and adoption should not be delayed or denied when parents of a different race or ethnicity are qualified, willing, and prepared to adopt. Often, Caucasian families serving as foster parents to African-American children develop great affection and emotional ties to them, and desire to adopt them both out of mutual fondness and because no comparably suitable placement in a same-race family is available to the child. Arguments against transracial adoption include the conviction that minority children belong emotionally, physically, and culturally with same-race families where they can develop a complete sense of themselves, their heritage, and what this means to their futures; minority children are best taught how to deal with a prejudiced society by same-race families; and living in white families precludes minority children from developing a healthy self-concept of themselves and their race, thus impairing relationships with others of their own race or ethnicity. This debate culminated in the Multiethnic Placement Act of 1994, prohibiting federally funded adoption and placement agencies from denying adoption to qualified candidates based solely on the race, ethnicity, color, or national origin of the prospective adoptive parents or the child. Statistically, the number of transracial adoptions has declined as the number of international adoptions has increased. The few long-term follow-up studies that do exist of children adopted transracially indicate that the majority do well. However, extra support and education for both child and family is advisable, especially for dealing with adolescent identity issues in this group of young people (Derdeyn and Lamps, 2002; Hollingsworth, 1998; McRoy and Grape, 1999; Sherry and Nickman, 1999).

Historically, foster parents were considered a rather neutral party in a child's transition from biologic to adoptive families, and the emotional ties of the foster parents and children entrusted to their care were under-appreciated and not fully acknowledged from a legal perspective. *Adoptions by foster parents* have increased as courts and agencies have recognized that the qualities desired in adoptive parents also hold true for foster parents, and as all involved in the process have recognized the strength of a child's attachment to his or her foster family, especially when the child was placed there as an infant or toddler. Because foster parents frequently have contact with the biologic families of the children during foster care, especially at the beginning, a higher percentage of adoptions by foster parents are open. Another common situation is known as kinship foster care. Children whose biologic parents are unable to care for them are often taken in by other biologic relatives, who are often officially approved as foster parents. Instead of completing the formal adoption process, these arrangements of kinship foster care become permanent care. The dynamics and outcomes of such arrangements are usually favorable, and share many dynamics with adoptions by unrelated foster parents (Derdeyn and Lamps, 2002; Hollingsworth, 1998; Silverstein and Roszia, 1998).

Adoption professionals and courts have come to agree that children can have their physical, emotional, and other needs met quite well by unmarried adults, hence the increase in single parent adoptions in the past 20 years. Another form of adoption, usually considered as part of divorce and blended family issues, is the *adoption of a spouse's child from a previous marriage or relationship*, either after the death or termination of parental rights of the same-sex biologic parent. In surrogacy, a woman agrees to be impregnated by a man's sperm, carry the baby to term, then at birth give the infant to the man to raise. The man's wife then adopts the child. Contractual arrangements vary, but the biologic mother is usually given a sum of money and her medical and living expenses are paid for by the father and adoptive mother. Considerable difficulties may be encountered with this arrangement if details are not carefully considered and legalities and finances formalized in advance (Sherry and Nickman, 1999).

Life cycle and developmental considerations

Adoptive children and families grow through developmental and life cycle stages just as traditional nuclear families with biologic children do. Most features are the same or similar to non-adoptive families, yet adoption does lead to some notable differences. Based on the work of Erik Erikson and Friedman, Peterson has offered the following schema for the developmental stages of the adoptive family (Peterson, 1997).

Pre-adoption period

A married couple establishes their life together, and after a period of time find themselves deciding not to conceive a biologic child or are unable to do so secondary to infertility. Variables include the length of time in this phase and the extent of fertility work-up and treatment. After deciding to adopt, the couple face uncertainty about approval, time until they receive a child, and in many cases, significant financial investment in the process.

Post-placement period

The newly adopted child must be accepted by and integrated into nuclear and extended families, and the other social communities to which the parents and other siblings, if present, belong. The family and child work at getting to know each other on an intimate basis, an especially important task if the adoptive child is not an infant and has been formed and influenced in untoward ways by his or her past experiences and environments. This is a time of profound emotion and changes for both child and family. Families are often caught off guard by feelings of anxiety and disappointment if their expectations before the child arrived were unrealistic. Parents, siblings, and the new child in the family need to be reassured that few parents and children "fall in love" with each other immediately, but that the hard work and tears of the first several weeks to months will pay off for all.

Preschool period

The family and child deal with the ramifications of biologic differentness. The fact of the adoption is introduced to the child in an age-appropriate fashion and parents are well-advised to field the preschooler's questions about where he came from, his biologic parents, and how he or she came to be with them as simply and honestly as possible. Attention should be focused on helping him to feel as safe and secure in the adoptive family.

School-age period

The child's place in the adoptive family continues to be solidified as new experiences are navigated together. The child deals with social stigma and prejudices he or she may encounter about adoption, as well as fantasies about her biologic family and what his or her life might have been like with them. Adoptive parents need reassurance that these questions, and even reactions and rebellion against them that they may start to see during these years, may be expected and do not negate the strength of the attachment and love formed between adoptive family and child.

Adolescent period

In addition to the usual emotional, physical, cognitive, and social tasks of adolescence, adopted teens continue the struggles of differentness, loss, and rejection that usually begin emerging in the late latency developmental period. They may begin to talk openly about searching for their biologic parents, a process that adoptive families may find hurtful and threatening. Some adopted adolescents may be forced to deal with long-term residuals of prenatal maternal substance abuse, inadequate or lack of prenatal care, the sequela of pre-adop-

tive physical and emotional abuse or neglect, and physical and cognitive deficits that may affect educational and vocational achievement. Both adoptive families and teens may benefit from individual and family therapies during these years (Lears et al., 1998; Peterson, 1997; Stevenson-Moessner, 2003).

Searching

In older adolescence or young adulthood, many adopted children try to locate their biologic parents for the first time, or increase in frequency and intensity what has been minimal contact with their birth families up until that time. The process of looking for and making contact with biologic parents for the first time is called "searching." Searching is motivated largely from a need to solidify the adopted person's identity and sense of self and one's own physical and psychosocial origins. Searching rarely reflects dissatisfaction, poor attachments or relationships with adoptive parents and families, or a lack of gratefulness and appreciation of the parents and families who raised them. Though the process may be lengthy, expensive, and emotionally draining, most adoptees and biologic mothers deem finding each other a beneficial experience, and research to date indicates that relationships with the adoptive family are rarely harmed – they may even improve when the adopted individual becomes more at peace about his or her origins and the circumstances under which the adoption occurred. Clinicians should recognize, however, that even if the outcome of searching is positive, it is an extremely stressful process for both the adopted individual and adoptive parents (Derdeyn and Graves, 1998; Derdeyn and Lamps, 2002).

Physical health and medical care of adopted children

In recent years, availability and accuracy of birth and medical records and the general health and well-being of infants and children being adopted has improved, largely due to federal and state regulations and requirements imposed by welfare and adoption agencies. However, all adoptions, domestic and international, demand hypervigilance concerning the physical condition and medical records for each child. For all adoptions, including those transpiring entirely within the United States, parents should be instructed to obtain as much information regarding the biologic parents' medical and psychiatric health, their extended family histories, the circumstances of the pregnancy and why the child was entered into the adoption process, the type and extent of prenatal care, pregnancy, labor, and delivery complications, the child's medical assessments at birth, and all records of medical care provided from birth until the time of adoption. Adoptive parents should be encouraged to review this information thoroughly with the child's new primary care physician. Though one hopes medical records are accurate, physicians should be aware of the possibility of inaccuracies or even completely falsified information. If physicians or parents suspect problems in this regard, they should contact the adoption agency and appropriate state authorities immediately.

Most internationally adopted children from developed countries will meet prevailing requirements for immunizations, physical examinations, and sick and well child care, but again, parents and physicians do need to maintain a high index of suspicion, especially if physical examination findings are inconsistent with written information about the child. Occasionally, birth dates are inaccurate, with older children misrepresented as being younger to attract greater interest for adoption. If at all possible, children arriving into the United States from other countries should be evaluated within 24 hours, especially if they were ill just before, during, or immediately after the trip. Within the first week, a checkup for baseline measurements of growth and development and a thorough physical examination should be done, looking for signs of developmental delays or chronic illness gone undetected or unreported. All accompanying medical records should be reviewed thoroughly with the adoptive parents. Children should be examined naked in good light to look for musculoskeletal and skin abnormalities. The following screening tests may be indicated for children of foreign adoptions, though not all on the same visit: complete blood count with differential, electrolytes, blood urea nitrogen, creatinine, blood glucose, urinalysis, hepatitis screens, thyroid and liver function tests, serologic test for syphilis, HIV testing, TORCH (toxoplasmosis, other agents, rubella, cytomegalovirus, herpes simplex) screening, urine for heavy metals, urine culture for cytomegalovirus, phenylketonuria (PKU) screen, three rounds of stool testing for ova and parasites, TB screen with chest x-ray. All immunizations should be updated to United States standards, then continued to be administered at appropriate ages. As soon as possible, children should be assessed by a dentist and have hearing and vision screens. Children from particular ethnic groups and geographical areas of the world may require screening for specific disorders such as thalassemias, hemoglobinopathies, glucose-6-phosphate dehydrogenase deficiency, lactase deficiency, sickle cell disease, and rickets, scurvy, and other nutritional deficiencies. Growth rates should be monitored regularly and carefully, especially during the first 2 years in the United States. Infants and children small for their ages upon arrival frequently catch up to their genetic growth curves with proper nutrition and emotional care. Detailed, comprehensive guidelines for the physical care of adoptive infants and children are available from the American Academy of Pediatrics (Lears et al., 1998; Mitchell and Janista, 1997a, 1997b; Sherry and Nickman, 1999).

Psychosocial and behavioral issues

A most important point to remember for parents, physicians, teachers, and others in the lives of adopted children is that the vast majority of adopted children grow into adulthood with very few problems of any kind, and are indistinguishable from their nonadopted peers. However, it is also true that a higher percentage of adopted children are seen in inpatient and outpatient psychiatric populations than other children who are not adopted. Though 2–3% of children in the United States are adopted, 4–5% of children in psychiatric outpatient programs and 10–15% of children in residential treatment are adopted. Relevant considerations are that adopted children may carry higher genetic risks for psychiatric disorders, substance abuse, learning problems, and mental retardation. Secondly, the medical histories of adopted children include inadequate prenatal, perinatal, and early childhood medical care more often than nonadopted children. Early life situations can put them at higher risk for physical, emotional, and sexual abuse and neglect before they are adopted. Finally, the concept of "goodness of fit" between adoptive parents and children is very important. As temperament and many aspects of personality and behavior are affected by genetics, a poor goodness of fit between adults and children in adoptive homes can be quite stressful.

While studies show that behavioral problems are more prevalent in adopted than nonadopted children, this discrepancy is more significant for girls than for boys. For adoptive children and adolescents fortunate enough to work through the emotional issues of their adoption in psychotherapy, several themes are common. These topics include abandonment, loss, grief, anger; lack of identity or a sense of not being permanent; worry about being rejected by or not good enough for their adoptive parents; autonomy, independence, separation and individuation for adoptive parents; and what being adopted might mean for future romantic and subsequent family relationships. Common behaviors seen in adoptive children that may or may not be concerning enough to adoptive parents to seek treatment include isolation from others, hoarding food, clothes, and toys, overeating, excessive and indiscriminate friendliness with strangers, difficulty communicating preferences and feelings, and stereotyped behaviors such as rocking and head banging. In general, adopted children show higher rates of attention-deficit/hyperactivity and learning disorders, mood and psychotic disorders, running away and conduct problems, and substance abuse (Bimmel et al., 2003; Derdeyn and Lamps, 2002; Mitchell and Janista, 1997b; Sherry and Nickman, 1999; Stevenson-Moessner, 2003).

"Doctor, how do I talk with my child about the adoption?"

Certainly, children do need to know that they are adopted and as much information about the particular circumstances of their adoption as possible. However, it is important to remember that sharing this information is best conceptualized as a process spanning many years. Children should be given information in developmentally appropriate ways at the times and in the amounts and detail as they become ready to understand and deal with that knowledge. Many suggest introducing the concept of "being adopted" between the ages of 2 and 4 years of age, especially as the child and others outside the household begin to notice and comment on differences between the adopted individual and the rest of the family. The most common mistake made by adoptive parents is telling too much in too great a detail before the child is cognitively and emotionally ready to handle the complete story. Many parents find it helpful to let the child's own questions guide the timing and complexity of explanations. Waiting until late school age or beyond to reveal the news of adoption risks necessitating dishonesty if the child asks about it earlier, perhaps subjecting the child to uncomfortable stares and rumors if he or she looks different from members of the adoptive family, or the child overhearing comments about his or her adoption from siblings, grandparents, teachers, physicians or others. Most importantly, parents need to be honest and non-defensive, give developmentally appropriate explanations, and reassure the child verbally and physically that he or she is wanted, loved, and accepted by the adoptive family just as he or she is (Derdeyn and Graves, 1998; Lears et al., 1998; Sherry and Nickman, 1999).

Caring for adopted children and their families

Helpful hints for working with these patients and their families have been sprinkled throughout this section. The importance of going over the available medical records in great detail, performing a thorough physical examination, and ordering a complete laboratory work-up has already been discussed. Never make assumptions about adoption and how adoptive parents and adopted children "should" look, feel, or behave. Such preconceptions may limit a clinician's ability to detect adoption-related concerns during visits or over the telephone. Remember that adoption has long-term implications for the child's physical and emotional health, and that dealing with the implications of being

---

CONSIDER CONSULTATION WHEN ...

- Any concerns arise about the psychiatric, behavioral, or academic health and progress of an adopted child and/ or his or her siblings.
- Adoptive parents or the adopted child or adolescent require more time than a primary care physician can provide in the outpatient office setting.
- Strange or unique illnesses or medical signs and symptoms arise that cannot be explained by disease exposure or whatever medical and biologic family histories are known.

KEY CLINICAL QUESTIONS

- *How are you and your child talking about his or her adoption these days?*
  Unlocks the parent's ability to talk about the adoption process and related matters with the child in a developmentally appropriate fashion.
- *What concerns do you have for your child in the next year related to his or her adoption?*
  Unlocks new parental concerns related to the adoptive process as the child or adolescent matures.
- *What is it like to be 12 and in the 7th grade now and adopted, too?*
  May unlock new or growing concerns about his or her adoption on the part of the child.

---

adopted is a lifelong process. Physicians are well advised to become familiar with the basics of the adoption process in the geographical area in which they practice – including domestic, international, special needs, foster care, and single and nontraditional family adoptions. Allowing extra time at routine well child appointments for anticipatory guidance with adoptive parents is essential, especially if they have no other children, biologic or adopted, or if they have little family or social support. Knowing competent behavioral health clinicians for referral is a necessity when psychiatric, behavioral, or cognitive concerns arise. Familiarity with local support groups for adopted children, adolescents, and their parents and families is quite useful. In summary, the pediatrician, via regular and consistent contact with the adopted child and his family over the years, is in a unique position to follow not only medical issues, but emotional and developmental concerns, adjustment, and coping, and make appropriate referrals should more expert attention be desired or indicated (Derdeyn and Graves, 1998; Mitchell and Janista, 1997a; Peterson, 1997; Sherry and Nickman, 1999).

Bereavement in childhood and adolescence

Although at least 5% of children in the United States lose a parent to death by their 16th birthday, and many others experience the loss of siblings, grandparents, friends, pets, and important others in their lives, the significance of bereavement and grief in childhood and adolescence is still under-appreciated by families and physicians alike.

The fourth edition of the Diagnostic and Statistical Manual of the American Psychiatric Association (1994) lists bereavement as a V code, or a condition meriting clinical attention but not rising to the level of a psychiatric disorder. According to the DSM-IV, bereavement may overlap with common symptoms of a major depressive episode, including sadness, insomnia, and decreased appetite with result-

DIAGNOSIS

Table 16.10 Bereavement

Discriminating features

1. All physical and emotional changes or symptoms following the death or loss of a significant loved one (parent, sibling, grandparent, close friend, or beloved pet) are most intense in the first 2–3 months following the death, then gradually subside in intensity by 6–12 months after the death.

Consistent features

1. May resemble depressive symptoms, including sad mood, crying, appetite and sleep disturbances, weight loss, withdrawal from usual activities and interactions for a time limited period.

Variable features

1. "Hearing" the voice of or "seeing" images of the deceased, survivor guilt, guilt about what the survivor did or did not say or do before the loved one died, temporarily feeling like life is not worth living without the deceased loved one.

ant weight loss (Table 16.10). Many would not think their sadness to be unusual given the circumstances of losing a loved one, and are more inclined to seek help for sleep and appetite disturbances, or other physiologic symptoms that they might not immediately recognize as part of their grief reaction. DSM-IV suggests these six findings that may be helpful in distinguishing bereavement from a major depressive episode: (1) guilt regarding matters other than what the survivor did or did not do at the time of the death; (2) thoughts about death other than that the survivor would be better off dead than without the deceased or that the survivor should have died with the loved one; (3) feelings of extreme worthlessness; (4) extreme psychomotor retardation; (5) severe functional impairment lasting for an extremely long period of time after the death; and (6) hallucinations other than the fleeting experiences of hearing the voice of or seeing the form of the deceased (APA, 1994; Doka, 2004; Stuber and Mesrkhani, 2001; Weller et al., 2002).

Several terms commonly are used interchangeably, though defining and distinguishing them can be helpful for this discussion. Bereavement denotes the objective, factual state of losing a loved one to death, or the physical separation from the loved one because of death that evokes emotion and particular behaviors and customs. Grief is the emotional response of a survivor to losing someone, or the very personal meaning of a loss to the individual remaining alive. Anticipatory grief refers to the emotional state of an individual between the time they learn that death will most likely occur and the actual time of death, such as the period between the diagnosis of a terminal illness and the

death itself. Mourning describes the intrapersonal process of grieving, the initial stages of trying to make meaning of the life and death of the loved one, as well as the behaviors and cultural, religious, and spiritual customs that accompany death. Bereaved individuals must usually navigate a mourning process as part of saying goodbye to the deceased (Doka, 2004; Weller et al., 2002).

Common emotional elements of grief for adults include sadness, anger, shock, helplessness, guilt, numbness, relief, and blaming self and others. Cognitive aspects of grief may include poor concentration, confusion, impaired memory, disbelief, experiencing illusions or other sensory associations of the deceased, and even depersonalization and derealization. Typical behavioral manifestations of grief are crying, withdrawal, over-activity or excessive engagement in work or social activities, either avoiding reminders of the deceased or latching on to objects, activities, or people that remind the bereaved of the person they are missing, and changes in relationships with others who are still living. Physical concomitants of grief include acute aches and pains, fatigue, dizziness, sleep and appetite disturbances, physiologic changes affecting sexual activity, minor neurologic symptoms such as tremors and sensory irregularities, and bowel, bladder, and menstrual irregularities. For some, losing a loved one creates a religious and/or spiritual crisis, while for others bereavement fosters spiritual growth and awakening. For adults, these signs and symptoms of grief are influenced by the importance of the relationship with the deceased, the circumstances around the death, cultural and religious background, family and social support available for the survivors, the baseline physical and emotional health of the bereaved, and prior experiences with death, dying, and loss (Doka 2004). This material is valuable for clinicians working with bereaved children to understand, for more likely than not the significant adults in a grieving child's life will be dealing with significant loss themselves even as they are trying to care physically and emotionally for the child. This also provides a helpful background for understanding developmental implications for bereavement and loss in childhood and adolescence.

Developmental perspectives on bereavement and grief

Infants and toddlers understand their world in terms of their direct physical and emotional experiences. Extremely young children are touched by death as it affects the immediate physical and emotional care they are provided and as their caregivers are influenced by loss, grief, and ability to nurture. Even babies can tell if they are in a distressed environment or if a caregiver to whom they are attached either disappears because they have died or is upset because another has died. Toddlers relate events in the world around them to what they may or may not have said and done. They need reassurance that they did nothing wrong to cause the absence and disappearance of an attachment figure. They tend to ask the same questions over and over again, and respond best to brief, simple, and honest explanations that may need to be repeated often. Preschoolers, or 3–5-year-olds, tend to understand death as a long trip taking the loved one away for ever or as a form of sleep. They have difficulty understanding the permanence of death, manufacture their own explanations for what they may not understand, and can annoy grieving adults around them with endless questions and what seem to be inappropriate or insensitive behaviors. Sensing that death is a sad or distressing event, they may be fearful of catching the illness or befalling the same accident that took away their loved one. They need patient and understanding reassurances from other trusted adults that they and others they love who are still living will be cared for adequately. Early elementary school-age children understand more completely the finality of death when it does occur, though they may not understand that they and others they know will all die eventually. Their timetable for grieving is different from adults and rather unpredictable, laughing and playing as if nothing unusual has happened when adults around them are sad and in tears, or crying uncontrollably over an unrelated slight. By age 9 or 10, children understand that death is inevitable and that they will die some day. Accompanying these realizations may be a new or intensified fear of death and dying. Adolescents may approximate adult understandings of death, including emotional, cognitive, and religious, spiritual, and cultural aspects. They can alternate between anxiety and denial about death as it relates to themselves, family, and friends, mirroring the unpredictable vacillations between dependence and autonomy characteristic of this age group. Depending on their level of maturity and other considerations in their lives at the time of a death, reactions may vary from being indistinguishable from adults to unpredictable and similar to younger children. Denial, anger, and recklessness are behaviors seen in grieving adolescents more often than in other age groups (AACAP, 1999; Boyce and Goldstein, 1999; Stuber and Mesrkhani, 2001; Weller et al., 2002).

Explaining death to a child

Research has shown that children who are introduced to the concept of death by supportive parents or caregivers in a calm, relaxed way before a death occurs are better prepared for additional explanations on the occasion of a significant loss. In the case of young children, encounters with dead birds, goldfish, or animals hit by vehicles and lying dead by the side of the road can be fine opportunities to introduce simple concepts of injury, loss of life, and inability to move, eat, play, and interact with other animals again. Comparing death to sleep is not advisable, for children may fear falling asleep in addition to misunderstanding death. The

concept of death as the condition in which the heart stops beating, the eyes and ears stop working, and a person no longer moves, eats, and talks is helpful to many children. Children need to be told directly that the dead person will not return and what has been done with the body, whether prepared for cemetery burial or cremated. It is important that explanations regarding religious and cultural aspects of death be consistent with what the child has already been taught and experienced within his or her family and community. Enough medical details about the terminal illness or accident should be given in an age-appropriate fashion to answer the child's questions, yet care should be taken not to burden him or her with too much detail and technical information. If true, reassurances that he or she was loved by the deceased and that survivors will be cared for are always comforting and worth repeating (Boyce and Goldstein, 1999; Stuber and Mesrkhani, 2001; Weller et al., 2002).

Responses to a parent's death

When a child loses a parent to death, life as he knows it totally changes. How it changes depends on many factors, including the emotional and physical availability of the other parent; other relatives, friends, and community supports; the age, cognitive and emotional maturity of the child; the quality of the child's relationship with the deceased parent, how news of the death is handled, what information is shared, and how the days immediately around the death are handled; and opportunity for healthy, open grieving. The child's temperament influences coping and adaptation after the death. Those who have difficulty with change in general, those with poorer impulse control and trouble handling frustration will have more trouble than others adapting after losing a parent.

Regression and physical aches and pains are common to all age groups, but especially preschoolers and latency age children who are not as fluent discussing their emotions with words and abstract language. The importance of the surviving parent to a child's adjustment cannot be over-emphasized. Surviving parents need encouragement and support in finding a healthy balance of outward, observable grieving themselves versus immersing themselves completely into work or children's activities as socially acceptable ways to avoid dealing with their own personal loss of a spouse. Indeed, the emergence of depressive and anxiety disorders in bereaved children is directly related to psychiatric disorders, past and present, in the surviving spouse and parent. Adolescents with a family history of depression may be at greater risk for depression during their bereavement period. While most children come through the bereavement period without significant psychiatric disturbance, mild depressive symptoms are common for up to a year after parental death. Though anxiety rarely rises to the level of a disorder, bereaved children do experience increases in their baseline levels of anxiety regarding potential future losses and the changes following parental loss. Academically, some children do better in school after parental death, almost as a tribute to or in honor of the lost parent. Others have difficulty concentrating, do not care, or struggle with depressive symptoms or ambivalence, especially if aspects of the school environment remind them of the deceased parent.

Birthdays and holidays may evoke renewed grief, especially when celebrations and rituals for those occasions have strong associations in the child's memory with the deceased parent and the family as it was before the death. Developmental rites of passage, such as young adolescent girls purchasing their first bra or adolescent boys beginning to shave, may be sad or stressful, especially if the same-sex parent is now absent.

The changes coming after a parental death, as opposed to continuing acute grief reactions to the death itself, may be the sources of greatest stress in the first 2–3 years without the deceased parent. Decreased financial income may necessitate moves, lifestyle changes, or increased hours at work and out of the home for the surviving parent. The child may be required to change schools, decrease extracurricular activities, with resultant changes in friends, academics, and other opportunities. Older adolescents may have to take on part-time jobs that they otherwise would not, and may be forced to alter post-high school educational and vocational plans. Younger children must adjust to different babysitters or longer hours with caregivers other than a parent. All these changes constitute threats to a child's stability, the continuity, consistency, and predictability in his or her life. All adults should be aware of these stressors, including grandparents, educators, clergy, and others significant in his or her life (AACAP, 1999; Boyce and Goldstein, 1999; Dowdney, 2000; Weller et al., 2002).

Sibling loss

When a child's brother or sister dies, the experience can be just as traumatic, or maybe even more so, than if a parent had died. Attention and sympathy tend to focus on the parents, leaving the child alone to deal with a mixture of grief, sadness, confusion, anger, and guilt without the emotional presence and stamina of a non-bereaved parent to help him or her through the experience. If the death was sudden and traumatic, especially if it was witnessed by the sibling, the surviving child may be at risk for both an acute stress reaction and posttraumatic stress disorder, in addition to weathering the age-appropriate, expected elements of grief and bereavement. If the brother or sister died after a long illness, the surviving siblings may have been functioning without full parental attention and involvement in their lives for several months preceding the actual death. Common to all children who lose a sibling, regardless of the circumstances, is the fear that the same tragedy could befall them, other

siblings, or parents. Siblings may feel guilty or even ambivalent about the death if they were jealous of the attention the dying child received or if significant sibling rivalry existed. There may be real or perceived pressure to be perfect or compensate for the lost child, especially if he or she was older, talented in a particular area, or believed to be favored by one or both parents. Siblings may also be left to cope in a household in which marital stress is increased or parents become overprotective of their remaining offspring. Surviving children need the physical and emotional support of their parents at the very time when parents are least able to attend to anything outside the realm of their own overwhelming grief. Despite this, parents should be supported in their efforts to grieve openly with surviving children, though not to the extent that the adult expressions of loss frighten the siblings. Parents should also be encouraged to let go of or relinquish some or all worry and involvement in whatever non-family matters they can to maximize time caring for themselves and the rest of the family in the early stages of the bereavement process. Though the few long-term follow-up studies about sibling loss indicate that the majority of surviving brothers and sisters do well, and no worse than children who have lost parents to death, parents should be encouraged to plan their schedules to include more time with their remaining family members. Family sessions with a qualified therapist are helpful for support and guidance as parents and siblings mourn the deceased child and establish a new equilibrium within the family and home (AACAP, 1999; Boyce and Goldstein, 1999; Weller et al., 2002).

Grandparent loss

Just as the levels of emotional and physical involvement of grandparents in the lives of their grandchildren vary, clinicians will encounter a range of child and adolescent reactions to grandparent deaths. In many families today, grandparents and other relatives live many miles away or have active retirement lives themselves that preclude significant involvement in the everyday lives of their grandchildren. In these situations, the death becomes significant in how it affects the parent who has lost his or her own parent, and how that loss in turn affects emotional and physical interactions with the child. The death of a grandparent is often the first experience a child has with serious illness and death, presenting an opportunity to talk about these matters in an intimate, significant way when and if the bereaved parent is able to do so. The grandparenting role is heavily influenced by cultural considerations, so that in many ethnic and racial minorities, certain geographical locations, and perhaps in some lower socioeconomic settings, grandparents are truly a second set of parents and integral to what is in reality an enlarged nuclear family. In these families, the child is affected significantly emotionally and experiences reminders of the loss many times a day. Grandparents often serve as major sources of encouragement and as special confidantes for their grandchildren, and the younger family members may grieve these deaths more deeply than is commonly appreciated (Boyce and Goldstein, 1999; Stuber and Mesrkhani, 2001).

Deaths of pets

Some grown-ups may be tempted to minimize, or even chuckle, at a child's reaction to the death of a pet, but many adults retrospectively report the loss of a childhood pet as one of their most poignant memories, and often the saddest. When the animal is an older, long-lived family pet, the child may not have known or cannot remember life without the dog, cat, or other beloved creature. Children may also be surprised or frightened by the strength of adults' reaction to the pet's death, doubling the emotional angst of the event. Parents should be reminded that emotional and/or behavioral regression after the death of an important pet is just as likely as it might be after the loss of a family member or friend. Parents should provide short, simple, yet honest answers about the death, and refrain from the temptation to bring in another animal to replace the deceased one before the child has adequately grieved and is ready for another. Just as with the death of a human being, telling the child that the dead animal is "sleeping" may cause the child to fear sleep, increase nightmares, and perpetuate an incorrect understanding of death. Similarly, if a sick or injured animal is "put to sleep," that event should be re-explained to the child using other words, perhaps stating that the animal was expected to die soon anyway, and that the veterinarian helped the dying process be less scary and painful for the pet. A simple memorial service and burial in which the child plays a role can solemnize the occasion and acknowledge the importance of the pet and the significance of the death in the lives of the child and family.

"Doctor, should we let our child attend the funeral?"

In general, children and adolescents benefit from the opportunity to participate in the ritual remembrance and solemnization of the life of the deceased, just as adults and other members of a family and community who knew the individual and are now grieving the death. Certainly, by the time a child is 10 years of age or older, he or she has a good enough comprehension of the meaning of death that funeral attendance is often quite helpful and even therapeutic for the grieving process. Along with funeral attendance, however, should come proper preparation and accompanying opportunities to discuss and ask questions about the event and its meaning. Though the decision about whether younger children attend funerals must be individualized, even preschoolers may benefit from attending a viewing,

the service itself, or a graveside memorial before burial. Attendance and seeing the body of the lost loved one concretizes the fact that the person is indeed dead, and lessens the need of the child to fantasize or imagine answers about what has happened, where the body is, and whether or not the deceased is coming back. When children attend funerals, they may benefit from the presence of a familiar, caring adult staying with them and monitoring the child's emotional state who, though they may know the deceased, is not so close that they are overcome with grief themselves. In many instances, seeing very upset, openly grieving adults is more upsetting to children than seeing the body of the deceased or the funeral itself. Though some adults are offended by this practice, taking photographs of the deceased, the funeral setting, and graveside may be helpful later for the child's adjustment, especially if the child is very young at the time of death or is unable to attend the funeral (Boyce and Goldstein, 1999; Dowdney, 2000; Stuber and Mesrkhani, 2001).

The role of the physician

A general knowledge of child development and an appreciation for how different age groups of children and adolescents respond to and cope with stress and changes in their lives is the most helpful foundation for working with bereaved youths. Familiarity with the different cultural and ethnic groups in the geographical area in which one practices and how such families typically handle and respond to significant deaths is also helpful. Balancing these general considerations with the particular circumstances, temperaments, resiliencies, and vulnerabilities of individual children should be the desired goal of clinicians caring for bereaved children and their families.

Physicians' greatest contributions are in the areas of monitoring the child's medical condition and educating parents about what they might expect as their child grieves and adjusts to life without their loved one. Especially if a parent has died, the surviving parent may be so overwhelmed with grief and assuming the roles and responsibilities of their spouse that signs and symptoms of illness, routine well child check-ups, and even bereavement-related symptoms such as weight loss, sleep disturbance, and depressive symptoms may go unnoticed. Newly bereaved children may benefit from some extra appointments intentionally and strategically scheduled between usual well child visits for the purposes of monitoring physical and emotional adjustment and coping and providing anticipatory guidance to the surviving parent. This is also true of children who have lost siblings. Parents, in their own grief, unintentionally may "lose track" of where their surviving children are medically and emotionally.

Physicians should not be shy about referring children and families for psychiatric consultation or therapy if con-

PEARLS & PERILS

- Physicians need to be hypervigilant about the physical health and medical needs of bereaved children, especially if the parent(s) and caregivers are also grieving the same loss, distracted, and unable to give full attention to surviving children.
- For older children and adolescents, funeral or memorial attendance is usually helpful for their mourning process; younger children may also benefit from attendance, especially when accompanied and tended to by a familiar adult less affected by the loss and grief personally so they can assist the child during the services.
- Children's reactions to death and their grief process vary developmentally and are different than an adult's or older adolescent's – it is helpful if these differences are explained to adults so they will not misunderstand children's reactions and behaviors.
- Children benefit from consistent and predictable routines, surroundings, and caregivers immediately after the death and during the bereavement period.

cerns arise about the intensity or duration of intense grief reactions in any child or parent. Even if the expressions of bereavement are understandable and adjustment is going as well as can be expected, a few sessions of family work may be valuable for helping members to understand how the other surviving loved ones are mourning and coping with the loss and how they can be more supportive of each other. Older children and adolescents may benefit from bereavement groups, and children and youth of all ages may benefit from individual therapy to help process and integrate the loss, whether at the time of the death, in the months and years to follow, or both. Once again, primary care physicians are in a unique position to monitor and advocate for the individual needs of these children and families (AACAP, 1999; Boyce and Goldstein, 1999; Stuber and Mesrkhani, 2001).

CONSIDER CONSULTATION WHEN ...

- The child or adolescent manifests severe or prolonged depressive symptoms or there is impairment of functioning at home, school, or in social settings.
- The surviving parent(s) or adult caregivers are so overwhelmed with their own grief that they cannot care adequately for the emotional, physical, and medical needs of the bereaved children.
- Family members are grieving at different rates, at different times, and in different styles, leading to tensions and misunderstandings at home and among family members.

KEY CLINICAL QUESTIONS

For the child:
- *Do you have any worries about your parents or other brothers or sisters since the death?*
  May unlock information about other family members struggling with their grief.

For the parent:
- *Do you have any worries about how your child is handling the death?*
  May unlock information about how the child is progressing through the bereavement period.

For the child:
- *What do you miss most about the way things were before the death?*
  May unlock clues about how home life can be adjusted to make the bereavement period and coping after the death easier for the child.

For child and parent:
- *Tell me about _____ (name of the deceased) and what you miss the most.*
  Lets the child and parent know that the deceased is not forgotten, that their feelings about their loved one are important to the physician, and gives them the opportunity to talk with a skilled, caring person about their lost loved one.

Cultural, religious, and spiritual aspects of child and family life

Any assessment of a child or adolescent's religion and spirituality must begin with a consideration of his or her family context and background. While faith tradition, denominational affiliation, and attendance and participation in organized religious institutions and rituals are important and formative, it is helpful to know what roles religious faith and practice play in the everyday lives of the family members. Is there family prayer, readings of sacred texts, discussion of religious values in relationship to choices children and adolescents must make regarding extracurricular activities, sex, or substance use? Are children exposed to religious books, music, videos, and television programming? Do family members turn to religious faith and spirituality for routine matters of daily living, for comfort and guidance in times of adversity, or both? How does religious faith influence how parents prioritize time and money? To what extent are discipline and core moral and ethical values influenced by religious belief? Have parental and family religious attitudes and practices been relatively stable over time, or have various life events or stresses weakened or strengthened the roles of personal spirituality and/or institutional religion over time? These are just a few questions that may yield helpful insights into the religious and spiritual life shared by children and adolescents with siblings, parents, and even

PEARLS & PERILS

- Clinicians should take the time to get to know a wide variety of religious professionals and resources in the geographical area in which they practice. This includes not only leaders of churches, synagogues, and mosques, but also hospital chaplains, pastoral counselors, and directors of charitable organizations. This cultivates a rich referral and consultation network for cultural, religious, and spiritual questions as they arise when working with children and families.
- Remember to be as nonjudgmental as possible – the goal is to understand the child and family and what is important to them, not to change their beliefs, practices, or be perceived as critical or prejudiced.
- Remember that religion and spirituality are not confined to religious affiliation, attendance at services, observance of religious holidays, or even prayer. Health attitudes and behaviors may be influenced by cultural, religious, and spiritual factors that the patient and family may be unaware of.

extended family members, friends, and other significant individuals in their lives (Josephson and Dell, 2004).

The religious and spiritual life of a child is inextricably linked to cognitive and emotional development. This has been described by several developmental theorists, and perhaps most eloquently in the faith development theory of James W. Fowler (Fowler and Dell, 2004). Relationships with caregivers during the first 2 years of life, adequate care of basic physiological needs, and the quality of emotional interactions provide the backdrop for not only the child's future human relationships, but also his or her ability and inclination for future engagement and relationship with God, supreme beings, or other forms of divine or religious/spiritual beings. Toddlers and preschoolers are learning very straightforward, concrete images and categories of good and evil. The "good" typically includes God as creator of nature, sunshine, happy families, and angels that watch over their safety. The "bad" includes devils, death, and events and people that cause pain and illness. They are beginning to understand cause and effect, and understand the value families and religious organizations place on love, companionship, and caring for others. School-age children know and understand the need for and helpfulness of rules and guidelines for just societies, fair treatment of individuals, and general ethical and moral behavior. They understand the role religion and spirituality play in the formation and maintenance of fair and just systems. They accept and internalize tenets of religious and other belief systems they have been taught or exposed to, and use the symbols, rules, and stories of their faith communities both to make sense of their world and maintain its order and predictability. By early adolescence and beyond, coincidental with the acquisi-

tion of abstraction and critical, reflective thinking, the young person re-examines the beliefs and stories taught to them by their families and faith communities. They may choose to accept, reject, or put on hold the teachings of the religious traditions of their earlier youth and families of origin. Often to the surprise or disappointment of their parents, they may explore other faith traditions or even reject God and religious belief altogether. Older adolescents are not afraid to question the status quo and the beliefs of their parents and religious communities and faith traditions.

For all age groups, it is important to understand what the child or adolescent has been taught by family and religious community about God and religious faith, what God means to them as individuals, and what role, if any, they believe God has in what is going on in their lives and the world around them. Depending on the age of the child and the issues bringing them to the attention of a mental health professional, the answers to these general inquiries may be very different, even unpredictable. Themes in psychiatric assessment and treatment with religious and spiritual overtones and implications may include, but are not limited to: why bad things happen, guilt, forgiveness, abandonment, shame, hopelessness, pain and suffering, various forms of abuse by trusted others, obsessions, rituals, generalized anxiety, pessimism about the future, and general purpose and meaning in life. In all these issues, the clinician must pay close attention to the developmental stage and tasks the individual child or adolescent is negotiating at that particular time within their family, educational, and faith community systems (Josephson and Dell, 2004; Moncher and Josephson, 2004; Sexson, 2004).

In view of the increasing religious and ethnic diversity in nearly every country and geographical area, and the political and religious climates of the world, it is becoming more important that mental health professionals and primary care physicians be aware of the influences of culture, religion, and spirituality in the lives of children, adolescents, and their families. For instance, practices and attitudes about diet, seeking medical attention, well child care and immunizations, taking medicines for pain and relatively common pediatric ailments, seeking psychiatric care, taking psychotropic medication, sexuality and sex education, birth control, caring for seriously ill and dying children, and many medical ethical considerations are profoundly influenced or even dictated by cultural customs and religious beliefs (Al-Mateen and Afzal, 2004; Black, 2004; Mercer, 2004; Murrell, 2004; Rube and Kibel, 2004; Stuber and Houskamp, 2004). It behoves all clinicians to be aware of basic beliefs and practices of the largest ethnic and religious communities they serve, and to become comfortable asking their patients and their families how their particular faith and culture contributes to their health and routines of daily living. In view of the diversity of thought and practice even within groups that self-identify themselves with similar or identical names (for instance, the 11th edition of the *Hand-*

book of Denominations in the United States lists 19 organized, self-governing Baptist denominations alone!), clinicians are also well advised to develop a network in their geographical areas of religious professionals of varied backgrounds to consult when religious, spiritual, and cultural issues important to patient care arise.

Cultural and religious groups also serve children, adolescents, and families in other ways that complement the mission of pediatric care. In this age of budget deficits, third party payer cuts, and skyrocketing numbers of children without adequate health insurance, nutrition, clothes, books, and other necessary and desirable items, religious and charitable organizations are wonderful resources for our patients. Examples of services provided by religious organizations and institutions include: emergency cash assistance, food pantries, thrift shops, clothing closets, emergency counseling or crisis hotlines, emergency hospital or nursing care, home health services, transportation assistance, emergency shelters and low-cost housing, child daycare and before and after school programs for children with working parents, substance abuse treatment programs, literacy and tutoring programs, migrant and immigrant support, support for abused women and children, well child clinics, prenatal care, organized recreation, music and arts programs, adoptive grandparent programs, day camps, summer overnight camps, many types of support groups, English as a Second Language (ESL) courses, and worship and religious education opportunities in many languages. Indeed, the concerns and missions of medicine and religious groups have much in common, and children and their families benefit immediately and in the years to come when medical and religious professionals and groups cooperate for the sake of all who need their services (Dell, 2004).

CONSIDER CONSULTATION WHEN ...

- For the clinician: whenever a particular child or family's presentation or situation has cultural, religious, or spiritual aspects that you wish to understand more completely to provide better, more complete care of the medical and family needs at hand.
- For the child, adolescent, and family: (1) whenever the family expresses or you believe they might benefit from discussing their cultural, religious, and spiritual beliefs and lives with a supportive, knowledgeable individual, especially if concerns or questions are arising in the context of medical care and medical decision-making; (2) whenever the family expresses interest in developing social, religious/spiritual, or supportive relationships with others in the community; (3) whenever the clinician suspects that a cultural/religious/spiritual belief or practice is outside the mainstream for the faith or cultural group the family claims, or when such a belief or practice is contributing to a child's illness or medical problem, or restricting healthy growth and development.

KEY CLINICAL QUESTIONS

Helpful questions for gauging the role of religion and spirituality, in person or on paper, include:
- *Is religious belief or practice important in your family life? Do you now attend a particular house or place of worship? Have you in the past? Do you have any cultural or religious beliefs that I should understand so that I can help care for you and your family the very best I can?*
  May unlock the key to understanding child-rearing practices and family values, beliefs, and practices that affect health, illness, and growth and development
- Religion and spirituality are not confined to church attendance, affiliation, reading of sacred texts, or public and private celebration of holy days. Do not forget to ask about nonbiblical inspirational literature, religious music, radio and television programming, religious books, tapes, and videos for children, religious parenting books, and books on tale and motivational recordings. These questions may unlock family attitudes about parenting, dating, sex education, contraception, discipline, and other issues relevant to parenting children and adolescents.

Annotated bibliography

Books for clinicians

Canino IA, Spurlock J (2000) *Culturally Diverse Children and Adolescents*, 2nd edn. New York, The Guilford Press.
  A thorough treatise on culture and implications for assessment and therapeutic work with children, adolescents, their families, and the societal systems with which all are involved.

Ferber R, Kryger M (eds) (1995). *Principles and Practice of Sleep Medicine in the Child*. Philadelphia, W.B. Saunders.
  Though nearly 10 years old, this remains the most exhaustive reference book in child and adolescent sleep medicine. Key topics include normal sleep and pathophysiology, assessment, and treatment of a broad array of specific sleep disorders.

Josephson AM, Dell ML (eds) (2004). Religion and spirituality. *Child and Adolescent Psychiatric Clinics of North America*, 13(1).
  An entire volume devoted to religion and spirituality in clinical work with children, adolescents, and families. Topics include assessment, religious/spiritual considerations in pathology and treatment, and specific concerns that may arise when working with children and families of specific major world faith traditions.

Mindell JA, Owens JA (2003). *A Clinical Guide to Pediatric Sleep: Diagnosis and Management of Sleep Problems*. Philadelphia, Lippincott, Williams, and Wilkins.
  More recent but less detailed than the Ferber and Kryger text. A user-friendly clinical manual, with helpful charts, algorithms, and a CD-ROM.

Pruett KD, Pruett MK (eds) (1998). Child custody. *Child and Adolescent Psychiatric Clinics of North America*, 7(2).
  A collection of review pieces on custody and related forensic aspects of marital separation, divorce, and remarriage; the roles of fathers and grandparents in visitation and custody; crisis placement; special custody

considerations for maltreated children; foster care; adoption; and cultural and ethical considerations affecting child custody in these situations.

Webb NB (ed) (2002) *Helping Bereaved Children: A Handbook for Practitioners*, 2nd edn. New York, The Guilford Press.

A compilation about loss and bereavement in childhood and adolescence. Includes chapters on assessment; deaths of parents, grandparents, siblings; family suicides and other violent deaths; deaths in the school and community; deaths from terrorism; and interventions and grief work with bereaved youth.

Books for parents

Kroen WC (1996) *Helping Children Cope with the Loss of a Loved Ones: A Guide for Grownups*. Minneapolis, Free Spirit Publishing.

Thorough and concise, this guide coaches adults on ways to help children after a significant death, even as the adults around them are also grieving.

Melina LR (1986) *Raising Adopted Children: A Manual for Adoptive Parents*. New York, Harper Publishers.

A perennial favorite with parents, this book strikes a good balance between reference information and offering helpful recommendations.

Swedo SA, Leonard HL (1999) *Is It Just a Phase?* New York, Broadway Books.

Written for parents, the authors review 24 concerns and problems of childhood adolescence, with tips and guidelines for watchful waiting, medical and behavioral management, and indications for professional consultation and intervention.

Watkins M, Fisher S (1995) *Talking with Young Children about Adoption*. New Haven, Yale University Press.

With a more specific focus than Melina's book, many parents find this helpful to read as they consider how to talk with their adoptive child about his or her individual adoption situation.

Books for children

Evans MD (1984) *This Is Me and My Two Families: An Awareness Scrapbook/Journal for Children Living in Stepfamilies*. New York, Magination Press.

This book remains one of the best for children in stepfamilies. Additional benefits are gained when the book is read with parents and stepparents or used in individual or family therapy.

Galvin MR (1991) *Clouds and Clocks: A Story for Children Who Soil*. New York, Magination Press.

One of the first books written especially for encopretic children, it is still one of the most helpful and popular.

Levy J (2004) *Finding the Right Spot: When Kids Can't Live with Their Parents*. New York, Magination Press.

Considers situations other than traditional infant adoption in which children find themselves living with adults and families other than their own biologic parents.

Nemiroff M, Annuaziata J (2003) *All About Adoption*. New York, Magination Press.

A thorough, upbeat book for adopted children, great to be read with adoptive parents.

Ransom JF, Finney KK (2000). *I Don't Want to Talk about It: A Story about Divorce for Young Children*. New York, Magination Press.

Targeted to children ages 4 to 8 years, this book consistently receives positive feedback from parents.

Willner-Pardo G (1996) *Hunting Grandma's Treasures*. Boston, Houghton Mifflin.

A book for helping a child between the ages of 4 and 8 with feelings after the death of an important person in his or her life.

CHAPTER 17

Chronic Illness in Children and Adolescents

Arden D. Dingle, MD and Sandra B. Sexson, MD

OUTLINE	
Introduction	Assessment
Child	Treatment
Family	Summary
Disease issues	

Introduction

Having a chronic illness as a child or adolescent has become increasingly common, with estimates that 10–20% of children are affected. Chronic disease refers to conditions that require at least 6 months of continuous medical care and behavioral adaptation with permanent alterations in lifestyle. While disease or disorder refers to the presence of a pathologic process and an illness describes being in an unhealthy state (Feldman, 1996), for the purposes of this chapter these terms will be used interchangeably. With the improvements in early detection, diagnosis, and management, many of these young people will survive for many years, with illnesses previously considered fatal. The overwhelming majority will become adults.

Most affected children and families appear to manage well, demonstrating resilience and effective adaptation. However, chronic illness usually has a significant effect, with some of the mediating variables being the child's age, sex, cognitive abilities, family functioning, type of illness, and the impact on daily life (see Pearls & perils). Chronically medically ill children have a higher risk of having a psychiatric disorder than the general population and their families often experience considerable distress.

Unfortunately, much of the research on the impact of illnesses and effective interventions is hampered by a lack of well-controlled studies. Obtaining an accurate view of psychologic and social variables such as intrapsychic distress, the emotional impact of the disease, self-esteem, social functioning, and peer relationships has been difficult. Many of the studies have not obtained information directly from the involved children. Much of the information available on children with chronic diseases and their families has focused on describing the problems and interventions associated with particular diseases. There has been more of a trend to examine chronic illness in general, based on the belief that the similarities across diseases, such as the onset and course, potential fatality, degree of incapacitation, visibility, and social issues are significant factors in understanding the impact of chronic illness. Also, recent research has focused on understanding the personal and environmental factors that impact adjustment to chronic illness and functioning (Perrin et al., 1993; Knapp and Harris, 1997, 1998; Tarnowski and Brown, 2000; Brown et al., 2003; Geist et al., 2003; LeBlanc et al., 2003; Lewis and Vitulano, 2003; Mrazek, 2003a; Stewart, 2003; Vitulano, 2003).

PEARLS & PERILS

- Medical assessments should explore psychosocial issues routinely.
- Treatment adherence is a significant problem and should be assessed at every opportunity.
- Children should take increasing responsibility for the care of their illness as they develop with continued appropriate supervision and monitoring.
- While most children and families do well, subclinical psychologic symptoms are common and should be addressed.
- Optimal age-appropriate activities and functioning should be the goal for most chronically ill children.
- Chronically ill children should attend school, homebound instruction is rarely necessary.
- Treatment planning consistently should consider and target psychosocial issues.
- Psychiatric involvement is beneficial, but needs to be carefully approached and implemented and should be tied to ongoing medical care.
- Collaboration and integration of care among disciplines, providers, and institutions is essential.

Child

Development

Children's concepts of health and illness vary with their developmental stage. They appear to follow a progression, which is consistent with typical cognitive development. Working effectively with a child requires an understanding of development in general, as well as knowing what level a particular child is at and how previous experiences have enhanced or impeded understanding of the disease and its treatment. Generally, children's concepts are more concrete, egocentric, and personal than adults. Children who are chronically ill appear to develop a better understanding of their disorders based on their experiences with being ill than would be expected developmentally.

Preschoolers may view their illness or treatment as a punishment or consequence for misbehavior. Magical thinking and the idea of immanent justice allow children to believe they have some control rather than that the illness is due to chance. There is evidence that children acquire a more accurate comprehension of illness and personal control with personal experience as well as age. Older children tend to explain disease using theories of contagion, first including all illnesses and then developing an understanding of the difference between contagious and non-contagious illnesses. Research shows that even preschoolers can comprehend the causes of illness if explained appropriately.

School-aged children generally can have a clearer understanding of their disease and its treatment, though they may be confused or have mistaken ideas if specific, concrete explanations are not given. Typically, by this age, children acquire an understanding of germs but still have difficulty with what happens once germs are in the body. By age 12 or 13, children view illness as having multiple causes, with an appreciation of the role and interaction between hosts, agents, and recovery. They obtain a better understanding of their bodies and its processes. With the development of abstract thinking, older school-aged children and adolescents can obtain a more rational understanding of their disease and treatment.

By early adolescence, many children can comprehend physiologic explanations of illness and treatment. The process for understanding the intent of medical procedures and treatment is similar and parallel. Accurate perceptions depend on the child's cognitive abilities and current emotional factors (Burbach and Peterson, 1986; Crisp et al., 1996; Davidow, 1996; Schonfeld, 2002). Normandeau and colleagues (1998) found that school-aged children assessed health based on dimensions of functionality, mental health, and adherence to a healthy lifestyle.

The illness, treatment, and hospitalizations may interfere with the age-appropriate needs of toddlers and preschoolers to be active, explore their environments, and learn to socialize. Hospitalizations may lead to separations and impact attachment in primary relationships. Being ill can affect the school-age developmental tasks of mastery and becoming acclimated to school and other environments outside the family. Boys appear to be more sensitive to interference with physical activities, while girls are stressed by the impact on peer and social relationships. In addition to managing their illness, adolescents must negotiate the normal developmental tasks of adjusting to physical changes and appearance, resolving social, identity, and sexual issues, choosing a peer group, becoming self-sufficient and independent, and planning for the future. Illness in adolescents can impact autonomy and the development of independence, peer interactions, and intimate relationships. Continued dependence on parents and other adults can be significant. Delayed physical and sexual maturation or physical disfigurement may affect peer relationships and identity formation. The development of appropriate self-esteem in chronically ill children may be negatively impacted by the physical and psychologic stresses associated with being ill (Garrison and McQuiston, 1989; Meijer et al., 2000; Stoddard, 2002; Brown et al., 2003; Lewis and Vitulano, 2003; Mrazek, 2003a; Vitulano, 2003).

A number of studies have found that most chronically ill children achieve a sense of normalcy defined as school participation, self-definition as an ordinary person, reduced sense of difference from peers, focus on daily routines with the illness kept in the background, and more responsibility for illness self-care. Generally, children with earlier onset of illness have better psychosocial outcomes (Admi, 1996; LeBlanc et al., 2003; Stewart, 2003).

Personality traits and coping styles

Resilience factors such as temperament, intelligence, and coping styles appear to moderate psychosocial functioning through an impact upon risk factors and an association with adaptive functioning. Generally, individuals with higher intelligence, adaptable temperaments, and flexible coping strategies do better. Children tend to use various psychologic defense mechanisms based on experience, modeling, developmental level, and innate capacities. Individuals often require time and support to be able to accommodate to having an illness and its impact on daily life and function. Learning about and dealing with having a chronic illness is psychologically equivalent to mourning or grieving a significant loss. Even if not fatal, chronic illnesses usually mean significant alterations in expectations for the child's present and future functioning.

While certain styles, defenses, and personality factors are considered more effective than others, it is important to assess each child, family, and situation individually to determine their level of function and distress. For example, the psychologic strategy of denial is considered a lower level defense. It is commonly seen, in the initial stages of dealing with an illness. As long as it co-exists with reasonable treatment adherence and functioning of the child, it may be the most adaptive approach for that child at that time, providing a protective function and minimizing overt emotional distress.

Coping styles appear to be associated with most aspects of functioning. Problem-centered approaches emphasize attempts to change the situation, while emotion-based ones concentrate on improving negative reactions connected to specific stresses. Attitudes emphasizing seeking social support and active problem solving to manage specific illness demands tend to predict positive adjustment. Additional productive approaches include using strategies such as comparison to others, relaxation, distraction, emotional ventilation, selective attention, reframing, and positive thinking to alter one's response to stresses that cannot be controlled. Other coping strategies include reliance on faith and a hopeful outlook for the future. Children with better adjustment tend to choose strategies based on the type of stress. Those who employ only a limited range of strategies or rely on avoidance tend to do worse. Additional work needs to be done to examine further the relevance of context, amount of control by the child, and the impact of maturation (Ryan-Wenger, 1992; Olsen et al., 1993; Davidow, 1996; Thies and Walsh, 1999; Luthar et al., 2000; Yeh, 2001; Meijer et al., 2002; LeBlanc et al., 2003; Lewis and Vitulano, 2003; Stewart, 2003; Vitulano, 2003).

Psychopathology

Chronic illness in childhood is a major risk factor for the onset of psychopathology, with chronically ill children having a significantly higher risk for emotional and behavioral disorders as well as school-related adjustment difficulties. Typically, psychosocial adjustment is the poorest the first 6–12 months after diagnosis. Common difficulties include adjustment problems, anxiety, school phobia, depression, social withdrawal, aggression, and other externalizing problems. Often, the level of symptoms is subclinical and does not meet the criteria for a psychiatric disorder. A number continue to be psychiatrically symptomatic in adulthood. Rates of substance abuse in adolescents with chronic illness appear to be similar or lower than those of healthy teenagers. It may be that delays in physical and psychosocial maturation may mean that certain risk-taking behaviors are postponed until adulthood. Chronically ill adolescents may be at higher risk for adverse effects of substance use such as worsening their disease, interacting with prescribed medications, and decreasing treatment adherence.

Considerable evidence exists that events related to illnesses or treatments can be significant enough to produce post-traumatic stress symptoms or disorders in the ill children or their parents. Several studies report that parents often have more symptoms than the children. Besides the psychologic distress, these types of symptoms may worsen adherence to treatment regimes. Chronically ill children with internalizing (i.e. anxiety, depression) and to a lesser extent, externalizing (i.e. oppositional, defiant behavior) utilize health-care more frequently than chronically ill children without these symptoms.

However, there is a wide variation in the psychosocial functioning of chronically ill children, with the majority doing well. There have been little data to suggest that the risk of developing psychosocial difficulties is related to having a specific disease except for the increased risk of psychopathology associated with conditions affecting the brain. Numerous research studies suggest that child characteristics, family/parent variables, and life stress are more important in predicting the emotional outcome of ill children than the type, severity, and duration of the illness. Better functioning families tend to have children with better adjustment and coping. Genetic influences appear to be important mediators of both resilience and risk factors (Cadman et al., 1987; Jellinek et al., 1988; Lavigne and Faier-Routman, 1993; Thompson and Gustafson, 1996; Wallender and Varni, 1998; Weinberg et al., 1998; Tarnowski and Brown, 2000; Wamboldt and Wamboldt, 2000; Geist et al., 2003; LeBlanc, 2003; Lewis and Vitulano, 2003; Mrazek, 2003a).

Family

Most families cope well with having a child who is chronically ill. Perrin and Thyen (1999) have proposed a model of emotional responses to the diagnosis of chronic illness in a child. The hierarchy of responses that the family goes through is shock, disbelief/denial, grief and anger, stabilization, and acceptance. Family response to and coping with a child with a chronic illness is a significant factor in the adaptation of ill children. Family adjustment to having a child with a chronic illness depends on prior functioning, coping styles, and experiences of disease. Other issues include the family's ability to modify their parenting styles, as the child becomes older, allowing more independence and autonomy. Family religious and cultural beliefs as well as its perspectives on illness also significantly modify adaptation and functioning. Feelings of guilt, anger, fear, and loneliness are frequent. Common issues include marital strain, uncertainties of diagnosis and treatment, possible social stigma and relative neglect of siblings.

Having a chronically ill child produces several burdens upon the family, which vary in their impact depending on the family's functioning and resources. These challenges can include economic impact (medical costs, decreased ability to work, restricted mobility due to need for insurance or access to medical facilities), decreased social interactions outside the home and compartmentalized parental roles, with the mother generally being the caretaker and the father the provider. Parents usually share similar views of the disease and its impact, though mothers tend to express more concern about the illness impact and the effective management of the treatment regime. Many parents have subclinical psychiatric symptoms, often depression in the mothers and higher stress in fathers. Symptoms were associated more with behavioral demands and perceived competence to manage the demands rather than disease severity (Davidow, 1996; Knafl and Zoeller, 2000; Brown et al., 2003; Mrazek, 2003a).

There has been a paucity of research examining family conceptions of illness and wellness when a child is chronically ill. Jutras and colleagues (2003) found that diabetic children, their siblings and mothers had comprehensive definitions of wellness for both healthy and chronically ill children that focused on mental and social aspects with less emphasis on observable physical cues. Mothers considered positive attitude and emotional considerations more important than did the children. They also mentioned illness constraints on daily living and the need for adaptation.

There are no data that family or parental behavior predicts the onset of medical illness in children genetically predisposed to particular diseases. A number of studies have documented that childhood chronic illness can impact family dynamics and functioning, either positively or negatively. Childhood illness also appears to increase parental vulnerability to depression and marital problems, though the effects on mental health appear to be primarily mediated through how well the family functions in general (Wamboldt and Wamboldt, 2000). Studies have found that perceived social support is positively related to parental coping (Tak and McCubbin, 2002).

Parents

Families with ill infants can have difficulty distinguishing between problems related to illness or normal behaviors. Parental guilt and shock can impact the bonding relationship (Brown et al., 2003).

Parents of children with chronic pulmonary diseases and rheumatological diseases who perceived their children as vulnerable tended to have more socially anxious children. Physician disease severity ratings and parental vulnerability ratings had small to medium correlations (Anthony et al., 2003). Manne and colleagues (2003) found that mothers of children undergoing bone marrow transplantation who had greater acceptance and use of humor had decreases in depressive symptoms over the 6 months after the procedure. Positive framing, use of emotional support, and use of religion were associated with depressive symptom course with differences depending on the use of the coping strategies at the time of transplantation. Mothers' fears at transplantation predicted maternal depressive symptoms (Manne et al., 2003).

Siblings

A meta-analysis of the literature (Sharpe and Rossiter, 2002) on siblings of children with chronic illnesses found that siblings tend to do worse than comparison participants or normative data, though the effect sizes were heterogeneous. Parental self-reports tended to be more negative than child reports. Siblings had lower peer activities and cognitive development scores as well as higher anxiety and depression compared with controls. Chronic illnesses with daily treatment requirements had more negative associations than those illnesses that did not impact daily functioning. Williams and group (2002b) found that the well siblings' knowledge of illness, attitude toward the illness, mood, self-esteem, and feeling of social support were interrelated and connected to their behavior. Feelings of jealousy, overprotectiveness, and survival guilt were common. Socioeconomic status (SES) and family cohesion were connected to parental reports of the well siblings' behavior. The mother's mood impacted family cohesion and was influenced by SES. Siblings of children receiving bone marrow transplants have different problems depending on whether they are donors or not with significant rates of posttraumatic stress disorder (PTSD) symptoms in both groups (Packman, 1997; Brown et al., 2003).

Disease issues

The stresses associated with being chronically ill can be grouped as those that are common to most diseases, those specific to certain illness, and those due to conflict between illness demands and those of normal development tasks. Stresses associated with most diseases include the intrusiveness of disease symptoms and their integration into daily life. Other issues include restrictions and limitations on activities as well as having to perform medical care tasks in front of peers. Examples of problems connected to specific illnesses include the stigma with HIV/AIDS and the frequent, painful procedures occurring during oncology treatment. Competing illness and developmental demands often occur for school-aged children and adolescents especially in the context of school and peers. The section below describes a number of the general issues as well as those related to some specific illnesses (Admi, 1996; Sartain et al., 2000; Stewart, 2003).

General

Communication
Maintaining effective and reciprocal communication with chronically ill children and their caretakers is challenging, especially in situations of grave and potentially fatal illnesses. Parents often function as the gatekeepers of information and may withhold information from their children, believing that such behavior is protective. However, children may

then feel on the periphery of treatment planning and participation due to incomplete data or not directly communicating with their medical providers (Young et al., 2003). The literature indicates that parents and chronically ill children have greater agreement about the child's problems and function than parents with healthy children. Agreement is best for physically observable functioning, while there may be less agreement about the impact of an illness (Eiser and Morse, 2001).

Ogden Burke and colleagues (2000) found that one-third of parents differed with medical professionals on their child's illness trajectory (life-threatening, declining, or stable, optimistic). Communication about the diagnosis, treatment, and other medical issues can be a major factor in effective management of the disease by the family and child (Mrazek, 2003a).

Most chronically ill children require care from multiple providers of different specialties, in different settings and often, different institutions. Additionally, other systems involved with the child (i.e. the school) are integrally involved in some aspect of the child's treatment. Effective and on-going communication between all of the health providers and other involved individuals is essential, but often is fragmented and incomplete (Knapp and Harris, 1997; Sexson and Dingle, 2001; Mrazek, 2003a).

Disability

The extent and predictability of illness and treatment effects on function and impact on physical well-being and appearance can be significant factors in the ability of children and families to cope and adapt. General symptoms such as lethargy, nausea, weakness, fatigue, and pain often impair the child's ability to function and effectively participate in activities at home, school, and elsewhere. Illness- or treatment-induced physical alterations may compromise children's capabilities as well as their tolerance for being in social situations. The impact of various disabilities may vary depending on the child's age and development. Altered physical appearance can negatively affect self-esteem and social functioning (Cadman et al., 1987; Sexson and Dingle, 1997, 2001; Mrazek, 2003a).

Dying/death

Caring for a dying child is difficult for all involved, especially since our society generally does not consider death in childhood to be a typical phenomenon even for children with chronic conditions. Despite incredible medical advances in early detection and management of medical disorders, chronically ill children do die, and they and their families benefit from continued involvement with the health team, especially the primary care physician. Ongoing communication is essential. Failure to acknowledge and discuss the emotions, thoughts, and fears of the child and family leave them isolated. Learning about, understanding, and respect-

ing the family's personal, religious, and cultural beliefs are important. However, typically being truthful with children is crucial, since not acknowledging the reality of the situation leaves children isolated and fearful without being able to talk about their concerns and obtain help and comfort.

Children's response to dying depends partially on their concept of dying. Generally, children understand the irreversibility, finality, causality, and inevitability of death by 5–7 years of age. There is a wide range of reactions, but typical emotions include anxiety, anger, and depression on the part of the child, family, and medical providers. With an adequate period of time, most can achieve acceptance, though obviously sadness and grief persist. Continued active participation by the physician provides support and comfort as well as the necessary oversight so that the child does not suffer needlessly from pain and other problems (Lewis and Schonfeld, 2002).

Hospitalization

Single hospitalizations, especially if managed appropriately, do not appear to negatively impact a child's long-term development. Multiple hospitalizations may be more problematic, particularly if these occurrences interfere with the child achieving optimal functioning, especially in terms of maintaining peer relationships and school performance. Several influential factors should be considered: the illness, hospital experience, social and cultural hospital environment, family's adaptive abilities, and the child's capability to cope with the illness. Children under the age of 5 may be especially sensitive (Mrazek, 2002). Kelly and Hewson (2000) reviewed hospital admissions for chronically ill children and found that major psychosocial issues were primarily responsible for the admission for two-thirds of the children. The most significant issues were medical dependency, family members with medical or psychologic problems, discord between the family and medical providers about the treatment, lack of more intensive community supports, and medical debate about the best plan.

Medication

Taking medications can cause difficulties due to their effects or side-effects, causing embarrassment if taken at school or in other public arenas as well as being a constant reminder of illness. Additionally, parental supervision may interfere with the development of age-appropriate autonomy and decision making (Brown et al., 2003).

Adherence

Adherence to treatment is a major problem in this population. The literature organizes the relevant factors into categories of treatment characteristics, disease considerations, and child and family variables. Participation in treatment declines as the demands increase or are aversive. Relevant aspects of medical care include length of treatment, number and severity of side-effects, complexity, and effectiveness. Illness issues include age of onset, disease course and pattern of symptoms. Other characteristics that have been demonstrated to be relevant to adherence have included parent health, parenting style, child and parent knowledge of disease and treatment, family functioning, available resources, satisfaction with medical care, provider-parent relationships, and child emotional or behavioral problems. Despite considerable study, there is no clear understanding of the specific psychologic or personality factors that account for the ability of individuals and families to cooperate with and perform prescribed treatment recommendations. For adults, compliance is likely when they perceive themselves to be vulnerable to an illness or serious complications and if they anticipate benefits from treatment. For young people, there has not been demonstrated any clear link between their health beliefs and adherence. Issues that may affect adolescent compliance include treatment expectations that are incompatible with the normal developmental tasks such as loss of personal control and autonomy, restriction of age-appropriate activities, and promotion of dependency. Additionally, treatment side-effects may embarrass adolescents or make them feel unwell. Family functioning and structure has been found to be very important, especially for younger children (Rapoff, 1999; Kyngas et al., 2000; Lemanek et al., 2001; Geist et al., 2003).

Peers

Depending on the disease and the child's functioning, developing and maintaining peer relationships can be challenging. Prolonged periods of significant symptoms and hospitalizations can prevent children and adolescents from participating in activities such as school, sports, and extracurricular events where peer contact and interaction is predominant. Additional barriers can be ill children's fears of acceptance by their peers based on disease factors such as physical deformity, embarrassing symptoms, or attached social stigma. Alderfer and colleagues (2001), in a study using vignettes, found that children indicated more acceptance of healthy peers than chronically ill ones. Compared to healthy children, chronically ill children benefited more from demonstrating prosocial behavior and were less impacted by aggressive behavior. A study in the Netherlands (Meijer et al., 2000) compared the peer functioning of chronically ill children. There were no differences between groups with different illnesses. Compared to healthy peers, chronically ill children reported (both self and parent) less aggressive behavior. Parents also reported more submissive behavior in the chronically ill children. Physical restrictions and pain were associated with limited social activities but not with other measures of social functioning.

School

Successful school functioning depends on a child having reasonable psychologic functioning, interaction with peers, and attendance in addition to adequate academic performance. Children with chronic medical illness tend to have poorer academic functioning than that of their healthy peers, with a significant number having identified school problems. Many of these children may not be recognized because problems may be minimized or attributed to the medical illness or treatment. Often, there is a tendency to excuse problems or deficits in performance or behavior secondary to concern about the child's medical status or due to lower expectations. The reasons for problematic academic performance are not clear, though missing school and psychosocial factors have been implicated. Increased rates of school absence have been found in children with chronic illness, though it is not clear whether the cause is primarily related to physical or psychologic factors. There is marked variability in school attendance that is not clearly associated with disease type or severity. Treatment requirements (i.e. appointments) often are significant issues. Some data indicate that parents may keep their children home if the parents are anxious, overprotective, or have beliefs about the relative unimportance of academia. Other reasons include illness effects, minor infections, the child's response to the illness, the involved adults' attitudes, and the extent and type of school resources available. Fears about fitting back into the school mileu and with peers are common. Additional identified school difficulties have included keeping up with schoolwork due to absences, maintaining peer relationships, drug side-effects, limited access to medications, and exclusion from beneficial physical activities. Often, these children have been underserved in the educational system, either through dropping out or failing to achieve due to inadequate help. Most children with chronic illness do not require special services, but many require some level of intervention to optimize their school attendance and performance (Fowler et al., 1985; Sexson and Dingle, 1997, 2001; Geist et al., 2003).

Lightfoot and colleagues (1999) interviewed chronically ill children and adolescents and found that they valued school and had difficulties with school absence, not being able to participate fully without specific services or accommodations, teachers' reactions to their conditions, and peer relationships. Efforts by health professionals to schedule around school and to encourage school attendance were appreciated, as were individual relationships with supportive teachers. Concerns about school re-entry voiced by parents and school personnel included: the process by which the school was informed, the child's transition back to school, the ongoing monitoring of the child, teaching school personnel to manage unexpected medical difficulties, and the school's expectations of the child (Kliebenstein and Broome, 2000). Olson and peers (2004) found that school professionals viewed having chronically ill children at school positively. Diseases were rated differently in terms of their impact at school, with asthma having the least and acquired immunodeficiency syndrome (AIDS) the most. They were most concerned with the child's need for extra time or attention, possible medical emergencies and potential liability issues. Concerns about death or emergencies were discrepant with the clinical risk for conditions such as epilepsy and congenial heart disease.

Course and outcome

Diseases vary in the pattern of their symptoms as well as their prognosis. Often dealing with unpredictable symptoms (i.e. pain crisis in sickle cell syndromes) can be more difficult than illness with constant symptoms or medical demands (i.e. diabetes mellitus). A number of illnesses like asthma and epilepsy can have long periods of remission, while others like cancer have periods of intense symptoms with the potential for permanent recovery. Disorders with persistent and unremitting symptoms would be expected to have a more negative impact on emotional coping, though there is little research in this area. It may be that having a positive attitude is more important. Dealing with an uncertain outcome or a known terminal disease is difficult and it is important for children to remain hopeful (Mrazek, 2003a).

Specific

Acquired immunodeficiency syndrome (AIDS)

While the rates of children becoming HIV infected through maternal transmission has been declining with increased perinatal treatment in the United States, adolescents remain one of the highest risk groups for becoming infected. Adolescents at high risk include those who are minorities, poor, substance abusers, homosexual or bisexual, psychiatrically ill, on the street, or homeless. These adolescents have a higher risk for psychopathology due to the factors that make them at risk for HIV as well as having the disease itself (CDCP, 1999; Havens et al., 2003).

Numerous studies have documented significant neurologic, developmental, cognitive, and language abnormalities in HIV infected children which generally are more severe as the disease worsens. Two neuro-developmental patterns have been observed, progressive or static encephalopathy. Specific areas of vulnerability have been demonstrated in expressive language, attention, and motor functioning. Secondary infections and medication effects also can impact cognitive functioning. Societal attitudes and behavior also can interfere with school attendance and performance (Wolters et al., 1995; Sexson and Dingle, 1997, 2001; Havens et al., 2003).

There are limited data on the emotional and behavioral disorders in HIV infected children. Studies have found higher rates of anxiety disorders, depressive disorders, guilt, low self-esteem, and behavior problems. High rates of ADHD have been found, though some research has

found rates that were not different from a control group with similar backgrounds. None of the research has demonstrated direct associations between psychiatric symptoms and the HIV infection. These children tend to have complex circumstances and backgrounds, with other risk factors for psychopathology besides chronic illness (such as poverty, prematurity, parental psychopathology, prenatal drug exposure, disrupted living situations, inter-city environments) which may be as significant or more significant predictors of mental health problems. Additional stressors for these children include issues of secrecy, stigma, and other ill family members. Younger children often are not told of their diagnosis. Additionally, the demands of the treatment regime may be quite demanding and non-adherence often is a significant issue. Additional issues include potentially long periods without significant physical manifestations, educational issues, maintaining peer relationships, dealing with developmental challenges, and dealing with death once the disease has progressed enough (Boyd-Franklin et al., 1995; Moss et al., 1998; Havens et al., 2003).

Autoimmune disorders

Systemic lupus erythematosus (SLE) causes considerable morbidity, as does its treatment. Major depression, psychosis, and cognitive impairment are among the neuropsychiatric complications associated with this condition and its treatment (Mrazek, 2003a).

Cancer

Children with cancer may have emotional responses that affect their functioning due to the intense and often painful and unpleasant therapies as well as having to deal with a life and death struggle with the fear of recurrence. They have periods of intense symptoms often produced by the treatment with changes in physical appearance. Treatment usually requires multiple invasive, painful procedures and hospitalizations, making usual daily activities difficult to accomplish. Identified problems have included adjustment difficulties, anxiety, depression, PTSD, peer and social issues (Slater, 2002; Brown et al., 2003; Mrazek, 2003a).

Problems with school attendance and academic performance are common in these children due to the actual malignancies as well as the required treatment and vulnerability to infections. For example, survivors of leukemia demonstrate lower intellectual and academic functioning when compared to healthy children and those with other illnesses, with the greatest impairment in those children receiving central nervous system (CNS) irradiation and intrathecal chemotherapy. Compared to their siblings, these children were more likely to have emotional disturbances, be in special education, and have more school difficulties (Brown and Madan-Swain, 1993; Sexson and Dingle, 1997, 2001; Raymond-Speden et al., 2000).

Cardiac disorders

Children with congenital cyanotic heart defects may be at increased risk for CNS and intellectual impairments, as well as those who undergo open-heart surgery or extracorporeal membrane oxygenation (Mrazek, 2002).

Dermatologic disorders

Severe atopic dermatitis can cause children problems due to the intense itching and disfigured appearance. Such symptoms can interfere with physical activities, self-esteem development, and peer relationships. Some studies indicate that skin symptoms can be exacerbated with life stresses and that individual children can improve with psychologic interventions (Mrazek, 2003a).

Endocrine disorders

Children with insulin dependent diabetes require daily medications, often several injections, frequent blood testing, and diet restrictions. Stresses and family styles have been found to impact diabetic control, with parents often struggling with how involved they should be in the supervision and administration of care. Diabetic preadolescents with parents who had a style of warmth and support had better glucose levels. Poor control has been correlated with having a psychiatric disorder, difficulties in reading, and adverse psychosocial factors. Specific cognitive problems have been identified in diabetic children, and consistent evidence indicates that these children have an increased risk for developing learning problems. Cognitive changes such as decreased efficacy in making decisions and impaired attention have been found with mild hypoglycemia which may precede or occur without physical symptoms and thus not be recognized. Children at highest risk are those with preschool onset or severe fluctuations in metabolic control. A variety of psychiatric disorders have been found in these children with affective disorders being most common. Behavior disorders tend to be more common in school-aged boys. Children with persistent psychiatric disorders tend to have more problems with their diabetes (Holmes et al., 1995; Sexson and Dingle, 1997, 2001; Northam et al., 1998; Davis et al., 2001; Brown et al., 2003; Mrazek, 2003a).

Gastrointestinal disorders

Gastrointestinal disorders often have dietary requirements, medication, and possible surgery. Those affected may have significant pain as well as embarrassment due to symptoms such as flatulence, frequent bathroom use, and abdominal sounds (Brown et al., 2003).

Hematologic disorders

Hemophilia and sickle cell syndromes usually are diagnosed early in life and require ongoing, often intensive medical management. An added complication for a number of he-mophiliacs has been the generation that was infected with the HIV virus. In both conditions, physical symptoms and complications increase with age. Hemophiliacs have been found to develop a significant discrepancy between intellectual potential and academic achievement as they progress in school, with reading skills most impacted (Colegrove and Huntzinger, 1994). A study examining coping styles in children with hemophilia and their families found that there were no group gender differences in coping styles, parents in the same family tended to use the same strategies, most used all strategies at least some of the times, and the children with hemophilia tended to use resignation and distraction more than the healthy ones (Miller et al., 2000).

Those children with sickle cell syndromes have been observed to have a number of psychosocial and behavioral problems with increased adjustment difficulties in older individuals. Those children sustaining cerebrovascular accidents and other neurocognitive complications will have difficulty academically. However, others also may be at risk for more subtle cognitive problems related to anemia, ischemia, or nutritional deficits (Brown et al., 1993; Sexson and Dingle, 1997). Children with sickle cell syndromes have been found to have decreases in cognitive functioning compared to controls even in the absence of strokes. Data demonstrated lower IQ scores when compared to controls and siblings and greater effect with increasing age (Schatz et al., 2002).

Liver diseases

Pediatric patients with end-stage liver disease may be at risk for delays in cognitive and motor development, with earlier onset increasing the risk. Whether liver transplant improves cognitive function remains unclear (Hobbs and Sexson, 1993; Slater, 1994; Mrazek, 2002).

Neurologic disorders

Children with epilepsy can have learning difficulties either related to brain pathology or medication effects with age of onset, type, frequency, and severity of seizures, and type of medication being important variables. Unrecognized seizures can significantly impact cognitive functioning. Children with seizures have a higher rate of psychopathology compared to children with other medical conditions and the general population. Common diagnoses include attention, behavior, anxiety, and depressive disorders. Stress can exacerbate seizures, and a number of children with epilepsy can have non-epileptic seizures induced by psychologic factors. Additional issues include fear of injury and loss of control when having a seizure as well as the reactions of others. Having epilepsy also may mean limitations on activities such as driving or participation in sports. Other neurologic conditions include a spectrum of neurodegenerative and neuromuscular diseases with variable cognitive and psychiatric symptoms (Williams et al., 2002b; Brown et al., 2003).

Pulmonary disorders

Depending on the severity of asthma, there may be limitations on the child's activity and significant side-effects from the medications. A number of these medications can impact academic performance, as can school absences and potential neurologic consequences of hypoxia. Problems with academic performance are consistent with the general findings in children with chronic illness and are exacerbated by the presence of other risk factors such as poverty, family problems, and pre-existing psychologic difficulties. A number of studies have documented that asthmatic children have a significant rate of anxiety and depression. A recent hypothesis about the association between asthma and psychiatric symptoms is that asthma, depression, and anxiety are all conditions that are due to dysfunction in biochemical processes with genetic regulation. Attention-deficit/hyperactivity disorder symptoms appear to be moderately increased in asthmatic children (Biederman et al., 1994; Sexson and Dingle, 1997, 2001; Ortega et al., 2002; Mrazek, 2003a, 2003b).

Most children with cystic fibrosis now live into adulthood and often have prolonged periods of minimal symptoms. An involved treatment regime is required, which can include medication, dietary recommendations, physical therapy and exercise. Often, sustained parental involvement is necessary, for example, with the physical therapy. In addition to problems with adherence and dependency, adolescents often have delayed sexual and physical maturation. Additionally, they have to deal with the deaths of similarly affected peers and knowledge of their own mortality. Severity of disease has been found to be a primary predictor of psychiatric disturbance in these children with a better quality of life associated with positive coping strategies. A review of studies on children with cystic fibrosis found that issues included problems with communicating with medical professionals and school personnel, restrictions on activities, and difficulties developing and maintaining peer and social relationships. Coping styles tended to be similar to those of healthy children. When compared to healthy peers, variable differences have been found in self-esteem, self-concept and self-efficacy, and psychiatric symptoms. A spectrum of psychiatric disorders has been reported, particularly eating disorders and anxiety. A significant proportion achieve below grade level in math and reading (Brown et al., 2003; Christian, 2003; Mrazek, 2003b).

Renal diseases

In a study of adjustment, mothers of children with end-stage renal disease reported that their children were at greater risk for psychologic problems, though the children reported no more problems than the normative sample. The coping styles and mental health of the mothers explained some of the variance in their ratings, but were not predictive of the children's self-ratings. Disease severity was not found to predict adjustment. Children with renal failure demonstrate deficits in basic language and mathematical skills, with some studies suggesting that renal transplants may improve cognitive functioning (Hobbs and Sexson, 1993; Sexson and Dingle, 1997, 2001; Madden et al., 2002).

Rheumatoid disorders

Juvenile rheumatoid arthritis has been associated with behavioral problems and depression. Berry and colleagues found a significant lack of understanding of the illness and treatments among children with this disease (Berry et al., 1993; Mrazek, 2003a).

Sensory impairments

Visual and hearing impairments commonly are associated with each other and other problems such as cognitive deficits, cerebral palsy, epilepsy and hearing impairments. However, children can be blind or deaf for genetic, infectious, or traumatic reasons without other associated deficits. Multisensory impairments most commonly are due to genetic syndromes or as a result of prematurity or low birth weight. Parents with intact senses often react with shock upon discovering their child's condition. Persistent parental distress may impact family communication and functioning. Particularly with deaf children, parents may struggle with the view of deafness as a difference rather than a disability (Young, 1999; Hindley and van Gent, 2003).

Deafness

Language development of deaf children with deaf parents is similar to that of hearing children, while those with hearing parents often have impoverished communication. Earlier identification and intervention are associated with better receptive and expressive spoken language development, and children with cochlear implants can demonstrate significant language improvement. Some controversy still exists about the appropriateness and benefits of cochlear implants within the deaf community. Deaf children can exhibit deficits in cognitive development and performance that appear to be related to their language abilities and tend to underachieve academically. In mainstream settings, in the early years of school, there appear to be few peer issues, though later deaf children tend to be socially isolated. Most deaf children do not have psychiatric disorders, though there appears to be a higher rate of psychopathology than in the general population. Psychiatric conditions are more likely in children with additional impairments. The spectrum of disorders is the same as in the general population. Pervasive developmental, emotional, and disruptive disorders are common (Hindley, 1997; Meyer et al., 1998; Hindley and van Gent, 2003).

Blindness

Blind children without other significant difficulties have essentially normal development, though there are some data that they may have difficulties in processing visuospatial information and understanding interpersonal relationships due to a lack of visual interaction. There is limited and inconclusive information on academic achievement. Studies on emotional and social development have been contradictory, with variable impressions of social and peer relationships. Blind children appear to have a higher rate of psychiatric disorders than the general population, with those with additional medical impairments having the highest rate. Identified problems have included mental retardation, developmental disorders, adjustment disorders, personality disorders, sleep problems, peer difficulties, social withdrawal, loneliness, self-injurious behavior, and anxiety. Autistic behaviors appear more frequent in children with congenital blindness, especially if they also are mentally retarded. Congenital blindness may have a greater pervasive impact on psychologic development, but acquired blindness may produce more of a sense of loss (Hindley and van Gent, 2003).

Trauma

Traumatic injuries as well as the outcomes of medical illnesses and interventions significantly influence a child's life experience. Lengthy convalescence, altered mobility, and disfiguring injuries can impact educational, social, and psychologic functioning. Studies of pediatric burns patients suggest educational and vocational impairment. Burned children have demonstrated a range of psychologic symptoms, with a number having impaired social relationships, behavioral problems, depression, anxiety, PTSD and personal relationship difficulties (Blakeney, 1994; Tarnowski and Rasnake, 1994; Stoddard, 2002).

Assessment

Relevant psychologic and social issues should be assessed routinely during the child's medical evaluations and care. Any chronic illness can have associated psychosocial difficulties, which vary in their importance and impact. All chronically ill children, adolescents, and families experience psychologic and social reactions and issues connected to the illness. However, there are significant differences in how these issues are perceived and managed. Psychiatric assessment should identify the relevant intrapsychic and environmental factors that may affect medical problems and what interventions if any, are necessary. Psychologic factors may be significant even if the child does not have symptoms that meet the criteria of a major psychiatric disorder. It is also essential to determine if the psychologic or cognitive symptoms are caused by the medical condition or treatment and require additional medical evaluation and reassessment of treatment such as psychotic symptoms in a child with SLE who is on steroids.

The child's past history should be obtained, with information from previous providers. Obtaining information on functioning during and views of the illness at various ages and stages of disease as well as a chronology of the relationship between exacerbation of the disorder and any emotional or environmental stresses are helpful. It is essential to acquire information on how all the involved individuals (child, caretakers, involved family, school personnel, health providers, and others) understand and view the illness and treatment in terms of etiology, responsiveness, prognosis, treatment requirements, and expected impact on functioning. Specific questions should be asked to elucidate knowledge of disease and treatment, view of expected future, coping strategies, academic and social functioning, adherence, and family functioning.

Support for the connection of psychologic or environmental factors can include: onset of symptoms after specific trauma or stress; disability or handicap out of proportion to reported symptoms; clear secondary gain; and exacerbation linked to stressful events.

Other possible indications of poor functioning may include poor adherence to treatment regimes, refusal to participate in age appropriate behavior (school, peers, and activities), or engagement in risky behaviors. Possible psychologic or psychiatric symptoms such as depression should be identified and treated, and not considered just a natural consequence of being chronically ill.

Having a psychiatrist as part of the treatment team and involved early in the process can be helpful. Having the caretaker, child, and family evaluated by the psychiatrist may aid in the diagnostic process, especially in terms of trying to understand family relationships, psychologic attributions about the illness, contributing psychologic and environmental issues, and relevant psychosocial information. The psychiatric evaluation should be presented to the family as an integral aspect of the medical evaluation, since stress and chronic illness often are comorbid. It should focus on the physical problems and their impact with questions about psychologic and psychiatric functioning included in that framework. A psychiatric evaluation of the caretakers can be helpful in elucidating their attributions about the illness, view of treatment and heath-care, relationships to the child, as well as information about their backgrounds, parenting, emotional functioning and access to resources. The psychiatrist also can assess the child and family to provide information on their functioning, level of distress, and potential sources of support. Children, school age and older, should be seen individually with an emphasis on exploring their understanding of their illness and psychologic functioning. Clinical interviewers should emphasize open-ended questions, but evaluations particularly with the children also may require multiple narrower questions, which cover all likely possibilities (see Key clinical questions).

KEY CLINICAL QUESTIONS

Attributions/beliefs about the disease

- *Who else do you know with this type of problem?*
- *What happens to individuals with your disease?*
- *What is going to happen to you?*
- *What is the worst aspect of having this illness?*
- *What is the treatment for your illness? What does it do? Does it work?*
- *What do your parents/siblings think?*

Understanding the disease/treatment; possible adherence issues

- *What is your understanding of your disease and treatment?*
- *What are your medications/diet/other requirements? What are they supposed to be doing?*
- *Do your medications help? With what?*
- *Do your medications bother you? How?*
- *How do you take your medications/keep to your diet? Who helps you remember?*
- *What times do you take your medicine? Where is it kept?*
- *How many times have you missed taking it in the last week? What do you do then?*
- *Does it make any difference if you miss taking it/don't keep to your diet/exercise?*
- *What other treatments would be more helpful?*
- *Who knows that you have to take medication/be on a diet/exercise?*
- *What happens when you are with friends and you are supposed to take your medication?*
- *What happens if your friends are eating/doing something you are not supposed to? What do you do?*

Functioning

- *How is your life different since you got ill? What can/can't you do?*
- *How would things be if you did not have this illness?*
- *How are things different at home?*
- *Who helps you manage your illness?*
- *Who are your friends? What do you do with them?*
- *How is school? What problems has being sick caused? What kind of help do you get?*
- *How much school have you missed? Why? How do you keep up?*
- *What fun activities do you do? When? With whom?*

Potential psychologic or environmental factors

- *What happened right before you became ill/got worse?*
- *Who knows about your illness? Who told them? What was said?*
- *What do your friends think about your illness? What do your classmates say?*
- *What happens when you miss school?*
- *How do others treat you differently since you became ill?*
- *What would you think if the team told you that you do not need additional medical interventions right now?*
- *What is good/bad about being in the hospital/your doctor/being ill?*
- *How long do you think you are going to be ill/in the hospital?*

Observations of the child's and family's behavior and interactions in medical settings should be considered, as well as information from other involved agencies or institutions such as schools, child protective services, or the juvenile justice system.

During the assessment, it is important to consider and accommodate any limitations that the child has that may impact the evaluation. Issues can include physical and sensory impairments so that room arrangements and assessment techniques may have to be modified. Other issues can include fatigue, medical treatments, or physical symptoms (Costello et al., 1988; Brown et al., 2003; Geist et al., 2003; Hindley and van Gent, 2003; LeBlanc et al., 2003; Mrazek, 2003a).

Children with chronic medical illnesses who meet the criteria of a psychiatric disorder are diagnosed using a psychiatric classification system, either the DSM-IV or ICD-10. The DSM-IV system has several possible diagnostic categories. If the psychologic symptoms are primarily related to adjustment issues related to the physical condition, a diagnosis of psychologic factors affecting a general medical condition is given (Table 17.1). This disorder is in the category of other conditions that may be a focus of clinical attention and is coded on axis I. The psychologic factor (i.e. anxiety, depression) and medical condition (i.e. diabetes mellitus) are specified. Often, these psychologic factors lead to problems with adherence. This set of disorders is diagnosed when children

---

DIAGNOSIS

Table 17.1 Psychologic factors affecting a medical condition

Discriminating features

- General medical disorder is present
- Psychologic factors adversely affect the general medical condition (one of following)
  - Close temporal relationship between the factors and development, exacerbation, or delayed recovery of medical condition
  - Factors interfere with medical treatment
  - Factors constitute additional health risks
  - Stress-related physiologic responses precipitate or exacerbate medical condition

Consistent features

- Coded by nature of psychologic factors
- For example, major depressive disorder affecting asthma

Variable features

- Subtyping
  - Mental disorder (axis I disorder)
  - Psychologic symptoms
  - Personality traits or coping style
  - Maladaptive health behaviors
  - Stress-related physiologic response
  - Other or unspecified psychologic factors

Table 17.2 Psychiatric disorder due to a general medical condition

Discriminating features

- General medical disorder is present
- From history, physical exam, or laboratory results, psychiatric symptoms appear to be a direct physiologic consequence of a general medical condition
- Not delirium

Consistent features

- Coded by nature of psychiatric symptoms/disorder
- For example, major depressive disorder due to hypothyroidism

Variable features

- Various psychiatric disorders

CONSIDER CONSULTATION WHEN ...

- There is concern about excessive utilization of medical care.
- Treatment non-adherence is significant.
- Repeated education about the disease and treatment has not been effective.
- Impairment of function exceeds the level expected.
- Psychologic issues or environmental stressors appear to be associated with exacerbation.
- Psychiatric symptoms in child or caretaker are significant.

and adolescents with previously identified medical problems have persistent or recurrent symptoms related to their medical illness for which the underlying organic abnormality is not an adequate explanation for the frequency or severity. The symptoms appear to be temporally associated with psychologic issues or environmental events, to be related to behaviors, which increase the patient's vulnerability to illness, or to be the consequence of non-adherence to treatment recommendations. If the psychologic symptoms are considered to be a direct physiologic or anatomic consequence of the medical condition, the diagnosis is a psychiatric disorder due to a general medical condition (Table 17.2). The psychiatric disorder and medical condition are specified. This disorder is coded on axis I and each one is classified based on the psychiatric disorder. An example is depression due to hypothyroidism. If the child's psychiatric condition is considered to be co-existing with the medical condition, the psychiatric disorder (i.e. ADHD) is coded on axis I and the medical condition is placed on axis III. Other relevant factors may be diagnosed as V codes and placed on axis I (i.e. parent-conflict) or as a stress (i.e. failure to attend school and placed on axis IV (APA, 1994; Brown et al., 2003).

Treatment

Treatment approaches should be individualized for each unique patient. However, for most of these children, designing a treatment plan should include coordination between medical providers, usually with the primary care physician as the coordinator and integration of a psychiatrist either as a provider or consultant (see Consider consultation when ... box). Many chronically ill children see multiple medical providers as well other specialists providing rehabilitative and nutritional services. Agencies such as the schools and other community institutions should be involved to access resources and optimize the child's functioning and activities. For some children, other agencies such as child protective and juvenile justice systems need to be accessed for additional resources.

Important components of treatment include concentrating on increasing function, identifying stress and problematic areas, and implementing interventions to improve coping strategies. Pain should be adequately managed with medication and appropriate behavioral interventions. Behavioral management is essential to reinforce appropriate coping behavior, increase adherence to the treatment plan, and decrease secondary gain related to being sick. Education on the treatment approach and its rationale, clarification about symptoms to be concerned about, systems of communication with medical providers, and possible problem solving strategies are important. If the child has significant psychologic symptoms or a psychiatric disorder, the appropriate psychotherapeutic and if necessary, psychopharmacologic interventions should be utilized. Children should be actively involved in their care, with responsibilities appropriate for their developmental abilities. Treatment plans should consider family resources and abilities to increase adherence (Brown et al., 2003).

Children with particular disorders may benefit from specialized services such as those developed to work with the deaf, which include clinicians with sign language proficiency and a social and cultural emphasis (Hindley and van Gent, 2003). Other examples include programs developed to treat children with asthma, diabetes, HIV/AIDS, sickle cell disorders, and cancer.

Education

It is essential to correct any gaps in knowledge or misunderstandings that the child or family may have about the child's illness and treatment. Much of the morbidity of pediatric disease is the result of inaccurate or inadequate information or knowledge, problems with adherence and difficulties in communication. While rarely sufficient, repeated, ongoing assessment of disease knowledge and education is key. Use of ancillary resources such as educational programs, written and verbal materials, taped information, support groups and the internet can be useful (Brown et al., 2003). Children and families, especially those affected by rare diseases, can find information and support from national associations for specific diseases as well as the information and sharing opportunities available on the internet.

Adjunct interventions

Encouraging healthy lifestyle behaviors such as nutritional eating, exercise, and recreation can be helpful. Often, children benefit from participating in formal physical or occupational programs (Mrazek, 2003a).

School

Though home-bound instruction can maintain a child's academic achievement, the loss of participation in the school milieu may limit opportunities to learn informally, socialize with peers, experience a wider world, and develop independence and autonomy. Thus, school attendance and active participation should be encouraged and facilitated. Medical providers can be helpful by encouraging school attendance, providing information on the relevant health issues, including what the child can and cannot do, identifying necessary resources and services as well as communicating consistently with school personnel. Often, children need help preparing to return to school with suggestions on how to explain their situation and who to tell what. It is essential that teachers and other school personnel understand the child's condition so that they can handle medical issues that may occur at school and develop appropriate expectations for the child's school performance. Having the health team and parents discuss the child's medical issues in advance is beneficial, as can speaking to the child's classmates. Accessing and utilizing special education services either through traditional categories (i.e. learning or behaviorally disordered) or alternative ones such as "other health impaired" or "orthopedically handicapped" typically requires intensive coordination between the family, school, and healthcare providers. Chronically ill children often are absent for multiple, brief periods, so developing a system to provide the child with ongoing educational experiences during the absences is essential (Sexson and Dingle, 1997, 2001; Lightfoot et al., 1999).

Psychiatric interventions

Most chronically ill children with psychosocial difficulties do not receive mental health services (Cadman et al., 1987). A major goal of psychosocial care is to help children and families effectively cope with their disease and obtain the highest possible level of age-appropriate functioning and activities

as possible (Mrazek, 2003a). Generally, a multidisciplinary approach is necessary (Lewis and Vitulano, 2003). There are few data on the effectiveness of psychosocial interventions for children with chronic illness and their families with very few randomized controlled treatment trials. Kibby and colleagues (1998) did a meta-analysis of psychologic interventions and found that these interventions for disease-related, emotional, or behavioral problems were effective with effects lasting at least 12 months. Children who received treatment did better than those who did not. Behavioral therapy was the most common modality. Disease type, severity, and duration did not appear to be significant. Children with sensory, physical or cognitive impairments may need accommodation to participate in therapy (i.e. room arrangement, sign language interpreters) or modifications of therapeutic techniques to emphasize either verbal or non-verbal interventions.

Individual

Psychologic or pharmaceutical treatments to minimize the distress associated with frightening or painful procedures have been shown to reduce the development of posttraumatic symptoms. Cognitive behavioral therapy has been shown to decrease anxiety in adolescents with cystic fibrosis, as have medically and emotionally supportive strategies. Cognitive behavioral therapy is helpful for procedure-related pain. Relaxation training has been used with children with a range of diseases with variable results. The combination of relaxation training and biofeedback may be more effective. Behavior therapy with continent reinforcement can enhance adherence and improve functioning (Kazak et al., 1996; Hains et al., 1997; Powers, 1999; Brown et al., 2003).

Family

Most prevention and intervention studies suggest a family approach and a number of studies have demonstrated positive results (Wamboldt and Wamboldt, 2000). Educational interventions with a family focus and an emphasis on strengthening adaptation, identifying and treating psychiatric conditions, and improving the family's perception of support from the health system and others can be helpful. An emphasis on education and adherence issues from the beginning of treatment with the consistent involvement of family can help improve treatment success (Geist et al., 2003). There has been recent interest in developing comprehensive models of interventions to support families with chronically ill children. One model employed in Australia is based on the principles of family-centered, non-illness specific, preventative, non-linear, and flexible care. It offers a spectrum of services as necessary: individual, couple, or family therapy; physical and emotional support during crisis or interactions with medical systems; therapeutic projects by families and patients to share their stories with the community; facilitated peer group therapy; parent mentor program; facilitated social events; and community education (Morison et al., 2003).

Group

Typical types of group interventions for chronically ill children include emotional support, psychoeducation, adaptation/skill development, symptom reduction, and summer camps. Groups can provide opportunities to improve social functioning, peer relationships, disease and treatment knowledge, problem solving skills as well as a forum for modeling, helping others, and sharing similar circumstances. Most of the literature on this intervention focuses on disease-specific groups. There has been no systematic attempt to examine how important homogeneity or disease specificity is for the effectiveness of group interventions.

Plante and colleagues (2001) reviewed the literature on group interventions from 1970 to 2000. They found that there have been no well-controlled studies on the psychologic or physical impact of emotional support groups. Psychoeducational groups appeared comparable to education only groups in improving attitudes towards medical services and treatment adherence and to family-based behavioral therapy in decreasing global family conflict. These groups do not appear to be effective in ameliorating symptoms. Multi-family groups targeting adaptation/skill development had positive results for adolescents with diabetes and cancer survivors, as did groups focused on diabetes management. Groups concentrating on coping and disease management skills to improve physical symptoms and psychologic functioning in diabetic and asthmatic children have demonstrated positive results in controlled studies. Symptom reduction groups have exhibited positive results in decreasing physical symptoms in several controlled studies for a variety of specific diseases. Studies on summer camps for specific diseases have shown improvements in disease knowledge/management, self-esteem, anxiety, and attitudes towards illness, but there has been no comparison to control groups, and generalization of these effects is unclear. Several studies have utilized nurses to teach cognitive and behavioral strategies in small groups to improve control over disease stresses (Stewart, 2003).

Psychopharmacology

Psychiatric conditions are treated with the same medications used in children without chronic medical conditions. Treating psychiatric symptoms or syndromes should be approached cautiously with low starting doses, slow titration, and close monitoring. Many of the medications used to treat medical conditions have the potential to interact with psychotropic medications. For example, many medical and psychiatric medications are metabolized by the P450 isoenzyme systems. Medication side-effects may exacerbate or impact the patient's existing symptoms.

Summary

Considering the psychosocial issues that commonly affect chronically ill children and intervening to promote optimal functioning is an essential component of good medical care. While most of these children and families manage well, monitoring these factors to provide early identification and treatment will enhance their quality of life. Most chronically children can lead productive and satisfying lives with active participation in the usual range of developmentally appropriate activities.

Annotated bibliography

Geist R, Grdisa V, Otley A (2003). Psychosocial issues in the child with chronic conditions. *Best Practice and Research: Clinical Gastroenterology*, 17:141–152.
Article summarizing some of the major issues faced by chronically ill children and their families.

Lewis M (ed.) (2002). *Child and Adolescent Psychiatry: A Comprehensive Textbook*. Philadelphia, Lippincott Williams Wilkins, pp. 1239–1245.
A major child and adolescent textbook with chapters on several medical diseases as well as on collaboration between pediatrics and child and adolescent psychiatry

Kibby MY, Tyc VL, Mulhern RK (1998). Effectiveness of psychological intervention for children and adolescents with chronic medical illness: a meta-analysis. *Clinical Psychology Review*, 18:103–117.
Overview of the research on psychologic interventions with chronically ill children

LeBlanc LA, Goldsmith T, Patel DR (2003). Behavioral aspects of chronic illness in children and adolescents. *Pediatric Clinics of North America*, 50:859–78.
Overview of behavioral issues in chronically medically ill children

Morison JE, Bromfield LM, Cameron HJ (2003). A therapeutic model for supporting families of children with a chronic illness or disability. *Child and Adolescent Mental Health*, 8:125–130.
Interdisciplinary model of support for chronically ill children and their families

Normandeau S, Kalnins L, Jutras S, Hanigan D (1998). A description of 5- to 12-year old children's conception of health within the context of their daily life. *Psychology and Health*, 13:883–896.
Overview of chronically ill children's concept based on interviews with variously aged children and adolescents

Sexson SB, Dingle AD (2001). Medical disorders. In: Kline FM, Silver LB, Russell SC (eds) *The Educator's Guide to Medical Issues in the Classroom*. Baltimore, Paul H Brookes Publishing Co, pp. 29–45.
Overview of various medical illnesses and how the illness and/or the treatment and caretaker response may impact school functioning.

CHAPTER 18

The School's Role in the Psychosocial Development of Children

Graeme Hanson, MD

OUTLINE

Introduction

In most societies, children are expected to attend some type of formal education beginning around age 6 or 7. In the United States, children spend an average of 5½–6 hours a day in a structured school setting, generally with same-age peers and in a group format. The prime task of the school is to impart knowledge, to promote an interest in learning, and to encourage the development of cognitive-intellectual skills that will assist the child in everyday living and ultimately, in attaining mastery in an occupation. In addition, the school environment, including peers, the teachers, the structure, and the educational programs, has a significant influence on the psychosocial development of children.

This chapter will focus on the key components of this psychosocial influence – how the components of this influence bring about change, positive or negative, in the growing child's sense of self, and adaptation to his/her world, to the family, and to the cultural and social environment. Clearly, there are a variety of powerful influences on child development including genetic endowment, parents, siblings, and extended family, ordinal position in the family, culture and environment, socioeconomic status, peers, and importantly, the school and the school environment. Looking at the development of a child from an ecological perspective involves looking at the family, the school and the community as places where the child's values and behaviors are influenced through interactions with others (Bronfenbrenner, 1986). "These relationships are reciprocal – families, schools, and communities influence children just as children influence the tone of the family, school, and community. These interactions are also developmental – they change and mature" (Smith et al., 2004, p. 214).

For physicians and mental health providers working with children, it is necessary to understand the myriad and important influences the school setting brings to the lives of their patients, both positive and negative. A clinician's recognition of the powerful role that the school plays in the lives of children facilitates a better understanding of the information that the child or parent brings to the clinician's office and, especially, to the therapy hour, related to the school and the child's experiences in the school (Hanson, 1997). Using this understanding of the role of the school environment in their patients' lives, clinicians can effect beneficial changes in a child's daily experience at school through active involvement with the school.

This chapter will address such issues as the role of learning and the development of knowledge and skills as well as the nonacademic aspects of schools, such as peer relationships, extracurricular activities, the physical structure of the school, and, importantly, the role of teachers and other school personnel in the lives of children. The focus in this chapter will be primarily on elementary and middle school children with some discussion of the influence of school in early adolescence. The role of the school in adolescent psychosocial development, including identity formation and development of a sense of competence, peer relationships and re-negotiating relationships to authority, etc. is an enormous topic which would require a separate chapter unto itself.

There is little in the child and adolescent psychiatry literature that addresses the psychosocial influence of the school on the developing child. In the education literature, the focus is mainly on how to improve the school's role in the psychosocial development of children. One of the difficulties in addressing this topic is the divergence of research and literature into sub-specialty categories. Each specialty involves a piece of the pie, so to speak, or a section of the child's life, but it is unusual to find an occasion where the perspectives from the various fields are brought together. Erik Erikson in his writings does seem to have a comprehensive overview of the importance of school and learning to the young child's emotional and social development, and especially of the teachers' role in shaping children's lives.

Another difficulty in writing a chapter on the role of the school in the psychosocial development of children is that there is such remarkable variability among school districts, between individual schools, and even among classrooms, making it difficult to generalize on this topic. Kozol, in his 1991 book *Savage Inequalities* demonstrated that, for students of color and for poor children in general, schools are grossly substandard in terms of physical facilities and resources. "Because funding for most public schools is based in part on local property taxes, 'inner city' schools are typically grossly under funded for their facilities in comparison to suburban schools. Poor children face the worst of poor-quality schools … For both male and female students, the quality of the school environment is related to exposure to, involvement in, and victimization by violence" (Smith et al., 2004, p. 220). Fiscal and budgetary characteristics account for much of this discrepancy. There is a troubling disparity between districts, with a more affluent population having many more resources than districts in low socioeconomic environments.

The impact of school on an individual child is not simply a matter of physical plant and resources. Rutter found that a number of factors in individual schools make a significant difference in the overall outcome of students, and especially in minimizing the development of pathology in at risk students. In this study, it was not simply the number of different resources available in the school, but more importantly, the overall quality of the school setting, especially characteristics like approaches to discipline, student involvement in their own educational activities, the teachers as positive role models, and an emphasis on academics, etc. (Rutter, 1980).

Because of this remarkable variability from school to school, this chapter will focus on a rather general picture of some of the key aspects that the school experience brings to the social and psychologic development of children, looking at both the potential for positive influence on the child's development as well as negative or interfering influences on the child's adaptation. "Schools, along with families and communities, are important influences that can contribute to the development of healthy and successful young people, even those thought to be at risk. Schools can serve as a negative influence to perpetuate the status quo, or use the opportunity to serve as a positive, transforming influence in the lives of children and youth" (Smith et al., 2004, pp. 213–214). Another confounding issue is that children in this country change schools frequently. They typically change teachers

every year as they move upward through the grades, and, this being a very mobile culture, usually change schools when the family moves. These changes obviously affect the way in which the school experience influences any one child's development and make it difficult to generalize.

Clinicians need to be familiar with the structure of the school system in order to know how best to intervene on behalf of their patients. There is considerable variability from district to district. In addition to public schools, there are schools run by private organizations, including religious orders. Parents elect to send their children to these non-public schools for a variety of reasons. Most private and parochial schools charge tuition. Many of these schools do have scholarship programs. Families who can afford private schools choose them for a variety of reasons. Most private schools can afford to have enhanced services and programs for students that are not available in many public schools, e.g. sports, music, drama and art classes, smaller class sizes and often, but not always, more highly qualified teachers. Also, since parents are paying for their child's tuition, there is potential for more active parental involvement in the running of the school. Some parents of private school students also want their children to be in a more homogeneous social and economic group. Many parents choose parochial schools for their children, in part, because they wish an education for their child consistent with their, the family's, religious beliefs, for the child to be schooled with like-minded children and because there is an assumption that parochial schools have more strict moral and disciplinary structures. However, depending on the school, some private schools have fewer support services for children with special needs than do public schools. Although the public system is responsible for providing supportive services for all children with special needs (see below), in many public systems these services are provided through the public sector and may not be available in the private school.

In most districts the principal of the school is a key person to contact. Clinicians who wish to consult with school personnel about a patient could be well served contacting the principal first to introduce themselves, give the reason for the call and then inquire of the principal who would be the most appropriate person in the school with whom to discuss the case. It is essential to obtain consent from the parents to gain information from and to give information to the school. The child's primary teachers may be the best source of information. However, there may be other school personnel who have more useful information about the child and the family, e.g. the guidance counselor, school nurse, physical education instructor, or school social worker. In addition to their knowledge of the individual child, teachers and other school personnel often have remarkably good insight into the family dynamics. One needs to be aware that school personnel vary in their capacity to observe and evaluate children in their

KEY CLINICAL QUESTIONS

When gathering information from the school, important questions include:
- *What is the nature of the child's relationships with and acceptance by peers?*
- *What is the ability of the child to attend to and concentrate on academic work?*
- *What is the nature of the parents' involvement/collaboration with school personnel?*
- *What is the child's overall academic achievement, estimates of overall intelligence, areas of particular strength or weakness, both intellectually and socially?*

care. A clinician consulting with school personnel needs to inquire about the child's relationships with and acceptance by peers, the child's ability to attend to and concentrate on academic work, differences between the child's adaptation in the classroom and the non-academic settings, especially playground, lunch room, coming and going to school, etc. How the child relates to adults vs. other children, and what is the nature of the parents' involvement/collaboration with school personnel are important questions. Basic information concerning the child's academic achievement, estimates of overall intelligence, areas of particular strength or weakness, both intellectual and social, including any formalized testing accomplished, can be very revealing.

Some parents do not want the school to know that their child has psychologic or physical problems. This can be a difficult situation for the clinician, since in many cases the school's participation in an overall treatment/remediation plan can be crucial. Helping parents understand the key positive role the school can play is important. Exploring with the parent their reluctance to involve the school can be informative and may reveal important, and hopefully surmountable, psychologic resistance to involving the school, e.g. some negative experience the parent had as a child, or a general suspicion of bureaucracies. The clinician's willingness to intervene on behalf of the family can be very beneficial. In many instances, it can be helpful for the clinician to explain to school personnel that some children have characteristics and interpersonal styles that are constitutional and that affect the child's relationships and adaptation to school. Temperamental differences and characteristics, e.g. shyness, idiosyncratic thinking, inability to understand or read social cues, extreme impulsivity, etc., are most likely inborn, and school personnel can adapt their approaches to such children, taking into account these characteristics while being supportive to the family.

Erik Erikson's observations in his concept of stages of development are pertinent to this chapter, especially his observations on the so-called "latency" phase as outlined

in 'Identity and the life cycle', the phase of industry versus inferiority. "While all children at times need to be left alone in solitary play (or later in the company of books and radio, motion pictures, and video) … and while all children need their hours and days of make-believe and games, they all, sooner or later, become dissatisfied and disgruntled without a sense of being successful, without a sense of being able to make things, and make them well and even perfectly; this is what I call the *sense of industry* … He, the child, develops the pleasure of *work completion*, attention, and persevering diligence" (p. 86). The opposite of this sense of successful sense of industry is a sense of inadequacy and inferiority. The child who is not successful in mastering the tasks of everyday life, especially those in the school, develops a sense of inadequacy and inferiority. Clearly, the school environment has a major influence on the development of this "sense of industry."

Role of academic learning and development of a sense of mastery

The process of formal education with its structure, rules, encouragement of concentration, "work," and cognitive problem solving accompanied by directions/instruction in organizational skills and study habits greatly assists the child in developing knowledge and skills that promote a sense of industry. Also, exposure to a variety of modes of understanding/comprehending the world, such as language, mathematics, geography, history, art, music, etc., can reveal or uncover strengths/talents, and special capacities in individual children, which leads to the sense of individual success and may help shape future occupational choices. "Academic achievement and interest in school are critical factors related to young people being less likely to be involved in violence, delinquency, substance abuse, and teenage parenthood … Academic achievement contributes to higher levels of occupational attainment and the avoidance of negative life courses" (Smith et al., 2004, p. 216).

Non-academic aspects of school that play an important role in the child's psychosocial development

Peers

Beginning in the first grade, the child begins to measure him/herself against peers. The child is no longer the first or second child in the family or simply belonging to this mother and father in this family, but is now one of several peers, often of the same age and socioeconomic or cultural background. Also, the child's sense of self and self-appraisal now begins to include his/her peers' assessment or evaluation of the child's perceived strengths and weaknesses.

Not uncommonly, physical attributes, talents, or lack of talent, become important as the child compares him or herself to peers and, likewise, as peers perceive characteristics of the child. Attributes such as height, weight, hair color, physical dexterity, or lack thereof, take on special psychologic and social meaning for the first time. Talents (such as musical, artistic, athletic, leadership) also take on a significant role in the child's development of a sense of self. How these attributes and talents are supported, recognized, or negated in the school setting by school personnel, peers, and the family can have a powerful influence on the child's sense of self.

Children learn key aspects of social interaction and adaptation to a social system through trial and error in negotiation with peers, and by observing and identifying with the various methods their peers use in the busy hustle and bustle of everyday life at school – in the classroom, at recess, comings and goings, and even in after-school activities.

The role of the teacher

For many students in the early years of grade school, the teacher can be a particularly important person in that student's social and academic adaptation as well as in his or her developing sense of self. "Until I became involved in schools, I didn't understand that children need to form emotional bonds with their teachers and see healthy social relationships among adults in their lives to function well in school" (Comer, 2003, p.11). Rutter, in the study cited above, emphasizes that teachers serve as important role models for students, and the children tend to identify with people in authority and people they admire and like. (Rutter, 1980) The day-to-day involvement with the classroom teacher offers the young latency-age child an opportunity to develop a relationship with an adult that is not encumbered with the infantile, toddler, and preschool history of complex parent-child interactions, with both positive and negative memory traces of the developmental transactions that affect mutually the child and the parent and that color the nature of that relationship. The relationship with the teacher offers to the child an opportunity to initiate with a clean slate a relationship with a potentially caring adult, an adult who is interested in the child's development but not involved with the day-to-day, sometimes regressive, caretaking of the child. The teacher's attitude toward, and acceptance of, the child can have a powerful influence on that child's developing sense of him/herself as an individual who transcends the family and who is increasingly now a participating member of society. "Perceived teacher support is a protective factor contributing to students' feeling competent and understood, especially when other areas of support are less available for students" (Smith et al., 2004, p. 217).

In the literature, there is considerable research on teacher attitudes towards individual students and the influence of that attitude on pupil success. However, as Allan Fromme said, in his introduction to John Holt's important book *How Children Fail* (1964, pp.11–12), "Another relationship of great importance to the growth of the individual – and to even greater importance to the good of society – still cries out for study but remains generally neglected. Despite the fact that millions of children and thousands of adults are daily pressed into a student-teacher relationship, we know very little about their interactions and the influences they have on each other. Of course, there is a great deal of material available on learning theory and general educational practice, but none of this tells us what actually happens when a teacher asks a child a question in the classroom." Since the writing of that book there has been research on certain aspects of teacher-pupil interactions; yet much of the nature of that interaction is idiosyncratic to that individual dyad and what each party brings to that interaction. "Children who feel labeled by teachers and believe that teachers have negative expectations of them do not achieve or behave at the same levels as students who have a more positive relationship with their teachers … A teacher with high expectation of a particular student gives that student opportunities to think and problem solve and correct initially incorrect responses, opportunities teachers do not give to students about whom they have pessimistic attitudes" (Smith et al., 2004, p. 217). For many students, because the teacher comes to the student's life relatively free of the preschool emotional history and "baggage," the teacher can easily become an idealized positive identification figure, and an important person who offers to the child an alternative model of adulthood perhaps close to, or sometimes quite distant from, the model presented by the parents. Clinicians should be sensitive to the psychologic role and meaning that particular teachers have in their child patient's lives. This influence can also be problematic, especially when there is not a good fit between pupil and teacher, or especially when a child vulnerable to feeling inferior encounters a teacher who, for his/her own psychologic reasons, takes a dislike to the child, a kind of negative transference. In other situations, a teacher may have a dislike of the child's parents or have unrealistic expectations of the child. It is not uncommon, especially in small cities, to have several siblings from the same family in sequence in the same classroom with the teacher. The teacher's experiences with the older sibling may influence their attitude and expectations of the younger sibling. A recent example from practice involved a 14-year-old girl who was the second child in a family where the older sibling was a very intelligent and successful brother. The patient, the girl, had the same teachers that the brother had had. Unfortunately, the teachers would from time to time make comments to the girl comparing her to her older brother in an unfavorable light, which left this girl, who already had some vulnerability to feeling inferior, with an even more severe inferiority complex and a reluctance to go to school.

As Erik Erikson so eloquently observed, "Good teachers, healthy teachers, relaxed teachers, teachers who can feel trusted and respected by the community, understand all this and can guide it. They know how to alternate play and work, games and study. They know how to recognize special efforts, how to encourage special gifts. They also know how to give a child time, and how to handle those children to whom school, for a while, is not important and rather a matter to endure than to enjoy; or the child to whom, for a while, other children are much more important than the teacher" (Erikson, 1959, p.87).

Extracurricular activities

In the average school environment, there usually are an array of extracurricular activities that can serve as positive forces in the child's social development and identity formation. As mentioned above in the elementary school years, budding talents, e.g. artistic, musical, or athletic talents, become more apparent and also contribute to the child's evolving identity and his/her role in society. Certain talents in one area may help to offset limitations in another. For instance, an 8-year-old boy with diagnosed reading/language difficulties was musically talented and also quite adept at spatial relationship problems. His enlightened school teacher, after consultation with the child's psychiatrist, found ways for the child to demonstrate his areas of strength (e.g. playing a musical piece in class) instead of having to compete in his areas of greatest weakness, writing reports.

Potential leadership skills recognized and encouraged through various school-related activities, e.g. a science club, newsletter editor, class officer, etc. can highlight a student's skill/talent in that particular direction and, for the student, offer a kind of "training ground" in a protected environment to exercise these special skills and talents.

Various club activities sponsored by the school offer a child an opportunity to learn about group functioning, political activity, e.g. advocacy, how to negotiate with authorities, pride in membership, etc. Most school-related "clubs" or groups have faculty advisors/mentors or preceptors who serve as role models for the child.

The school and family interface

The influence of the school on the developing child is profoundly influenced by the family's relationship to the school and to education in general. There is a considerable literature regarding the role of the family in the child's academic engagement and achievement. Parental attitudes towards the acquisition of knowledge, problem solving, intellectual curiosity, and study/work habits will shape a child's approach to the learning environment, which will, in turn, affect a child's integration/adaptation to the overall social environment of the school. Robert-Jay Green makes the observation, "… the family is the *original* and *primary* classroom experience in a child's life. A child's cognitive functioning and behavior in school reflect family interaction patterns – especially in task-orientated, instructional, and intellectual/achievement situations at home" (1995, p. 208).

Obviously, the child whose parent had a negative experience at school and whose parent, therefore, sees the school environment as hostile, nonsupportive, and/or irrelevant, will approach going to school with a very different attitude than the child whose parents have presented a positive, encouraging view of the school experience. Negative parental attitudes toward the school, from whatever source, dilute and undermine the child's ability to embrace the total school experience as a significant force for social development.

In addition, the parent/family's approach to education, to the value of mastering skills, academic achievement, using one's mind for problem solving, and most importantly, valuing intellectual curiosity, will have an influence on the child's interest in taking advantage of the academic setting. For many children, the parents' interest in or investment in their child's school experience is powerfully important. Parents who attend teacher-parent conferences, who visit school, who simply show interest in their child's school experience provide a framework for successful and enthusiastic involvement of the child throughout the school years. In addition, parental attitudes toward teachers often colored by their, the parents', own experience of school, is important to the child's relationship to his or her teacher. A parent's attitude toward teachers in general may help solidify one side of whatever ambivalence a child has toward school, either positive or negative. Additionally, if there is a bad match between parental expectations or personality and the particular teacher's expectations and personality, that conflict can put the child in a difficult position and affect the child's comfort in the classroom and in dealing with his/her teacher.

How parents deal with other parents of children in the same school affects a child's adaptation to school. When a child observes their parent becoming involved in parent/teacher association type meetings or collaborative efforts by parents to have influence on the school's structure (on its extracurricular activities, such as clubs, sports, etc., or on its curriculum directly), this observation can give a message to the child that the parents take the child's school experience very seriously. This behavior demonstrates that adults in general are supportive of this educational experience and that adults are collaborating in the best interests of their children. Parent participation, for instance, in the thorny and sometimes controversial issues such as sex education, politics, history, science, etc., is another way that children can see that adults are actively involved in their child's education. In some specific instances, parents as a group collaborating with schools can have a profound influence on major issues. For instance, the common problem of bullying in the school setting is best managed when parents and teachers collaborate to develop specific intervention plans to minimize harassment and bullying at the school.

Bullying at school

In the last decade, there has been increasing recognition of and research on bullying in schools, with a growing understanding of the long-term negative sequelae for both the victim and the perpetrator of bullying. In addition, the recognition that, in many cases, the perpetrators of serious violence in schools had been subjected to bullying by their peers, e.g. in the Columbine massacre, has promoted public awareness of the potential seriousness of bullying. This awareness has led to increased attention to the problem, e.g. research on epidemiology and causative factors, the development of prevention programs, and recommendations for the treatment of victims as well as perpetrators. Also, there has been increased public awareness and concern for early identification and intervention for the victims by bringing this public health issue to the attention of teachers, pediatricians and other childcare providers.

After Columbine, an investigation by the U.S. Secret Service of 41 school shootings, involved with 37 incidents (including Columbine), revealed that two-thirds of the perpetrators described feeling bullied or threatened by their peers. Another recently published study in the *Journal of the American Medical Association* examined all school associated violent deaths in the United States between 1994 and 1999 and found that homicide perpetrators in school were twice as likely as homicide victims to have been bullied by peers (Anderson et al., 2001).

Definition

Dan Olweus, in his seminal study, *Bullying at School: What We Know and What We Can Do* (1993, p. 9), defines bullying or victimization as "A student is being bullied or victimized when he or she is exposed, repeatedly and over time to negative actions on the part of one or more students." He elaborated that "… a negative action is when someone intentionally inflicts, or attempts to inflict, injury or discomfort upon another" (op. cit., p.9). This can be accomplished by direct physical means, e.g. hitting, punching, tripping, pinching, or through verbal or other non-directly physical means, e.g. shunning, making faces, spreading rumors, making hostile or negative gestures.

The prevalence estimates vary with age. Rates of victimization tend to decrease from elementary school through high school. Some studies show that approximately 8–10% of fourth to sixth graders report having been bullied very frequently, with as many as 25% having been bullied several times.

Gender differences

Boys tend to be bullied by other boys, whereas girls report being bullied by both boys and girls. In bullying between boys, physical assault is the most common mechanism whereas with girls, the bullying behavior tends to be less physical and more verbal/social. Girls tend to use name-calling, exclusion from the group (shunning), malicious gossip, and other forms of social rejection, e.g. reputation smearing. In general, bullying tends to be a one on one or at most two to three on one experience, often with many passive onlookers, who in most circumstances, do not intervene.

Children who are bullied do not tell teachers or other school personnel about their being bullied in part out of fear of reprisal. If they talk about it with anyone, they confide in parents or friends. Teachers, therefore, may not be aware that bullying is occurring.

Most bullying episodes take place at school, in the playground, at lunch, at study hall, recess, etc., and less so on the way to school or after school.

Characteristics of victims of bullying

Many victims of bullying are so-called "passive victims" who are often socially isolated, insecure, sensitive, and cautious. They have few friends and feel lonely. Having few friends and being socially isolated unfortunately denies the child the support and protection of peers, who often can prevent or intervene on behalf of the student. Children who have been victims of abuse or physical maltreatment are more at risk for being bullied, as are boys who are physically weaker. Although physical characteristics in general, e.g. wearing glasses, being overweight, red hair, freckles, etc., do not necessarily put a child at higher risk for being bullied, certain disabilities do appear to be associated with high risk, e.g. stammering, motor disturbances, especially cerebral palsy, muscular dystrophy, and other pareses.

Another category of victim is the "bully-victim," similar to the passive victim but who additionally shows more ADHD-like symptoms … impulsivity, motoric hyperactivity, problems with concentration, and quickness to retaliate. They also tend to bully younger students. This sub-group comprises a high-risk sample of youth, with a combination of characteristics of both passive victims and active bullies (Limber, 2000).

Characteristics of children who bully include impulsivity, short temper, difficulties dealing with frustration, social dominance, and the use of physical aggression as a problem solving technique. The school structure and atmosphere also play a role in the prevalence of bullying. Schools that have insufficient adult supervision, especially during recess, lunchbreak, playground, etc. are at increased risk for

Warning signs of victimization

Possible warning signs of bully victimization include:

- Returns from school with torn, damaged clothing, books, or belongings.
- Has unexplained cuts, bruises, and/or scratches.
- Has few, if any, friends.
- Appears afraid to go to school.
- Has lost interest in school work.
- Complains of headaches, stomach-aches.
- Has trouble sleeping and/or has frequent nightmares.
- Appears sad, depressed or moody.
- Appears anxious and/or has poor self-esteem.
- Is quiet, sensitive, and passive.

(from Limber, 2002)

problems with bullying. Additionally, if a school's culture is to deny or tolerate the negative impact of bullying, or if the school has no clear guidelines and instruction on the handling of pupil to pupil aggression, more episodes of bullying are likely to occur.

There are some significant associations between long-term outcomes for both victims of bullying and for bullies. Victims of bullying tend to have lower self-esteem and depression, even after the active bullying has ceased. How much the bullying contributes to this outcome and how much is related to pre-existing traits is not clear. Bullies, especially male bullies, tend to have higher rates of anti-social behavior, more encounters with the law, and more conduct disturbances.

A clinician evaluating or treating either a victim or a perpetrator of bullying is in a good position to collaborate with the school in promoting bullying prevention strategies, like the successful program developed by Olweus (1999). Since a high percentage of children who are bullied do not report the incident to school personnel, the child's clinician is in an excellent position (after obtaining consent from the parent and/or child) to discuss the situation with appropriate personnel at the child's school.

There are several excellent resources to help the clinician help the school:

1 The American Medical Association (2002) *Educational Forum on Adolescent Health: Youth Bullying*.
2 Olweus D, Limber S, Mihalic S (1999) *The Bullying Prevention Program, Blueprints for Violence Prevention*.
3 The Respect for All Project (2004) *Let's Get Real*, a video on bullying in middle schools, www.respectforallproject.org.

Violence in the school setting

Although there has been much publicity regarding violence in schools, and there have been episodes of serious violence in some schools, e.g. at Columbine, severe or mass violence in school settings is still relatively uncommon, and in the past few years has actually decreased. However, the level of violence in a particular school needs to be carefully assessed by the child's clinician. Schools in neighborhoods where there is considerable violence as a part of the culture most likely will reflect the neighborhood ethos. Again, because there is such variability from district to district and school to school it is extremely difficult to generalize about the role of violence in the school setting. For the clinician, getting to know the patient's school environment is very important when trying to develop an intervention plan for that patient. Some children appear to be able to adapt successfully to an environment where physical threats, force, and aggressivity are a part of the everyday culture. Other students, in part related to individual vulnerabilities, sensitivities or prior victim experience, will have a more difficult time adapting to more physical and aggressive atmospheres. Clinicians do need to be on the alert for those children who may be at risk for becoming seriously violent, e.g. research shows that victims of bullying who have few friends may have a tendency to become not only bullies, but potentially perpetrators of serious violence.

Of course, a child attending a school where there is a significant concern about violence on site will have a very different school experience from that of a child attending a school with little concern. The presence of police, metal detectors, and weapon searches creates an atmosphere of potential danger and restriction of freedom. This could be particularly problematic for the teenager, who typically and developmentally appropriately wants to feel free of adult constraint or interference. Alternatively, on the positive side, students may feel that the authorities in the adult world are trying to protect the students from harm and create a safe learning environment.

Children with handicaps and with special education needs

It is important for clinicians to have a general knowledge of the provisions for accommodating students with special needs, children with physical or emotional handicaps that interfere with the student's ability to learn in the regular school setting. All children in the United States are entitled to an appropriate, publicly financed education. In 1974, an important piece of federal legislation was passed, Public Law 94–142, which guaranteed that all children, regardless of handicap, are entitled to a free and public education, and that schools are responsible for making accommodations and providing support services that would enable the handicapped child to take advantage of this education. Since that time there have been a number of revisions and updates to this federal regulation. In 1990, Congress enacted the Individuals with Disabilities Education Act (IDEA). The following is a brief summary of the current (2005) status, presented here to help the clinician understand and navigate the system on behalf of the patient and the family.

The basic concepts supporting P.L. 94–142 remain intact, and all school districts are responsible for the implementation of the regulations. It is important to note that children in private schools are equally eligible for the benefits under these provisions, although the private schools are not responsible to provide the evaluation of the individual student for eligibility or to provide the services and accommodations necessary to enable that child to take advantage of the educational setting. The requirement is only in the public setting.

Basically, any child who has a physical/emotional problem that interferes with his/her ability to learn in the educational program is entitled to 1) an assessment of the child's difficulties that interfere with learning to determine if the child is eligible for services/special accommodations, and if eligible, 2) a comprehensive evaluation of the child's needs and then the development of an Individualized Education Plan (IEP) that is implemented by the school. The parent or school personnel can request an evaluation for an IEP. Once the request is initiated, schools have a prescribed time limit in which to evaluate the request, provide an assessment of the child and to develop and implement an IEP. Not all requests for a full evaluation are granted. There needs to be a clear indication that the child's difficulties significantly interfere with his/her learning, or that there is a discrepancy between the child's innate capacity to learn and his/her achievement. The clinician can play a significant role by alerting parents to this entitlement for their child and by encouraging parents to request an evaluation for an IEP. The clinician can be even more helpful by providing input into the IEP process or by attending the IEP meeting itself. Although the federal mandates apply to all age children (now 0–18), each school district has its own implementation strategy and the zero to three population is handled differently from state to state. Therefore, it is important for clinicians to acquaint themselves with the workings of the school administration in their area. Often, in the school district there is a department of special education that oversees this process.

In addition to the above-mentioned federal mandate, there are other federal and local regulations that require school districts to make accommodations for children with handicapping disabilities in order for the child to benefit from the school setting. One of the important aspects of the federal regulation is that children with handicaps must be schooled in the least restrictive environment. This has been interpreted to mean that, whenever possible, children with handicaps should be schooled in "regular" or mainstreamed classrooms. There has been a movement to move children who have been in separate, special classes, back into regular classrooms, a movement called "mainstreaming," or more recently, "inclusion." This movement has not been without controversy. Proponents of "mainstreaming" advocate that it is beneficial for students with handicaps to be placed with non-handicapped students, providing the handicapped students with more "typical" role models. Opponents contend that "mainstreaming" is detrimental to both groups, in that regular students are held back by having to accommodate to the needs of handicapped students, and that handicapped students feel out of step and stigmatized when they are not able to keep up with or perform at the same level as "typical" students. Clinicians for the individual student can play a role in advocating for what the clinician and family think is best for the child.

Children who are eligible for special education services may be provided an array of interventions ranging from individual tutoring, to special help within the regular classroom, to some part of the day in a "special education" classroom, to full-time special education class, including enrollment in non-public schools that specialize in the teaching of children with certain handicaps. These options represent progressively restrictive methods of interventions. Support services, e.g. speech and language therapy, psychotherapy, occupational therapy, etc. may also be provided under the regulations, if such therapy is deemed necessary to allow the child to benefit from the educational experience. The requirement to provide the education in the "least restrictive environment" applies in all cases.

Again, as is emphasized throughout this chapter, clinicians providing services to children can benefit significantly in the evaluation/diagnostic process through an understanding of the day-to-day school environment surrounding that child. Knowledge of this environment can then inform the clinician as to how to intervene to optimize the academic and psychosocial influence of the school on each individual child.

Annotated bibliography

Comer J (2003) Transforming the lives of children. In: Elias MJ, Arnold H, Steiger-Hussey C (eds.) *EQ+IQ = Best Leadership Practices for Caring and Successful Schools.* Thousand Oaks, Corwin.
An excellent review, by a national expert, on the role that schools play in the lives of children and what can be done to enhance the school environment, bringing in parents, community leaders and changing the atmosphere in the school.

Mattison, RE (2000) School consultation: a review of research on issues unique to the school environment. *J Am Acad Child Adolesc Psychiatry*, 394(4):402–413.
This review complements this chapter in that it looks at the research over ten years in four areas important to school functioning and specific student school problems … absenteeism, disciplinary issues, retention (non-promotion), and dropping out.

Olweus D (1993) *Bullying at School: What We Know and What We Can Do.* Oxford, Blackwell.

A thorough review, with research on epidemiology, demographics, victim and perpetrator characteristics, and with suggestions for prevention, by one of the international researchers in the field of bullying.

Smith EP, Boutte GS, Zigler E, Finn-Stevenson M (2004) Opportunities for schools to promote resilience in children and youth. In: Maton KI, Schellenbach CJ, Leadbeater BJ, Solarz AL (eds) *Investing in Children, Youth, Families and Communities: Strength-based Research and Policy.* Washington, American Psychological Association.

An excellent discussion of the role of schools on the development of children, and the important connections between social and emotional factors in the learning process. An extensive and useful bibliography.

CHAPTER 19

Child and Adolescent Sexuality

Debbie R. Carter, MD and Sarah Herbert, MD

Overview of sex and gender

Sexuality is an essential aspect of human development that is expressed in varying ways throughout the lifespan, including in childhood and adolescence. Yet, childhood sexuality, and even adolescent sexuality have not been subjects easily discussed or researched until recent years. This chapter will focus on significant issues and problems in child and adolescent sexuality in the context of what is known regarding normative development during these years.

Influences on the expression of child and adolescent sexuality are multiple, including biologic, psychologic, social, and cultural. The development of child and adolescent sexuality must be understood in the context of all of these influences.

Sexual differentiation

The biologic or intrinsic influences on sex and gender begin with the difference in sex chromosomes. In the first few weeks after conception, the anatomic structures that will become the internal and external genitals (the gonadal ridges, internal ducts, and external genitals) are the same in both male and female embryos (Cohen-Kettenis and Pfafflin, 2003). When a Y chromosome is present, the SRY gene, located on this chromosome, induces the undifferentiated gonadal ridge to become a testis. In the absence of a Y chromosome, the embryonic gonadal ridge develops into ovaries provided both X chromosomes are present. Around 7 weeks of gestation, the testes will start to produce testosterone and anti-Mullerian hormone. Without this, the fetus would develop along phenotypically female lines. These hormones lead the Wolffian ducts to differentiate into the internal male genitalia. In the absence of functional testes, the Mullerian ducts will develop into the uterus, fallopian tubes, and the upper part of the vagina. The external genitals also develop from identical structures in the male and female. In males,

after 3 months' gestation, testosterone and dihydrotestosterone (DHT) direct the genital tubercle to develop into the penis and the genital swellings to fuse to form the scrotum. In females, without testosterone, these same structures become the clitoris and labia.

In most cases, this development proceeds normally and results in a neonate who is clearly male or female. When there are abnormalities in this process of sexual differentiation, the child's biologic sex may be ambiguous and clarification needed at birth. For example, in the case of a female child with congenital adrenal hyperplasia (CAH), the fetus has normal chromosomes, but has been exposed *in utero* to adrenal androgens that masculinize her external genitalia. An enlarged clitoris or fused labia may lead to some confusion at birth as to her biologic sex. There are other situations where a disorder of sexual differentiation may not be recognized at birth and only become evident at puberty. Such an example might be complete androgen insensitivity syndrome. At birth the infant, even though genetically XY, looks phenotypically completely female. However, when she does not go through menarche at puberty, it becomes obvious something is different and further evaluation is needed.

Development of gender identity and gender role

It is clear that gonadal hormones in mammals influence the development and programming of the central nervous system. While the extent to which this occurs in humans is still unclear, these hormones may well have a significant impact. The development and expression of sexuality result from the complex interaction of both intrinsic (or biologic) factors and extrinsic factors. The extrinsic influences include the family environment, responses of peers, racial/ethnic views of sexuality, and the ways in which our society and culture view sex and gender. Thus, there are many ways in which children learn what are considered to be typical expressions of gender.

The biologic factors noted in the previous section on sexual differentiation, along with information from the external world, are then incorporated by the child into a self-perception of being male or female. This is referred to as gender identity. An initial awareness of gender can be observed in children at an average age of 18 months. Gender identity in most children is established by 2½–3 years of age (Money and Ehrhardt, 1972; Cohen-Kettenis and Pfafflin, 2003). Gender constancy, however, develops in stages. First, children learn to identify their own or others' sex (gender labeling or gender identity). Then they learn that gender is stable, or unchangeable, over time (gender stability). Finally, they learn that gender is permanent and not dependent on appearance or activities (gender consistency) (Cohen-Kettenis and Pfafflin, 2003). There is some controversy regarding at what age children reach this last stage. Some have found that children by age 3 or 4 have completed gender constancy, while others have found that even 7-year-olds may not have completed this stage. For the most part, there is agreement that 5- to 7-year-olds will make consistent and systematic use of genital information as a criterion for classification (Goldman and Goldman, 1982).

Younger children, even those as young as 3 years and up, are aware of gender stereotypes. This knowledge accumulates rapidly. Children's thoughts about sex-typed traits and behavior are fairly rigid initially, but they begin to have more flexibility after age 7 (Cohen-Kettenis and Pfafflin, 2003).

Gender role identity is the child's psychologically constructed self-image of his/her femininity or masculinity. This identity is dynamic and thought to be altered by the child's growth and development. The various groups and environments with which the child comes into contact, including the family, peers, and cultural institutions, are believed to enhance or challenge the individual's expression of this gender role identity by accepting or rejecting roles the child performs. For example, some activities and careers in the United States have been viewed as primarily male pursuits. Women who wished to engage in these careers were either not allowed or discouraged from doing so. Another example would be the cultural imperative that women athletes appear feminine.

Gender identity and gender role behaviors were previously believed to be largely determined by interactions with the environment. Thus, they were considered to be subject to alteration at least up until the age of 3. Evidence from children with disorders of sexual differentiation, among others, suggests that gender identity and gender role behaviors may not be as completely determined by extrinsic factors or as malleable as was previously thought (Diamond and Sigmundson, 1997; Reiner and Gearhart, 2004). Girls exposed to androgens *in utero* and postnatally clearly have a higher energy level and behaviors that may be more stereotypically associated with boys. They do not, however, appear to question their gender as female.

PEARLS & PERILS

Knowing appropriate definitions of sexuality helps the physician approach sexuality with children and adolescents from a developmental perspective.

- Biologic sex – chromosomes, gonads, internal genitalia, external genitalia, sex hormones, secondary sex characteristics.
- Gender identity – person's basic sense of self as male or female; generally consistent with biologic sex.
- Gender role – person's behaviors, attitudes, and personality traits that a society in a particular culture and historical period designates as masculine or feminine.
- Gender role identity – person's self-designation as masculine or feminine.
- Sexual orientation – pattern of a person's erotic responsiveness to persons of the same, opposite, or either sex.
- Sexual identity – person's self-identification as gay, lesbian, heterosexual, or bisexual; sexual behaviors may not be consistent with self-identification.

Male pseudohermaphrodites with 5-alpha-reductase deficiency do not have the enzyme necessary to convert testosterone to dihydrotestosterone, and thus their external genitalia are not masculinized *in utero*. They do, however, have testes, demonstrating they have been exposed to normal levels of testosterone *in utero* and postnatally, and they have normal internal male genitalia. At puberty, with the increase in testosterone, they begin to develop male secondary sex characteristics. Many of these individuals reportedly change from having a female identity as their gender of rearing to a male identity once their bodies begin to masculinize in the presence of testosterone produced by the testes at puberty (Imperato-McGinley et al., 1979). Likewise, in a recent follow-up report, Reiner and Gearhart (2004) reported that a significant number of biologic males with cloacal exstrophy who were being reared as girls, declared themselves to be male or chose to revert to a male identity during later childhood or adolescence. Both examples provide evidence that intrinsic factors, along with extrinsic factors, play a role in gender identity and gender role behaviors.

Normative aspects of sexual behavior in children

There have been few studies of normative sexual behaviors in children. The reasons for this observation are multiple. First, our culture does not readily acknowledge that sexuality is a normal part of childhood. Therefore, getting permission to observe the sexuality of children or to ask them questions about sex has been a daunting task (Bullough, 2004). Often, sexual behaviors in this age group are described only as pathology or evidence of previous sexual abuse. Since very young children may not be as articulate or aware of their behavior, mothers have been questioned about their children's sexual behaviors. This may be helpful in assessing the youngest children, but parent reports are not as useful for determining normative sexual activities for school-aged children. Children learn quickly what their families consider to be unacceptable sexual behaviors and are adept at hiding these activities as they get older. Retrospective reports of childhood sexual behaviors gathered from adults may provide useful information, but also may suffer from the limitations of memory that limit most retrospective reports (Friedrich et al., 1998). What little information is available on normative sexual behavior in children will be described below.

Infants and children can be observed exhibiting what appears to be pleasure when engaged in self-stimulating activities such as thumb sucking and masturbation. During diaper changes, children seem to enjoy having their genitals cleaned and may explore their genitals and anus on their own. Children exhibit genital pride in play activities such as "doctor." Activities considered to be evidence of normative sexual behavior in preschool children may be seen in Pearls & perils .

When children enter elementary school, same-sex peer groups tend to enforce gender role behavior boundaries. There is little tolerance for individuals, particularly boys, who do not fit gender stereotypes. Sex play may occur with one or several peers or may occur in groups that engage in games such as "truth or dare." Normative sexual activity in children is generally consensual and most often occurs between peers of the same age with ongoing friendly relationships. The range of behaviors is wide and may include touching, peeking, kissing, hugging, and even pretending intercourse (Friedrich et al., 1998; Friedrich and Barbesi, 2002). Up to 3% of children under age 12 engage in intercourse. Although children may be embarrassed if they are discovered by an adult, they do not always experience shame or guilt. Emotions attached to the experiences are generally lighthearted and playful. Furthermore, when they are directed by the adult to stop the behavior, children generally do stop, at least in the presence of the adult. Children involved in these exploratory sexual activities do not seem overly preoccupied with sexual issues, and show evidence of having other interests.

The household emotional and sexual climate in which children are being reared may contribute to the expression of children's sexual behaviors. Households vary in how freely they discuss sexuality, how uninhibited they are about touch and nudity, how much respect there is for physical and emotional space, and how much power and sexuality are linked (Johnson 1993, 2000). Activities considered to be evidence of

normative sexual behavior in school-aged children may be seen in Pearls & perils.

Pearls

It is important to know what sexual behaviors are normal at various developmental stages to adequately deal with sexuality in children and adolescents. The following are sexual behaviors that one would expect to see at various stages of development.

Preschool

- Genital exploration.
- Penile erections and vaginal lubrication.
- Touching of others' sex parts.
- Masturbation for pleasure; may experience orgasm.
- Sex play with peers and siblings, including exhibition of genitals, exploration of own and others' genitals, attempted intercourse.
- Enjoyment of nudity, taking off clothes in public; watching people who are nude.
- Use of elimination words with peers.
- Asks about genitals, breasts, intercourse, babies.
- Plays house, acting out Mommy and Daddy roles.
- Puts objects in own genitals or rectum for curiosity and exploration.

School-aged

- Sex games with peers and siblings.
- Role plays with sex fantasy.
- Kissing.
- Mutual masturbation.
- Simulated intercourse.
- Playing "doctor."
- Masturbation in private.
- Modesty, embarrassment, attempts to hide sex games or masturbation from adults.
- May fantasize or dream about sex.
- Interest in media sex.
- Use of sexual language with peers.
- Talks about having boyfriend/girlfriend.
- Interest in breeding behavior of animals.

[Gordon and Schroeder (1995) *Sexuality: A Developmental Approach to Problems*; Johnson TC (2000) *Understanding Children's Sexual Behaviors: What's Natural and Healthy*.]

Perils

- Pathologizing normal sexual behaviors is a common problem in medicine.
- Attitudes toward child and adolescent sexuality vary widely.
- The clinician's beliefs about what is normal and healthy with respect to issues of sex and gender may vary dramatically from those of the families who come to them with concerns.

Special issues in child sexuality

Inappropriate sexual behaviors

At times, children exhibit sexual behaviors that may indicate a problem. The Consider consultation when … box reviews sexual behaviors in children that may indicate the need to seek the assistance of a mental health clinician. While they are not necessarily pathologic, they may indicate a need for

CONSIDER CONSULTATION WHEN …

- The children engaged in the sexual behaviors do not have an ongoing mutual play relationship.
- Sexual behaviors which are engaged in by children of different ages or developmental levels.
- Sexual behaviors which are out of balance with other aspects of the child's life or interests.
- Children who seem to have too much knowledge about sexuality and behave in ways more consistent with adult sexual expression.
- Sexual behaviors which are significantly different than those of other same-sex children.
- Sexual behaviors which continue in spite of consistent and clear requests to stop.
- Children who appear unable to stop themselves from engaging in sexual activities.
- Children's sexual behaviors which are eliciting complaints from other children and/or adversely affecting other children.
- Children's sexual behaviors which are directed at adults who feel uncomfortable receiving them.
- Children (4 years of age and older) who do not understand their rights or the rights of others in relation to sexual contact.
- Sexual behaviors which progress in frequency, intensity, or intrusiveness over time.
- When fear, anxiety, deep shame or intense guilt is associated with the sexual behaviours.
- Children who engage in extensive, persistent mutually agreed upon adult-type sexual behaviors with other children.
- Children who manually stimulate or have oral or genital contact with animals.
- Children who sexualize non-sexual things, or interactions with others, or relationships.
- Sexual behaviors which cause physical or emotional pain or discomfort to self or others.
- Children who use sex to hurt others.
- When verbal and/or physical expressions of anger precede, follow, or accompany the sexual behaviour.
- Children who use distorted logic to justify their sexual actions ("She didn't say no").
- When coercion, force, bribery, manipulation or threats are associated with sexual behaviour.

KEY CLINICAL QUESTIONS

The following questions can elicit specifics of sexual concerns that a parent or caretaker has about a child.
- *Describe the behavior about which you are concerned.*
- *Where, when, and with whom does it occur?*
- *What are your expectations of your child in the area of sexuality?*
- *Has anything stressful been going on in your child's life?*
- *How are sexual issues and behaviors handled in your family?*
- *Are there behavior problems in areas other than sexual behavior?*
- *What have you done so far to try to deal with these problem behaviors?*
- *How closely are you or others able to monitor your child?*

(adapted from Friedrich and Barbesi, 2002)

further evaluation to determine if there is a significant problem.

When there is concern regarding sexual behaviors in a child, the physician can begin with questioning the parents or caretakers using the key questions outlined in the box above.

When there is concern about a child's inappropriate sexual behavior with others, it is important to gather as much collateral information as possible. Information from the following list should be included.

- Number and types of sexual behaviors (past and current) (alone and others).
- History of sexual behavior problems.
- Motivation for sexual behavior.
- Other child's description, response to, and feelings about the activity.
- Use of trickery, bribery, coercion, force.
- Affect of the child regarding sexuality.
- Full developmental history (history of abuse, placements outside the home, protective services involvement).
- All legal involvement, with records from court, probation officers, and other institutions or authorities.
- Behavior in school or daycare.
- Psychiatric, legal, abuse, and substance abuse history of all family members.
- Emotional and sexual climate in home.

Sexual behaviors in children that appear to indicate reason for concern may be divided into four different groups (Johnson, 1993). In group I, children are involved in sexual exploration that would be considered natural and healthy in our culture. In group II are behaviors that are described as sexually reactive. Group II behaviors are generally seen in children who have a history of exposure to pornography, live in households with excessive sexual stimulation (including watching parents, older siblings, or too much explicit sex on television), or are victims of sexual abuse. These children focus on sexuality to a degree that is out of proportion to the attention their peers give to sexuality. There is a compulsive quality to their sexual behaviors, either alone or with same-age peers. They may not stop behaviors in the presence of an adult when asked, but they do not force or coerce. These children may feel shame, guilt, or extreme anxiety about sex.

In group III, children are mutually engaged in the full gamut of adult sexual behaviors. Children in this group use sexual behavior to relate to their peers. Their behavior is more extensive than that of children in group II. Preoccupied with sex, these children generally engage in sexual behaviors with same-age peers and purposefully keep their activities secret from nearby adults. They may entice or persuade their peers to become involved in sexual behaviors. Their affect is matter of fact and without shame, guilt, or aggression. These children feel distrustful of adults, most likely because of a history of severe physical, emotional, and sexual abuse (Johnson, 1993).

Children in Group IV are sexual offenders. They are preoccupied with sex and coerce or aggressively force others of any age into sexual activity. Sexual behaviors may be impulsive and compulsive, increasing in severity over time. Additionally, these children usually have numerous other behavior problems. It is rare that these individuals feel empathy for their victims. They often experience rage, loneliness, and fear. Because of their life experiences, these emotions are associated with sex and aggression. Roughly 25% of these children and adolescents are girls (Johnson, 1993). They are at great risk for continuing to develop as sexual perpetrators, as they generally will not stop their behaviors without specialized, intensive treatment.

Gender variant behaviors in childhood/gender identity concerns

Gender variant behaviors and identity may become evident in children as young as 18–36 months of age. These children may show significant preoccupation with gender identity and gender role behaviors associated with the opposite gender. Manifestations may include choice of toys, fantasy roles assumed in dress-up and role-playing behaviors, choice of playmates, choice of name, and type of clothing. Boys with gender variant behaviors may avoid rough-and-tumble play, while girls may show a higher level of activity more traditionally associated with boys. The child may verbalize a wish to be a member of the opposite sex, may believe he or she is a member of the opposite sex, or believe that this will occur when he grows up. Both boys and girls may wish to have genitals of the opposite sex or may wish to be rid of the ones they have.

Children who engage in cross-gender behaviors and articulate discomfort in the assigned biologic sex have been labeled as having gender identity disorder (GID) (DSM-IV,

2000). This diagnosis has become quite controversial in recent years, with some individuals calling for its removal from DSM-V. The rationale for its removal is because only a very small percentage of these children actually persist in their desire to be or live as the opposite sex, despite articulating this when much younger. It appears that the gender identity issues resolve with time for the majority of these children. When they have been followed into their adolescent or adult years, very few have a transgender identity. Instead, they appear to have a homosexual or bisexual sexual orientation (Minter, 1999; Pleak, 1999; Zucker and Bradley, 1995).

Boys are referred for treatment for GID more often than girls. Thus, more information is available about boys with GID. Parents may not seek assistance for girls until they are older, perhaps because our culture tolerates more latitude in gender role behaviors for girls than for boys. All children with gender identity disorder or gender variant behaviors do not verbalize a desire to change gender. Older children and adolescents, because of their recognition of the stigma involved, are less likely to do so.

The etiology of gender identity disorder or gender variant behaviors is unclear. Biologic and psychodynamic factors have been explored. There is some research in the area of prenatal effects of hormones including evidence from the study of girls with congenital adrenal hyperplasia and boys with androgen-insensitivity syndrome. It has also been noted that some extremely feminine boys are quite physically attractive and are often described as having the potential to "make a beautiful girl" by strangers. It is possible that parents may subtly change the child's appearance to be consistent with the other gender, although studies find that parents do not do this because of an explicit wish for a child of a specific gender. Children with GID may have difficulties in their relationships with their parents. However, it is not clear what the etiology of the disturbance is. Traditionally, mother and son have been described as "enmeshed" and the son's femininity has been ascribed to maternal closeness. However, others have postulated that the son's femininity comes first, and the father's discomfort with having a feminine son results in the father's (and others') rejection or withdrawal from the child. This then leads the mother to step in and try to compensate for the rejection or withdrawal of the father and others.

The evaluation of a child with gender issues should include attention to the following information: statements the child makes about his/her gender, cross-dressing, choice of toys, role play, peer relations, mannerisms and voice, anatomic dysphoria, and rough-and-tumble play.

Treatment for children who show signs of cross-gender identification is controversial. Initially, treatment was directed at prevention of homosexuality or transgenderism. There was little evidence to support this since the gender issues resolved in children diagnosed in childhood whether

Gender identity issues
- The majority of children with gender identity issues in childhood will not be transgender.
- The gender identity issues generally fade in the school-age years.
- The most common outcome by adolescence or early adulthood is homosexuality or bisexuality.

or not they received treatment. Some now argue that there should be no reason for treatment based on this, diagnosis since the outcome is generally homosexuality or bisexuality, and homosexuality is no longer considered evidence of psychopathology. Others have suggested that treatment is beneficial in helping children cope with emotional responses to rejection or other psychopathology (Zucker and Bradley, 1995). Menvielle (1998) has suggested other equally important goals of treatment. He recommends that professionals do not contribute to these children's struggles with self-esteem by conveying the message that their identity is unacceptable. The focus in this intervention is primarily on the parents. Parents are helped to grieve the loss of the ideal child they had hoped for, and they are encouraged to develop a positive parenting style with information, guidance, and emotional support. They are given guidance in helping their child negotiate social pressures, and encouraged to foster their child's unique interests and talents even though gender variant (Menvielle, 1998).

Sexual differentiation disorders

When sexual differentiation disorders occur, choices may have to be made regarding assignment of gender. Medical professionals and parents make the best decision possible, but in some cases it may be wrong. Later in the child's school years or adolescence it may become obvious that the gender assigned at birth was not the most appropriate for that particular child. Professionals involved in the care of these children should be aware of this possibility and available to assist the child and parents with issues regarding sex or gender that arise. Such issues may involve what to do if the child is clearly unhappy with his/her gender, declares that he/she is the gender opposite the one assigned, or if the child shows gender role behaviors much more stereotypically assigned to the opposite gender (Cohen-Kettenis and Pfäfflin, 2003; Diamond and Sigmundson, 1997; Meyer-Bahlberg, 1993).

In the past, secrecy about the child's status at birth was the norm, but today there is more openness. Professionals who work in this field now suggest that children be told about their status in childhood in developmentally appropriate ways (Herbert, 2001). There is a role for medical professionals to assist parents and children in talking about these issues and planning how to cope with problems as they arise.

Puberty and adolescent sexual development

Intrinsic and extrinsic factors clearly play important roles as children develop at puberty and into their adolescent years. The major intrinsic influences are the hormonal changes associated with sexual maturation. Increased production of adrenal sex steroids (adrenarche) begins approximately 2 years before the maturation of the hypothalamic-pituitary-gonadal axis (Joffee, 1999). Adrenal androgens are responsible for the development of pubic hair and linear growth in both boys and girls (Joffee, 1999).

Next, the hypothalamus and pituitary gland begin to secrete increased amounts of gonadotropin releasing hormone (GnRH), follicle-stimulating hormone (FSH), and lutenizing hormone (LH). As a result of the increased secretion of pituitary hormones, testosterone in boys and estradiol in girls increase progressively. Growth hormone secretion becomes established mid-puberty. On average, puberty lasts 3 to 4 years. For girls, the average age for the onset of breast buds, the first sign of pubertal development, is approximately 10 years of age, with a range of 8–13 years. Breast buds before age 8 used to be considered precocious puberty, but a study of 17,000 girls from MDs' offices revealed that 15% of African-American girls and 5% of Caucasian girls had breast bud development by age 7 (Joffee, 1999). In response to the effect of FSH, ovarian growth occurs approximately 1 year earlier than breast budding. Ovarian estrogen stimulates breast development, thickening of the vaginal mucosa, vascularization and pigmentation of the labia majora, uterine and clitoral enlargement, as well as an increase in body fat (Joffee 1999).

Boys enter puberty approximately 1 year after girls, with enlargement of the testes at age 11 years, with a range of 9–14 years. In boys, pituitary gonadotropins and growth hormone lead to greater muscularity. Testosterone secretion in boys leads to enlargement of the epididymis, seminal vesicles, and prostate gland, penis, and scrotum. It also contributes to the growth of pubic, axillary, and facial hair, deepening of the voice, increased libido, and increased muscle mass (Joffee, 1999).

Learning how to cope with these physical changes emotionally and psychologically is one of the tasks of adolescence. Early puberty in girls and delayed puberty in boys can be associated with psychologic and social difficulties. The adolescent girl may feel as if she is receiving undue attention from potential romantic objects, thus setting her apart from peers. Delayed puberty in a boy may leave him feeling inadequate and having lower social status than male peers developing more quickly.

Adolescence is the time when young people begin to explore more intimate relationships with peers. It is not unusual for this exploration to involve sexual activity. This is the age at which many individuals begin to understand their sexual orientation. While attraction to the opposite sex proceeds as expected for many young people, sexual orientation becomes more of an issue when it is not what the adolescent expected.

Sexual orientation refers to the gender to which the individual is attracted for the development of intimate attachments. Cognitions, affects, fantasies, and behaviors are all components of sexual orientation. Heterosexual is used to refer to individuals primarily oriented toward members of the opposite gender; homosexual if they are oriented toward members of their same gender; and bisexual if they are oriented toward individuals of both genders. Straight, gay, lesbian, and bisexual are terms by which individuals come to identify their sexual orientation, which is also sometimes referred to as sexual identity or sexual orientation identity. How individuals identify may not be entirely consistent with their orientation, particularly during the adolescent years when young people are still coming to understand their identities. There may be some confusion or experimentation about sexual orientation at this time. However, some young people are very sure of their homosexual orientation during adolescence. They are likely to feel alienated from their health-care providers if awareness is not taken seriously.

Clearly, there is a genetic component to sexual orientation, since twin studies have shown that same-sex orientation occurs more often in identical twins than in fraternal twins or in non-twin brothers. Similar heritability has also been shown in female homosexuality. Studies have also explored the effects of prenatal exposure to sex hormones, enzyme deficiencies in steroid synthesis pathways, or neuroanatomic differences in addition to the role of genetics. However, no conclusion has been reached as to the origin of homosexual orientation.

Normative aspects of adolescent sexuality

Adolescent sexual development and sexual behavior occur in the context of all the changes that are going on in the realms of physical, cognitive, and emotional development. This is a time of significant self-discovery for teenagers.

Early adolescence (ages 11–14 years) is a time of psychosocial change when separation from parents begins and peer group norms begin to exert more influence. With all the pubertal changes, it is not surprising that adolescents of this age focus on bodily changes and compare their changes with those of same-sex peers. Young adolescents are preoccupied with the normality of their sexual thoughts, feelings, impulses, and behaviors. Since formal operational thinking is just beginning, they may not be good at considering

the potential harmful consequences of their behaviors. At this stage, there is an increase in sexual drive and sexual behavior, presumably related to the increases in gonadal hormone levels that occur at puberty. Masturbation may become a more significant activity. Curiosity may spark sexual experimentation with peers, sometimes with same-sex peers. There may be crushes on important adult figures in the adolescent's life, some of whom may be adults of the same gender. While conversations may involve a good deal of sexual innuendo, the majority of very young adolescents are not having sexual intercourse. According to the latest data (CDC, 2004), only 7.4% of teenagers surveyed in the Youth Risk Behavior Survey (YRBS) had had intercourse before the age of 13. By 9th grade, however, approximately a third of high school students had had intercourse. These statistics varied widely depending on gender and ethnicity (CDC, 2004).

As puberty progresses, masturbation may be (re)discovered. Many older children and adolescents masturbate. In an Australian study of high school students, 58.2% of boys and 42.7% of girls reported having masturbated. A much higher percentage of boys reported masturbating three or more times a week than was seen with the girls (Feldmann and Middleman, 2002). Yet cultural and religious opposition to masturbation may create significant feelings of guilt and fear. Thus, this safe, developmentally normal form of sexual expression may be rejected in favor of sexual intercourse, especially when surrounding adults are ambivalent or intolerant about masturbation. A recent study looked at how parents and adolescent children communicate about sex (Miller et al., 1998). The researchers noted that masturbation was the least likely sexual subject to be discussed between parent and child. Yet masturbation may help an adolescent learn valuable information about his/her own sexual responses and relieve sexual urges while postponing sexual intercourse.

In middle adolescence (ages 14–17), puberty is generally complete. Although the adolescent is already physically mature and able to reproduce, psychosocial development is still progressing. Major issues at this time include conflicts with parents around limits and a need for independence. Peer influence and conformity to peer norms reach their peak, and adolescents focus on gaining peer approval. Sex-

---

Masturbation

Pearl
- Masturbation is a safe, developmentally normal and educational sexual activity.

Peril
- Avoidance of discussions about masturbation may actually contribute to earlier sexual intercourse.

PEARLS & PERILS

ual behaviors increase significantly at this stage; yet there is no permission for the teenager to express sexuality in an adult manner. Risk-taking behaviors such as driving, substance use (nicotine, alcohol, and drugs) and sexual activity increase and may be fostered by the adolescent's feeling of invulnerability and need to experiment.

According to the Youth Risk Behavior Survey (CDC, 2004), 46.7% of high school students surveyed nationwide had had sexual intercourse during their lifetime, with small differences reported between boys and girls. The percentage of students who had had sexual intercourse increased from a low of 32.8% of ninth graders to a total of 61.6% of 12th graders. The percentage of high school students who had had sexual intercourse in the 3-month period preceding the survey, and thus were classified as currently sexually active, was less: 34.6% of girls and 33.8% of boys. Thus, a significant percentage of young people have engaged in intercourse, but the frequency of doing so varies with age and gender.

Late adolescence begins at age 17 or 18 and lasts through the early 20s. Generally, by this stage of adolescence, the young person's sexual identity is well-established and he/she has developed an ability to form and maintain mutually satisfying intimate relationships. Since formal operational thinking may be established by this age, the young person may have a better ability to plan for his/her future and act in ways that involve less risk-taking.

Most of the data regarding sexual activity in the adolescent years have focused on sexual intercourse. Unfortunately there are few data on other types of sexual behavior, such as masturbation, oral sex, and anal sex. For boys, sexual intercourse or active anal intercourse may be viewed as an enhancement of their masculine image. Girls may tend to view sexual activity as an expression of greater intimacy in a romantic relationship. Other areas of attention regarding adolescent sexuality should include information about sexual fantasies, sexual curiosity, sexual health and education, and the process of developing a healthy sexual identity (Ponton and Judice, 2004). Adolescents may be unaware of the range of normal human sexual responses or of the common occurrence among adults and adolescents of less-than-satisfactory sexual encounters. They may tend not to discuss these concerns because of embarrassment about revealing something they consider a personal failure.

The child's family and ethnocultural heritage also significantly impact sexual development in the adolescent years. An example may be useful in illustrating the effect of family and cultural norms on sexuality. For many children reared in African-American families, sexuality is viewed as a positive and natural part of life. Damaging myths about African-American sexuality may, however, promote antagonistic relationships. Black men may be portrayed as animalistic and oversexed. Black women may be portrayed in conflicting stereotypes. Sometimes they appear loose and exotic, and at other times they are shown to be domineering or nur-

turing but sexless. Children and adolescents exposed to such negative models often struggle to establish a self-identity in which sexuality is a positive aspect of the personality.

Another significant influence on adolescent sexual activity is the way in which sex has been represented in our media-driven culture. Images of young people and movie stars in sexually provocative poses are highly popular advertising ploys.

Assessment of adolescent sexual behavior

The assessment of a young person's sexual behavior first involves the usual history gathering. Routine visits should include questions about sexual development and sexuality concerns. Particularly with adolescents, it is important to ensure accurate and appropriate levels of confidentiality. It is reasonable to promise that private information will not be shared with parents. However, confidentiality cannot be promised in situations where child protective services (CPS) must be notified. It is important to rule out sexual abuse and sexual assault with adolescent patients of either gender.

"Am I normal?" is a question that is common to most adolescents, even if it is not readily verbalized to parents or health professionals. Knowledge and understanding about puberty and human reproduction should be assessed, and misinformation corrected. Reassurance is often greatly appreciated. Adolescents should be allowed to express any concerns about physical developmental changes, masturbation, dating behavior, sexual feelings, and pressures related to intimacy. Health professionals should determine the adolescent's usual sources of sexuality information, the extent of communication about sexuality within the family, and opportunities for formal sexual education.

Questions about sexuality should be asked in an orientation-neutral manner, and they should be repeated if the patient is seen on an ongoing basis. Questions such as, "Have you had sex with another person?" and "Are you involved with males, females, or both?" indicate a willingness to discuss homosexual as well as heterosexual activity. Furthermore, the recognition that heterosexuality is not assumed can decrease the fear many gay and lesbian adolescents feel about revealing their sexual orientation to a physician. Gay and lesbian adolescents are at a higher risk for poor developmental adjustment as they go through the process of coming out. Almost all gay and lesbian adolescents are at least initially spurned by their families when they disclose their sexual orientation. Many also lose friends and are the victims of verbal or physical abuse from their peers. There may be a decline in school performance. If these teenagers feel unsupported, they are ultimately at risk for substance abuse, running away, and suicide attempts. Gay and lesbian youth are statistically overrepresented in the homeless population.

Assessment of the extent of adolescent sexual risk-taking should include questions regarding not just sexual intercourse, but the kinds of intimate sexual behaviors in which they have been involved. How frequently they have engaged in sexual behaviors and with how many partners of each gender are relevant to assessing risk. Potential exposure to sexually transmitted diseases, knowledge and use of any preventive measures (both boys and girls), and a history of any health consequences are all relevant in taking the history. Health consequences of risky sexual behaviors such as infections, pregnancy, genital injury, or abuse should be elicited. Those who have had health consequences should be asked about treatment outcome as well as their own and their parents' response to the problem.

Interviewing should be done privately once some degree of rapport has been established. The adolescent and the interviewer should also understand each other's terminology, including street language and ethnocultural variations. There is evidence that some adolescents do not understand the terminology used by physicians. In one study (Ammerman et al., 1992), over 50% of the young people sampled either were incorrect or did not know what the physician meant by words relevant to sexual history taking such as venereal, sexually transmitted disease, sexually active, and confidential. Likewise, the physician should be sure he or she understands what the teenaged patient means. Teens may use terms with which physicians may not be familiar, such as "hooking up," "snowballing," "bumpin' uglies," "getting jiggy with it," or "being on the down low." Physicians should not hesitate to clarify what the young person means when they are not familiar with words or phrases used (Denizet-Lewis, 2004). In fact, clarification may be generally indicated since such wide variability in the understanding of colloquial terms abounds.

Special issues in adolescent sexuality

Adolescent sexual risk taking

Each year, 25% of sexually active teenagers contract a sexually transmitted disease. Overall syphilis, gonorrhea, and chlamydia disproportionately affect adolescents and young adults. Teens in the United States have higher STD rates than teenagers in other developed countries (for example, England, Canada, France, and Sweden) (Alan Gutmacher Institute, 2002a). STDs are under-reported and under-diagnosed in this population, yet there may be serious consequences for untreated gonorrhea or chlamydia. They may lead to pelvic inflammatory disease, which may then be related to infertility or ectopic pregnancy.

Adolescents who often perceive themselves as invulnerable are less likely to use preventive methods when engaging in sexual behaviors. United States teenagers have more sexual partners and are less likely to use condoms than teens in

Interviewing adolescents about sexual orientation
Pearls
- Use orientation-neutral questions that indicate a willingness to discuss homosexual as well as heterosexual activity.
- Ask questions about sexuality and sexual orientation at each visit.

Peril
- Avoidance of discussions about sexual orientation or assumption of heterosexuality may cause increased trauma for the gay or lesbian adolescent.

other developed countries. In fact, it appears that the primary reasons why US teens have the highest rates of pregnancy, childbearing, and abortion among developed countries is less overall use of contraceptives and in particular lower use of the most effective methods such as long-acting hormonal methods. When comparisons are made among developed countries, differences in contraceptive use appear to be related to negative societal attitudes toward teenage sexual relationships, restricted access to reproductive health services, ambivalence toward contraceptive methods, and a lack of motivation to delay motherhood or to avoid unintended pregnancy (Alan Gutmacher Institute, 2002b).

Data from the latest Youth Risk Behavior Survey (CDC, 2004) described the risk behaviors of United States high school students (Table 19.1). A nationally representative sample of students from grades 9 through 12 who attended both public and private schools were surveyed regarding some of their sexual behaviors. Risk behaviors related to sex

TABLE 19.1

Percentage of high school students who have ever had sexual intercourse

Category	Female %	Male %	Total %
Race/ethnicity			
White	43.0	40.5	41.8
Black	60.9	73.8	67.3
Hispanic	46.4	56.8	51.4
Grade			
9	27.9	37.3	32.8
10	43.1	45.1	44.1
11	53.1	53.4	53.2
12	62.3	60.7	46.7
Total	45.3	48.0	46.7

CDC (2004) Youth Risk Behavior Surveillance – United States 2003. *MMWR* 53: SS-2.

addressed by the survey included dating violence, forced sexual intercourse, sexual intercourse before age 13, four or more sex partners, current sexual activity, condom or birth control pill use during last sexual intercourse, alcohol or drug use before last sexual intercourse, pregnancy, and AIDS/HIV infection education.

Condom use during the last sexual intercourse was reported by 57.4% of girls and 68.8% of boys. Interestingly, condom use was reported less frequently by the 12th grade girls than by the 9th grade girls. The meaning of this observation was not clear. A very high percentage (87–89%) of the young people surveyed reported that they had received education at school about AIDS/HIV infection. Having four or more sexual partners during the adolescent's lifetime was another measure of risk. The survey found that 11.2% of the girls and 17.5% of the boys had had four or more partners. These percentages increased steadily with age both for boys and girls over the 4 years of high school.

Risk behaviors related to drinking alcohol or using drugs prior to last sexual intercourse among the currently sexually active young people was 21% of girls and 29.8% of boys. Interestingly, the rate for girls decreased, while the rate for boys increased from the 9th to 12th grade. Dating violence had been experienced equally by boys and girls, but girls had been forced to have sexual intercourse twice as frequently as boys (11.9% of girls vs. 6.1% of boys).

Trends were noted over the previous 12 years (1991–2003) of the Youth Risk Behavior Survey. The percentage of students who had had sexual intercourse and had four or more sexual partners decreased significantly from 1991 to 2003. Likewise, the percentage of currently sexually active students who used a condom during the last sexual intercourse increased significantly, suggesting a decrease in high-risk behavior over that period of time. However, there was also a significant increase in young people who drank alcohol or used drugs before the last sexual intercourse, thus indicating an increase in risky sexual behavior (CDC, 2004).

According to the results of the National Youth Risk Behavior Survey, high-risk sexual behaviors reported by high school students coincide with reports of alcohol, marijuana, cocaine, and other illicit drug use. Adolescents who do not engage in substance use are least likely to report having sexual intercourse. Other studies link a risk for sexually transmitted disease to substance abuse and use. D'Angelo studied HIV prevalence rates in adolescents across several populations. The HIV rate is highest in adolescents from cities in which AIDS is endemic who engage in high-risk sex and abuse illicit substances or alcohol.

Data from the Youth Risk Behavior Survey (CDC 2004) indicated that pregnancy occurred for 4.9% of girls currently in 9th–12th grades, ranging from 2.3% of 9th grade girls to 7.6% of 12th grade girls. These statistics, however, did not include girls who were not in high school, thus excluding a group of girls who may well have had a greater rate of preg-

nancy, having dropped out of school to parent their infants. The teenage pregnancy rate has dropped over the past 10–12 years; likewise the teenage birth rate and abortion rate have also dropped.

Levels of sexual activity and the age at which adolescents become sexually active do not vary significantly across comparable developed countries such as Canada, Great Britain, France, and Sweden (Alan Guttmacher Institute, 2002). Yet it is well known that the adolescent pregnancy rate in the United States is significantly higher than many comparably developed countries. Japan and most Western European countries have a low rate of pregnancy (40 per 1000), whereas the United States, Belarus, Bulgaria, Romania, and the Russian Federation have the highest rates (70+ per 1000).

Adolescent birth rates have declined over the past 25 years, but are still quite high in the United States where the birth rate is 54.4 births per 1000 women aged 15–19 years. Birth rates range from being low in 10 countries (3.9 per 1000 in Japan is the lowest) to a high in five countries of which one is the United States (54.4 per 1000) (Alan Guttmacher Institute, 2002a). Abortion rates among teenagers have declined significantly in the United States from 46 per 1000 to 29 per 1000 in the period of time between 1985 and 1996. However, the rate in the United States remains one of the highest among developed countries.

For some adolescents, pregnancy provides an opportunity to move to a more adult status. Motivation for pregnancy may not just be due to a lack of access to appropriate contraception. A girl may be at particular risk for pregnancy if she has limited academic or social success. She may see a pregnancy as a potential bright spot in an otherwise difficult life. She may see a baby as someone she can love or someone who will love her. Other risk factors for teen pregnancy include a family history of early, unwed pregnancy, experience of early losses through divorce or death and a subsequent search for replacement of broken relationships, feelings of being unloved, abuse of drugs or alcohol that decreases the likelihood of using contraception, and a life of poverty in an unstable family.

Given the ambivalent attitudes toward teenage sexuality in this country, the lack of sexual education that offers substantive information regarding STD protection and pregnancy prevention, and the lack of easily accessible methods of preventing STDs and pregnancy, teens are more likely to be frightened to discuss issues of sexuality with their primary care physicians or their mental health clinicians. They may deny symptoms of infection or pregnancy, thus delaying effective treatment. Most adolescents will benefit from conversation regarding sexuality with their physicians. Education about how to make appropriate and responsible decisions about sexual activity, incorporation of safer sex practices, and education about sexually transmitted diseases should be included in adolescent assessments at medical or mental health visits.

Sexually transmitted diseases and pregnancy

PEARLS & PERILS

- The adolescent who feels invulnerable is less likely to take appropriate precautions.
- Young people involved in substance use are more likely to engage in intercourse, contract STDs, or get pregnant.
- Education of the adolescent is key.
- Parent-child discussions can be effective in promoting use of contraception and protection from STDs.
- Lack of adult supervision is associated with higher rates of STDs.

Chronic illness

PEARLS & PERILS

- Illness or treatment that affects body size or shape will likely have an adverse impact on self-esteem and body image during adolescence.
- Society may view the chronically ill child or adolescent as asexual.
- Parents may be more protective of their chronically ill child and interfere with developmentally appropriate strivings for independence, including dating and sexual activity.
- The adolescent may combat these responses to chronic illness with provocative sexual behaviour.

A pregnant teen will benefit from a discussion about her feelings. She can be expected to progress through a cycle of reactions, including shock, denial, and anger, before arriving at acceptance. Immediate attention to the pregnancy must be encouraged, since adolescents typically receive less prenatal care and place their infants at risk for prematurity. The vast majority of teenagers who decide to have their babies keep them rather than surrender them to adoption or foster care. The physician can help the patient think realistically about how she will accomplish this goal. The patient should be encouraged to consider how she will continue her education, both before and after the baby is born. Some larger communities have special school programs for pregnant teenagers and their partners that offer health-care, nutrition programs, job preparation, parenting education, daycare after the baby arrives, and follow-up information about contraception. It is recommended that physicians who work with adolescents develop a network of resources, including clinics, educational programs, and early parenting programs to which they can refer their adolescent mothers.

Adolescents who have HIV must consistently use safer sex practices in order to prevent spread of the disease. Given adolescents' sense of invulnerability, it may be difficult for these teenagers to anticipate the impact of their actions. Even more difficult for HIV positive teens is the necessity to confront impending mortality, something that is not a usual developmental task for this age group. Therefore, HIV positive teens would benefit from having a good relationship with their primary physician and the opportunity to talk about issues important to their situation. Many large cities with significant HIV positive populations have specialized programs for HIV positive teens.

Chronic illness and sexuality

Chronic illness may affect sexual development in several ways. The child's caregivers may inhibit the child's attempt at separation and individuation due to concern about the child's fragility caused by medical or mental illness. The adolescent with physical disabilities may be seen as asexual by society at large. The adolescent who is restricted by chronic illness, disability, or hospitalization may use sexually provocative language or behavior to reassure him or herself and others that she is a normal teenager. The child may be excluded from peer interactions concerning sexuality. Thus, sexual development may be hampered by delays in psychosocial development (Joffee, 1999).

The physician can assist children and their families by addressing developmental issues regarding sexuality along with concerns about management of the illness. Some of the chronic illnesses most likely to be associated with sexual problems are: endocrinopathies (congenital adrenal hyperplasia or Klinefelters syndrome); chronic physical illnesses (HIV, cystic fibrosis, sickle cell disease, juvenile rheumatoid arthritis); genital anomalies (micropenis, hypospadias, vaginal agenesis); and oncologic diseases (Lock, 1998, 2001).

Adolescent homosexuality

Most adolescents are aware of their sexual orientation, although some gay, lesbian, or bisexual individuals are not sure of this during their teen years. Others are aware, but deny it, wait for it to go away, or wait until they are away from home to allow expression of their orientation. "Coming out" refers to the process by which gay, lesbian, or bisexual individuals come to understand their sexual orientation and then to disclose it to others. This may take place in the teen years or later during the adult years.

Some young people who will come to identify as gay or lesbian in their adult years may identify as bisexual in adolescence, since this label is less stigmatized than the homosexual or gay/lesbian label. However, it appears that among the youth of this generation there is more acceptance of sexual behaviors that are not "heteronormative" (Herdt, 2001). There may be less hesitance to come out as gay, lesbian, or bisexual in the adolescent years. Recent community-based surveys suggest that there are as many young people who identify as bisexual as there are ones who identify as gay or lesbian. There are also equal numbers of male and female young people who identify as gay or lesbian, something not reported in adult surveys where there are frequently only half as many women who identify as lesbian as there are men who identify as gay.

In understanding adolescent homosexuality, it is important for the physician to recognize three major domains of sexuality: sexual orientation, sexual behavior, and sexual identity. In adolescents, there may be a complex relationship among all three domains. For example, more adolescents may have a homoerotic orientation than engage in same-sex behavior or who accept a gay identity. There is also more resistance among the youth of today to accepting sexual identity labels, preferring to describe their behavior, attractions, and relationships (Savin-Williams and Cohen, 2004).

There is evidence that young people who come out during their adolescent years may be aware of their sexual orientation for years before they first disclose this to anyone else. Several researchers (Table 19.2) have found an average of 3 or more years between the teen coming to terms with his/her sexual orientation and the disclosure of this to others. This may be due to fear of rejection or the stigma associated with homosexuality in this culture. This time between coming out to oneself and then coming out to others is considered a time of increased risk for gay and lesbian youth.

Adolescent homosexuality is not considered a pathologic condition, but the stigma associated with homosexuality may lead to significant distress for the teenager. Self-identified gay, lesbian, and bisexual young people in a community-based survey of high school students experienced more problems in the areas of mental health, sexual risk-taking, and general health (Lock and Steiner, 1999). Convenience studies and clinical samples found the same results, but also have reported significant problems with runaway behavior, truancy, and drug use. The societal stigma associated with homosexuality may lead

> ### PEARLS & PERILS
>
> ### Gay and lesbian youth
> **Pearls**
> - The time between coming out to oneself and coming out to others can be a time of significant isolation and potential risk.
> - Coming out to others can be a time of significant risk.
> - Rejection by family and/or friends is likely.
> - Physical or verbal abuse may follow disclosure of sexual orientation to others.
> - Depression, suicide, truancy, homelessness, and substance abuse are risks.
>
> **Peril**
> - Fear of rejection may lead young people to fear coming out to physicians or other potentially supportive adults.

the adolescent to have a significant fear of disclosing sexual orientation to a mental health professional as well. However, if this occurs with a trusted and knowledgeable health professional, there is then the opportunity to decrease the isolation, correct inaccurate cognitions regarding homosexuality, and assist the teen in dealing with family and peers.

Gay and lesbian individuals go through a process of coming to terms with their sexual orientation. This process has been conceptualized by several different authors. Stages decribed by Cass (1990) are: 1) pre-coming out, 2) coming out, 3) exploration, 4) first relationship, and 5) integration. Modifications of this model to more appropriately reflect the experience of women put the first relationship before the stage of exploration. (See Savin-Williams and Cohen, 2004 for a discussion of the complexities of sexual orientation in adolescents.)

TABLE 19.2

Developmental milestones in gay and lesbian youth

	D'Augelli & Hershberger 1993		Herdt & Boxer 1993	
	Females	Males	Females	Males
Milestone	(n=52)	(n=142)	(n=55)	(n=147)
First same-sex attraction	11+/-4	10+/-4	10+/-4	10+/-4
First same-sex self-label	n/a	n/a	12+/-3	11+/-3
First same-sex sexual activity	15+/-3	15+/-3	n/a	n/a
First opposite-sex sexual activity	15+/-4	12+/-4	14+/-4	14+/-4
First disclosure to someone else	16+/-2	17+/-2	16+/-2	16+/-2

Gay and lesbian adolescents who are in the process of developing their sexual identities must also contend with ethnocultural heritage. Those who grow up in orthodox religious homes, in homes where the children are expected to live with the family until marriage, in homes where everyone is expected to marry and have children, or in homes with polarized gender role expectations will be the most in conflict with their families. Members of certain ethnic groups feel that it is impossible for other members of their group to be homosexual. Belonging to a specific ethnic culture and being homosexual may be perceived as mutually exclusive. Parents may blame the dominant culture for their child's sexual orientation. For example, a 20-year-old Indian-American may explain that his parents are hurt because they believe homosexuality is against the Muslim faith. For his parents, homosexuality is an aspect of the dominant culture: their son learned to be gay from his white friends. To them, homosexuality is the result of a decadent, Western, urban society.

Transgender teens

There has been little attention paid to transgender adolescents compared to that given to gender dysphoric children and transsexual adults. Yet depression, suicidality, rejection, and violence may bring them to mental health providers. While gender identity or gender role issues frequently resolve in childhood, transgender issues that persist into the teen years are much less likely to resolve with acceptance of the gender identity associated with the young person's biologic sex. Consequently, complex dilemmas face young people, their families, and the professionals who treat them. There is generally little acceptance of cross-dressing or using pronouns appropriate to the adolescent's perceived gender in institutional settings for minors, such as schools, psychiatric hospitals, or residential facilities. Further, there are no consensus guidelines on how to handle these issues. This situation inevitably evokes difficult discussions among mental health professionals and requires thoughtful interventions.

Therapeutic intervention for transgender adolescents may take several different forms. In the past, treatment might have involved trying to alter the adolescent's gender identity to be congruent with his/her biologic sex either through a psychoanalytically oriented psychotherapy or behavior therapy. With few exceptions, efforts to change an adolescent's gender identity have not proven to be effective. (Swann and Herbert, 1999; Zucker and Bradley, 1995).

Another typical approach might be to engage the teenager in supportive psychotherapy as a way to alleviate the psychologic distress and strengthen ego functioning. Psychopathology is seen as inherent in the condition. Intrinsic to this kind of therapy is the belief that decisions regarding gender identity change require greater maturity and thus the teen should wait until adulthood. The clinician's role would be to help the adolescent explore the conflict between biologic sex and gender identity while assessing sexual orientation and possible confusion between gender identity and sexual orientation (Swann and Herbert, 1999). A successful outcome of treatment would be resolution of the cross-gender identification with either a heterosexual or homosexual orientation.

A more recent approach to treatment permits cross-gender identification as a viable outcome. The therapist acknowledges the impact that society has on an individual's psychologic functioning and development, but does not conceptualize the only successful or healthy outcome as being resolution of the gender identity issues. This approach is best for young people who have long-standing histories of cross-gender identification that have persisted from childhood into adolescence.

It is no longer acceptable to equate transgender issues in the teen years with severe psychopathology or to ignore the issue until the teen becomes an adult. Psychiatrists and other mental health clinicians along with health-care professionals who are knowledgeable about the issues facing transgender young people should be able to provide appropriately respectful evaluation and treatment.

Paraphilias

A person with a paraphilia is compulsively responsive to and obligatorily dependent on an unusual and personally or socially unacceptable stimulus. The stimulus may be perceived or it may be in the ideation and imagery of fantasy, but it is necessary for optimal initiation and maintenance of sexual arousal and for the facilitation or attainment of orgasm. Paraphilic imagery may occur in fantasy during masturbation or during intercourse with a partner. Although they are usually thought of as occurring in adulthood, the paraphilias have forerunners in childhood (as a protoparaphilia) and adolescence. Paraphilias are reported more often in males. They generally become a focus for treatment when there are legal consequences for the behavior. There are over 40 paraphilias, but only a few come under the province of the judicial system. Studies of adults with paraphilias have shown that traumatic events with erotic implications may have occurred in the lives of these adults prior to puberty.

The paraphilias include exhibitionism, fetishism, frotteurism, pedophilia, transvestic fetishism, voyeurism, sexual sadism, and sexual masochism. In exhibitionism, there is exposure of one's genitals to an unsuspecting stranger for sexual arousal. Fetishism occurs when an animate or an inanimate object is required for sexual arousal. Frotteurism involves touching or rubbing a nonconsenting

Paraphilias

- The paraphilias generally begin in adolescence, although precursors may be seen in childhood.
- Prepubertal traumatic events with erotic implications may be a precursor to a paraphilia.
- Treatment includes CBT and/or behavior therapy.

person, and pedophilia occurs when there is sexual arousal involving children. In transvestic fetishism, a person has recurrent fantasies or persistently cross-dresses in order to achieve sexual excitation. In voyeurism, an unsuspecting individual is observed while disrobing, naked, or engaging in sexual activity. In sexual sadism and masochism, acts of causing or experiencing humiliation are found sexually stimulating.

The paraphilias are treated through the use of psychotherapy, in particular cognitive behavioral therapy (CBT), or behavior therapy. Pairing a noxious stimulus such as an ammonia capsule with inappropriate sexual arousal has been an effective technique. Medications such as medroxyprogesterone acetate (Depo-Provera) that lower circulating androgens have been used to decrease the desire for sexual expression. However, other psychotropic medications, including lithium, the antidepressants and certain antipsychotics (clozapine and thioridazine) have been found helpful. All medications are used in conjunction with psychotherapy, including cognitive behavioral therapy (CBT).

TABLE 19.3 Report of aggression by adolescent sex offenders

Type of aggression	Adolescent report (%)	Referral source report (%)
No violence	42	08
Verbal coercion	15	10
Threatened physical violence	06	07
Physical violence	25	61
Threatened with weapon	03	07
Used weapon	0.5	01
Excessive physical violence	1.5	03

Becker JV and Hunter JA (1993) Aggressive sex offenders. *Child Adolesc Psychiat Clin NA* 2(3):480.

Sexually aggressive youth

Violence has become an issue of major concern in this country (Table 19.3). Young males are frequently the victims of violence. The homicide rate for young males in the US is higher than for any other developed country. In particular, homicide is the leading cause of death for young African-American males (Becker and Hunter, 1993). However, young males are not just victims of violence, but are also perpetrators of violence, including sexual abuse and violence. A study of adult sex offenders found that 58% of those interviewed reported becoming sexual offenders prior to age 18 (Abel et al., 1985, cited in Becker and Hunter, 1993).

Sex offending behavior may be classified as *hands off* (voyeurism and exhibitionism) and *hands on* behavior (fondling, oral, anal, and vaginal penetration). Victims may be children, peers, adults, and animals. (Becker and Hunter, 1993). Characteristics of adolescent sex offenders are not significantly different from those of violent, but nonsexual offenders. Factors identified include lack of social competence skills, prior delinquent behavior, psychopathology, low academic performance, and lack of impulse control (Becker and Hunter, 1993). Family characteristics of adolescent sex offenders include unstable or unhealthy home environment, overt family violence, and history of abuse.

Assessment of adolescent sex offenders should include a detailed history, including family, educational, psychosocial, and psychosexual aspects. A history of neglect and of being a victim of sexual or physical abuse themselves should be elicited. Parental psychopathology, criminal history, and level of functioning are relevant in this assessment. Of particular importance is the extent to which the adolescent was exposed to violence in the home, was the recipient of this violence, and what his or her reaction was to witnessing or experiencing this violence. Medical information should include any previous history of head trauma. Diagnostic assessment should include information regarding other psychiatric disorders such as conduct disorder, attention-deficit/hyperactivity disorder (ADHD), learning disabilities, mood and psychotic disorders, posttraumatic stress disorder (PTSD), substance abuse, and personality traits such as narcissistic and anti-social. Information should be obtained on victim selection and the extent of force and violence. Whether verbal coercion, physical force, sadistic behavior, and/or a weapon were used should be determined along with the extent of damage done to the victim. It is very important to include corroborative data from the referral source, as it is clear that many youth under-report the extent of violence utilized in the commission of the sex offense (see Table 19.3, Becker and Hunter, 1993). It is important to determine the degree to which the young person accepts responsibility for his or her actions, the degree of empathy for the victim, and the extent of cognitive distortions that sup-

Sexually aggressive behaviors

- The majority of sex offenders committed assaults during adolescence.
- Sex offenders who have the capacity for empathy have a better prognosis.

port aggressive sexual behavior. The American Academy of Child and Adolescent Psychiatry "Practice parameters for the assessment and treatment of children and adolescents who are sexually abusive of others" (1999) serves as a comprehensive resource for anyone evaluating or treating these young people.

The ability to treat aggressive adolescent sex offenders varies depending on the severity of the psychosexual disorder and the degree of impairment in the individual's personality. Early life experiences of abuse and neglect have left these young people with anger, bitterness, and impairment in their ability to form attachments to others. Treatment requires a combination of therapeutic approaches including cognitive behavioral approaches to improve their self-control skills. If these young people are able to understand the antecedents of their current behaviors, including an understanding of their own past experiences of abuse and past emotional pain, and if they are able to develop a capacity for empathy, the prognosis is better. There may be little motivation for change in young people who have significant character disorders and lack genuine remorse for their aggressive sexual behaviors. They are only minimally responsive to therapy (Becker and Hunter, 1993).

Prevention

If it were possible for most adolescents to refrain from early sexual activity, many of the negative biopsychosocial consequences could be avoided. Many adults believe that adolescents should refrain from sexual intercourse until marriage, or until they have a mature committed relationship in which both partners are able and willing to take responsibility for any consequences. Many professionals believe that sexual intercourse should be postponed at least until the reproductive system is fully mature (late teens) and until there is sufficient psychosocial maturity for responsible behavior. Since data from the YRBS (CDC, 2004) continue to suggest that the majority of youth in this country are sexually active in their teens, and the average age of marriage is now in the mid to late twenties, it may be unrealistic to expect adolescents to abstain from all physical expressions of sexuality.

Adolescents need to be well informed about the risks of all forms of sexual intimacy. They must be provided with the knowledge and methods for preventing sexually transmitted diseases, pregnancy, and premature parenthood. Instructions about "safer sex" may require a description or at least mention of practices that increase the risk of serious infections or injuries, such as anal intercourse. Sexually active teenagers, even those who consistently use barrier methods of contraception and have a single partner, should be screened yearly for infections. More frequent screening should be considered for high-risk adolescents such as homeless youth, substance users, youth with conduct disorders or psychiatric disorders, and youth with many different partners.

Pregnancy prevention is an appropriate preventive medical task. A physician may help a teen appreciate the potential impact of a pregnancy on her life by asking specific questions. These questions could be what the patient's plans are for the next 5 years, how these plans might be affected by a baby. Likewise, if the teen has a friend with a baby, then the questions might involve how much this young mother is able to do with her baby. This may help her plan more effectively for her future.

Sex education or family life education does not guarantee prevention of consequences. It will not ensure abstinence, but contrary to what many think, it has not been shown to increase sexual experimentation. The sex education of children and adolescents is a responsibility shared by parents, schools, health professionals, and other adults who provide services to young people. All contribute positively or negatively to each young person's understanding of and attitude toward human sexuality. Parents and other family members begin this process at birth and provide the primary influence in the development of personal values and beliefs. Society's unresolved debate about the content and timing of sexuality education and parental reluctance to discuss sexuality topics often leave young people uninformed or misinformed. They turn to friends, the media, and available written materials that range from dictionaries to sex-oriented adult magazines where they may receive incomplete or inaccurate sexual information.

As children reach adolescence, the normative efforts at distancing from parents may interfere with open communication and effective education in even the most enlightened and comfortable families. Health professionals can be important allies of young people providing accurate information to them and giving them the opportunity to discuss their dilemmas and concerns in the area of sexuality. Likewise, health professionals can assist parents with educating their children, utilizing developmentally appropriate communication about sexuality. There is also a role for the physician in helping the community appreciate the importance of family life education for all children and families.

Summary

Children and adolescents are sexual beings from the time of birth. Providing good comprehensive care requires that this aspect of development be incorporated into any assessment of a child or adolescent's health or mental health. Sensitivity to racial, ethnic, and cultural differences is essential in doing this assessment. Clinicians working with children and adolescents should have knowledge and competence in dealing with individuals whose expressions of gender and sexuality are atypical as well as typical. Much remains to be learned about this important and vital aspect of human development. It has been difficult to secure permission and funding for research regarding sexuality in children. Information obtained from such research would prove important in assisting children, families, and society to appreciate differences between normative sexual development, atypical or variant sexual behaviors, and sexual behavior problems requiring intervention.

Annotated bibliography

Child Adolesc Psychiatric Clin N Am, 13, 2004.
> *This entire volume is devoted to issues of sex and gender as they pertain to children and adolescents. It is an up-to-date review of some of the contemporary and controversial issues today.*

Richardson J, Schuster MA (2003). *Everything You Never Wanted Your Kids to Know About Sex (but Were Afraid They'd Ask): The Secrets to Surviving Your Child's Sexual Development From Birth to the Teens.* New York, NY, Three Rivers Press.
> *Excellent book for parents who have questions about how to approach issues of sexuality with their children. How to talk with children in developmentally appropriate ways is addressed.*

Bell R et al. (1998). *Changing Bodies, Changing Lives: A Book for Teens on Sex and Relationships*, 3rd edn. New York, NY, Random House, 1998.
> *This is an excellent reference for teens. The book addresses not just the physical changes that come with puberty and adolescent development, but includes a range of issues such as masturbation, attraction to same sex peers, and sexual decision-making.*

CHAPTER 20

Risk-taking and Dangerous Behavior in Children and Adolescents

David J. Mullen, MD and Robert L. Hendren, DO

Introduction

Behavior that risks injury to self and/or other persons is a ubiquitous feature of human behavior, particularly in adolescence. Adolescents are well known for behaving as if they are invulnerable to potential harm. They ride bicycles diagonally across busy intersections, drive fast and under the influence of substances, participate in high-risk sexual activities, and engage in a variety of illegal activities at a higher rate than adults. Adolescents are frequently involved in accidents with injury. Suicidal and homicidal behaviors as well as violence continue to be of significant concern in adolescents. In 2001, suicide was the third leading cause of death for young people ages 15–24 after accidents and homicide (NIMH, 2003). In 1994, males aged 14–24 committed 48% of reported homicides while constituting only 8% of the population in the United States (Fox, 1996).

Although the majority of teens do not become involved in these very dangerous activities, some elevation in risk-taking behavior appears to be a feature of normal development, and should, like all potential problem behaviors, be evaluated from a developmentally informed perspective. Part of normal adolescent development may include experimentation with sexual behaviors, alcohol use, and minor risk-taking that may result in minor difficulty like a traffic ticket. It is clear, however, that many young people become excessively involved in a variety of high-risk activities with resultant increases in morbidity and mortality (Pickett et al., 2002). Repeated unprotected sex, drug use that goes beyond experimentation or more than one traffic ticket may be a sign of crossing over the line of normalcy. Adolescents with psychiatric disorders, in particular those with conditions associated with poor impulse control, are at special risk for engagement in potentially dangerous behaviors.

This chapter focuses on excessive risk-taking behaviors and the epidemiology of these behaviors, including what is known regarding associated psychosocial features. The relationships between specific psychopathology and risk-taking are then elucidated followed by an exploration of potential etiologic factors. Finally, potential interventions targeting excessive risk-taking as well as suicide and violence are discussed.

A full understanding of risk-taking and dangerous behaviors among young people requires careful consideration of the motivation for such behavior, and its potential role in the child's development. As suggested above, high-risk behaviors may be characterized by the presence or absence of intention to cause harm to self or others. It is likely that the majority of adolescent risk-taking behavior, while involving potential for harm, is not engaged in for the purpose of producing injury to self or others. However, in some situations, such a clear distinction may be difficult. For example, some para-suicidal behavior may be less designed to actually result in injury but more to affect some social influence.

The variety of types of behavior engaged in by young people that are considered of potentially high risk is considerable. Some behaviors create increased risks due to their potential to result in serious bodily harm. These activities include high-speed driving, climbing in or around construction areas or bridges, skateboard riding, especially involving dramatic stunts, and particularly if no protective padding is worn. For example, a recent very high-risk "stunt" type behavior with some popularity among teens is "car surfing" in which a youth rides atop a moving vehicle as if it were a skateboard. This practice can be particularly dangerous primarily due to the risks associated with falling from the vehicle, with one small study reporting that of 26 reported episodes of injury, 85% required long-term

CONSIDER CONSULTATION WHEN ...

- There seems to be a pattern of escalating risk-taking behavior present that does not seem to respond to repeated family or physician redirection, even if neither the patient nor others have as yet been harmed.
- More serious psychiatric comorbidity such as depression or psychosis appears to be accompanying the risk behavior, particularly if there is concern about possible suicidal or homicidal intent.
- Risk-taking behavior is associated with an escalating or serious substance use pattern.
- Serious medical morbidity appears to be associated with risk-taking behavior that might otherwise be considered minor, such as may occur with unstable or brittle insulin dependent diabetes

KEY CLINICAL QUESTIONS

- *Are you impulsive? Do you do things without thinking that you later regret?*
  This question asks indirectly about risk-taking behavior and can be the start to a conversation about potentially dangerous behavior
- *Are you moody? Do you ever feel really depressed for more than a short time, sometimes for no reason? Have you ever felt so bad that you thought you wanted to die? Do you ever feel really good; so good that other people want you to calm down and say you are extreme?*
  This question begins to get a history of major depression, affective instability, mania, and risk for suicide. More questioning is needed if these questions yield results, but this is a good way to get started.
- *Are you a risk taker? Tell me about some "risky behavior" you or some of your friends have done lately. Do either you or your friends use alcohol or drugs? If not, why not? Does or has anyone in your family engage(d) in risky behavior?*
  This question asks about the adolescent's own risk-taking behavior and that of his or her friends. If their friends are engaged in risk-taking behavior but they say they are not, asking why not can often reveal if they are being candid with you. Asking about family history of risky behavior may reveal more than asking about specific diagnoses, although you should also ask about family history of mental disorders.
- *Do you have good friends? Do you feel odd or different from most people? Are there some people that you think are out to hurt you? Do you ever see or hear things that others do not see or hear such as scary people or noises?*
  This series of questions are intended to start in a less threatening way to learn if a youngster has some thought disorganization and may be delusional or psychotic. If the first question is negative or the later questions are positive, more directed questioning is necessary.
- *Do you have a lot of accidents? Do you take any medication? Have you ever seen a mental health professional?*
  This line of questioning is intended to learn about additional risk factors and if answers are affirmative, additional questioning is indicated.

cognitive rehabilitation (Geiger et al., 2001). Other behaviors involve relative neglect of appropriate safety precautions or placing oneself in situations that may result in more chronic or cumulative harm as well as sudden injury. Many behaviors may involve both of these elements. Unsafe sex, use of street drugs, and neglect of medical care are behaviors of this type. The Consider consultation when ... and Key clinical questions boxes contain several examples of how to get the information to help the physician decide the seriousness of the adolescent's risk-taking behavior. It is sometimes difficult to decide how serious the behavior is, especially when an adolescent is minimizing the risk. If answers to key questions lead to continued concerns in either the parent or the physician, it is appropriate to ask for an additional opinion from a child and adolescent psychiatrists or other mental health specialist about the need for a more aggressive intervention.

Violence and suicidal behavior have been correlated with other types of risk-taking behavior but may involve some features, such as depression, that are more specific to these particular types of behavior. However, the evidence supports that children who engage in high-risk behaviors generally are more likely to become involved in violent or suicidal behavior, and participation in one type of high-risk behavior appears to increase the likelihood of involvement in others (Flisher et al., 2000). Violence is closely related to the disruptive behavior disorders, particularly conduct disorder and substance abuse and factors such as a family history of anti-social behavior, prior exposure to violence as either victim or witness, and availability of weapons may increase the risk of violent behavior (Elliott and Tolan, 1999). Further, although both sexes become involved in high-risk behavior, males appear to be more involved in risk behaviors that involve being the perpetrator of violence.

In addition to an association with mood disorder, suicidal risk appears to be elevated by the presence of a specific family history of suicide and some patient characteristics, such as anorexia nervosa, seem to be correlated less with a generalized disposition to high-risk behavior and more with a specific wish to die (Apter et al., 1995).

As already noted, high-risk behavior and psychopathology are often closely associated. The following section will explore some of more common forms and features of psychopathology that appear to contribute to elevations in risk-taking behaviors.

Associated symptoms and psychopathology

Risk-taking is a complex behavior and is associated with a number of mental disorders and with one or more underlying symptoms. Risky behavior can best be understood by breaking this complex behavior down into associated diagnoses and, most importantly, to the underlying "primary symptoms" that can then be targeted by more specific interventions. These primary symptoms of high-risk behavior can range from impulsive behaviors to behavior associated with sadness, rage or exuberance directed toward others or toward themselves, to poor cognitive processing and poor judgment.

High-risk behavior ranging from excessive exposure to danger to self and other directed destructive behavior can be associated with a number of DSM (Diagnostic and Statistical Manual IV-TR) defined mental disorders. The impulsivity, hyperactivity, and inattention associated with attention-deficit/hyperactivity disorder (ADHD) can lead to greater than expected accidents and injuries (Barkley, 2002). The affective instability in bipolar disorder, borderline disorder, and intermittent explosive disorder can lead to emotionally charged risk-taking and aggressive behavior. The irritability associated with major depressive disorder and dysthymia can lead to risky and self-destructive behavior including suicide. Excessive anxiety associated with post-traumatic stress disorder (PTSD), pervasive developmental disorders (PDD), and other developmental disabilities can result in low frustration tolerance and risky behavior. Young people with conduct disorder often seek the arousal, novelty, and stimulation of high-risk behavior leading to dangerous and destructive results (Schmeck and Poustka, 2001). Substance abuse and thought disorder (psychosis, schizophrenia) impair judgment and may lead to inadvertent risk-taking and exposure to danger due to misperceptions and distortions. However, while a DSM diagnosis may help guide interventions for associated risky behavior, a diagnosis by itself is often not enough to lead directly to effective treatment due to comorbidity, the overlapping of symptoms between disorders.

Designing effective treatments for risky behavior often takes time and usually involves some trial and error when directed toward the non-specific risk-taking behavior even when the DSM diagnoses is correctly identified. Intervention may be more productive when directed toward the underlying primary or target symptom.

First on the list of primary risk-taking symptoms is impulsivity. Impulsivity is the failure to resist an impulse, drive or temptation resulting in rapid, unplanned reactions to internal or external stimuli. It is the inability to delay reward where the individual is unable to modify his or her behavior according to the context of the situation or to reflect on the consequences of the behavior, thus impairing judgment.

With impulsivity, there is an associated underestimated sense of harm and lack of regard for the negative consequences (Moeller et al., 2001).

Subjects who demonstrate impulsive choice choose small or poor rewards that are immediately available over larger but delayed rewards (Cardinal et al., 2001). They are unable to calculate future risks or consequences and unable to delay acting on an impulse. Impulsive aggressive traits appear to mediate the familial transmission of suicide attempts (Brent, 2003).

An example of a primary symptom of impulsivity resulting in risk-taking behavior might be a boy who pulls down the pants of a girl in his school on a dare, or an adolescent driving an automobile who recklessly passes in a no passing zone. Intervention targeted at impulsivity aims to prolong the thinking before action phase with either cognitive behavioral techniques, removal from high-risk situations or pharmacologic intervention.

Novelty or sensation seeking is often associated with impulsivity but there are differences. Novelty seeking as a means of stimulation seems more likely to occur in "antisocial" or conduct disordered young people with low autonomic arousal (Herpertz et al., 2001). It can also occur in young people who are experiencing a stressful time or are over-stimulated and are seeking distractions. This might occur with PTSD, depression and/or substance abuse. Interventions are targeted at finding less dangerous, stimulating activities, decreasing over-stimulation if present, and, at times, reflective therapies and pharmacologic intervention.

Affective instability is emotional disregulation that in children and adolescents usually occurs rapidly and is highly reactive. Emotional state fluctuates widely and rapidly and is out of proportion to the circumstances (Bhangoo and Leibenluft, 2002). Affective instability may be combined with impulsivity to result in risky and aggressive behavior (Vitiello, 1997), but the two are not the same as a person can be impulsive with or without an affective component. Both affective instability and impulsivity are related to poor attention and attention shifting and to little or no verbal self-control (Rothbart and Posner, 2000; Liebenluft et al., 2003).

Mood lability, rages, euphoria, and rapid cycling or mixed moods are increasingly diagnosed as bipolar disorder (BPD) in young people (Wozniac, 1997). However, children with a number of psychiatric disorders manifest emotional dysregulation in the form of exaggerated reactions to negative or frustrating stimuli (Bhangoo and Leibenluft, 2002). They may not meet the full criteria for BPD because they do not have grandiosity, decreased need for sleep, increased goal-directed activity but do have hyperarousal, abnormal baseline mood, and extreme responses to frustration. Children with BPD may be unique in having increased responsiveness to positive emotional stimuli.

Depression and irritability can lead to risk-taking and aggressive behavior that can be directed toward others or toward the self. Factors that increase impulsivity such as substance abuse or the availability of weapons can increase the risk of harm, but treatment needs to be directed not only toward these factors but also to the underlying depression (American Academy of Child and Adolescent Psychiatry, 2001).

Anxious hyperarousal is due to over-stimulation and may result in risk-taking behavior as a means of avoidance or because of poor judgment and impulsivity. Young people who are hyperaroused from anxiety and/or fear may be quick to startle and defensively strike out at others or place themselves in potentially dangerous situations.

Cognitive disorganization from delusions, psychosis or substance abuse can also result in risk-taking behavior. While the behavior may appear impulsive to the outside observer, closer inquiry may reveal more long-standing, distorted perceptions or impaired reasoning as the precedent to the risky behavior.

Identifying the underlying, primary target symptom or combination of symptoms is usually the most productive focus for treatment and can inform the neurodevelopmental origins of the risky behavior discussed in the next section of this chapter.

Etiology

The etiology of risk-taking behaviors, like most complex behaviors, is multifactorial. The pervasiveness of high-risk behaviors suggests that it is at least to some extent normative and therefore plays a role in normal development in much the same way as oppositional behavior does in younger children. Etiologic factors likely include biologic, psychologic, as well as social components.

Biologic factors

From the perspective of evolutionary biology, humans as a species are born in a markedly immature and dependent state with a prolonged juvenile period following birth. This in part is due to the expanded size of the brain relative to the limited size of the birth canal, thus necessitating an early birth. Although the extent to which childhood has been defined as a truly separate stage of development may have varied historically, cultures have generally recognized to some extent the existence of the relatively immature state of the child and have accorded children a dependent status. In addition, the majority of cultures contain one or more rituals designed to mark the entrance of the maturing young person into adulthood and include the recognition of new rights and responsibilities. Of course, with these responsibilities has generally come an expectation of greater economic and social competence and independence, all of which entail a risk of failure. In addition, humans, like our nearest primate relatives, have a strong disposition to form status hierarchies and compete for dominance, especially among males. Therefore, it would seem that a psychologic disposition to minimize the risks/dangers inherent in the developmental stage might facilitate the adolescent's willingness to embark upon the transition to adulthood (Weisfeld, 1999).

The neurobiologic contributions to risk-taking behavior include the large contribution of temperament, as such temperamental characteristics as novelty seeking as well as aversion to the same are both described as normal temperamental variations, while extremes are associated with psychopathology and biologic abnormalities. Cloninger describes novelty seeking as an important underlying temperamental variable that he postulates relates to dopaminergic activity. Harm avoidance, another variable described by Cloninger and believed to be related to serotonergic activity, is also likely to be related to risk-taking behavior (Cloninger et al., 1999; Taylor, 1993). Individuals who are high in harm avoidance are unlikely to engage in significant risk-taking behavior due to anxiety about potential harm, while those with novelty seeking temperamental variables are at increased risk.

Behavioral genetics has linked genetically based differences in dopamine receptor structure to an increased rate of novelty seeking, though this work is not consistently replicated. In addition, dopamine is theoretically linked to ADHD, a condition that includes impulsivity as one of its primary features, and the psychostimulants – prima-

---

PEARLS & PERILS

Pearls

- Marked or severe risk-taking behavior may be a form of suicidal behavior in some patients. For example, one adolescent male admitted entering the "territory" of a rival gang and antagonizing members of that gang in the hope that he would be shot.
- Severe generalized irritability may lead to high-risk behavior in patients with mania and may be associated with psychotic thought disturbances.
- Avoid moralizing when inquiring about adolescent behaviors, and avoid making explicit references to adolescent dependency issues in order to optimize rapport.
- Always inquire about the potential role of substances of abuse in adolescent risk-taking behavior.

Perils

- Do not forget to inquire about suicidal ideation.
- Do not assume that an escalating pattern of risky behavior is simply a facet of normal adolescent development.
- Do not neglect to obtain collateral information about the young person's behavior when it is available.
- Do not make a confidentiality promise that you cannot keep to an adolescent, i.e. tell a suicidal teen that you will not share the information concerning suicidal intent with anyone.

rily dopaminergic agents – are effective in the treatment of ADHD.

Abnormalities in serotonin activity are also extensively implicated in the etiology of impulsivity, particularly in impulsive aggression and violence (Kreusi et al., 1992). Low serotonergic levels are also associated with depressive disorder, which is associated with suicidal behavior and is frequently comorbid with conduct disorder.

As noted above, young people and adults with anti-social behavior syndromes are noted to demonstrate autonomic hypo-reactivity. This relatively reduced level of reactivity seems to be related to impairments in passive avoidance learning and an overall elevated level of sensation seeking (Raine, 1996).

Changes in hormonal activity in adolescence, particularly in levels of testosterone, may be associated with increases in risk-taking behavior and may contribute somewhat to the observed differences in some types of risk behavior between males and females, i.e. violence. Susman et al. (1987) found that higher levels of androstenedione are related to higher levels of acting out problems in boys. Olweus and colleagues (1988) found that high levels of testosterone caused boys to be more impatient and irritable, resulting in an increased propensity to engage in aggressive-destructive behavior. High doses of anabolic steroids have been associated with marked increases in irritability and episodic aggression (Pope, Kouri, and Hudson, 2000). However, the association between testosterone and aggression in adolescence is not a simple one. Contextual factors and underlying personality dimensions appear to be significant (Rubinow and Schmidt, 1996). In one study, the quality of parental supervision and relationship seemed to play a significant role in reducing testosterone-linked aggression (Booth et al., 2003).

Orbito-frontal functioning has been extensively associated with executive functioning and impairments in functioning, whether traumatically induced or otherwise, have been associated with increases in risk-taking behavior and impaired impulse control (Dolan and Park, 2002; Mitchell et al., 2002). Interestingly, the specific difficulties associated with orbito-frontal impairment may not be readily identifiable using methods aimed at verbal or cognitive performance (Bechara et al., 1996). Some have argued that perceived invulnerability may play a role in adolescent risk-taking, but studies that sample the adolescent's ability to cognitively estimate risk have not strongly supported a cognitive impairment in risk appraisal (Quadrel, Fischhoff, and Davis, 1993). However, given the relative immaturity of the adolescent frontal cortex, it may well be that they are disposed to take increased risks despite an apparent intact capacity to cognitively estimate risk.

Dysfunction of the basal ganglia has been associated with impulsivity in ADHD patients (Casey et al., 1997), and patients with Tourette syndrome often demonstrate problems with impulse regulation (Comings and Comings, 1987). Temporal lobe structures including the amygdalae are also associated with impulsive behavior and affective instability (Bechara et al., 1999; Perrine, 1991).

In addition to more endogenous sources of central nervous system dysfunction, substance abuse, in itself a risky behavior tends to result in further exposure to other sources of risk that may be mediated by either the direct pharmacologic effects of the substance (further degradation of impulse control) or indirectly through association with deviant peers and engaging in drug-related illegal activities.

Psychologic factors

Adolescent development normally entails a significant element of separation and individuation, with the eventual development of a relatively stable and autonomous adult identity. This process is likely to contribute to the observed limit testing in adolescence with respect to parents, but may result in a more general disposition for increases in exploratory behavior with respect to the social and physical environment as well as the limits of the sense of self. For instance, the natural history of adolescent-onset conduct disorder often involves the admiration by a previously fairly socially normal teen of a more seriously involved adolescent due to the more anti-social child's relatively high level of apparent "independence."

Risk-taking behavior may also be conceptualized as a response of the personality to conditions in which there is a disparity between the desired goals of the individual or the stresses with which the person is attempting to cope and the perceived resources available for coping (Flisher et al., 2000). In this model, one of the potential responses for the adolescent is growth involving the development of the needed personal resources. Another response, however, may be a sense of desperation and the adolescent may attempt by more direct, risky means to use the limited existing resources to meet the current demands.

The above model may well contribute to an understanding of the elevations observed in risk-taking seen in the varieties of psychopathology, as these conditions are typically associated with evidence of functional impairment and consequently with reductions in personal resources available to cope with a given stressor.

Trauma spectrum conditions are frequently associated with increases of risk-taking behavior, probably related to increased affective instability and an associated degradation of impulse control. Psychologically, the patient's sense of a foreshortened future and possible process of identification with the aggressor may facilitate aggressive behavior. Chronic trauma also appears to have an adverse impact on the hippocampus and thereby may impair the individual's ability to appropriately and accurately assess relevant context-related cues and thus lead to an excessive response (Tanev, 2003).

The potential etiologic relationships between mood disorders and risk-taking behavior are likely to include components that are more general, such as increasing the disparity between stress and available coping resources as well as the more specific impacts of hopelessness and suicidal ideation in depression and increased irritability, impulsivity/pleasure seeking and grandiosity in mania. Cognitive disorganization as an element in risky and dangerous behaviors of course obviously impairs coping resources and may result in significantly increased threat perception.

Finally, the psychologic role of peer relationships and risk-taking in adolescence is likely to be quite significant. In some adolescent subcultures such as street gangs, a willingness to take certain types of risks – engage in highly aggressive behaviors, participate in a variety of criminal behaviors including both person and property crimes as well as drug use and distribution – may translate into increases in the young person's status.

Social factors

A number of social correlates with high-risk behaviors are identified. Poor parental monitoring, a known risk factor for conduct problems, has been associated with studies of high-risk behaviors (Li, Stanton, and Feigelman, 2000). Poverty, high levels of family conflict, limited parental knowledge of adolescent risk-taking, and association with deviant peers appear to be associated with increased risk-taking (Petridou et al., 1997; Young and Zimmerman, 1998; Ary et al., 1999). All of these features may also in part be related to the concept of limited coping resources as a contributor to risk-taking behavior.

Obviously, these factors are unlikely to operate in isolation for a given patient and many may be adversely affected to one extent or another by several resulting in a very high level of vulnerability to risk-taking behavior. In addition, these factors are likely to interact with each other actively.

Assessment

Assessment of a child demonstrating high levels of risk-taking requires, as do all evaluations of children, an assessment of the patient's characteristics in terms of both liabilities and strengths as well as an evaluation of the resources and limitations of the psychosocial context. First, the clinician must establish the presence or absence of immediate dangerousness. Is the youngster acutely homicidal or suicidal and in need of emergency intervention? Depending upon the setting, the clinician may need to seek hospitalization of the patient, and certainly extensive utilization of available social supports will be critical in such a situation. As mentioned above, there are grey areas about what constitutes serious risk, but a good rule of thumb is that if either the physician or the parent (not necessarily both) are concerned, ask for a child and adolescent psychiatry or other mental health consultation about the need for and extent of intervention.

As noted earlier, an understanding of the role of risk-taking behavior in the youngster's life and development is crucial. A careful evaluation of the patient, including the establishment of adequate rapport that will allow sufficient sharing of important material, is therefore paramount. Of course, in many young people who are extensively involved in high-risk behavior, establishing a positive rapport with an authority figure will be a true clinical challenge! Is the young person engaging in high-risk behavior as part of a gang-related lifestyle with associated attempts to capture and maintain status? Could the behavior be considered para-suicidal in quality and be associated with an underlying depressive disorder?

The presence of specific psychopathology and an understanding of both differential diagnosis as well as associated symptoms will also be central to treatment planning. While some elements of a treatment plan may be specific to the diagnosis, adequately addressing high-risk behavior will often require an understanding of target symptoms that cut across diagnostic categories, such as impulsivity. The clinician should attend particularly to clinical features known to exacerbate risk-taking behavior such as mood disorders, substance use disorders, disruptive behavior disorders including ADHD, history of sexual or physical trauma, and poor parental supervision with high levels of family discord.

As above, an understanding of the resources and liabilities of the child's psychosocial situation will be necessary in the construction of an intervention plan. The physical and emotional availability of caregivers, including parenting and limit setting skills, are key elements in this context. An assessment of current stressors including the involvement of the patient in an ongoing abusive relationship, either sexual or otherwise, is important as the clinician may need to engage in specific interventions designed to terminate the abuse situation including the involvement of child protective services. The presence of any family history of psychiatric and behavioral disorders should be noted to assist both with clarification of the differential diagnosis as well as a more complete understanding of the extent of risk.

In addition to an assessment of the family situation, it is important to understand the nature of the child's involvement with other systems/institutions. The child's academic performance, including possible disciplinary actions as well as any juvenile justice system involvement, may provide both levers for intervention as well as sources of systemic stress.

Interventions

Due to the heterogeneous nature of young people who demonstrate significant levels of high-risk behavior, appropriate intervention and treatment requires substantial individualization. Effective treatment will likely target a range of relevant variables depending upon the specific patient presentation. For example, a patient with bipolar disorder who has comorbid conduct disorder and ADHD and who has extensive gang and legal involvement, is likely to require interventions targeting issues of mood instability and irritability, chronic inattention and impulsivity, as well as deviant peer associations and quite likely parental demoralization and family conflict. Such a patient may also need specific treatment for ongoing substance abuse given the extensive comorbidity of substance use disorders with both bipolar disorder and conduct disorder.

Furthermore, given the resource constraints that are often present in a managed care environment, considerable skill in prioritizing interventions and marshalling available resources is required. Available interventions are generally divided into psychosocial and pharmacologic interventions.

Psychosocial

The spectrum of psychosocial interventions targeting the range of behaviors discussed in this chapter is quite broad and a full explication is beyond the scope of this chapter. However, psychosocial intervention programs that have been successful with conduct disordered young people, a diagnostic group that demonstrates substantial high-risk behavior, are generally characterized by broad systemic approaches that include family as well as peer interventions. Multisystemic therapy is an example of a broad-based approach that utilizes a combination of "nested" treatments that target specific features of the disorder and may include individually based therapies such as cognitive behavioral therapy as well as family and peer-based treatments (Henggeler, Melton, and Smith, 1992; you might consider Henggeler, Schoenwald, Rowland and Cunningham, *Serious Emotional Disturbance in Children and Adolescents: Multisystemic Therapy*, 2002). Parental monitoring and interventions designed to increase parental awareness of risky behaviors have demonstrated significant effectiveness in reducing high-risk behaviors (Wu et al., 2003).

Pharmacologic

While there are no specific medications indicated for risk-taking behaviors, a number of medications are utilized for the core features associated with elevated risk-taking. Impulsivity – especially in the context of aggression, affective reactivity, mood dysregulation, and cognitive disorganization – has been the target of pharmacotherapy involving drugs from several classifications.

Antipsychotic medications, both typical and atypical agents, are utilized in the treatment of impulsive aggression and cognitive disorganization. Typical agents that are utilized in aggressive patients include haloperidol and chlorpromazine. Atypical agents utilized in this population include risperidone, olanzapine, and quetiapine (Pappadopulos et al., 2003).

The mood stabilizers, valproic acid, lithium carbonate and carbamazepine have been studied in impulsive, aggressive young people (Weller et al., 1999; Steiner, 2002). Lithium was also effective in reducing aggressive and explosive behavior in a subgroup of children with behavior disorder who had symptoms of an affective disorder (DeLong and Aldershof, 1987). In the same study, another subgroup of children who had behavior disorder and neurologic and medical disease also had decreased rage and aggressive outbursts after lithium treatment.

The sympatholytic agents propranolol, clonidine, and guanfacine may have some utility in risk-taking populations. Propranolol has proven to be effective in the treatment of aggressive behavior in children and adolescents with chronic brain dysfunction and in a few young people with conduct disorder refractory to other pharmacologic approaches (Kuperman and Stewart, 1987).

The selective serotonin reuptake inhibitors may be theoretically helpful for the treatment of impulsive aggression although the data in adolescents for this indication are not robust (Carlson and Mick, 2003) and there has been some recent increased concern about the potential of these agents for increasing suicidal ideation (Healy, 2003).

The psychostimulants – methylphenidate and the amphetamines – have been widely and successfully used in the treatment of ADHD, a disorder for which impulsivity is a core symptom. There is also some indication that these agents may ameliorate the aggressive behaviors seen in conduct disorder (Klein, 1997).

Research

Clearly, much more research is needed to understand the etiology and treatment of aggression in young people. One important area for further inquiry concerns the core symptoms/features that seem to give rise to high risk and dangerous acting out behaviors, and the relationship between those behaviors and the normal limit testing of the developing adolescent as well as the normal ranges of temperament of which novelty and sensation seeking may be a part. Greater clarification of underlying neurodevelopmental abnormalities is necessary, and improved neuroimaging techniques may assist in this process. Early identification and intervention for children identified as being at high risk based on neurodevelopmental understanding has the potential to alter the long-term trajectory and eventual outcome of aggressive behavior. In addition, much more needs to be learned concerning treatment strategies in terms both of method effectiveness (psychosocial and pharmacologic) as well as cost containment in these times of resource constraint. While pharmacogenomics is not yet applicable to clinical decision making, it is likely to play an important role in the not-too-distant future.

Summary

Part of normal adolescent development may include experimentation with risky behavior that does not carry significant risk or does not happen repeatedly. However, it may be difficult to decide how serious the behavior is, especially when an adolescent is minimizing the risk. Asking key questions can help. After this, a good rule of thumb is that if either the physician or the parent feels concerned (not necessarily both), it is likely time to ask for an additional opinion from a mental health specialist about the need for a more aggressive intervention. The etiology of risky behavior involves interplay between biologic and psychologic predispositions and the strength of the social supports surrounding the adolescent. Interventions can include psychosocial and pharmacologic interventions in an outpatient or inpatient setting. Making a decision about which intervention is necessary might be another reason to seek consultation.

Annotated bibliography

American Academy of Child and Adolescent Psychiatry (2001) Practice parameter for the assessment and treatment of children and adolescents with suicidal behavior. American Academy of Child and Adolescent Psychiatry. *J Am Acad Child Adoles Psychiatry*, 40 (Suppl 7):24S–51S.

A comprehensive review of suicidal behavior from etiology to assessment and treatment based on a consensus child and adolescent psychiatry work group and extensive reviews from consultants and practicing clinicians.

Henggeler SW, Schoenwald SK, Rowland MD, Cunningham PB (2002) *Serious Emotional Disturbance in Children and Adolescents: Multisystemic Therapy*, 1st edn. Guilford Press, New York.

An excellent summary of the extensive research supporting the usefulness of multisystemic therapy and practical guidelines for how to use this intervention.

Raine A (1996) Autonomic nervous system factors underlying disinhibited, antisocial, and violent behavior. Biosocial perspectives and treatment implications. *Ann N Y Acad Sci*, 20(794):46–59.

One of the best summaries of the groundbreaking studies supporting the interplay of biology and psychosocial factors in the etiology of violent behaviors.

Weller EB, Rowan A, Elia J, Weller RA (1999) Aggressive behavior in patients with attention-deficit/hyperactivity disorder, conduct disorder, and pervasive developmental disorders. *J Clin Psychiatry*, 60 (Suppl 15):5–11.

A thoughtful, practical review of clinical interventions for aggressive behavior across several disorders that highlights how to tailor an approach for an individual.

CHAPTER 21

Evaluating and Managing Attachment Difficulties in Children

Shannon Croft, MD and Marianne Celano, PhD

Background

As early as the 1930s, pediatricians and child psychiatrists took an interest in children who had suffered from maltreatment and deprivation (Karen, 1994). At that time, concern for sterility led most pediatric wards and institutions responsible for the long-term care of children to minimize any unnecessary physical contact between children and staff. Babies' bottles were often propped so they wouldn't have to be held when fed. Older children had few social contacts and almost nothing to play with. In such settings, infants developed "hospitalism" (which now is known as "failure to thrive"), leading to failure to gain weight, irritability, listlessness, lack of normal vocalizations, and often ultimately to death. Children who grew up in these institutions were noted to be retarded and had delayed speech and hyperactive behavior. Child psychiatrists Loretta Bender and Stella Chess (in Karen, 1994) described these children as "affectionate to everyone" but unable to sustain relationships with families, even when later put into reasonably good foster care.

These observations led some clinicians to look past the child's need for nutrition and other physical needs and begin to consider the child's need for a loving close relationship with a consistent mothering person. In 1939, Harold Skeels, at the Iowa Child Research Welfare Station, placed institutionalized toddlers with older teenaged girls who were themselves residents in a home for feeble-minded girls. Within 2 years the toddlers' average IQs rose from 64 to 92 (in Karen, 1994). Many of these children went on to be adopted by outside families, and one of these children actually presented Dr Skeels the Joseph P. Kennedy award for his research more than 30 years later. In 1947 Rene Spitz made a film called *Grief: A Peril in Infancy* (Spitz, 1947) documenting the effects of maternal deprivation on infants. This film, as well as a subsequent film documenting the effects of maternal deprivation inherent in normal hospital procedures at the time, would popularize these ideas, and eventually catalyze changes in pediatric ward policies.

The mother-infant bond

John Bowlby, a British psychiatrist considered by most to be the father of attachment theory, proposed that the disruption of the mother-child bond (either by physical separation or emotional unavailability) led to mental disorder. In a paper entitled "Fourty-four juvenile thieves," he found that early maternal deprivation was the key factor that discriminated between these delinquents, especially those he found to be "affectionless," and other clinic children (Bowlby, 1944). These clinical findings were reinforced by primate research showing that monkeys who were socially deprived when young would develop significant pathology when they became adults (Harlow, 1961).

Bowlby went on to describe the normal infant's reaction to separation: protest leading to despair, and then ultimately detachment (Fonagy, 2001). This in turn led him to postulate an attachment system of behaviors whose purpose is to maintain proximity to a caregiving adult. In infants such behaviors include smiling, cooing, and crying. Older toddlers use speech and movement to draw the attention of caregivers. In Bowlby's model, as a child develops, he or she is biologically impelled to become attached. Depending on the environment, the child will either become "securely" or "insecurely" attached. Children who are "securely attached" will see themselves as safe and caregivers as generally reliable, while children who become "insecurely attached" develop an internal working model of themselves as unlovable and will expect their caregivers to reject them (Fonagy, 2001).

Mary Ainsworth took Bowlby's work and developed a research method for testing attachment hypotheses empirically (Ainsworth et al., 1978). To test her belief that children's attachment styles would be associated with their mother's styles of parenting, she designed "the strange situation" (see Box 21.1). In addition to home observation, a lab visit observed the infant's behavior during the introduction of the child to a stranger, and two brief separations and reunifications with the mother (Wilson, 2001). After analyzing the behavior of the children, she was able to classify them as "securely attached" or "insecurely attached" with further distinctions described in subgroups A-D.

Secure attachment in children is thought to teach basic trust and reciprocity in relationships, facilitate cognitive development, protect children against the effects of future trauma by increasing resilience, and promote the development of self-worth, empathy, and conscience, and allow for the ability to control impulses and emotions (Levy and Orlans, 1999).

Consequences of insecure attachment

Subsequent research using the strange situation looked specifically at differences in attachment behavior between children who had been abused and neglected and children who had not been abused. Abused and neglected children were more often found to be insecurely attached, and seemed to have ineffective ways of seeking closeness to their mothers (Hanson and Spratt, 2000). In a similar study, more than 80% of children with verified maltreatment showed an insecure/disorganized pattern of attachment (Boris and Zeanah, 1998).

There is also increasing evidence that children with disordered attachment (particularly those with disorganized attachment) are at significant risk of later emotional and behavioral problems. Studies (Boris and Zeanah, 1998; Levy and Orlans, 1999) have found associations between insecure/disorganized attachment at 18 months and aggressive and disruptive behavior at 7 years. Similarly insecure/avoidant attachment at 18 months was associated with anxious withdrawal and sadness at 7 years of age. In another study (in Wilson, 2001), an attachment classification as insecure/resistant as an infant was predictive of anxiety disorders in late adolescence. Measures of attachment behaviors in adolescents and adults (Bender et al., 2001; Sund and Wichstrom, 2002) have demonstrated associations between attachment difficulties and depression, character pathology, conduct disorders, and substance abuse. Some have suggested that insecurely attached children may grow up to become parents incapable of establishing healthy attachment relationships with their own children, thereby leading to intergenerational transmission (Levy and Orlans, 1999).

Recent studies of institutionalized children

While the body of research looking at insecure vs. secure attachments has grown, another group of researchers have been examining children who may have never developed a selective attachment at all. These studies have recently focused on children reared in institutions in Romania, where scant resources and rotating shift workers left children with few opportunities to form attachment relationships with caregivers. Studies in Bucharest show that children raised in these institutions showed patterns of indiscriminate behavior, inhibited/withdrawn behavior, and a decreased response to comfort (Smyke et al., 2002). Other studies have looked at children adopted from these Romanian orphanages and placed into UK homes. After up to 4 years of placement in homes in the UK, these children continued to show elevated rates of attachment disturbances, and the severity of their disordered attachment behavior was correlated to the duration of their deprivation (O'Connor and Rutter, 2000). When compared with UK adoptees who did not suffer deprivation, these Romanian adoptees showed increased rates of inattention and over-activity associated with attachment difficulties (and these problems were not otherwise accounted for by malnutrition or cognitive deficits) (Kreppner et al., 2001). Studies in other countries have

---

BOX 21.1

Ainsworth's Strange Situation attachment patterns

Group A: insecure/avoidant
- Avoided reunification with the mother.
- Might turn away from the mother on reunion, showing little distress.
- Easily consoled by a stranger.

Group B: secure
- The majority of all infants tested (two-thirds).
- With mother in room explores environment securely.
- More easily consoled by the mother than the stranger.
- Attempts to get mother's attention on reunion by reaching or crying.

Group C: insecure/resistant/ambivalent
- With mother in room had less active exploratory behaviour.
- On reunion might initially seek contact, but would then resist contact and interaction with mother, seeming angry.
- Might push away or squirm if mother tried to hold infant on reunion.

Group D: insecure/disorganized
- Behaviors toward mother seem confused and apprehensive.
- During separation display no coherent pattern of coping strategies.
- Behavior appears to be contradictory.
- Might move backwards toward parent on reunion.

found similarly disturbed attachment behaviors in children reared in orphanages who have been deprived of stable attachment figures (Minnis, 2001).

Reactive attachment disorder (RAD)

Consistent with findings from these children deprived of possibilities for attachment, *The Diagnostic and Statistical Manual of Mental Disorders*, 4th edition (DSM-IV) (American Psychiatric Association, 1994) presents reactive attachment disorder (RAD) as one of the most severe disturbances of attachment (Table 21.1). RAD is described as "markedly disturbed and developmentally inappropriate social relatedness in most contexts, beginning before age 5 years" (p. 116). To be given this diagnosis, children must have experienced pathogenic care as evidenced by disregard for emotional or physical needs or repeated changes of primary caregivers. Two subtypes are delineated, the inhibited and the disinhibited. In the inhibited subtype, children fail to initiate and respond to social interactions in an age-appropriate way. These children may resist comforting by caregivers. The disinhibited subtype is characterized by excessive familiarity with strangers, demonstrating a lack of discrimination. Such children may appear superficially charming and inappropriately quick to express affection to adults they have just met.

While not specifically discussed in the DSM-IV, some authors have suggested that infants may display behaviors that may indicate risk for RAD including a weak cry and suck, inappropriate tone (either too stiff or too limp), lack of social smiling and little attempt to make eye contact (Wilson, 2001). While these behaviors will not by themselves make a diagnosis of RAD, they certainly warrant further clinical evaluation. At this time there are no good prevalence data, however, the DSM-IV describes RAD as "uncommon." It

KEY CLINICAL QUESTIONS

- *Does the child indicate a stable preference for a caregiver over strangers, even given the presence of disordered behavior?* Insecure attachment may represent a disorder of selective attachment relationships, but insecurely attached children should still show evidence of some selective attachment. RAD, on the other hand, may be understood as a disorder of non-attachment, and children with this disorder may not show any selective attachment behavior.

has been suggested that rates of RAD could be inferred from available data about the prevalence of child maltreatment, but most researchers are convinced that this approach is problematic (Hanson and Spratt, 2000).

While not part of the DSM criteria, there are a number of associated features commonly shared by children diagnosed with RAD. Some of these include a lack of empathy and conscience, aggressive and self-destructive behavior, cruelty to animals, destruction of property, lying, poor impulse control, abnormal speech patterns, unstable peer relationships, and reduced eye contact (Levy and Orlans, 1999; Wilson, 2001). Parents report children who have been diagnosed with RAD have more problems with behavior, emotions, attention, and aggression than parents report of their non-RAD diagnosed children (Hall, 2003). Additionally, parents rate their children with RAD as having less empathy, while children with RAD tend to rate themselves so highly that it appears they may be consciously trying to present themselves in the most socially desirable manner possible (Hall, 2003).

Given this long list of associated pathology, it is clearly important to identify cases when a child may meet criteria for another condition not based solely on disturbances in attachment. While institutionalized children may develop inattention and overactivity (Kreppner et al., 2001), most children with attention-deficit/hyperactivity disorder do not have a history of institutional care or poor parenting. In posttraumatic stress disorder (PTSD) a child may experience symptoms after experiencing a trauma, but in most cases this will not lead to disturbed attachment (unless the trauma occurred within the primary attachment relationship as may be the case in intrafamilial physical or sexual abuse, and domestic violence). Conduct disorder and oppositional defiant disorder may be discriminated from RAD, as children with simple behavioral disorders may have some problematic relationships, but do not show the same level of disturbance of attachment. Children with RAD tend to be more socially competent than autistic children, but have more relationship problems than do children with simple language disorders (Hanson and Spratt, 2000).

DIAGNOSIS

Table 21.1 Reactive attachment disorder (RAD)

Discriminating features

1. Always associated with pathogenic care.
2. Disturbance must be evident before the age of 5.

Consistent features

1. Developmentally inappropriate social relationships.

Variable features

1. May present as inhibited: fearful and restricted in relationships with caregivers.
2. May present as disinhibited: shallow, facile, and indiscriminate relationships.

Limitations of DSM diagnosis (alternate conceptualizations)

The current DSM-IV criteria for RAD are not without their critics. Some feel that the requirement that a child must have evidence of pathogenic care to be diagnosed with RAD should be removed from the DSM (Boris et al., 1998; Minde, 2003a), citing case examples of children who exhibited behavior consistent with a RAD diagnosis without any evidence of neglect or bad parenting. It is also important to point out that not all children who receive pathogenic care develop RAD. In fact, about 70% of children in Romanian institutions who were subject to social deprivation of 2 years' duration or greater did not develop severe attachment disorder (O'Connor et al., 2000). Others point out that using current criteria there are problems differentiating disorders of non-attachment like RAD from disordered (often disorganized) attachment, yet these two entities appear to be different, even if they both fall in the spectrum of attachment disorders (Minde, 2003a; O'Connor and Zeanah, 2003). It will be necessary in the future to elucidate this wider spectrum of attachment disorders. Future diagnoses will also benefit from expanded qualifiers for children of different ages (from infancy to adolescence), as well as the addition of cultural variables.

Clinical assessment of attachment disturbances

When assessing a child who is suspected of having RAD, one must first consider the child's current safety. Children with histories of social deprivation may have been exposed to other kinds of abuse and neglect. Children who have been abused may develop a wide range of pathology, including PTSD, mood and anxiety disorders, as well as problems with aggression and attention. Some children may have been emotionally neglected by unavailable depressed parents, whose style of parenting may lack warmth and encouragement, often focusing on hostility and criticism with harsh but inconsistent discipline (Scott, 2003). Other risk factors or "challenges to attachment" that need to be assessed include death of a parent, maternal substance abuse, marital discord, poverty, and multiple out of the home placements and foster care (Boris and Zeanah, 1998). If children with attachment difficulties are themselves still living in an abusive neglectful environment, then treating their "attachment" problems may actually cause them some trauma by forcing them into closer relationships with abusive caregivers (Scott, 2003).

At this time, there is no agreed upon comprehensive strategy for the evaluation of RAD. Most authors (Sheperis et al., 2003; O'Connor and Zeanah, 2003) agree that multiple methods of assessment are needed. By combining careful observation, interviews of the caregivers and the child, and occasional self-report measures, the clinician will hopefully arrive at a point of convergence of information regarding the child's attachment relationships and behavior. Observations of the child's behavior are especially important in assessing attachment difficulties. As DSM criteria include a description of the child's behavior toward strangers (especially in the "indiscriminant" subgroup), a visit to a new doctor's office provides an opportunity to observe this behavior first hand (Boris and Zeanah, 1998). Still, clinicians are cautioned that some children who show signs of disinhibited behavior with strangers may have normal attachment behaviors with caregivers, and that all children with disrupted attachment with caregivers may not exhibit indiscriminate behavior with strangers (O'Connor and Zeanah, 2003). There have been attempts at developing more structured functional family assessments where children and their families are observed under various conditions designed to elicit symptoms of RAD (Sheperis et al., 2003), but to date these methods have not been validated for the diagnosis of RAD.

Detailed clinical interviews are also essential to make the diagnosis of RAD. It has been demonstrated that comprehensive interviews are sufficient to ascertain the presence of disinhibited and inhibited symptoms (O'Connor and Zeanah, 2003). More importantly, a clinical interview needs to assess the detailed history of these symptoms, including when the symptoms were first noted and any changes in symptom profile noted over time. This is especially important in cases where children are in foster care or have been adopted, as it is possible that the child attachment behaviors may change as they form relationships with their new caregivers. It is also important to find out for each child what situations tend to "bring out" disturbed attachment behavior, and what factors tend to diminish this behavior. For example, one child might only demonstrate fearful withdrawal and inhibited behavior in situations where he or she was already anxious, but in other situations he or she might exhibit disinhibited interactions with strangers. This kind of detailed assessment is only possible if caregivers themselves are interviewed in depth. Clinical interviews or some other method of gathering historical information will also be needed to demonstrate pathogenic care, currently a criterion of the RAD diagnosis. It is also important to find out about associated pathology that might be seen in children with RAD and evaluate for the comorbid conditions discussed above.

General parent questionnaires may be useful as aids in evaluating the full range of a child's functioning. Some authors have espoused attachment specific questionnaires like the Randolph Attachment Disorder Questionnaire, a 30-item self-report instrument for use in children aged 5 to 18, and the Reactive Attachment Disorder Questionnaire, a 17-item parent instrument (Sheperis et al., 2003). Unfortunately, only the Reactive Attachment Disorder Questionaire is based on DSM-IV criteria, and it has not been normed for children in the United States. Questionnaires may ultimately prove of limited usefulness in the assessment of RAD, as the pen and paper format may not lend itself to the sensitive

Assessing RAD

- Observation looks at child's behavior with both strangers and familiar caregivers, in particular examining the quality of the child's current relationship with caregivers.
- Clinical interviews focus on the history of attachment disturbances and specific details about the context and course of these symptoms.
- Comorbid conditions such as behavioral, attentional and mood disturbances need to be evaluated.
- Self-report questionnaires may be useful to evaluate overall levels of functioning, but at this time are less useful for purposes of clinical assessment.

evaluation of complex social relationships (O'Connor and Zeanah, 2003).

Treatment approaches

Despite the fact that attachment disorders have been recognized in children for over 20 years by clinicians, there is no known effective treatment for children with RAD. The development of interventions for RAD has been complicated by several factors. First and perhaps most important, there are unresolved questions about how attachment disturbances are conceptualized. According to the DSM-IV and ICD-10, RAD consists of two subtypes, disinhibited and inhibited. However, some authors (Boris and Zeanah, 1999) have suggested a spectrum of disturbance with secure attachment on one end and disorders of non-attachment (approximating RAD) on the other. Ordinary forms of insecure attachment, disorganized attachment, and secure base distortions would occupy the middle portions of the spectrum. Second, there is no "gold standard" for assessing attachment disorders or monitoring symptom course, with considerable variability in assessment methods across clinicians and researchers. In general, research on attachment disturbances has not used the diagnostic criteria defined by the DSM or ICD, relying instead on concepts and measures from the field of developmental psychology. Without a consensus about how to define and operationalize attachment disturbances, it is difficult to determine the appropriate target for treatment.

Third, there is no consensus about the mechanisms by which pathogenic care influences various symptom patterns in children. Even the metaphors for understanding attachment disturbances have been questioned. Consistent with concepts such as "developmental arrest" and "regression" borrowed from the psychoanalytic literature, some authors have argued that development in children with RAD has been delayed or "frozen" (e.g. Keck and Kupecky, 1995). However, current theory and research in developmental psychopathology suggests that disturbance is best conceptualized as development that has followed a mala-daptive pathway. Thus, development is derailed rather than frozen. Although it is widely agreed that pathogenic care, often in the form of protracted neglect or deprivation, is the primary etiologic factor in the development of RAD, it is not known how pathogenic care interacts with other variables to produce symptoms associated with RAD. Nor is it clear why some children known to experience pathogenic care do not exhibit attachment disorder behaviors (Richters and Volkmar, 1994). The effects of pathogenic care may be mediated by individual child characteristics (such as child temperament) and by aspects of the sociocultural context in which child-rearing is embedded. There is some evidence to suggest that attachment disturbances are related to the quality of early caregiving (Smyke et al., 2002 in Minde 2003a), the duration of institutionalizaton (O'Connor et al., 1999) and the age of the infant at the time of the caregiving disruption (Albus and Dozier, 1999). There are no well controlled studies examining the natural course of RAD in children which would clarify the interplay between pathogenic care, child characteristics, and environmental characteristics over time.

Finally, the short- and long-term consequences of pathogenic care are dynamic and wide ranging, resulting in significant variability in symptom presentation over time. As already discussed, comorbid features of RAD include a wide variety of emotional and behavioral symptoms. Some of these behaviors may be classified more correctly under other diagnoses, such as PTSD, adjustment disorders, or anxiety disorders. In fact, there is considerable diagnostic overlap between RAD and PTSD in infancy and early childhood (Hanson and Spratt, 2000). It is unclear whether externalizing behavior problems are a comorbid symptom of a neglectful upbringing (Minde 2003a), a manifestation of a core disturbance of attachment, or a developmental consequence of physical abuse. For example, children with attachment disturbances may exhibit the reactive aggression observed in abused children (Shields and Cicchetti, 1998). Reactive aggression is believed to be a learned behavioral response to abuse in which children perceive threat in neutral or friendly situations, resulting in inappropriate aggressive outbursts. This conceptualization of aggression suggests a very different treatment approach than aggression presumed to reflect an underlying attachment disturbance.

The literature on RAD treatment lags far behind the growing bodies of research on other psychiatric disorders of childhood. Existing studies of RAD are retrospective in nature, utilize very small samples, and have not included adequate control groups. The most researched interventions involve very young children in parent-child therapy. Most of the studies are with formerly institutionalized children, usually from a single orphanage, rather than with children with more heterogeneous experiences of pathogenic care. Thus, our knowledge of and competence in administering interventions for attachment-disordered children is quite limited, particularly for older children. In recent years, a number of treatments for RAD, some controversial, have been proposed at conferences and in the literature. However, none of these treatments has been subjected to randomized clinical trials to assess their efficacy and safety.

Psychodynamically informed individual psychotherapy

Historically, treatment for RAD has consisted of individual therapy for the child informed by both psychoanalytic and attachment theory. It is assumed that what takes place in the therapeutic situation is a partial reenactment of what the child experienced in the original bond with his or her mother. That is, the therapeutic situation activates a working model of approaching attachment relations with others, specifically the mother or father. The patient's inner working models of self and attachment figure are presumed to mature as a result of changes in affect, cognition, and behavior sustained within the context of the patient's attachment relationship with the therapist. A fundamental prerequisite is a strong therapeutic alliance between the therapist and the child. Brisch (2002) has suggested some modifications of Bowlby's (1988) guidelines for the therapeutic application of attachment theory with children. According to these guidelines, the therapist should: (1) serve as a reliable emotional and physical base for the child so that a secure attachment relationship can develop, (2) facilitate play that promotes play enacting material relating to the child's experience with early attachment figures, (3) interpret attachment-related interactions verbally or symbolically, (4) foster emotional expression related to attachment issues in the transference, relating them to past attachment experiences; (5) promote an environment in therapy where the child can develop a secure attachment with the therapist; (6) when appropriate, dissolve the therapeutic bond carefully to model a way to cope with future separations. Concurrent therapy of parents plays an important role in psychodynamic treatment of children with attachment disturbances. The child's therapist educates the parents about the theory underlying treatment, the therapeutic process, the specific treatment plan, behavioral changes parents might see in their child, and insights that develop as the work progresses. The therapist must also provide a secure emotional base for the parents, showing sensitivity to their attachment needs, so that the parents will feel free to discuss their own experiences of trauma and loss in their concurrent therapeutic work (Brisch, 2002). However, parenting behavior or the parent-child relationship is not typically the focus of psychodynamically informed individual therapy for children with attachment disturbances.

Although psychodynamically informed individual treatment has been the dominant intervention for individuals with attachment disturbances for over 20 years, there have been very few studies examining whether attachment strat-

egies (assessed with the Adult Attachment Interview) become more secure as a result of new attachment experiences in the course of psychotherapy. Studies with adults (Fonagy et al., 1996) and case reports (Brisch, 2002) provide the only evidence of the efficacy of psychodynamic therapy for children with RAD. Case reports indicate that this therapy has been successfully applied to children and adolescents with no signs of attachment behavior, with undifferentiated (disinhibited) attachment behavior, or with inhibited attachment behavior. In addition, psychodynamically informed treatment attentive to attachment dynamics has been reported to be successful in cases of aggression, psychosomatic symptoms, school phobia, underachievement, addictive symptoms, and anti-social behavior in children and adolescents.

Individual therapy for the parent

In cases in which the child's pathogenic care is due in part to the parent's psychiatric illness, the parent is often referred for individual treatment. Depression may cause parents to be physically and psychologically unavailable to their infants, which in turn negatively affects the developing attachment relationship (Cummings and Cicchetti, 1990). Individual psychotherapy and pharmacotherapy can help parents to manage the depressive symptoms interfering in their optimal availability and responsivity to their children.

Parent-child psychotherapy

Treatment models focusing on the parent-child dyad are among the most studied interventions for children with attachment disturbances. Attachment interventions have been developed specifically for high-risk infants (Lieberman and Zeanah, 1999), where high risk is defined in terms of infant irritability, adverse psychosocial conditions, psychiatric disorder in the parent, or insecure attachment. Infant-parent psychotherapy, built on attachment and object relations theories, was initially developed by Fraiberg and colleagues (1975) three decades ago to improve emotional synchrony and empathic attunement of parents toward their high-risk infants, including those with attachment disorders. Fraiberg's initial model highlighted the role of parental emotional baggage, termed "ghosts in the nursery," in contributing to the development of parent-infant relationship disturbances. The "ghosts" refer to the parent's unresolved conflicts arising from his or her own early attachment relationships which impede the parent's ability to be emotionally and physically available to the infant because of the tendency to re-enact these conflicts within the parent-infant relationship.

In cases when the caregiver demonstrates resolved attachment, the therapist can facilitate the parent-child relationship through modeling and directly coaching interactions congruent with attachment security. If the parent is not resolved with respect to his or her own attachment history, an initial period of separate individual treatment for parent and child is recommended (Hughes, 2003). Subsequently, the aim of parent-infant therapy is to assist the parents in becoming aware of the ways in which they re-enact their own unresolved childhood experiences in the relationship with the infant. Therapeutic techniques include interpretation of parent-child interaction, practical nondidactic developmental guidance, and direct support and advocacy. Typically, the therapist addresses the parent's verbalizations to the infant and the parallel nonverbal communications, tracking both the parent's and infant's responses, and pointing out how the parent's subjective responses to the infant are related to the infant's immediate concrete experience. Parents are then coached to become more attuned with their infant's emotional and developmental needs, leading to more appropriate and attentive infant responses.

Parent-child therapy has also been applied to families with toddlers (Cicchetti et al., 1999). In addition to the goals of improving emotional reciprocity between the parent and child, and increasing maternal attunement to the child's cues, toddler-parent therapy aims to increase the toddler's comfort in leaving the attachment figure for brief periods to explore the surrounding environment. Although the primary goal is to improve the attachment relationship, the toddler's confidence in exploring his/her environment while using the parent as a secure base contributes to the acquisition of normal developmental milestones and may reduce his or her risk for depression, even if the parent is depressed (Cicchetti et al., 1999).

For children of all ages, a key component of parent-child therapy is the active intersubjective stance by the caregiver in which their experience of the child's affect is made clear and is used to help the child eventually regulate and construct meaning regarding his or her inner life. This is based on the notion that in secure attachment dyads the child understands his or her inner life in part by experiencing the reflected response of the parent to his or her nonverbal expressive behaviors. In therapy, the caregiver and therapist clarify their subjective experience of the child through obvious and even exaggerated nonverbal expressions of responsiveness in a manner similar to what is exhibited by a parent to an infant. Essentially, the caregiver and therapist maintain an interpersonal emotional tone that is consistent with the acceptance, empathy, curiosity and playfulness, sensitivity, responsiveness and availability exhibited by parents in secure attachment dyads. Conflicts and misattunements between parent/therapist and child are directly addressed and repaired. Parental interventions are congruent with attachment theory. For example, a child in distress is brought closer to the parent so that the parent can co-regulate the child's affective state. Parents also respond to the child's affective dysregulation by providing a structured routine, reducing the child's choices when the choices lead to repetitive failure.

According to a recent meta-analysis of attachment interventions in early childhood (Bakermans-Kranenburg et al., 2003), interventions offering direct coaching of specific behaviors by the caregiver are effective in improving infant attachment security. However, the mechanisms underlying the treatment response are unclear, and few studies compare attachment-based intervention with an intervention based on an alternative theoretical perspective (O'Connor and Zeanah, 2003).

The appeal of attachment-based infant-parent psychotherapy is its concordance between attachment theory and therapeutic technique. Interventions target the very factors hypothesized to cause the child's attachment disturbance: the parent's pathogenic internal models of attachment and related pattern of interacting with the child. This model works better for infants who have shown some type of attachment to the parent than for infants who fail to develop a selective attachment, such as children adopted from foster care institutions. Indeed, the persistence of attachment disorder in formerly institutionalized children adopted by "adequately sensitive" parents poses a challenge for this treatment model (O'Connor and Zeanah, 2003). Other authors (Lieberman, 2003) have suggested that even in cases in which the cause of the child's attachment disorder preceded the adoption, the child's lack of trust in the reliable availability and protectiveness of the attachment figure remains a core problem after adoption and influences the developing relationship with the adoptive parent.

In cases of adoption, the child brings to the adoptive relationship his or her expectations, fears, and behavioral patterns developed in the context of interactions within the early child-rearing environment (e.g. context of pathogenic care), and the adoptive parents bring to their relationship with the child their own idiosyncratic hopes, fantasies, expectations, and vulnerabilities (Lieberman, 2003). Even parents considered sufficiently sensitive and responsive to children may discover that they are ill equipped to cope with their adopted child's emotional distance, refusal to be comforted, sudden mood shifts, indiscriminate sociability, and, in some cases, noncompliance and aggression. In the worst cases, the ongoing failure of emotionally satisfying reciprocity in the parent-child relationship can cause parents to give up on the challenge of raising the child, which in turn reinforces the child's perception of him or herself as unlovable as well as the futility of finding a consistent and emotionally available attachment figure.

In their study of children adopted before the age of 4, Lieberman (2003) observed that adoptive parents tended to overlook or minimize the child's expressions of anxiety, and that their responses often were not attuned to the child's attachment cues. For example, they responded with disciplinary measures when they perceived the child's behavior as inappropriate rather than with firm but comforting behavior assuring the child of the parent's ongoing availability. Similarly, Marvin and Whelan (2003) attribute the failure of emotional reciprocity between parent and child to the child's tendency to miscue their caregivers regarding their underlying attachment and/or exploratory needs. For example, an avoidant child may communicate his/her need for soothing by sending a cue that he wants to explore, making it difficult for the parent to respond appropriately.

To prevent failed adoptions and the ensuing persistence of attachment disturbance, Lieberman (2003) suggests modifications to parent-infant psychotherapy with children showing attachment disorder behaviors following adoption: (1) educate adoptive parents about the likely psychologic and behavioral problems of children deprived of a consistent attachment figure in early life, (2) offer emotionally supportive, child-focused developmental guidance to help the parents become more responsive to the child's complex and contradictory attempts to gain reassurance, (3) direct parents to overemphasize their emotional response to the child's attachment needs, demonstrating sadness upon separation and joy upon reunions.

Holding therapies

A novel therapy specifically designed to treat the serious difficulties experienced by older children with attachment disorders is holding therapy, also called attachment therapy or rage reduction therapy. Its defining feature is the close physical contact between the child patient and the therapist or therapists for long periods of time (45 minutes or longer) on a daily basis over a period of typically 2 weeks (Keck and Kupecky, 1995), with bimonthly to monthly follow-up over the course of a year (Minnis and Keck, 2003). The child typically lies across the lap of one or two therapists (or the therapist and the parent), while the adults provide noxious stimulation (e.g. tickling, yelling, poking in the ribs) and interfere with the child's bodily functions. The child may initially resist by screaming and fighting, but eventually surrenders. At this point, the child is reunited with the caregiver, to whom he or she allegedly instantly attaches. This treatment is based on the assumption that children with attachment disorders have repressed rage that needs to be released before they can form healthy attachments. The prolonged restraint (i.e. holding), noxious stimulation, and interference with bodily functions are hypothesized to release children's rage and teach them that adults will control and protect them. Holding is considered the central therapeutic mechanism for change because of its intensity and because the prolonged physical contact mimics the touch/holding experiences that are part of the normative attachment process between caregiver and infant.

Proponents of holding therapy claim that holding therapy is the only treatment sufficiently intense to break though the child's defenses and contain the child's distress and rage. Similarly, a neurobiologic perspective (Minde 2003a) states that resolution of attachment-related memories may require them to be re-experienced in the presence of high emotional arousal, since this is how they were first experienced. Anecdotal reports claim that attachment therapy is effective where all other clinical interventions have failed. However, its detractors argue that holding therapy is contrary to fundamental attachment theory principles (Lieberman and Zeanah, 1999), inconsistent with current notions in developmental theory (O'Connor and Zeanah, 2003), and might be viewed as intrusive, countertherapeutic, or even traumatizing (James, 1994) to the already traumatized child. Further, there are concerns about the safety of this technique. In the US there have been six reported deaths of children attributed to holding therapy or its variants (e.g. "rebirthing therapy" or "compression holding") or to parental practices consistent with these techniques. To date, there is little empirical evidence for the efficacy of holding therapy. Existing studies (O'Connor and Zeanah, 2003) are limited by small samples, lack of reliable and valid measures of attachment between child and caregiver, and failure to compare holding therapy with less costly and invasive forms of treatment. Even if holding therapy is shown to be effective in reducing emotional and behavioral problems of children believed to have attachment disturbances, there are less intensive, less expensive and more effective treatment models available to target these symptoms. Although holding offers some hope to parents of children with severe disturbances often misunderstood by clinicians, systematic and rigorous empirical inquiry into the efficacy, effectiveness, and safety of holding therapy is needed before it can be recommended as a form of treatment. Proponents of holding therapy agree that systematic intervention research is needed, but admit that human investigation committees are hesitant to support a study including physical contact with children in one of its treatment arms (Minnis and Keck, 2003).

Parent training, family support, and family therapy

A number of family interventions have been proposed as effective in enhancing the attachment relationships between parent and child (Sexson et al., 2001). Parent-child interaction therapy (Eyberg et al., 1995), a treatment model developed primarily for families with oppositional preschoolers, can be modified to target the parent-child bond. This therapy includes two phases. In the child-directed interaction phase, the parents are coached in using traditional nondirective play techniques to facilitate a more accepting and rewarding interactional stance toward the child. In the parent-directed interaction phase, parents are taught to clearly communicate their involvement with the child, expectations for the child's behavior, and empathy and responsivity to the child's affect.

Filial therapy (Guerney, 1964; Van Fleet, 1994) is similar to parent-child interaction therapy in that it aims to promote positive attachment by fostering the parent's and child's ability to collaboratively engage in playful activities with one another. The therapist essentially teaches the parent how to use client-centered play therapy techniques such as reflection and empathic responding, and to recognize and understand the symbolism of the child's play. Parents observe the therapist play with the child, then "practice" play sessions in the therapist's office and at home, receiving feedback about their skill acquisition. Eventually, the parents and child engage in play sessions at home, returning to the therapist periodically for supervision. As in other treatment models, it is assumed that the empathic reflection of the child's feelings, needs, and conflicts as expressed through play fosters the child's sense of security and trust. Unlike other interventions, the parent is the explicit agent of therapeutic change. The parent is believed to be more effective than a professional therapist because of his or her emotional significance for and investment in the child.

Family therapists have also begun to integrate attachment theory into systemic theory and techniques to enhance attachments in families with children under 12 years of age (Sexson et al., 2001; Byng-Hall, 1995). A popular technique for addressing attachment issues is the creative use of play in family therapy. Play offers adults and children a common ground for communicating their needs and conflicts, lowers family members' resistances to change, offers a safe medium for expression of painful affect, and often provides a mutual and pleasurable activity to facilitate attachment. Rather than the therapist interpreting the play or coaching the parent to act in a responsive manner, the therapist and family jointly co-create a narrative understanding about the child's and family's play (Larner, 1996).

Parents caring for children with attachment disturbances often need support and training to cope with their confusion and frustration about their children's inappropriate behavior and seeming indifference to them. Unfortunately, parents' frustration and detachment from their attachment-disturbed child is sometimes interpreted by clinicians as a source of the child's disturbance rather than a result of it (O'Connor and Zeanah, 2003). Clinicians should demonstrate sensitivity in engaging parents in the treatment process, and offer considerable support and guidance. Although it is unclear to what extent parent support would promote their children's development and attachment, parents' feelings of confusion and rejection by the child are justifiable targets for clinical intervention (O'Connor and Zeanah, 2003). In recent years, a number of support groups have arisen specifically for adoptive parents of children adopted from institutions or foster care. Participation in parent support groups may be particularly helpful for parents who feel dissatisfied with or neglected by traditional mental health and social service agencies. These groups may provide parents with the emotional support, advocacy, and skills training needed to prevent adoption failure. For example, anecdotal reports suggest that parents may be able to reduce or control some of the disturbing features of disinhibited attachment disorder, such as wandering off. An important component of parent support is respite care for the child with attachment disturbance. Planned use of respite may provide parents with the support and "breathing room" they need to continue to work on difficult attachment issues with the child, and may also prevent costly hospitalization and unnecessary out-of-home placements. However, children with a history of negative attachment experiences may have difficulty coping with the repeated separations from the parent. Therefore, clinicians and parents should assess the impact of the separation caused by respite placement before incorporating it into the treatment plan (O'Connor and Zeanah, 2003).

Social-cognitive treatment approaches

Unlike treatment models derived from attachment theory, social-cognitive or cognitive behavioral interventions focus not on the attachment relationship per se, but instead on the social and cognitive disturbances underlying or accompanying the attachment disorder behavior. These interventions possess the advantage of greater evidence of efficacy for changing specific target behaviors, including peer rejection, aggressive behavior due to misattribution of hostile intent to others, PTSD symptoms, and depressive symptoms (Lochman et al., 1993; Yule, 2002). In addition, evidence-based and widely applied parenting training programs derived from social learning theory (e.g. Webster-Stratton and Hammond, 1997) can be implemented to reduce the oppositional and anti-social behaviors exhibited by some children with attachment disorder. Although some authors call for greater integration of non-attachment-based interventions with

Treating RAD
- Identify children with attachment disturbances at an early age.
- Determine that the child is in a nurturing and secure environment (i.e. no ongoing neglect).
- Engage parent in treatment without attributing blame to parent for child's attachment disturbance.
- Obtain referrals for the caregiver, if necessary (e.g. parental depression).
- Intervene directly with the child's caregivers to learn how to interpret child's signals and respond more appropriately.
- Beware of untested claims about the efficacy of specialized treatments that are costly, intense, or intrusive.
- Provide ongoing support to the parents.

PEARLS & PERILS

CONSIDER CONSULTATION WHEN ...

Consultation and collaboration with other colleagues is the rule when treating children with this difficult condition.

- The diagnosis is often difficult to make, and requires a thorough exploration of the child's behavior in multiple settings, a task that can be facilitated by collaboration with pediatricians, school staff, and therapists.
- Multimodal treatment may at times require separate family, parent, and child interventions.
- Families dealing with children with attachment disorders often benefit from various levels of support.
- Associated conditions may benefit from pharmacologic interventions.

treatment models derived from attachment theory (Scott, 2003), others (Hughes, 2003) recommend that cognitive behavioral treatment strategies be used only after the child has developed a more secure attachment relationship with the caregiver.

Annotated bibliography

Bowlby J (1988). *A Secure Base: Clinical implications of attachment theory.* London, Routledge.

This is an excellent book by one of the pioneers in attachment theory. It is recommended as a good place to start your reading on the topic of attachment.

Brisch KH (2002) *Treating Attachment Disorders: From Theory to Therapy.* New York, Guilford.

This is one of the best books to come out recently on the treatment of attachment disorders. Brisch brings cases to life with clinical vignettes that illustrate how he works with these children.

O'Connor TG, Zeanah CH (2003) Attachment disorders: assessment strategies and treatment approaches. *Attachment and Human Development*, 5:223–244.

This is a significant article reviewing the assessment and intervention of children with attachment disorders. In particular, the authors highlight the need for the development of treatment guidelines. There are a number of other papers on RAD in this same issue of Attachment and Human Development.

Hanson RF, Spratt EG (2000) Reactive attachment disorder: what we know about the disorder and implications for treatment. *Child Maltreatment*, 5:137–145.

This is a well-written review article that discusses the risks of controversial coercive techniques that have become popular recently. This article would be a good choice for trainees or an introductory course.

CHAPTER 22

Child and Adolescent Responses to Trauma

Michael D. De Bellis, MD, MPH and Anandhi Narasimhan, MD

Background

Children can experience traumatic events in many different forms. Trauma can include experiencing a one-time traumatic event, such as a dog bite, or the challenge of growing up with chronic adversity such as child maltreatment or witnessing domestic violence. The awareness of different types of abuse and violence toward and around children has brought about a curiosity of what kind of impact this has on growing children. In this chapter, we will address the following questions. What effect do traumatic events have on children? How are they affected emotionally, cognitively, behaviorally, and developmentally? What modalities can be used to identify mental illness that results from trauma and prevent and halt progression of maladaptive psychopathology?

Defining a traumatic event

To understand the potential effects of trauma on children and their responses to trauma, it is important to delineate what we define as a traumatic event. To categorically describe what we mean by trauma, we can divide trauma into subtypes, interpersonal trauma and non-interpersonal trauma, chronic or long-lasting trauma, and acute or one-time-only experiences. Interpersonal types of trauma are ones associated with a transactional model with other humans. Examples of these would include military combat, witnessing domestic or community violence, and violent personal assault (child abuse, physical and sexual, neglect, torture, robbery, terrorist attack). Non-interpersonal types of trauma include natural disasters (i.e. hurricanes, floods), disasters related to human causality, accidents, or diagnosis

with life-threatening illness. An example of a non-interpersonal single-event trauma is experiencing a dog bite that did not require extensive medical intervention. An example of a non-interpersonal long-lasting trauma is experiencing a dog bite that require extensive medical interventions over a period of years. An example of an interpersonal single-event trauma is witnessing a murder of a stranger while walking to school, while an example of interpersonal chronic traumatic events include abuse within families or witnessing domestic violence over several years.

Although historically it has been believed that child traumas are mostly associated with outrageous acts of violent injurious behavior toward children resulting in physical harm, it is important to note that a lot of trauma that children are subjected to can oftentimes not be life-threatening (e.g. sexual abuse), not isolated, and can be recurrent and associated with other forms of danger (e.g. children who experience chronic sexual abuse and also witness domestic violence against their mother). In the real world, war experiences, child maltreatment, and witnessing domestic and/or community violence are the most common causes of interpersonal trauma in children and adolescents. When trauma is of interpersonal origins, it is usually chronic and may cause more severe and long-lasting symptoms.

The relationship of stress to mental illness

The *Diagnostic and Statistical Manual of Mental Disorders*, fourth edition text revision (DSM-IV-TR) has four diagnoses in which an identified stressor precipitates the mental illness: adjustment disorder(s), acute stress disorder, reactive attachment disorder, and posttraumatic stress disorder (PTSD) (American Psychiatric Association, 2000). In this chapter, we will briefly discuss adjustment disorder(s) and acute stress disorder, but focus our attention on PTSD. Further information on reactive attachment disorder can be found in Chapter 21 of this book (Croft and Celano, 2005).

PTSD

As described in the *Diagnostic and Statistical Manual of Mental Disorders*, fourth edition text revision (DSM-IV-TR), the essential feature (criterion A) of posttraumatic stress disorder is exposure to an extreme traumatic stressor in which the person experienced, witnessed, or was confronted with an event or events that involved actual or threatened death or serious injury, or a threat to the physical integrity of self or others; and responded with intense fear, helplessness, horror or, in children, disorganized or agitated behaviors (American Psychiatric Association, 2000). The DSM-IV-TR diagnosis of PTSD is made when criterion A is experienced and when three clusters of categorical symptoms are present for more than 1 month after the traumatic event(s): 1) intrusive re-experiencing of the trauma(s) (criterion B), 2) persistent avoidance of stimuli associated with the trauma(s) (criterion C), and 3) persistent symptoms of increased physiologic arousal (criterion D).

Cluster B re-experiencing and intrusive symptoms can best be conceptualized as a classically conditioned response. An external or internal conditioned stimulus (e.g. the traumatic reminder) activates unwanted and distressing recurrent and intrusive memories of the traumatic experience(s) (e.g. the unconditioned stimulus). Intrusive phenomena take the form of distressing intrusions such as nightmares or night terrors, dissociative flashback episodes, and psychologic distress and physical reactivity on exposure to traumatic reminders. In young children, these intrusive thoughts may be part of repetitive play or trauma-specific re-enactment(s) or compulsive rituals. Criterion C symptoms represent both avoidant and dissociative behaviors, and can be thought of as ways to control painful and distressing re-experiencing of symptoms. These include efforts to avoid thoughts, feelings, conversations, activities, places, people, and memories associated with the trauma, amnesia for the trauma, diminished interest in others, feelings of detachment from others, a restricted range of affect, and a sense of a foreshortened future. Criterion D hyperarousal symptoms consist of persistent symptoms of increased physiologic arousal. These include difficulty falling or staying asleep, irritable mood or angry outbursts, difficulty concentrating, hypervigilance, and exaggerated startle response. PTSD symptoms are thought to be mediated by dysregulation of the neurobiologic stress systems, which mediate the fear or anxiety response.

It should be noted that there have been four major changes from the *Diagnostic and Statistical Manual of Mental Disorders*,

third edition-revised (DSM-III-R) (American Psychiatric Association, 1987). First, acute stress disorder (ASD) is a new DSM-IV anxiety disorder diagnosis. Making the appropriate DSM-IV diagnosis depends on the nature and severity of the stressor, severity of the symptoms, and length of time of the illness. Tables 22.1 and 22.2 list the DSM-IV criteria for PTSD and ASD. ASD is thought to distinguish acute and severe short-term from long-term posttraumatic stress reactions. Second, criterion A, the traumatic experience(s), is the same in both acute stress disorder and PTSD, and includes both objective and subjective features. In the DSM-III-R, criterion A, the traumatic experience was an event outside the range of usual human experiences that would be markedly distressing to almost anyone. The DSM-III-R did not include subjective reactions to the trauma, nor did it include more common events such as child maltreatment, witnessing domestic or community violence, or civilian war experiences.

The third change in the DSM-IV diagnosis of PTSD is that symptom 6 of criterion D in DSM-III-R (physiologic reactivity upon exposure to events that symbolize or resemble the traumatic event) was moved from criterion D (persistent symptoms of increased arousal), to criterion B, intrusive re-experiencing of the trauma(s). Fourth, in DSM-III-R, the duration of symptoms needed to be present for at least 1 month. In the DSM-IV, PTSD symptoms must be present for more than 1 month, whereas, acute stress disorder symp-

Table 22.1 Posttraumatic stress disorder

Discriminating features

1. Exposed to a trauma followed by a response of intense fear, helplessness or horror, or disorganized or agitated behaviour.

Consistent features

1. Recurrent and intrusive distressing recollections of the trauma.
2. Avoidance of traumatic reminders and numbing.
3. Increased arousal.
4. Impaired social and academic functioning.
5. Symptom duration of 1 month or more.

Variable features

1. Depressed or irritable mood.
2. Nightmares.
3. Aggression or sexualized behaviors.
4. Unexplained somatic complaints.
5. Sleep problems.
6. New fears.
7. Separation anxiety.
8. Unexplained somatic complaints.
9. Inattention.
10. In adolescents, risk-taking (substance abuse, sexual acting out).

Table 22.2 Acute stress disorder

Discriminating features

1. Exposed to a trauma followed by a response of intense fear, helplessness or horror, or disorganized or agitated behaviour.

Consistent features

1. At least three symptoms of dissociation.
2. Recurrent and intrusive distressing recollections of the trauma.
3. Avoidance of traumatic reminders.
4. Increased arousal.
5. Impaired social and academic functioning.
6. Symptom duration 2 days to a maximum of 4 weeks.

Variable features

1. Numbing.
2. Reduction in awareness.
3. Derealization.
4. Depersonalization.
5. Dissociative amnesia.

arousal (criteria B, C, D of DSM-IV PTSD). For children, sexually traumatic events may include developmentally inappropriate sexual experiences without threatened or actual violence or injury. The symptoms must cause clinically significant impairment in social or school functioning. In younger children, it is more common to see disorganized and/or regressive behavior (such as bedwetting) or agitated, oppositional, and irritable behavior in response to a severe stressor. If a child experiences acute stress disorder for more than 1 month, but less than 3 months, the DSM-IV diagnosis is then changed to PTSD, acute or an adjustment disorder, chronic depending upon whether all criteria of PTSD are met.

In studies of adults, the diagnosis of acute stress disorder has received limited support (Bryant and Harvey, 1997). In one study of children, a diagnosis of acute stress disorder predicted PTSD (Daviss et al., 2000). However, because of the high degree of overlap in symptoms between acute stress disorder and PTSD, it is questionable whether, as presently formulated, they represent distinct diagnoses (Brewin et al., 2003). Therefore, evidence-based PTSD treatment methods should be utilized when a child has acute stress disorder.

toms are present for 2 days to 1 month. Based on the DSM-IV criteria, PTSD may be acute (i.e. symptoms duration is less than 3 months after the trauma) or chronic (i.e. symptoms duration is more than 3 months after the trauma). PTSD may also have delayed onset (i.e. symptoms occur at least 6 months after the trauma).

However, a study found that most individuals who have delayed-onset PTSD suffered from subthreshold PTSD (e.g. an adjustment disorder) immediately after the trauma experience (Bryant and Harvey, 2002). This finding as well as other studies (North et al., 2002, 1999) challenges the notion of PTSD developing after a period of time without symptoms.

Acute stress disorder

As in PTSD, the essential feature (criterion A) of acute stress disorder is the development of characteristic symptoms following exposure to an extreme traumatic stressor in which the person experienced, witnessed, or was confronted with an event or events that involved actual or threatened death or serious injury, or a threat to the physical integrity of self or others; and responded with horror or disorganized behavior (American Psychiatric Association, 2000). The essential features of acute stress disorder are the presence of three or more dissociative symptoms such as numbing or detachment, "being in a daze," derealization, depersonalization, and dissociative amnesia as well as symptoms seen in PTSD such as intrusive thoughts of the trauma, persistent avoidance of traumatic reminders, and increased physiologic

Adjustment disorders

Differentiating normal adaptive symptoms from pathologic symptoms can be challenging. Traumatic events are usually external threats, but it is the subjective experience of these objective events that constitutes the trauma. Anxiety is a normal adaptive process regulated by the brain's emotional center (e.g. the amygdala and the limbic system) (for a review, see De Bellis, 2003). A review of the longitudinal course of PTSD suggested that PTSD symptoms are common within the first month of a trauma. These symptoms may be a normal response to severe stress, as these symptoms usually fade within 3 months (Blank, 1993). For example, one recent study showed that 80% of children and adolescents who were admitted to the hospital for injuries resulting from traffic or bicycle accidents had at least one symptom of acute stress disorder (Winston et al., 2002). Only one-third of this sample suffered from clinically significant distress. When emotional and behavioral symptoms develop in response to an identifiable stressor and entail disproportionate distress with significant impairment in social and academic functioning, a diagnosis of adjustment disorder is appropriate. The prevalence of adjustment disorder has been reported to range between 2% and 8% in community samples of children and adolescents.

Adjustment disorder is a diagnosis that is linked to an etiologic stressor (Table 22.3). Making the diagnosis results from a process of exclusion of other DSM-IV axis I disorders. In adjustment disorder, the stressor can be of any severity and may not necessarily be of traumatic origin, but in PTSD and acute stress disorder, the stressor must meet criterion A

Table 22.3 Adjustment disorder

Discriminating features

1. The development of emotional or behavioral symptoms occurring within 3 months of and in response to an identifiable stressor.

Consistent features

1. Marked distress.
2. Impaired social and academic functioning.

Variable features

1. Depressed or irritable mood.
2. Anxiety.
3. Disruptive behaviours.

of PTSD. Thus, the diagnosis of adjustment disorder arises from the preface of maladaptive coping responses (Hill, 2002). According to DSM-IV criteria, the symptoms or behaviors (not related to bereavement) cause marked distress that is in excess of what would be expected, and there is significant impairment in social, occupational, or academic functioning. An adjustment disorder is specified as acute if the disturbance lasts less than 6 months and chronic if the disturbance lasts for 6 months or longer. There are subtypes within the diagnosis, such as with depressed mood, where patients predominantly endorse symptoms of depressed mood, feelings of hopelessness, and tearfulness; with anxiety showing symptoms of worry, jitteriness, nervousness, fears of separation; with mixed anxiety and depressed mood (a constellation of above-mentioned symptoms); with disturbances of conduct (violation of rights of others, age-appropriate norms, and rules); mixed disturbances of emotions and conduct; and unspecified (maladaptive reactions to stressors that do not fit the above subtypes).

It should be noted that many children who experience trauma have clinically significant adjustment disorders. Because of this, PTSD may be better conceptualized as a dimensional process rather than a categorical all-or-nothing outcome, as complete and partial PTSD responses (e.g. adjustment disorders) are usually seen in many forms of trauma including victims of childhood maltreatment (Armsworth and Holaday, 1993; Hillary and Schare, 1993; Mannarino et al., 1994; Wolfe et al., 1994; Wolfe and Charney, 1991). Furthermore, even children with sub-disorder level PTSD symptoms (e.g. adjustment disorders) have substantial functional impairment and distress (Carrion et al., 2001b) requiring treatment. No complaints of PTSD symptoms after experiencing a severe stressor (i.e. lack of sleep disturbances, intrusive symptoms, or concentration impairments) may be associated with little psychopathology and be a marker of resilience.

The epidemiology of PTSD

PTSD is a serious and debilitating chronic mental illness with enormous societal costs (Kessler, 2000). PTSD may arise from a variety of traumatic events in both children and adults. The diagnostic picture of PTSD in children is similar to adults (De Bellis, 2001; Pynoos and Eth, 1985), with the exception of children less than 4 years where more objective criteria based on observable child behaviors are warranted (Scheeringa et al., 1995). These observable child behaviors include: new fears; aggression; recent onset of separation anxiety; fear of toileting alone; fear of the dark; and any other unrelated fear. Children are more vulnerable to developing PTSD as they are more likely to be diagnosed with PTSD, once traumatized, than adults who suffer from similar traumas (Fletcher, 1996).

According to the National Comorbidity Survey, the estimated lifetime prevalence of PTSD in persons aged 15–54 years is 7.8% (Kessler et al., 1995). The National Comorbidity Survey reported a lifetime history of at least one other axis I disorder (i.e. mood, other anxiety, and substance use disorders) in 88.3% of men and in 79% of women with PTSD. Although there are only a few studies, PTSD lifetime prevalence rates for children and adolescents are thought to be similar or even higher than those of adults. Hence, a recent community sample estimated a DSM-III-R PTSD prevalence rate using the NIMH Diagnostic Interview Schedule Version III-R (DIS-III-R) of 6.3% in adolescents (Giaconia et al., 1995). A recent review reports rates of 9–50% of PTSD in children who have experienced natural disaster(s) (Vogel and Vernberg, 1993). Severe burns were associated with PTSD rates of 30% (Stoddard et al 1989), and 1-year post-bone-marrow transplantation rate of 50% (Stuber et al., 1991). In clinically referred maltreated children, the reported incidence rates of PTSD resulting from sexual abuse range from 42% to 90% (Dubner and Motta, 1999; Lipschitz et al., 1999; McLeer et al., 1994), from witnessing domestic violence from 50% to 100% (for domestic homicide) (Pynoos and Nader, 1989), and from physical abuse to as high as 50% (Dubner and Motta, 1999; Green, 1985).

Only a few studies have focused on assessing PTSD in non-clinically referred maltreated children. A 39% incidence rate of PTSD in a non-clinically referred maltreated sample interviewed within 8 weeks of abuse or neglect disclosure was reported (Famularo et al., 1993). About a third of the PTSD subjects re-examined from the original sample continued to meet PTSD criteria at 2-year follow-up (Famularo et al., 1996). Recently, a prevalence rate of PTSD of 36.3% in non-clinically referred sexually abused children 60 days immediately following sexual abuse disclosure was reported (McLeer et al., 1998). Thus, PTSD is commonly seen in maltreated children, especially during the period immediately following maltreatment disclosure. Given that PTSD symptoms are common immediately after a traumatic experience, PTSD may be considered a disorder of recovery.

Risk factors associated with PTSD

Certain risk factors increase the probability that an individual will develop PTSD after a trauma. These factors are divided into three categories: (1) factors prior to, (2) factors relating to, and (3) factors following the traumatic experience(s). Factors that increase the risks of having PTSD prior to the traumatic experience include a prior history of poor social support and adverse life events, parental poverty, prior history of childhood maltreatment, poor family functioning, familial/genetic family history of psychiatric disorders, introversion or extreme behavioral inhibition, being female, and poor health and prior mental illness (Davidson and Fairbank, 1993). Of these, genetics and the trauma experience may play a critical role. In a twin study, genetic factors accounted for 13% to 30% of the variance in the re-experiencing cluster, 30% to 34% in the avoidance cluster, and 28–32% in the arousal cluster of PTSD symptoms in Vietnam veterans with combat-related PTSD (True et al.,1993). While symptoms in the re-experiencing cluster and one symptom in the avoidance and numbing cluster were strongly associated with trauma exposure, shared environment did not contribute to the development of the disorder. However, some authors believe that childhood trauma is causally and independently related to this increased risk for adult psychiatric and alcohol and substance abuse disorders. For example, a study of twins discordant for childhood sexual abuse exposure showed that even after controlling for family background and parental psychopathology, the exposed twin suffered from an increased risk for adult psychopathology (Kendler et al., 2000). Risk factors for PTSD associated with the trauma are the degree of trauma exposure and an individual's subjective sense of danger, and other related traumatic events (Pynoos and Nader, 1990). Chronicity of psychiatric impairment from PTSD also increases with the dose of traumatic exposure (Pynoos and Nader, 1990). Risk factors associated with PTSD after the trauma include lack of social supports and continued negative life events and lack of posttrauma interventions (Pynoos and Nader, 1990). Thus, effective clinical intervention posttrauma may alleviate the disability and chronicity associated with PTSD.

Limitations of the DSM diagnosis: the developmental consequences of childhood trauma

Children and adolescents are likely to be victims of trauma that is of interpersonal origins. Trauma in childhood may be more detrimental than trauma experienced in adulthood because of the added interactions between trauma and psychologic and neurodevelopment. The *Diagnostic and Statistical Manual of Mental Disorders*, fourth edition (DSM-IV) (American Psychiatric Association, 2000) states that the following constellation of symptoms occur more commonly in association with an interpersonal stressor: anxiety, a loss of previously sustained beliefs, depression, dissociation, feeling permanently damaged, hostility, hopelessness, self-destructive and impulsive behaviors, somatization, shame, personality and relational disturbances, and an increased risk for substance abuse/dependence. Another way of looking at this clinical picture is PTSD with comorbidity, complex PTSD, or the concept of disorders of extreme stress (DESNOS) (Herman, 1993).

PTSD in children is also associated with high rates of comorbid mood and other anxiety disorders (March et al., 1997; Pynoos et al., 1995). Children and adolescents manifest both externalizing and internalizing disorder symptoms after a traumatic experience (March et al., 1997). High rates of comorbid mood, other anxiety disorders, and substance use disorders are seen in adolescents with PTSD (Clark et al., 1997; Deykin and Buka, 1997). Hence, trauma in childhood may cause delays in or deficits of multisystem developmental achievements in behavioral, cognitive, and emotional regulation. For example, children who witness repeated domestic violence have lower social competence scores (Davis and Carlson, 1987), more conduct and personality problems (Hershorn and Rosenbaum, 1985), poorer empathic abilities such as role enactment, role taking, social inference (Hinchey and Gavelek, 1982), and potential for aggression and hostility predominantly in boys (Doumas et al., 1994). Domestic violence has also been shown to be related to suppression of IQ scores in young children, where children who were exposed to domestic violence had IQs which were on average eight points lower than IQ scores of children not exposed to domestic violence (Koenen et al., 2003). Other research has illustrated hypervigilance toward stimulus related to danger and violence in physically abused boys (Dodge and Frame, 1982; Reider and Cicchetti, 1989). There can also be responses of guilt and shame in the victims of sexual abuse (Wolfe et al., 1994). Furthermore, even if childhood trauma does not result in childhood PTSD it increases the risk for adult PTSD (Widom, 1999). Mood disorders without PTSD are commonly observed in children and adolescents exposed to trauma. Parental conflicts, physical, sexual or emotional abuse, and bullying can result in depressive disorders (Boney-McCoy and Finkelhor, 1996; Kaplan et al., 1998).

The clinical assessment of PTSD and trauma-related symptoms

Since PTSD and other psychiatric disorders are so common in traumatized children, all traumatized children and adolescents, once identified, should receive a medical and mental health screening by licensed professionals. The initial mental health assessment involves a structured interview for information gathering. Refer to Section 1 of this book for further information on assessment. When interviewing traumatized children and their families, special attention should be given to red flags that may give the interviewer clues to the child's trauma, age of onset, and severity of responses. Red flags include common stress symptoms, regression in developmental achievements, or new-onset behavioral symptoms. Examples may include a previously outgoing curious child who becomes sullen, irritable, and mute, a previously toilet-trained child who begins to have accidents, or a child who never had a problem sleeping alone, who has a period of months of night terrors. This is an important time to remind the reader that children and adolescents usually do not present with a chief complaint of PTSD. Typically, a child or adolescent is presented for assessment because of episodes of acting out. These episodes can be related to PTSD or other unrelated disorders such as attention-deficit/hyperactivity disorder or bipolar disorder, or an undiagnosed medical disorder. Children, adolescents, and their families may pathologically deny the impact of interpersonal traumatic experiences as a way of coping. Red flags only mean more details need to be gathered. Red flags indicate that the child may have experienced overwhelming stress at that point in time, but are not proof that a previously denied trauma occurred (such as child abuse). Some clinicians find it helpful to obtain the clinical information on a one page sheet to construct a time line of symptoms and life events. This time line usually helps orient clinicians, patients, and caregivers, and may also facilitate memory.

Sometimes a comprehensive medical evaluation must be done to appropriately make a differential diagnosis and before the beginning of psychotherapy and an appropriate medication trial. The medical health and well child care of traumatized children and adolescents is usually not optimal.

KEY CLINICAL QUESTIONS

Ask questions to identify these common symptoms of stress or red flags:

1. Sleep problems
2. Enuresis
3. Encopresis
4 Somatic complaints
5. New fears
6. Oppositionality and aggression
7. School difficulties
8. Problems with peers
9. Acting out (i.e. sexualized behaviors)
10. Somatic complaints
11. Withdrawal
12. Depressed or irritable mood
13. Anxiety or restlessness or poor concentration
14. Appetite disturbance
15. Hopelessness

These children and adolescents may have significant developmental delays. Thus, all traumatized children and adolescents should undergo a physical exam for general health concerns. Sometimes, PTSD, mood and/or disruptive behavioral symptoms are the results of physical illness(es) that may require more detailed medical work-up and treatment. Developmental delays and symptoms of dissociation, concentration problems, attentional deficiencies, impulsivity, hyperactivity, and irritability can result from environmental toxins such as lead poisoning or a partial complex seizure disorder or more rarely from a brain injury (i.e. subclinical shaken baby syndrome or prenatal exposure to alcohol or drugs). Some maltreated children and adolescents will need to undergo laboratory blood testing [including complete blood count with differential, thyroid function studies, electrolytes, blood urea nitrogen (BUN) levels, creatinine, urinalysis, urine toxicology screen, urine pregnancy screen], and an electrocardiogram as part of a general health assessment, to rule out medical causes for behavioral problems, and to screen for contraindications before starting psychopharmacologic treatment. It is also important to consider screening traumatized children who are at risk from sexual abuse or prenatal exposure for sexually transmitted diseases such as human immunodeficiency virus (HIV). Thus, more sophisticated blood tests or neurologic and neuropsychiatric testing such as a neurologic exam, a sleep-deprived EEG, and an MRI scan of the brain, as well as complete psychoeducational and neuropsychologic testing, may be indicated for children with significant developmental delays and attention and learning problems, or for children whose symptoms are resistant to treatment.

The identification of "traumatic reminders"

Since childhood trauma is not only the experience of trauma but also the impact of the trauma on development (e.g. physical abuse or sexual abuse) such as the relationship the victim has with the perpetrator of the trauma or long-lasting effects of the trauma (e.g. loss of a parent), clinical identification of traumatic reminders may involve identification of subtleties that can sometimes be difficult to assess clinically. For example, a child who witnesses domestic violence may experience a "fight or flight reaction" and either freeze or act out every time a teacher raises his/her voice. In this case, the traumatic reminder may be shouting, yelling, or verbal aggression. A physically abused child may be hypersensitive or fearful of perceived failures. In this case, the traumatic reminder may be fear of perceived punishment.

Traumatic reminders can also involve changes in facial expression, unpredictable environmental changes or visits with the perpetrator or other family members. Some children may not be aware of their traumatic reminders. The evaluator may need to identify these traumatic reminders from their understanding of the child's trauma, their review of multiple sources of information, and by a careful understanding of the objective events, which lead to a child's sudden change in feelings or behaviors. The evaluating clinician needs to be a bit of a detective in evaluating the traumatic reminders that may trigger school difficulties, peer rejection, and/or disruptive (oppositional or impulsive) behaviors. The use of a time line in which the clinician plots age of onset and frequency of common stress symptoms with important life events can be helpful in differential diagnosis and the identification of traumatic reminders. It is equally important for the assessing clinician to be very familiar with normal child development. The assessment and treatment of

traumatic stress responses in children and adolescents raises issues that transverse the disciplines of cognitive, psychologic, neurobiologic, psychosocial, behavioral, and social development. Practical experience with children in clinical and non-clinical settings as well as theoretical knowledge of child development will obviously enhance an interviewers' skill in obtaining the appropriate information, and in making accurate diagnosis(es), treatment recommendations, or recommendations for further evaluation and assessment(s).

Developmental issues also influence the child's and adolescent's clinical presentation, emotional and cognitive means of coping in their psychosocial environment, processing of treatment, and course of recovery. For the 3–8-year-old child, major issues related to being a victim of trauma are helplessness and passivity, generalized fear, cognitive confusion, difficulty identifying feelings, lack of verbalization, magical reminders of trauma (omens), sleep disturbance, separation anxiety, regressed behavior, and anxieties about death (Pynoos and Nader, 1993). For the 9–12-year-old child, major issues include responsibility and guilt, reminders that trigger fear response, traumatic play and retelling, fears of extreme feelings, difficulties with concentration and learning, sleep disturbance, safety issues, changes in behavior, somatic complaints, hypervigilance to parent's anxieties, overconcern with others' behaviors, and disturbing grief reactions (Pynoos and Nader, 1993). For the adolescent, major issues include detachment, shame, guilt, self-consciousness, acting out, life-threatening re-enactment behaviors, abrupt shift in relationships, desire for revenge, intense anger, changes in attitudes about life, and premature entrance into adulthood (Pynoos and Nader, 1993). These issues reflect the developmental stages that the child or adolescent is striving to achieve. Consequently, a clear understanding of the child's trauma and his/her symptoms and developmental issues will not only foster an appropriate diagnosis but will also help the child begin to feel understood and to trust authority figures.

Clinical approaches to evaluation and treatment

The major focus of this chapter is on the identification of PTSD symptoms, an outline of clinical assessment approaches, and the rationale for the use of medications. Self-report measures may aid in assessment when given as questionnaires or as interviews. The UCLA PTSD Reaction Index (Steinberg et al., 2004) is a 20-item child and adolescent report measure that is one of the most widely used instruments for the assessment of traumatized children and adolescents. The Reaction Index has been extensively used across a variety of trauma types, age ranges, settings, and cultures. It has especially been broadly used across the US and around the world after major disasters and catastrophic violence as an integral component of public mental health

---

PEARLS & PERILS

Common symptoms in 3–8-year-old children who have experienced trauma:
- Helplessness and passivity
- Generalized fear
- Cognitive confusion
- Difficulty identifying feelings
- Decreased verbalization
- Magical reminders of trauma (omens)
- Sleep disturbance
- Separation anxiety
- Regressed behavior
- Anxieties about death

Common symptoms in 9–12-year-old children who have experienced trauma:
- Feelings of responsibility and guilt
- Reminders that trigger fear responses
- Traumatic play and retelling
- Fears of strong emotions
- Difficulties with concentration and learning
- Sleep disturbance
- Concerns about safety
- Behavioral changes
- Somatic complaints
- Hypervigilance to parental anxiety
- Overconcern with the behavior of others
- Disturbing grief reactions
- Common symptoms in adolescents
- Detachment
- Shame and guilt
- Self-consciousness
- Acting out
- Life-threatening re-enactment behaviors
- Abrupt shifts in relationships
- Desire for revenge
- Intense anger
- Changes in attitudes about life
- Premature entrance into adulthood

Ignoring developmental issues in the evaluation of trauma in children often prevents appropriate diagnosis and makes it harder to help the child feel understood and trusting of authority figures.

response and recovery programs. The PTSD Reaction Index has an algorithm to determine DSM-IV PTSD diagnosis. Total severity score and subscale scores map directly onto DSM-IV criterion B (intrusion), criterion B (avoidance), and criterion C (arousal). This assessment is currently used in the National Center for Child Traumatic Stress as a brief measure for PTSD. The mission of the National Child Traumatic Stress Network is to raise the standard of care and improve access to services for traumatized children, their families, and communities throughout the United States.

Further information can also be found at http://www.nctsnet.org/. Additionally, practice parameters for the treatment of pediatric PTSD have been published by the American Academy of Child and Adolescent Psychiatry (Cohen and the Work Group on Quality Issues, 1998). The American Academy of Child and Adolescent Psychiatry practice parameters were written to aid clinicians and are a comprehensive overview of specific pediatric mental disorders. The reader is referred to these for further detailed information on the epidemiology, assessment, use of structured interviews and rating scales, clinical course, and treatment of PTSD.

Methods for elucidation of PTSD symptoms

Criterion B PTSD symptoms

Criterion B, re-experiencing and intrusive symptoms, can best be conceptualized as a classically conditioned response. An external or internal conditioned stimulus (e.g. the traumatic reminder) activates unwanted and distressing recurrent and intrusive memories of the traumatic experience(s) (the unconditioned stimulus). Intrusive phenomena take the form of distressing intrusions such as nightmares or night terrors, dissociative flashback episodes, and psychologic distress and physical reactivity on exposure to traumatic reminders. In young children, these intrusive thoughts may be part of repetitive play or trauma-specific re-enactment(s) or compulsive rituals. These compulsive rituals may resemble symptoms of pervasive developmental disorders. In eliciting these symptoms, it is important to try to reconstruct the child's state of mind and behavior prior to the symptom in an effort to isolate the traumatic reminder(s). The key to treating these symptoms is to identify and teach the child how to effectively deal with these traumatic reminders. Intrusive symptoms such as hearing the voice of a threatening perpetrator (particularly when a child is alone or feels afraid) can be easily misdiagnosed as psychotic behavior (auditory hallucinations). Intrusive symptoms can also involve acting out behaviors such as sexual acting out with dolls or other children, or when a child re-enacts the perpetrator's abusive behaviors toward him/herself. For example, a teenager may stare at the mirror, be unresponsive to staff, and repeatedly

voice emotionally abusive words (originally said to her by her father) to herself.

Criterion C PTSD avoidant and dissociative symptoms

Criterion C symptoms represent both avoidant and dissociative behaviors and can be thought of as ways to control painful and distressing re-experiencing of symptoms. These include efforts to avoid thoughts, feelings, conversations, activities, places, people, and memories associated with the trauma, amnesia for the trauma, diminished interest in others, feelings of detachment from others, a restricted range of affect, and a sense of a foreshortened future. In assessing for these symptoms, one needs to learn what changes occurred in the child's premorbid personality and psychosocial functioning. Avoidance of traumatic reminders of interpersonal trauma can cause a child to have difficulty handling strong emotions such as anger, joy, or intimate relationships because strong and out-of-control emotions may have precipitated the traumatic maltreatment act. In children who have suffered multiple aversive experiences, reconstruction of their premorbid personality may be very difficult and will involve careful and detailed information on their developmental history. One must also be aware that children may deny their trauma or their posttraumatic symptoms or say that they do not remember an event in an effort not to talk about it. It is important to clarify this with the child to ascertain whether or not they have avoidant symptoms.

Dissociative symptoms are commonly seen in traumatized individuals. These symptoms are defined as disruptions in the usually integrated functions of consciousness, memory, identity, or perception of the environment that interfere with the associative integration of information (Putnam, 1997). The Child Dissociative Checklist is a 20-item parent self-report measure that can be used to screen for dissociative symptoms (Putnam and Peterson, 1994). Detachment or numbing can be seen when a child has an absence of emotional responsiveness such as joy when given a favorite toy or lack of anger when insulted, teased at school, or threatened. Typically, children with restricted range of affect appear serious, are unable to tell the clinician three wishes, have difficulty voicing their wants and hopes for the future (e.g. holiday gifts, what they want to be when they grow up). Children with these symptoms usually have constricted affect and a limited sense of humor. Teachers may notice that children with this symptom "stare into space" and have difficulty paying attention in school. The therapist may notice that a child stares and becomes mute when aspects of the trauma are discussed in therapy. Derealization is a difficult symptom to elicit. Sometimes traumatized children will say their abusive experience "does not seem real." Emotional numbing and diminished interest in others, particularly during development, may result in lack of empathy, comorbid dysthymia, and an increased risk for self-mutilation (van der Kolk et al., 1989), personality disorders (Johnson et al., 1999), and/or anti-social behaviors (Luntz and Widom, 1994). Part of trauma-focused therapy for children with externalizing symptoms is to help them process their trauma exposure to traumatic arousal in tolerable doses. This process allows them to develop empathy and compassion for themselves, which can then be transferred to others, thereby decreasing their anti-social behaviors.

Criterion D PTSD hyperarousal symptoms

Criterion D hyperarousal symptoms consist of persistent symptoms of increased physiologic arousal. These symptoms include difficulty falling or staying asleep, irritable mood or angry outbursts, difficulty concentrating, hypervigilance, and exaggerated startle response. It is important to be specific when eliciting these symptoms, because children may minimize and caregivers may be unaware of these symptoms. For example, if you ask most children and adolescents how they slept last night, they will say "fine." It is better to ask: "What time do you get into bed and what time do you fall asleep? Do you feel rested when you wake up? How often do you have bad dreams?" Furthermore, most children and adolescents will tell you that they feel irritable or angry or mad. They will seldom tell you that they feel bad, sad, or depressed because they may perceive these questions as value judgments. Symptoms of increased arousal such as anxiety, insomnia, restlessness, and poor concentration are also included as symptoms in DSM-IV-TR major depressive disorder, dysthymia, and generalized anxiety disorder. These, as well as their shared psychobiology, are some of the important reasons for these disorders to be commonly comorbid with PTSD.

Child and adolescent psychiatrists, as well as other mental health professions, can work together in identifying and tracking these symptoms during treatment using standardized rating scales for PTSD and depressive symptoms as well as by helping the caregiver fill out a mood and sleep/wake cycle daily activity log on their child. A list of some of these measures are included in the American Academy of Child and Adolescent Psychiatry practice parameters for PTSD (Cohen and the Work Group on Quality Issues, 1998) and the American Academy of Child and Adolescent Psychiatry practice parameters for depressives disorders (Birmaher et al., 1998).

Evaluation and treatment approaches

Debriefing and psychologic first aid

Critical stress incident debriefing or psychologic debriefing immediately after an acute traumatic experience is the hallmark of adult trauma work. It is based on work with disaster workers and emergency personnel (Mitchell and Dyregrov, 1993). Debriefing may be done in individual sessions, but is usually undertaken in group formats with trained group leaders. Debriefing involves seven phases: introduction of ground rules and assurance of confidentiality; objective discussion of the traumatic experience(s); the individual's thoughts about the experience(s); individual's feelings about the experience(s); a review of signs and symptoms associated with the distress of the traumatic experience(s); education in the normal nature of stress, stress reactions, and the "fight-or-flight reaction," and a question phase to clarify any additional or unsettled issues. For individuals who are suffering from significant distress, information for further treatment and appropriate referrals are made. Pynoos and Nader (1988) adapted this technique for children in crisis centers and classrooms. It serves both as an intervention and screening tool for at-risk children. In the context of a classroom discussion of the traumatic experience(s), a drawing and storytelling technique is used to express feelings, clarify confusions, and identify needs. However, recently the clinical effectiveness of critical stress incident debriefing for the prevention of PTSD has been questioned (Bledsoe, 2003; Caine and Ter-Bagdasarian, 2003; van Emmerik et al., 2002). Debriefing is not a substitute for needed individual or family treatment. It should not be used to delve into highly emotionally charged issues, such as intrusive thoughts of grotesque images or revenge fantasies (Pynoos and Nader, 1988). A child should be redirected to draw a more pleasant picture to bring proper closure, and arrangements should be made with the child's guidance counselor and parent (or caretaker) for needed individual treatment (Pynoos and Nader, 1988).

The trauma consultation child interview

The trauma consultation child interview or technique was developed by Pynoos and Eth (Pynoos and Eth, 1986). It is highly recommended reading for individuals who treat traumatized children and its details are beyond the scope of this chapter. This interview was developed for children and adolescents aged 3–16 years. It is applicable for the child who has witnessed murder, suicide, rape, accidental death, assault, kidnapping, natural or human-made disasters, and school and community violence. It may be used for victims of child maltreatment or criminal assault with modifications. It differs from the usual child psychotherapy session or initial psychiatric or mental health assessment interview because it has a stated focus of discussing the traumatic experience(s) (Pynoos and Nader, 1993). It takes 1–2 hours to permit sufficient time to explore the child's traumatic experience(s). Prior to the interview, it is important to obtain information about the child's trauma, his or her behavior after the traumatic experience, as well as premorbid functioning from family members, medical and child protective service records, the police, the school, or other appropriate sources of information. This information is needed for this interview, which was intended for individual intervention and incorporates a review and reprocessing of the traumatic experience(s).

Briefly, the trauma interview involves a three-stage process: opening, trauma, and closure. In the opening stage, it is the interviewer's job to establish the focus and a working relationship (therapeutic alliance) with the child or adolescent in a non-threatening and empathetic manner. In the discussion of the trauma stage, the interviewer does not allow the child to digress from this task of mastery of the trauma. The interviewer may need to question the child to ensure that the circumstances are completely reviewed. It is important to pay attention to the details the child provides and ask about their significance. The interviewer needs to observe for traumatic reminders and their relationships to current symptoms and behaviors. The last stage of this trauma consultation interview is closure. The interviewer reviews with the child or adolescent what they have discussed and emphasizes how understandable, realistic, and universal the child's feelings and thoughts are. Since chronic PTSD symptoms may provide the mechanisms for the pervasive psychopathology seen in maltreated children, it is extremely important to identify the traumatic reminders to these symptoms during the trauma interview.

Trauma-focused cognitive behavioral psychotherapy

The trauma consultation child interview is a one-session interview method aimed to help a child reprocess their trauma. Many children are not able to tolerate this degree of traumatic exposure. Instead, retelling of the trauma narrative is processed over several sessions using gradual exposure techniques. In other words, the trauma consultation child interview process is carried out over several weeks and after a good working relationship is established with the child and their caregiver. The best available evidence for treating child/adolescent PTSD supports trauma-focused psychotherapy with cognitive behavioral therapy (CBT) approaches (Cohen and the Work Group on Quality Issues, 1998; Deblinger and Helfin, 1996; Kolko, 1996; March et al., 1998; Saunders et al., 2001). These approaches include: exposure strategies that allow: 1) trauma processing and exposure to traumatic arousal in tolerable doses so that traumatic feelings can be mastered and adaptively integrated into the child's experience, 2) establishing a coherent narrative to promote habituation of conditioned anxiety, 3) learning to cope with unpleasant affect and physiologic sensation, 4) revising maladaptive cognitive schemas, 5) correcting cognitive distortions, 6) learning stress-management and relaxation skills, and 7) facilitating cognitive/narrative restructuring. These components are identified as the pre-

ferred treatment for PTSD symptoms. CBT is typically provided in a brief (10–18 session) treatment model. Caregiver involvement is critical for successful treatment (Cohen and Mannarino, 1998a). Play therapy, the traditional mainstay of child mental health treatment, was traditionally developed as a non-directive psychodynamic intervention. However, play therapy is currently used as a tool to help foster communication of trauma-related issues (Gil, 1991). Play with drawings, dolls, toys, and games can be used to enhance the therapeutic relationship. Play can also be effective when used as a vehicle for communication of cognitive behavioral strategies.

At the end of a study which administered school-based treatment with CBT to children grades 4–9 who met DSM-IV criteria for PTSD, 57% of children no longer met criteria for PTSD, and 87% of the children did not meet criteria at a 6-month follow-up (Amaya-Jackson et al., 2002). Children were included if they met DSM-IV criteria for PTSD and excluded if there was evidence of chronic abuse-related PTSD symptoms, and conduct problem T-scores >65. They attended school-based CBT sessions and there were also noted improvements in symptoms of depression, anxiety, and anger. In the initial sessions, rapport was built, subjects were educated about symptoms of PTSD through visual aids and appropriate case scenarios, and taught to manage anxiety. The children were asked to give their own examples of symptoms they experienced. Patients were encouraged to see the symptoms of PTSD as separate from themselves, and label the symptoms as "bully" or "bossy," which enabled them to externalize their symptoms. They were also encouraged to keep a storybook (for younger children) or a journal (for adolescents). The goal of this was to enable them to narrate their experiences and thought process with the aim of strengthening coping skills. Relaxation exercises were taught to help modify responses and the intrusiveness of memories.

CBT treatment and CBT approaches are also effective for children who experience chronic trauma such as sexual abuse. CBT is superior to non-directive supportive therapy for the treatment of sexual abuse-related PTSD in children (Cohen and Mannarino, 1996, 1998a, 1998b; Deblinger et al., 1996). CBT is associated with a decrease in depressive symptoms and improved social competence (Cohen and Mannarino, 1998b). Treatment for child and adolescent sexual abuse may involve the following stages (for a review, see Cohen and Mannarino, 1993; Deblinger and Heflin, 1996a): 1) Skill building components (affective modulation: encourage appropriate feeling identification and expression, including "negative" emotions). 2) Stress inoculation skills (focused breathing, progressive muscle relaxation, positive imagery, thought stopping). 3) Cognitive coping skills (learning about the connections between thoughts, feelings, and behaviors (not only abuse-related, but also in the context of normal life), and how examining and changing a child's thoughts can lead to less distress and more adaptive behaviors). 4) Safety skills (optimize a child's decision making abilities in a variety of potentially dangerous situations). 5) Creating the trauma narrative ("gradual exposure") and cognitive processing of traumatic events by gradually encouraging the child to create a narrative (written or otherwise) of the abuse. This includes retelling the "worst moment." Greater details are revealed during each subsequent session to help the child identify traumatic reminders, undergo cognitive processing of the abuse in terms of identifying cognitive distortions (blame, responsibility, shame, and what it means about the child, other people, and the safety of the world), and to help the child fit the traumatic experiences into a larger context of the child's whole life. 6) Psychoeducation (e.g. to provide information about child sexual abuse (i.e. how commonly it occurs, to all types of children, why people abuse kids, common responses to abuse, why kids often don't tell right away, potential for long-term positive outcome with treatment)). 7) Parent components (parallel the above, in addition, to provide parenting skills such as positive praise, active ignoring, time out, and contingency reinforcement programs to manage behavioral problems including sexually inappropriate behaviors). 8) Joint parent-child sessions (to optimize parent-child communication about the abuse and the child's response to it, to foster parent child trust and communication, to model positive parenting strategies for parent, and to optimize the successful sharing of the child's trauma narrative with the parent in such a way that the parent will not be traumatized but be encouraged to support their child).

Variants of CBT have been successfully used in traumatized children. Eye movement desensitization and reprocessing (EMDR) and massage therapy, a form of relaxation therapy, decreased PTSD symptoms in children who were victims of a natural disaster (Chemtob et al., 2002; Field et al., 1996).

Family therapy

Family therapy may also be helpful after a traumatic experience(s). The primary goal is to educate family members about posttraumatic reactions and to validate and legitimize each other's psychologic distress, to work through the trauma, and to provide mutual support. The goals to assist the child are (1) restore the child's sense of security, (2) validate the child's affective responses rather than dismiss them, (3) anticipate and respond to situations in which the child will need added emotional support such as traumatic reminders and feelings of vulnerability, and (4) assist the family in minimizing secondary stresses and adversities (Pynoos and Nader, 1993).

Specific family therapy models have been developed for physically and emotionally abused children. A successful approach for physically abused children and their offending parents focuses on enhancing cooperation among family members, understanding coercive behaviors, teaching positive communication skills, and improving problem solving abilities among all family members (Kolko, 1996). Parent-Child Interaction Therapy (PCIT) has also been successful in the treatment of childhood physical abuse (Urquiza and Mcneil, 1996). A relationship-based model for conjoint treatment of emotionally abused young children of mothers (who were victims of domestic violence) has been successful in helping children regain a perspective of their mothers as reliable caregivers, as well as to help the mothers understand the children's internal world (Silverman and Lieberman, 1999). Family therapy focused on re-establishing appropriate boundaries and limits has been successful with children and their battered mothers (Harway and Hansen, 1994).

Group therapy

Group intervention can also be an important therapeutic agent during the immediate weeks or months after traumatic experience(s). It also offers the opportunity to reinforce the normative nature of the child's or adolescent's reactions and recovery, to share mutual experiences and concerns, to address common fears and avoidant behavior, to increase tolerance for disturbing affects, to provide early attention to more severe depressive or PTSD symptoms, and to aid recovery through age-appropriate and situation-specific problem solving (Pynoos and Nader, 1993). Group approaches utilize psychoeducational and CBT strategies and tend to lessen young people's sense of stigma and isolation by allowing them to share their experiences with peers. Group treatment is especially valuable for adolescents by permitting the therapeutic working through trauma-related conflicts in peer relationships. It is a successful treatment for sexually abused children (Berliner and Saunders 1996), and for children and adolescents who experience traumatic loss (Layne et al., 2001) or domestic violence (Peled and Davis, 1995).

Long-term therapy-pulsed intervention

Pynoos and Nader (1993) suggest a suspension of short-term therapy as an alternative to long-term therapy. It is based on the model of Wallerstein (1990), proposed to treat children of divorce. In such a strategy, an acute phase of treatment is followed by planned periods of consultation in accordance with the time trajectory of trauma recovery and projected achievement of developmental stages. It is designed to help maintain the child's normal development through ongoing communication with the family and the child. This treatment must be individually tailored and based on the treatment needs of the child and family. For certain children and adolescents, it may provide a cost-effective alternative to weekly individual long-term psychotherapy.

Long-term therapy

Indications for long-term treatment, or individual weekly psychotherapy for a period of 1 year or longer, include severe impact, intensity, and duration of traumatic experience(s). If a child experiences multiple traumas, massive violence, loss of family members, friends, and/or multiple personal assaults, life-threatening injuries, and personal or health losses, the therapeutic processing of trauma and bereavement often requires more extended treatment (Pynoos and Nader, 1993). Children with previous psychiatric problems will also likely require longer-term treatment. For interpersonal trauma(s) such as domestic violence, child maltreatment, or death of a parent by suicide, longer-term treatment is also recommended to address issues of the child's personality formation and to repair the ability to trust and form meaningful relationships. One major longitudinal concern is the dysregulation or impaired development of empathy and conscience that can accompany exposure to violence. There may be continued risk of life-threatening or violent behavior throughout adolescence. A major goal of therapy is to return the child to a normal developmental path with a mature conscience, and as a result, to alleviate dangerous self-destructive re-enactment behavior.

The psychobiology of childhood trauma

Trauma causes activation of behavioral and biologic stress response systems. This is called the "fight or flight reaction." Multiple densely interconnected neurotransmitter systems and neuroendocrine axes are activated during traumatic stress (reviewed by Charney et al., 1993). These neurobiologic stress response systems significantly influence physical and cognitive development and emotional and behavioral regulation. Traumatic stress may have negative effects on the development of these systems (for a review, see De Bellis and Putnam, 1994). Results from recent research suggest that the overwhelming stress of maltreatment experiences in childhood is associated with alterations of biologic stress response systems and with adverse influences on brain development (De Bellis, 2001; De Bellis et al., 1999b; De Bellis et al., 1999c; De Bellis et al., 2002a; De Bellis and Keshavan, 2003). The locus ceruleus – norepinephrine/sympathetic nervous system or catecholamine system, the serotonin system, and the hypothalamic-pituitary-adrenal axis are three major neurobiologic stress response systems that significantly influence arousal, stress reactions, physical and cognitive development, emotional regulation, and brain development.

A brief review of the major biologic stress response systems is important because (1) these are the major systems implicated in mood, anxiety, and impulse control disorders (for a review, see Charney et al., 1999); (2) there are pharmacologic treatments to target these systems; (3) alcohol and various illicit substances will also "self-medicate" or target these systems by damping down hyperarousal or dysregulated stress system(s); and (4) a hyperaroused or primed stress system may lead to behavioral manifestations of motor restlessness and learning and memory deficits that may be secondary to anxiety. Sometimes an intense anxiety reaction looks similar to attention-deficit/hyperactivity disorder. However, a child with ADHD has symptoms, which are pervasive, whereas a child with PTSD will usually manifest symptoms of inattention and restlessness only when they are anxious or faced with a traumatic reminder. An understanding of the psychobiology of maltreatment may lead to early psychotherapeutic and psychopharmacologic treatment(s). This may lead to secondary prevention of the psychiatric chronicity and comorbidity commonly seen in maltreated children and adolescents.

Traumatic stress is perceived by the body as overwhelming fear. Traumatic stress increases the activity of the locus ceruleus, the major catecholamine or norepinephrine-containing nucleus in the brain. Activation of locus ceruleus neurons increases norepinephrine in specific brain regions (locus ceruleus, hypothalamus, hippocampus, amygdala, and cerebral cortex). These brain regions are associated with regulation of stress reactions, memory, and emotion (reviewed by De Bellis, 2003). The locus ceruleus via indirect connections through the limbic system results in activation of the limbic-hypothalamic-pituitary-adrenal (LHPA) axis. During stress, the locus ceruleus stimulates the LHPA axis via indirect connections through the brain's limbic system. Intense fear or anxiety activates an important brain structure in the limbic system, the amygdala, which in turn activates the hypothalamus, and hypothalamic corticotrophin-releasing hormone (CRH) or factor (CRF) is released. CRH activates the LHPA axis by stimulating the pituitary to secrete adrenocorticotrophic hormone (ACTH). These events promote cortisol release from the adrenal gland, also stimulate the sympathetic nervous system, and centrally cause behavioral activation and intense arousal (for a review, see Chrousos and Gold, 1992).

The serotonin system is also part of the stress response systems. Serotonin regulation is interdependent with the catecholamine system (Sulser, 1987). In animal studies of unpredictable and uncontrollable stress (e.g. inescapable shock), brain serotonin levels decrease. Drugs that increase brain serotonin (serotonin agonists) prevent stress-induced behavioral changes in animal studies (Southwick et al., 1992). Serotonin plays important roles in compulsive behaviors, the regulation of emotions (mood) and behavior (aggression, impulsivity) and is dysregulated in individuals with major depression, impulsivity, or suicidal behaviors (Benkelfat, 1993). Depression, suicidal thoughts, self-destructive behaviors, and aggression are commonly seen behaviors in victims of childhood maltreatment trauma (National Research Council, 1993).

In summary, the direct effects of the "fight or flight reaction" or traumatic stress reaction include increases in catecholamine turnover in the brain, the sympathetic nervous system, and activation of neuroendocrine systems. Activation of these biologic stress systems results in behaviors consistent with anxiety, hyperarousal, and hypervigilance, which are the core symptoms of PTSD.

Biologic stress response systems and the developing brain

Traumatized children and adults manifest dysregulation of biologic stress response systems (for a review, see De Bellis, 2001). Hence it is not surprising that traumatized children and adults with and without PTSD evidence this dysregulation at baseline, when confronted with a traumatic reminder or when confronted by other life stressors. For example, depressed women with histories of child abuse evidenced autonomic hyperarousal at baseline and hypersensitivity of the LHPA axis in response to a social stressor (Heim et al., 2000). Furthermore, serotonin turnover was decreased in adult combat-related PTSD (Arora et al., 1993).

The limited data published to date suggest that biologic stress response systems are dysregulated in maltreated children who may suffer from depressive and PTSD symptoms, but who may or may not have a diagnosis of PTSD. This is important, because treatment for traumatized children with adjustment disorders may be just as important as treatment for those children with PTSD. Maltreated children with and without a diagnosis of PTSD have elevated catecholamines and cortisol when compared with non-maltreated children (Carrion et al., 2002; De Bellis et al., 1999a; De Bellis et al., 1994a; De Bellis et al., 1994b; Perry, 1994). Understanding the complexities of dysregulated or hyperactive biologic stress response systems is the key to understanding the brain development and cognitive functioning of maltreated children.

Birth to adulthood is marked by progressive physical, behavioral, cognitive, and emotional development. Paralleling these stages are changes in brain maturation. In the developing brain, elevated levels of catecholamines and cortisol may lead to adverse brain development through the mechanisms of accelerated loss (or metabolism) of neurons, delays in myelination, abnormalities in developmentally appropriate pruning, and/or by inhibiting neurogenesis (for a review, see De Bellis, 2003).

Unlike findings in adult PTSD where several studies reported hippocampal atrophy (for a review, see Sapolsky, 2000), magnetic resonance imaging (MRI) studies of maltreated children suggest that child abuse-related PTSD is associated with global adverse brain development. In one research study, 43 maltreated children and adolescents with PTSD and 61 matched controls underwent comprehensive clinical assessments and an anatomic MRI brain scan (De Bellis et al., 1999c). Maltreated subjects with PTSD had 7% smaller intracranial and 8% smaller cerebral volumes than controls.

The total midsaggital area of corpus callosum, and the middle and posterior regions of the corpus callosum, were smaller in abused subjects. In contrast, right, left, and total lateral ventricles and prefrontal cortical CSF were proportionally larger than controls, after adjustment for intracranial volume. In another study, which controlled for socioeconomic status, 28 psychotropic-naïve children and adolescents with abuse-related PTSD and 66 sociodemographically similar healthy controls underwent comprehensive clinical assessments and anatomic MRI brain scans (De Bellis et al., 2002a). Compared with controls, subjects with PTSD had smaller intracranial, cerebral and prefrontal cortex, prefrontal cortical white matter, and right temporal lobe volumes and areas of the corpus callosum and its subregions (2, 4, 5, 6, and 7), and larger frontal lobe CSF volumes than controls. The total midsagittal area of corpus callosum and middle and posterior regions remained smaller, while right, left, and total lateral ventricles and frontal lobe CSF were proportionally larger than controls, after adjustment for cerebral volume. In these two studies, the finding of positive correlations of intracranial and cerebral volumes with age of onset of PTSD trauma suggests that traumatic stress is associated with disproportionately negative consequences if it occurs during early childhood. The finding of negative correlations of intracranial and cerebral volumes with abuse duration suggests that childhood maltreatment has global and adverse influences on brain development that may be cumulative.

In another study from a separate research group, smaller brain and cerebral volumes were also seen in maltreated children with subthreshold PTSD (e.g. traumatized children with adjustment disorders) and threshold PTSD compared with archival controls (Carrion et al., 2001a). Interestingly, maltreated children and adolescents with PTSD or subthreshold PTSD showed no anatomic differences in limbic (hippocampal or amygdala) structures cross-sectionally (Carrion et al 2001a; De Bellis et al., 1999c; De Bellis et al., 2002a) or longitudinally (De Bellis et al., 2001a). Furthermore, findings in pediatric PTSD differ from those of children and adolescents who have no history of DSM-IV criterion A trauma and who suffer from generalized anxiety disorder. These children may have an inherent dysmorphometry of the neurobiologic structures implicated in fear and anxiety. Children with generalized anxiety disorder have larger and particularly right-sided amygdala (De Bellis et al., 2000) and superior temporal gyrus (De Bellis et al., 2002b) volumes.

There was some indication that maltreated males with PTSD may show more evidence of adverse brain development than maltreated females with PTSD (De Bellis and Keshavan, 2003). Thus, these findings may suggest that males are more vulnerable to the effects of severe stress in global brain structures than females. However, both males and females showed findings of adverse brain development. Interestingly, in a study of a large sample of adult survivors of child abuse who were followed from childhood in a long-term prospective study of early (< age 11 years) child abuse and/or neglect, compared with sociodemographically matched controls, maltreated males demonstrated lower levels of a comprehensive measure of resilience as adults than maltreated females (McGloin and Widom, 2001), indicating that males are more vulnerable to the long-term consequences of childhood trauma.

Findings of decreased intracranial volumes and cerebral volumes in maltreated children with PTSD are worrisome. Traumatic stress during childhood may be associated with disproportionately negative effects on brain maturation and be regarded as an environmental induced complex developmental disorder. This stress-induced enhancement of neuronal loss may be the mechanism causing such pervasive problems in children and adolescents who experience trauma.

Understanding the complexities of dysregulated or hyperactive biologic stress response systems is the key to rational psychopharmacologic therapies for traumatized children. Because dysregulated biologic stress response systems can have profound adverse effects on brain development and cortical functioning, it is extremely important to "down-regulate" catecholamines and cortisol, by damping down the activity of the "fight or flight reaction" and its indirect limbic (amygdala) activation. This can be done in many ways. Obviously, the first and most important approach is to assure the safety of the traumatized child's living environment. This may involve identification and removal of traumatic reminders (e.g. a cracked wall from an earthquake or the imprisonment of a perpetrator of maltreatment). Effective psychotherapy and use of anti-anxiety and antidepressant medications which target specific somatic symptoms can "down-regulate" hyperaroused biologic stress systems. A dampening down of stress response systems will hopefully alleviate the adverse physiologic effects of maltreatment stress on a child's development. For example, because of the maltreated child's baseline hyperarousal and history of traumatized attachments, the therapeutic alliance may be difficult to form and effective therapy will take more time to progress. In theory, the appropriate use of medications aimed at desensitizing the traumatized child's biologic stress response systems can assist in fostering this therapeutic alliance by decreasing posttraumatic stress symptoms. Moreover, it is now known that there is a capacity for primate neurogenesis in the frontal cortex and the hippocampus (Gould et al., 1997a; Gould et al., 1999). Environmental stress and adrenal steroids (i.e. cortisol) inhibit the rate of neurogenesis (Gould et al., 1997b; Gould et al., 1998; Tanapat et al., 1998). In theory, medications may improve global brain functioning and alleviate PTSD and depressive symptoms through removing the stress mediated inhibition on the rate of cortical neurogenesis. This can, in theory, lead to therapeutic reversibility of the adverse brain developmental effects of trauma. Medications alone will not "cure" or

"heal" the multiple problems associated with chronic childhood trauma, but are an important and sometimes overlooked tool in a traumatized child's treatment.

Medications for the treatment of symptoms of PTSD

Psychopharmacologic treatment and psychotherapy aimed at target symptoms of PTSD criterion B, C, and D symptoms provide for the rational treatment of PTSD symptoms. At the time of this writing, it must be noted that double-blind psychopharmacologic studies of PTSD in traumatized children are not available. Therefore, the information presented is based on double-blind studies of psychopharmacologic agents used to treat these disorders in non-traumatized children and adolescents, published case reports regarding the psychopharmacologic therapies for children with posttraumatic stress disorders, and the adult literature regarding posttraumatic stress disorders treatment.

When undertaking a mental health screening and making a referral for psychiatric evaluation, it is important to identify all presenting symptoms of psychiatric disorders. Traumatized children and adolescents usually meet DSM-IV-TR criteria for PTSD symptoms and other non-posttraumatic stress psychiatric disorders and for multiple psychiatric disorders. Effective treatments will depend on appropriately identifying these disorders and upon being able to distinguish confusing clinical presentations within a diagnostic framework. Since the clinical identification of traumatic reminders of trauma may involve identification of subtleties that can sometimes be difficult to clinically assess, we will first review the clinical symptoms of specific PTSD criterion symptoms and their psychobiologic basis before discussing specific types of medications for treatment.

Re-experiencing and intrusive symptoms

Intrusive PTSD symptoms most closely resemble another psychiatric disorder, obsessive-compulsive disorder, which is characterized by intrusive and recurrent and persistent thoughts, impulses or images. Obsessive-compulsive disorder is a disorder of serotonin regulation, and antidepressants, which enhance serotonin functioning, attenuate these symptoms (for a review, see Rosenberg and Keshavan, 1998). Because of serotonin's interdependence with the noradrenergic system, dysregulation of serotonin may not only play a major role in cluster B symptoms, but may also increase the risk for comorbid major depression and aggression in traumatized children. Consequently, it has been shown that the onset of major depression is markedly increased for trauma exposed persons who suffer from PTSD, but not in trauma exposed persons who did not suffer from PTSD (Breslau et al., 2000). Thus, PTSD may lead to major depression and be influenced by common genetic vulnerabilities to serotonin dysregulation and trauma-related factors in children. Thus, it is not surprising that results from recent studies show strong support for the efficacy of the serotonin reuptake inhibitor antidepressant and anti-obsessive-compulsive disorder medications, sertraline (Brady et al., 2000) and fluoxetine (van der Kolk et al., 1994) in adult PTSD. To date, there are no published reports of serotonin reuptake inhibitors or other antidepressants for the treatment of PTSD in traumatized children. However, in double-blind studies, fluoxetine, a serotonin agent, has been shown to be very effective in decreasing symptoms of major depression in children and adolescents (Emslie et al., 1997).

Avoidant and dissociative behaviors

Avoidant and dissociative symptoms are thought to be mediated by dysregulation of the endogenous opiate system (for a review, see Bremner et al., 1993). However, higher concentrations of urinary dopamine are associated with avoidant symptoms in adult PTSD (Yehuda et al., 1992) and with avoidant and dissociative symptoms in maltreated children with PTSD (De Bellis et al., 1999a). Endogenous opiate systems and their links with dopamine systems may be contributory to the restricted range of affect and high incidence of self-injury and violent behaviors reported in traumatized children and in adults who have experienced childhood trauma. The dopamine system is linked with the serotonin and noradrenergic (norepinephrine) systems. Antidepressant and anti-anxiety medications, which dampen down the activity of these biologic stress response systems, should, in theory, dampen the activity of dopamine and endogenous opiates, and thus decrease both avoidant and dissociative behaviors.

Persistent symptoms of increased physiologic arousal and catecholamines

These symptoms are part of the biologic stress response systems response or the "fight or flight reaction." These symptoms are thought to be mediated by increased activity of central CRH and enhanced sympathetic nervous system tone as discussed in detail in The psychobiology of childhood trauma section of this chapter (above).

CONSIDER CONSULTATION WHEN ...

- Stress symptoms have not responded to interventions.
- Psychoeducational impairment is moderate to severe.
- Re-traumatization has been ruled out.
- There are clear identified target symptoms that can be effectively treated with medications.

Pharmacotherapy

The majority of traumatized children with clinically significant psychiatric symptoms of PTSD would benefit from medications. Children and adolescents who have at least moderate psychosocial impairment from symptoms that have not responded to brief psychotherapy, or children and adolescents who are so severely affected as to require intensive outpatient or inpatient treatment may be helped with psychotropic medication. It should be noted that most behavioral and emotional problems in children are self-limited or situational. Behavioral management of symptoms can be very effective; for example, treating insomnia with relaxation tapes or anxiety with thought-stopping techniques. Therefore, one should not start a medication unless there are specific and clear target symptoms that the medication prescribed is designed to treat, behavioral approaches have failed, or the symptoms are so severe that psychopharmacologic treatment needs to be instituted before effective behavioral management can start. It is also important to rule out any medical or substance use problems that may be contributing to these psychiatric symptoms. For adolescent girls who are sexually active, birth control issues and pregnancy must be addressed before beginning a medication trial. Both the clinician and child and adolescent psychiatrist can work together in identifying and documenting the duration, onset, and frequency of these target symptoms as well as documenting their improvement or any medication side-effects associated with psychopharmacologic treatment. For example, many traumatized children and adolescents require anti-anxiety or antidepressant medications to target symptoms of hyperarousal or "fight or flight reaction," biologic stress response systems, dysregulation such as reduced attention and learning, sleep disturbance, nightmares, restricted affect, anxiety, and/or depression. These symptoms can be monitored with specific rating scales, sleep/wake logs and diaries, or medication side-effect rating scales. It is extremely important to educate the patient and their family about what medications will and will not do. In this discussion, giving the patient and their family a chart describing the medication, the symptoms that the medication is designed to treat, and common side-effects is helpful. It is important to help the family and the child understand that medication alone will not take care of all the problems that lead them into treatment, nor will it "change their personality," make them into "docile robots," or cause them to become "drug addicted." These discussions can take place as part of the informed consent procedure.

Physicians who prescribe medications to children and adolescents need to obtain informed consent for treatment from their parent or legal guardian. For children in foster care or state custody, informed consent may also be needed from child protective services. Adolescents aged 14 years and older may also be required to sign an informed consent form depending on state law. In order to obtain informed consent for medication treatment, a child and adolescent psychiatrist must discuss the following with the patient and/or their decision maker in understandable language. This includes a discussion of the psychiatric disorder and symptoms to be treated, the nature of the medication prescribed, the probability and types of side-effects and the other risks of a medication trial, the possible benefits of the treatment, the fact that the physician cannot predict the results of the treatment, the likely results of no treatment, and the risks and benefits of alternative treatments. The discussion of these issues needs to be documented in the patient's medical record as well as a statement that the patient and/or their decision maker voluntarily accepts the prescribed treatment. Parents and/or adolescents have the right to refuse treatment. This discussion must also be documented in the patient's medical record.

One should take particular care when prescribing medications to children and adolescents. It is important to choose the best drug for the treatment of the particular target symptoms described with the best side-effect profile. It is important to start at the lowest effective dose, minimize the drug maintenance dose and frequency of administration, and avoid using multiple medications if possible. However, children and adolescents metabolize drugs faster than adults. Therefore, children and especially adolescents may need a higher equivalent dose for maintenance than an adult for the drug to have a therapeutic effect. A medication trial should take 6–12 weeks before a decision can be made as to the effectiveness of the medication. The treating psychiatrist must also be aware of the mental status and the ability of the parent to comply with a medication trial. One way to handle this is to have the caregiver repeat back the medication instructions to you and/or to have them write it out on a medication record. For example, it may not be wise to keep a

child on medication if the parent has the potential to misuse it by giving a child a potentially toxic dose as a prn. When treating maltreated children who remain in their maltreating family, these types of issues will need to be addressed as part of a multidisciplinary team approach before beginning a medication trial.

We will now review specific classes of medications that can be helpful for the treatment of PTSD and their common side-effects. We will also discuss possible strategies for treating patients with complicated comorbidities in each section. This chapter is not meant to be a comprehensive assessment of all medications and their side-effects. The reader is referred to a comprehensive textbook on psychoactive drugs for children and adolescents for further information (Werry and Aman, 1999).

Anti-anxiety medications

Adrenergic agents

Adrenergic agents dampen down baseline biologic stress response systems (locus ceruleus-sympathetic nervous system) and are among the most commonly used anti-anxiety medications in traumatized children. Clonidine, a central alpha2-adrenergic partial agonist, dampens catecholamine transmission centrally by decreasing the activity of the locus ceruleus. Perry reported an open-label treatment trial of clonidine at relatively low doses (0.05–0.1 mg bid) in physically and sexually abused children with PTSD. Clonidine treatment was associated with general clinical improvement and decreases in the arousal cluster of PTSD symptoms and impulsivity (Perry, 1994). Harmon and Riggs (1996) reported the effectiveness of using an open trial of clonidine in the transdermal patch for effective reduction of PTSD symptoms in seven maltreated children aged 3–6 years (Harmon and Riggs, 1996). The author found that open trials of clonidine when given in the evenings 20 minutes before bedtime (usual dose of 0.05–0.1 mg po qhs) is particularly helpful in reducing initial insomnia and nightmares in maltreated preschool and school-aged children and in adolescents. Increasing effective sleep was also associated with decreasing daytime inattention and irritability.

In a case report, a maltreated boy with PTSD was followed prospectively using single voxel proton magnetic resonance spectroscopy measures of anterior cingulate N-acetylaspartate/creatine ratios, a marker of neural integrity. Clonidine treatment was associated with NAA/creatine ratios increase and improvement in sleep measures upon symptom remission, indicating that clonidine may improve anterior cingulate functioning and alleviate PTSD symptoms through removing the stress mediated inhibition on the rate of anterior cingulate neurogenesis (De Bellis et al., 2001b). Clonidine needs to be started slowly (initial dose of 0.025–0.05 mg po qhs) because it may cause sedation and hypotension. The

PEARLS & PERILS

- Psychotropic medication may benefit traumatized children and adolescents who have moderate impairment that has not responded to brief psychotherapy or whose symptoms are severe enough to prevent reasonable functioning.
- Medications should only be used for specific and clear target symptoms that are likely to be responsive.
- Medications should only be used when behavioral approaches have failed or the symptoms are so severe that behavioral interventions cannot be implemented.
- Medical contributions to psychiatric symptoms should be ruled out.
- While psychotropic medication may be helpful, medication alone is seldom, if ever, adequate treatment for the symptoms that bring traumatized children and adolescents to care.

maximum dose of clonidine is appropriately 3 to 5 µg/kg per day in divided doses. Some children cannot tolerate a morning dose because of sedation and doses over 0.2 mg total per day are associated with sedation. Guanfacine is a longer-acting central alpha2-adrenergic partial agonist that is more selective and thus less likely to be associated with side-effects and rebound adrenergic symptoms. Abruptly stopping clonidine or guanfacine treatment can cause rebound adrenergic symptoms such as headache, anxiety, tremors, abdominal pain, sweating, tachycardia. Therefore, these medications need to be tapered when discontinued. Guanfacine was found to be effective in decreasing nightmares in a single case study of a 7-year-old child (Horrigan, 1996). Guanfacine has been given in regimens of 0.5 mg at bedtime, increasing by 0.25 to 0.5 mg every 5–7 days to a mean effective dose of 1.25 mg (0.0225 mg/kg per day) given in two divided doses. However, smaller doses can be very effective for PTSD symptoms. Blood pressure and pulse rate should be monitored at baseline, routinely, and during dose increase of these medications. Patients may be screened with an electrocardiogram for pre-existing cardiac abnormalities before starting these medications. Common side-effects of clonidine and guanfacine are sedation and dry mouth. However, these side-effects are unlikely at these low doses.

Propranolol, a beta-adrenergic antagonist, also dampens down sympathetic nervous system arousal. It is frequently used in low doses for stage fright. Five weeks of an open treatment trial of propranolol, at a dose of 2.5 mg/kg/day, was associated with decreases in aggressive behaviors, intrusive symptoms, and insomnia in eight of 11 abused children with PTSD (Famularo et al., 1988). Common side-effects of propranolol include Raynaud's phenomenon, bradycardia, bronchoconstriction, sexual impotence, and depression. Propranolol should not be given to children with asthma. Clonidine, guanfacine, and propranolol appear to be relatively safe at the low doses described and effective for the treatment of PTSD symptoms in uncomplicated cases where the psychopharmacologic treatment of PTSD is of primary concern. It should be noted that a 10-day course of treatment with propranolol started within hours after a single-event trauma in adults presenting to the emergency department was associated with prevention of PTSD at 3 months post-trauma (Pitman et al., 2002). This type of preventive study is promising, but currently there are no data in children.

Antidepressant medications

Selective serotonin reuptake inhibitors

Selective serotonin reuptake inhibitors (SSRIs) act to increase serotonin at the level of the synapse. This mechanism of action may be particularly important in traumatized individuals, as our review detailed how trauma is associated with decreased serotonin levels. Low levels of serotonin may lead to depression, impulsivity, and aggression. Selective serotonin reuptake inhibitors (fluoxetine, sertraline, paroxetine, fluvoxamine) are efficacious for the treatment of major depression in double-blind studies of adults and youth. A recent survey of child psychiatrists indicated that 95% have used SSRIs to treat childhood PTSD (Cohen et al., 2001). These drugs have a relatively safe side-effect profile, very low lethality after overdose, and easy (once a day) administration. Currently, there is no indication for baseline laboratory tests before beginning an SSRI. Selective serotonin reuptake inhibitors are the first-line treatment for the traumatized child or adolescent with major depression and major depression comorbid with PTSD (Cohen and the Work Group on Quality Issues, 1998). However, one open-label study demonstrated that treatment of children and adolescents with the SSRI citalopram was associated with improvement of PTSD symptoms (Seedat et al., 2002). One should start these medications at a low dose and go slowly because SSRIs have a relatively flat dose-response curve, suggesting that maximal clinical response may be achieved at minimum effective doses.

Common side-effects are gastrointestinal symptoms, restlessness, sweating, headaches, bruising, and changes in appetite, sleep, and sexual function. Side-effects are dose-dependent and may subside with time or by decreasing the dose. Akathisia, a very distressing restlessness in the legs, is a common side-effect of SSRIs and can be very uncomfortable. Severe akathisia can resemble a manic episode. Lowering the dose, switching to a less selective serotonin reuptake agent, or adding very low doses of propranolol (10 mg po bid) may help alleviate the akathisia. Some children and adolescents will not be able to tolerate this side-effect and the medication will need to be discontinued. Some patients have an allergic reaction to the SSRIs and get a very red raised itchy rash on their trunk and extremities. If this happens, the medications needs to be stopped immediately and the pediatrician notified. The rash will usually subside in a few days after discontinuation of the SSRI. Children and adolescents can become manic or hypomanic while being treated with an antidepressant. Common symptoms include a change in behavior involving silliness, impulsivity, agitation, grandiosity, and recklessness. If this happens, the medications may need to be lowered or stopped. Hypomanic symptoms will usually decrease once the medication is stopped. However, if a full-blown mania occurs, appropriate intervention such as hospitalization may be indicated. Members of the treatment team should also monitor suicidal ideation in any depressed child or adolescent during the course of treatment and take appropriate action for the child's safety. Abrupt withdrawal from an SSRI due to discontinuation, missing doses or too rapid tapering can cause a short-lived serotonin discontinuation syndrome. The symptoms are dizziness, nausea, vomiting, fatigue, chills, increased anxiety, and depression. Using an SSRI with a longer half-life (i.e. fluoxetine or sertraline) or carefully tapering the medication will avoid this withdrawal syndrome. A rare effect of overdose of SSRIs is the serotonin syndrome. It has the following clinical features: confusion, agitation, myoclonus, hyperreflexia, sweating, shivering, tremor, diarrhea, incoordination, and fever. This can be fatal if not treated rapidly in a hospital or emergency room.

Selective serotonin reuptake inhibitors inhibit the cytochrome P450 isoenzymes. This means that a number of other medications can have their metabolism affected by the concurrent administration of an SSRI. The caregiver must always let their child's physician know that they are taking an SSRI before being prescribed another medication. Monoamine oxidase inhibitor (MAOI) medications should never be given with an SSRI. Selective serotonin reuptake inhibitors can also be used with low doses of clonidine (0.025 to 0.1mg po qhs) to target insomnia and nightmares during the initial course of antidepressant treatment. Selective serotonin reuptake inhibitors have been safely used with tricyclic antidepressants and stimulants when doses are adjusted (for a review, see Werry and Aman, 1999).

When treatment does not work

This circumstance can happen for several reasons. It is always important to review the case and re-evaluate your differential diagnosis and the target symptoms of treatment when this happens. Sometimes children who suffer from PTSD also have comorbidities that need to be addressed such as ADHD. Traumatized children may also suffer from cognitive problems such as inattention, deficits in executive function, learning disabilities or low IQ (Beers and De Bellis, 2002). Cognitive behavioral therapy strategies may need to be adapted for these children. In these cases, a formal neuropsychologic evaluation may be helpful. Recommendations concerning cognitive strengths and weaknesses can not only be of value for educational purposes, but can also help a therapist understand how to adapt evidence-based treatments to a particular child. An increase or new precipitating psychosocial stress, which is causing the child to feel unsafe and anxious, may result in new or a re-emergence of symptoms. Sometimes agitation and acting out may be the first indication of re-traumatization. CBT approaches require attendance of regular sessions, completion of homework assignments, and the cooperation of the caregiver and the child. Sometimes families need to be stabilized through family and psychosocial interventions before the child and caregiver can fully attend to treatment.

With regard to medications, caregivers may complain about ineffective doses of medications that were previously effective. One reason for this is non-compliance with the drug regimen as prescribed. The second reason is an unre-

alistic expectation of what a drug will and will not do for the child. The third is that the medication is causing significant side-effects. For example, the experience of akathisia can lead to restlessness and acting out behaviors. The fourth is an overlooked medical problem that is related to the increase in psychiatric symptoms. The fifth is normal growth and development. Growth may either mean that the dose will need to be adjusted (increased) for effectiveness or that, because of individual differences during pubertal development, the medication may need to be changed to another type or class of drug.

Summary

Trauma in childhood has psychopathologic and developmental consequences. Developmental consequences may include biologic changes in stress systems as well as failures to obtain important psychologic developmental achievements. A comprehensive mental health assessment that incorporates objective events and subjective experiences in a developmental fashion is the first step in the evaluation of childhood trauma and PTSD. Practice parameters are available as guidelines for treatment in the real world. Although trauma in childhood may have a profound and long-lasting impact on development, it is always hopeful to know that individual children strive toward growth. When rescued from extremely neglectful and abusive environments, profoundly traumatized children are capable of accelerated rates of catch-up growth, including remission of severe psychopathology and normalization of cognitive function (Koluchova, 1972, 1976; Money et al., 1983). Evaluation, evidenced-based psychotherapy and the appropriate use of medications are part of a comprehensive treatment plan that can enable this process.

Annotated bibliography

Cohen JA, and the Work Group on Quality Issues (1998) Practice parameters for the assessment and treatment of children and adolescents with posttraumatic stress disorder. *American Academy of Child and Adolescent Psychiatry*, 37(Suppl 10):4S–26S.
This reference outlines the latest evidence-based practice parameters accepted by the American Academy of Child and Adolescent Psychiatry.

De Bellis MD (2001) Developmental traumatology: the psychobiological development of maltreated children and its implications for research, treatment, and policy. *Development and Psychopathology*, 13:537–561.
This reference comprehensively and critically outlines the developmental psychobiology of childhood trauma.

Pynoos RS, Eth S (1986) Witness to violence: the child interview. *Journal of the American Academy of Child and Adolescent Psychiatry*, 25:306–319.
This seminal paper is a must read for all who interview children. This paper comprehensively outlines how to interview the traumatized child. Developmental and sensitive issues are carefully addressed.

Bibliography

Chapter 1

Achenbach TM, Rescorla LA (2001) *Manual for the ASEBA School-Age Forms and Profiles*. Burlington, VT, University of Vermont, Research Center for Children, Youth and Families.

American Academy of Child and Adolescent Psychiatry (1998) Practice parameters for the assessment and treatment of children and adolescents with language and learning disorders. *J Am Acad Child Adolesc Psychiatry*, 37(Suppl 10):46S-62S.

American Academy of Child and Adolescent Psychiatry (1997) Practice parameters for the psychiatric assessment of infants and toddlers (0–36 months). *J Am Acad Child Adolesc Psychiatry*, 36:21S-36S.

American Academy of Child and Adolescent Psychiatry (2001a) Practice parameter for the assessment and treatment of children and adolescents with suicidal behavior. *J Am Acad Child Adolesc Psychiatry*, 40(Suppl 7):24S-51S.

American Academy of Child and Adolescent Psychiatry (2001b) Practice parameter for the assessment and treatment of children and adolescents with schizophrenia. *J Am Acad Child Adolesc Psychiatry*, 40(Suppl 7):4S-23S.

American Psychiatric Association (2000) *Diagnostic and Statistical Manual of Mental Disorders, DSM III*, 3rd edn. Washington DC, 1980.

American Psychiatric Association (1994) *Diagnostic and Statistical Manual of Mental Disorders, DSM IV-TR (Text Revision)*, 4th edn. Washington DC, American Psychiatric Press.

Connors CK, Sitarenios G, Parker JDA, Epstein JN (1998) The revised Connors' Parent Rating Scale (CPRS-R) Factor structure, reliability, and criterion validity, *J Abnor Child Psychol* 26:257–68.

Jellinek MS, Murphy JM, Little M, Pagano ME, Comer DM, Kelleher KJ (1999) Use of the Pediatric Symptom Checklist to screen for psychosocial problems in pediatric primary care: a national feasibility study. *Arch Pediatr Adolesc Med*, 153:254–60.

King RA (1997) Practice parameters for the psychiatric assessment of children and adolescents. American Academy of Child and Adolescent Psychiatry. *J Am Acad Child Adolesc Psychiatry*, 36(Suppl 10):4S-20S.

Thomas JM, Benham AL, Gean M et al. (1997) Practice parameters for the psychiatric assessment of infants and toddlers (0–36 months) American Academy of Child and Adolescent Psychiatry. *J Am Acad Child Adolesc Psychiatry*, 36(Suppl 10):21S-36S.

Chapter 2

Achenbach TM, Edelbrock KC (1983) *Manual for the Child Behavior Checklist and Revised Child Behavior Profile*. Burlington, VT, University of Vermont Department of Psychiatry.

Achenbach TM, Rescorla LA (2001) *Manual for ASEBA School-Age Forms and Profiles*. Burlington, VT, University of Vermont, Research Center for Children, Youth, and Families.

Aman MG, Singh NN (1986) *Aberrant Behavior Checklist Manual*. East Aurora, NY, Slosson Educational Publications, Inc.

Barkley RA (1998) *Attention-Deficit Hyperactivity Disorder: A Handbook for Diagnosis and Treatment*, 2nd edn. New York, Guilford Press.

Baron-Cohen S, Gillberg C (1992) Can autism be detected at 18 months? The needle, the haystack, and the CHAT. *Br J Psychiatry*, 161:839–43.

Beck AT, Steer RA (1993) *Beck Depression Inventory: Manual*. San Antonio, Psychological Corp.

Bruininks RH, Woodcock RW, Weatherman RF, Hill BK (1997) *Scales of Independent Behavior – Revised*. Itasca, IL, The Riverside Publishing Company.

Collett BR, Ohan JL Myers KM (2003) Ten-year review of rating scales. V: Scales assessing attention-deficit/hyperactivity disorder. *J Am Acad Child Adolesc Psychiatry*, 42:1015–37.

Conners CK (1989) *Manual for Conners' Rating Scales*. N. Tonawanda, NY, Multi-Health Systems.

Cooper Z, Fairburn CG (1987) The eating disorder examination: a semi-structured interview for assessment of the specific psychopathology of eating disorders. *J Eating Dis*, 6:1–8.

Deluty RH (1979) Children's Action Tendency Scale: a self-report measure of aggressiveness, assertiveness, and submissiveness in children. *J Consult Clin Psychol*, 47:1061–71.

DuPaul GJ, Power TJ, Anastopoulos AD, Reid R, McGoey KE, Ikeda MJ (1997) Teacher ratings of attention deficit hyperactivity disorder symptoms: factor structure and normative data. *Psychol Assess*, 9:436–44.

Elliot DS, Huizinga D, Ageton S (1985) *Explaining Delinquency and Drug use*. Beverly Hills, CA, Sage.

Eyberg S, Pincus D (1999) *Eyberg Child Behavior Inventory and Sutter-Eyberg Student Behavior Inventory – Revised*. Odessa, FL, Psychological Assessment Rescources.

Garner DM, Garfinkel PE (1979) The eating attitudes test: an index of the symptoms of anorexia nervosa. *Psychol Med*, 9:273–9.

Garner DM, Olmsted MP, Bohr Y, Garfinkel PE (1982) The eating attitudes test: psychometric features and clinical correlates. *Psychol Med*, 12:871–8.

Garner DM (1991) *Eating Disorder Inventory-2. Professional Manual.* Odesa, FA, Psychological Assessment Resources.

Gilliam JE (2003) *Gilliam Asperger's Disorder Scale Examiner's Manual.* Austin, TX, PRO-ED.

Gordon M, Barkley RA (1998) Tests and observational measures, In RA Barkley (ed.) *Attention-Deficit Hyperactivity Disorder: A Handbook for Diagnosis and Treatment*, 2nd edn. New York, Guilford Press.

Goyette CH, Conners CK, Ulrich RF (1978) Normative data on the revised Conners' parent and teacher rating scales. *J Abnorm Child Psychol*, 6:221–36.

Jay SM, Ozolins M, Elliot C, Caldwell S (1983) Assessment of children's distress during painful procedures. *Health Psych*, 2:133–47.

Jellinek MS, Murphy JM, Burns BJ (1986) Brief psychosocial screening in outpatient pediatric practice. *J Pediatrics*, 109:371–8.

Katz ER, Kellerman J, Siegel SE (1980) Behavioral distress in children with cancer undergoing medical procedures: developmental consideration. *J Consult Clin Psychol*, 48:356–65.

Kazdin AE, French NH, Unis AS, Esveldt-Dawson K, Sherick RB (1983) Hopelessness, depression, and suicidal intent among psychiatrically disturbed inpatient children. *J Consult Clin Psychol*, 51:504–10.

Kovacs M (1985) CDI (the Children's Depression Inventory). *Psychopharmacol Bull*, 21:995–1000.

Kovacs M (1992) *Manual for the Children's Depression Inventory.* North Tonawanda, NY, Multi-Health Systems, Inc.

LeBaron S, Zeltzer LK (1984) Assessment of acute pain and anxiety in children and adolescents by self-reports, observer reports, and a behavior checklist. *J Consult Clin Psychol*, 52:729–38.

McGrath P, Vair C, McGrath MJ, Unruh E, Scjnurr R (1985) Pediatric nurses' perception of pain experienced by children and adults. *Nursing Papers*, 16:34–40.

Moos RH, Moos BS (1994) *Family Environment Scale*, 3rd edn manual. Palo Alto, CA, Consulting Psychologists Press, Inc.

Myers K, Winters NC (2002) Ten-year review of rating scales. II: Scales for internalizing disorders. *J Am Acad Child Adolesc Psychiatry*, 41:634–59.

Nihira K, Leland H, Lambert N (1993) *AAMR adaptive behavior scale-residential and community*, 2nd edn. Austin, TX, Pro-Ed, Inc.

Palmer R, Christie M, Cordle C, Davies D (1987) The Clinical Eating Disorder Rating Instrument (CEDRI): a preliminary description. *Int J Eating Dis*, 6:9–16.

Pelham WE Jr, Milich R, Murphy D, Murphy HA (1989) Normative data on the IOWA Conners Teacher Rating Scale. *J Clin Child Psychol*, 18:259–62.

Pfeffer CR (1986) *The Suicidal Child.* New York, Guilford Press.

Poznanski EO, Mokros HB (1995) *Children's Depression Rating Scale, Revised (CDRS-R) Administration Booklet.* Los Angeles, CA, Western Psychological Services.

Prout HT, Strohmer D (1991) *Emotional Problems Scales.* Lutz, FL, Psychological Assessment Resources, Inc.

Reich W (1997) *Diagnostic Interview for Children and Adolescents – Revised DSM-IV Version.* Toronto, Multi-Health Systems.

Reiss S (1994) *The Reiss Screen for Maladaptive Behavior: Test Manual*, 2nd edn. Overland Park, IL, International Diagnostic Systems Publishing.

Reynolds WM (1988) *Suicidal Ideation Questionnaire: Professional Manual.* Odessa, FL, Psychological Assessment Resources.

Reynolds WM (2002) *Reynolds Adolescent Depression Scale – 2.* Odessa, FL, Psychological Assessment Resources.

Reynolds CR, Richmond BO (1994) *Revised Children's Manifest Anxiety Scale Manual.* Los Angeles, CA, Western Psychological Services.

Robins D, Fein D, Barton M, Green J (2001) The Modified Checklist for Autism in Toddlers: an initial study investigating the early detection of autism and pervasive developmental disorder. *J Autism Development Dis* 31:131–44.

Rutter M, Bailey A, Lord C (2003) *Manual for the Social Communication Questionnaire.* Los Angeles, CA, Western Psychological Services.

Schopler E, Reichler RJ, Renner BR (1988) *Manual for the Childhood Autism Rating Scale.* Los Angeles, CA, Western Psychological Services.

Shaffer D, Schwab-Stone M, Fisher P et al. (1993) The Diagnostic Interview Schedule for Children – Revised version (DISC-R). I: Preparation, field testing, interrater reliability, and acceptability. *J Am Acad Child Adolesc Psychiatry*, 32:643–50.

Sparrow SS, Balla DA, Cicchetti DV (2004) *Vineland-II Adaptive Behavior scales.* Circle Pines, MN, American Guidance Services.

Spielberger CD (1973) *Manual for the State-Trait Anxiety Inventory for Children.* Palo Alto, CA, Consulting Psychologists Press.

Swanson JM, Lerner MA, March J, Gresham FM (1999) Assessment and intervention for attention-deficit/hyperactivity disorder in the schools: lessons from the MTA study. *Pediatr Clin North Am*, 46:993–1009.

Swanson JM, Kraemer HC, Hinshaw SP et al. (2001) Clinical relevance of the primary findings of the MTA: success rates based on severity of ADHD and ODD symptoms at the end of treatment. *J Am Acad Child Adolesc Psychiatry*, 40(2):168–79.

Ullman RK, Sleator EK, Sprague RL (1997) *ACTeRS: Teacher and Parent Forms Manual.* Champaign, IL, MeriTech, Inc.

Ysseldyke JE, Christenson SL (1987) *The Instructional Environment Scale: A Comprehensive Methodology for Assessing an Individual Student's Instruction.* Austin, Tx, Pro-Ed.

Chapter 3

American Academy of Child and Adolescent Psychiatry (2001) Practice parameter for the assessment and treatment of children and adolescents with schizophrenia. *J Am Acad Child Adolesc Psychiatry*, 40(Suppl 7):4S-23S.

American Academy of Pediatrics Committee on Substance Abuse (1996) Testing for drugs of abuse in children and adolescents. *Pediatr*, 98:305–7.

Anderson CM, Polcari A, Lowen SB, Renshaw PF, Teicher MH (2002) Effects of methylphenidate on functional magnetic resonance relaxometry of the cerebellar vermis in boys with ADHD. *Am J Psychiatry*. 159:1322–8.

Anfinson TJ, Kathol RG (1992) Screening laboratory evaluation in psychiatric patients: a review. *Gen Hosp Psychiatry*, 14:248–57.

Annas GJ (2001) Testing poor pregnant patients for cocaine – physicians as police investigators. *New Engl J Med*, 344:1729–32.

Anonymous (1997) Adolescents and anabolic steroids: a subject review. American Academy of Pediatrics. Committee on Sports Medicine and Fitness. *Pediatr*, 99:904–8.

Anonymous (1999) The American College of Rheumatology nomenclature and case definitions for neuropsychiatric lupus syndromes. *Arthritis Rheum*, 42:599–608.

Anonymous (1994) Fragile X syndrome: diagnostic and carrier testing, Working Group of the Genetic Screening Subcommittee of the Clinical Practice Committee. American College of Medical Genetics. *Am J Med Genet*, 53:380–1.

Arbelle S, Benjamin J, Golin M, Kremer I, Belmaker RH, Ebstein RP (2003) Relation of shyness in grade school children to the genotype for the long form of the serotonin transporter promoter region polymorphism. *Am J Psychiatry*, 160:671–6.

Becker AE, Grinspoon SK, Klibanski A, Herzog DB (1999) Eating disorders. *New Engl J Med*, 340:1092–8.

Bostwick JM, Philbrick KL (2002) The use of electroencephalography in psychiatry of the medically ill. *Psych Clin N Am*, 25:17–25.

Bukstein O (1997) Practice parameters for the assessment and treatment of children and adolescents with substance use disorders. *J Am Acad Child Adolesc Psychiatry*, 36(Suppl 10):140S-156S.

Casey BJ, Castellanos FX, Giedd JN et al. (1997) Implication of right frontostriatal circuitry in response inhibition and attention deficit/hyperactivity disorder. *J Am Acad Child Adolesc Psychiatry*, 36:374–83.

Caspi A, Sugden K, Moffitt TE et al. (2003) Influence of life stress on depression: moderation by a polymorphism in the 5-HTT gene. *Science*, 301:386–9.

Castellanos FX, Giedd JN, Hamburger SD, Marsh WL, Rapoport JL (1996) Brain morphology in Tourette's syndrome: the influence of comorbid attention-deficit/hyperactivity disorder. *Neurology*, 47:1581–3.

Castellanos FX, Giedd JN, Eckburg P et al. (1994) Quantitative morphology of the caudate nucleus in attention deficit hyperactivity disorder. *Am J Psychiatry*, 151:1791–6.

Castellanos FX, Lee PP, Sharp W et al. (2002) Developmental trajectories of brain volume abnormalities in children and adolescents with attention-deficit/hyperactivity disorder. *J Am Med Assoc*, 288:1740–8.

Committee on Substance Abuse, American Academy of Pediatrics (1996) Testing for drugs of abuse in children and adolescents. *Pediatr*, 98:305–7.

Courchesne E, Saitoh O, Yeung-Courchesne R et al. (1994) Abnormality of cerebellar vermian lobules VI and VII in patients with infantile autism: identification of hypoplastic and hyperplastic subgroups with MR imaging. *Am J Roentengenol*, 162:123–30.

Dallas JS, Foley TP (1996) *Hypothyroidism*. In: Lifshitz F (ed.) *Pediatric Endocrinology*. New York, Marcel Decker.

Dekker MC, Koot HM (2003) DSM-IV disorders in children with borderline to moderate intellectual disability. I: Prevalence and impact. *J Am Acad Child Adolesc Psychiatry*, 42:915–22.

Denckla MB (2000) Overview: specific behavioral/cognitive phenotypes of genetic disorders. *Ment Retard Dev Dis Res Rev*, 6:81–3.

Dening TR, Berrios GE (1990) Wilson's disease: a longitudinal study of psychiatric symptoms. *Biol Psychiatry*, 28:255–65.

Diaz-Olavarrieta C, Cummings JL, Velazquez J, Garcia de la Cadena C (1999) Neuropsychiatric manifestations of multiple sclerosis. *J Neuropsych Clin Neurosci*, 11:51–7.

DiMauro S, Andreu AL, De Vivo DC (2002) Mitochondrial disorders. *J Child Neurology*, 17(Suppl 3):3S35–47.

Durston S, Tottenham NT, Thomas KM et al. (2003) Differential patterns of striatal activation in young children with and without ADHD. *Biol Psychiatry*, 5:871–8.

Edgeworth J, Bullock P, Bailey A, Gallagher A, Crouchman M (1996) Why are brain tumours still being missed? *Arch Dis Childhood*, 74(2):148–51.

El-Youssef M (2003) Wilson disease. *Mayo Clin Proc*, 78:1126–1136.

Engel GL (1977) The need for a new medical model: a challenge for biomedicine. *Science*, 196:129–36.

Ernst M, Zametkin AJ, Phillips RL, Cohen RM (1997) Cerebral glucose metabolism in adolescent girls with attention-deficit/hyperactivity disorder. *J Am Acad Child Adolesc Psychiatry*, 36:1399–1406.

Estrov Y, Scaglia F, Bodamer OA (2000) Psychiatric symptoms of inherited metabolic disease. *J Inher Met Dis*, 23:2–6.

Filipek PA (1999) Neuroimaging in the developmental disorders: the state of the science. *J Child Psychol Psychiatry*, 40:113–128.

Filipek PA, Semrud-Clikeman M, Steingard RJ, Renshaw PF, Kennedy DN, Biederman J (1997) Volumetric MRI analysis comparing subjects having attention-deficit hyperactivity disorder with normal controls. *Neurology*, 8:589–601.

Frazier JA, Giedd JN, Hamburger SD et al. (1996) Brain anatomic magnetic resonance imaging in childhood-onset schizophrenia. *Arch Gen Psychiatry*, 53:617–624.

Gartner J (2000) Disorders related to peroxisomal membranes. *J Inher Met Dis*, 23:264–72.

Giedd JN, Rapoport JL, Leonard HL, Richter D, Swedo SE (1996) Case study: acute basal ganglia enlargement and obsessive-compulsive symptoms in an adolescent boy. *J Am Acad Child Adolesc Psychiatry*, 35:913–5.

Green WH (2001) *Child and Adolescent Clinical Psychopharmacology*, 3rd edn. Philadelphia, PA, Lippincott Williams & Wilkins.

Hariri AR, Mattay VS, Tessitore A et al. (2002) Serotonin transporter genetic variation and the response of the human amygdale. *Science*, 297:400–3.

Hauser P, Zametkin AJ, Martinez P et al. (1993) Attention deficit-hyperactivity disorder in people with generalized resistance to thyroid hormone. *New Engl J Med*, 328:997–1001.

Hendren RL, De Backer I, Pandina GJ (2000) Review of neuroimaging studies of child and adolescent psychiatric disorders from the past 10 years. *J Am Acad Child Adolesc Psychiatry*, 39:815–28.

Hendren RL, He XY (2003) *Laboratory and Diagnostic Testing*. In: Wiener J, Dulcan MK (eds) *Textbook of Child and Adolescent Psychiatry*, 3rd edn. New York, American Psychiatric Association Press.

Hodapp RM (1997) Direct and indirect behavioral effects of different genetic disorders of mental retardation. *Am J Ment Retard*, 102:67–79.

Ievers CE, Brown RT, McCandless SE, Devine DE (1999) Case studies: psychological test findings for two children with X-linked adrenoleukodystrophy. *J Dev Behav Pediatr*, 20:31–5.

Jacobsen LK, Giedd JN, Castellanos FX et al. (1998a) Progressive reduction of temporal lobe structures in childhood-onset schizophrenia. *Am J Psychiatry*, 155:678–85.

Jacobsen LK, Rapoport JL (1998b) Research update: childhood-onset schizophrenia: implications of clinical and neurobiological research. *J Child Psychol Psychiatry*, 39:101–13.

Jacobsen LK, Giedd JN, Vaituzis AC et al. (1996) Temporal lobe morphology in childhood-onset schizophrenia. *Am J Psychiatry*, 153:355–61.

Katzman DK, Lambe EK, Mikulis DJ, Ridgley JN, Goldbloom DS, Zipursky RB (1996) Cerebral gray matter and white matter volume deficits in adolescent girls with anorexia nervosa. *J Pediatr*, 129:794–803.

Katzman DK, Zipursky RB, Lambe EK, Mikulis DJ (1997) A longitudinal magnetic resonance imaging study of brain changes in adolescents with anorexia nervosa. *Arch Pediatr Adolesc Med*, 151:793–7.

Lancman M (1999) Psychosis and peri-ictal confusional states. *Neurology*, 53:S33–S38.

Lee DO, Helmers SL, Steingard RJ, DeMaso DR (1997) Seizure disorder presenting as panic disorder with agoraphobia. *J Am Acad Child Adolesc Psychiatry*, 36:1295–8.

Loo SK, Specter E, Smolen A, Hopfer C, Teale PD, Reite ML (2003) Functional effects of the DAT1 polymorphism on EEG measures in ADHD. *J Am Acad Child Adolesc Psychiatry*, 42:986–93.

Luna B, Minshew NJ, Garver KE, Lazar NA, Thulborn KR, Eddy WF, Sweeney JA (2002) Neocortical system abnormalities in autism: an fMRI study of spatial working memory. *Neurology*, 59:834–40.

Lyon GR, Rumsey JM (1996) *Neuroimaging: A Window to the Neurological Foundations of Learning and Behavior in Children*. Baltimore, Paul H. Brookes.

Maddalena A, Richards CS, McGinniss MJ et al. (2001) Technical standards and guidelines for fragile X: the first of a series of disease-specific supplements to the Standards and Guidelines for Clinical Genetics Laboratories of the American College of Medical Genetics. Quality Assurance Subcommittee of the Laboratory Practice Committee. *Genet Med*, 3:200–5.

Mehler PS (2001) Diagnosis and care of patients with anorexia nervosa in primary care settings. *Ann Intern Med*, 134(11):1048–59.

O'Connor P (2002) The Canadian Multiple Sclerosis Working Group. Key issues in the diagnosis and treatment of multiple sclerosis. An overview. *Neurology*, 59(6 Suppl 3):S1–33.

Peterson BS (1995) Neuroimaging in child and adolescent neuropsychiatric disorders. *J Am Acad Child Adolesc Psychiatry*, 34:1560–76.

Pipe A, Ayotte C (2002) Nutritional supplements and doping. *Clin J Sport Med*, 12:245–9.

Piven J, Saliba L, Bailey J, Arndt S (1997) An MRI study of autism: the cerebellum revisited. *Neurology*, 49:546–51.

Piven J, Arndt S, Bailey J, Havercamp S, Andreasen NC, Palmer P (1995) An MRI study of brain size in autism. *Am J Psychiatry*, 152:1145–9.

Poussaint TY (2001) Magnetic resonance imaging of pediatric brain tumors: state of the art. *Topics Magnet Resonance Imaging*, 12(6):411–33.

Prasad AN, Breen JC, Ampola MG, Rosman NP (1997) Argininemia: a treatable genetic cause of progressive spastic diplegia simulating cerebral palsy: case reports and literature review. *J Child Neurol*, 12:301–9.

Rapoport JL, Giedd J, Kumra S et al. (1997) Childhood-onset schizophrenia: progressive ventricular change during adolescence. *Arch Gen Psychiatry*, 54:897–903.

Rapoport, JL, Giedd J, Blumenthal J et al. (1999) Progressive cortical change during adolescence in childhood-onset schizophrenia: a longitudinal magnetic resonance imaging study. *Arch Gen Psychiatry*, 54:649–54.

Roman T, Szobot C, Martins S, Biederman J, Rohde LA, Hutz MH (2002) Dopamine transporter gene and response to methylphenidate in attention-deficit/hyperactivity disorder. *Pharmacogenetics*, 12:497–9.

Rosenberg DR, Keshavan MS, O'Hearn KM et al. (1997a) Frontostriatal measurement in treatment-naive children with obsessive-compulsive disorder. *Arch Gen Psychiatry*, 54:824–30.

Rosenberg DR, Keshavan MS, O'Hearne KM, Bagwell WW, MacMaster FP, Birmaher B (1997b) Frontostriatal measurement in treatment-naïve children with obsessive-compulsive disorder. *Arch Gen Psychiatry*, 54:824–830.

Rowe DC, Stever C, Chase D, Sherman S, Abramowitz A, Waldman ID (2001) Two dopamine genes related to reports of childhood retrospective inattention and conduct disorder symptoms. *Mol Psychiatry*, 6:429–33.

Semrud-Clikeman M, Steingard RJ, Filipek P, Biederman J, Bekken K, Renshaw PF (2000) Using MRI to examine brain-behavior relationships in males with attention deficit disorder with hyperactivity. *J Am Acad Child Adolesc Psychiatry*, 39:477–84.

Sheline Y, Kehr C (1990) Cost and utility of routine admission laboratory testing for psychiatric inpatients. *Gen Hosp Psychiatry*, 12:329–34.

Shevell M, Ashwal S, Donley D et al. (2003) Quality Standards Subcommittee of the American Academy of Neurology, Practice Committee of the Child Neurology Society. Practice parameter: evaluation of the child with global developmental delay: report of the Quality Standards Subcommittee of the American Academy of Neurology and The Practice Committee of the Child Neurology Society. *Neurology*, 60:367–80.

Sparks BF, Friedman SD, Shaw DW et al. (2002) Brain structural abnormalities in young children with autism spectrum disorder. *Neurology*, 59:184–92.

Steingard RJ, Renshaw PF, Yurgelun-Todd D et al. (1996) Structural abnormalities in brain magnetic resonance images of depressed children. *J Am Acad Child Adolesc Psychiatry*, 35:307–11.

Swedo SE, Leonard HL, Garvey M et al. (1998) Pediatric autoimmune neuropsychiatric disorders associated with streptococcal infections: clinical description of the first 50 cases. *Am J Psychiatry*, 155:264–71.

Walsh JM, Wheat ME, Freund K (2000) Detection, evaluation, and treatment of eating disorders the role of the primary care physician. *J Gen Intern Med*, 15(8):577–90.

Warner EA, Walker RM, Friedmann PD (2003) Should informed consent be required for laboratory testing for drugs of abuse in medical settings? *Am J Med*, 115(1):54–8.

Wenger DA, Coppola S, Liu SL (2003) Insights into the diagnosis and treatment of lysosomal storage diseases. *Arch Neurology*, 60:322–8.

Winsberg BG, Comings DE (1999) Association of the dopamine transporter gene (DAT1) with poor methylphenidate response. *J Am Acad Child Adolesc Psychiatry*, 38:1474–7.

Wyckoff PM, Miller LC, Tucker LB, Schaller JG (1995) Neuropsychological assessment of children and adolescents with systemic lupus erythematosus. *Lupus*, 4:217–20.

Wyllie E, Glazer JP, Benbadis S, Kotagal P, Wolgamuth B (1999) Psychiatric features of children and adolescents with pseudoseizures. *Arch Pediatr Adolesc Med*, 153:244–8.

Zametkin AJ, Ernst M, Silver R (1998) Laboratory and diagnostic testing in child and adolescent psychiatry: a review of the past 10 years. *J Am Acad Child Adolesc Psychiatry*, 37:464–72.

Chapter 4

Adnopoz J (2002) Home-based child and family treatment. In: Lewis M (ed.) *Child and Adolescent Psychiatry: A Comprehensive Textbook*, 3rd edn. Philadelphia, Lippincott Williams & Wilkins, pp. 1386–93.

Alessi N, Naylor MW, Ghaziuddin M, Zubieta JK (1994) Update on lithium carbonate therapy in children and adolescents. *J Am Acad Child Adolesc Psychiatry*, 33:291–304.

Aman MG, De Smedt G, Derivan A, Lyons B, Findling RL (2002) Risperidone Disruptive Behavior Study Group: double-blind, placebo-controlled study of risperidone for the treatment of disruptive behaviors in children with subaverage intelligence. *Am J Psychiatry*, 159:1337–46.

American Academy of Child and Adolescent Psychiatry (2002) Practice parameter for the use of electroconvulsive therapy with adolescents. *J Am Acad Child Adolesc Psychiatry*, in press.

American Academy of Child and Adolescent Psychiatry (1997) Practice parameters for the assessment and treatment of children and adolescents with schizophrenia. *J Am Acad Child Adolesc Psychiatry*, 36(Suppl 10S):177S-193S.

American Academy of Child and Adolescent Psychiatry (2001) Practice parameter for the assessment and treatment of children and adolescents with schizophrenia. *J Am Acad Child Adolesc Psychiatry*, 40(Suppl 7):4S-23S.

American Academy of Child and Adolescent Psychiatry (1998) Practice parameters for the assessment and treatment of children and adolescents with depressive disorders. *J Am Acad Child Adolesc Psychiatry*, 37(Suppl 10):63S-83S.

American Academy of Pediatrics Committee on Drugs (1996) Unapproved uses of approved drugs: the physician, the package insert, and the Food and Drug Administration: subject review. *Pediatrics*, 98:143–5.

American Diabetes Association (2004) Consensus development conference on antipsychotic drugs and obesity and diabetes. *Diabetes Care*, 27:596–601.

Anonymous (1998) Practice parameters for the assessment and treatment of children and adolescents with depressive disorders. *J Am Acad Child Adolesc Psychiatry*, 37(Suppl 10).63S-83S.

Anonymous: SSRIs (2003) suicide risk and withdrawal. *Lancet*, 361(9374):1999.

Armbruster P, Chock U, Tanner E, Holmes S (2002) Parent work. In: Lewis M (ed.) *Child and Adolescent Psychiatry: A Comprehensive Textbook*, 3rd edn. Philadelphia, Lippincott Williams & Wilkins, 1055–65.

Auiler JF, Liu K, Lynch JM, Gelotte CK (2002) Effect of food on early drug exposure from extended-release stimulants: results from the Concerta, Adderall XR Food Evaluation (CAFE) Study. *Cur Med Res Opin*, 18:311–16.

Baldessarini RJ, Tondo L (2000) Does lithium treatment still work? Evidence of stable responses over three decades. *Arch Gen Psychiatry*, 57(2):187–90.

Baldessarini RJ, Tondo L, Hennen J (2001) Treating the suicidal patient with bipolar disorder: reducing suicide risk with lithium. *Ann N Y Acad Sci*, 932:24–43.

Bernstein GA, Garfinkel BD, Borchardt CM (1990) Comparative studies of pharmacotherapy for school refusal. *J Am Acad Child Adolesc Psychiatry*, 29:773–81.

Biederman J, Lopez FA, Boellner SW, Chandler MC (2002) A randomized, double-blind, placebo-controlled, parallel-group study of SLI381 (Adderall XR) in children with attention-deficit/hyperactivity disorder. *Pediatr*, 110(2 Pt 1):258–66.

Birmaher B, Axelson DA, Monk K et al. (2003) Fluoxetine for the treatment of childhood anxiety disorders. *J Am Acad Child Adolesc Psychiatry*, 42:415–23.

Birmaher B, Ryan ND, Williamson DE, Brent DA, Kaufman J (1996) Childhood and adolescent depression: a review of the past 10 years. Part II. *J Am Acad Child Adolesc Psychiatry, 35*:1575–83.

Browne K (2003) *Child protection*. In: Rutter M, Taylor E (eds) *Child and Adolescent Psychiatry*, 4th edn. Massachusetts, Blackwell Science Ltd, 1158–74.

Cala S, Crismon ML, Baumgartner J (2003) A survey of herbal use in children with attention-deficit-hyperactivity disorder or depression. *Pharmacother*, 23:222–30.

Campbell M, Rapoport JL, Simpson GM (1999) Antipsychotics in children and adolescents. *J Am Acad Child Adolesc Psychiatry*, 38:537–45.

Campbell M, Armenteros JL, Malone RP, Adams PB, Eisenberg ZW, Overall JE (1997) Neuroleptic-related dyskinesias in autistic children: a prospective, longitudinal study. *J Am Acad Child Adolesc Psychiatry*, 36:835–43.

Carlson GA, Kelly KL (2003) Stimulant rebound: how common is it and what does it mean? *J Child Adolesc Psychopharm*, 13:137–42.

Committee on Safety of Medicines (2003) Use of selective serotonin reuptake inhibitors (SSRIs) in children and adolescents with major depressive disorder (MDD), www.mhra.gov.uk

Connor DF (2004) Paroxetine and the FDA. *J Am Acad Child Adolesc Psychiatry*, 43(2):127.

Correll CU, Leucht S, Kane JM (2004) Lower risk for tardive dyskinesia associated with second-generation antipsychotics: a systematic review of 1-year studies. *Am J Psychiatry*, 161(3):414–25.

Cramer-Azima FJ (2002) Group psychotherapy for children and adolescents. In: Lewis M (ed.) *Child and Adolescent Psychiatry: A Comprehensive Textbook*, 3rd edn. Philadelphia, Lippincott Williams & Wilkins, pp. 1024–36.

DelBello M, Schwiers ML, Rosenberg HL, Strakowski SM (2002) A double-blind, randomized, placebo-controlled study of quetiapine as adjunctive treatment for adolescent mania. *J Am Acad Child Adolesc Psychiatry*, 41:1216–23.

Demb HB, Nguyen KT (1999) Movement disorders in children with developmental disabilities taking risperidone. *J Am Acad Child Adolesc Psychiatry*, 38:5–6.

DeVeaugh-Geiss J, Moroz G, Biederman J et al. (1992) Clomipramine hydrochloride in childhood and adolescent obsessive-compulsive disorder – a multicenter trial. *J Am Acad Child Adolesc Psychiatry*, 31:45–9.

Eberle AJ (1998) Valproate and polycystic ovaries. *J Am Acad Child Adolesc Psychiatry*, 37(10):1009.

Efron D, Hiscock H, Sewell JR et al. (2003) Prescribing of psychotropic medications for children by Australian pediatricians and child psychiatrists. *Pediatr*, 111:372–5.

Elia J, Ambrosini PJ, Rapoport JL (1999) Treatment of attention-deficit-hyperactivity disorder. *New Engl J Med*, 340:780–8.

Elia J, Borcherding BG, Rapoport JL, Keysor CS (1991) Methylphenidate and dextroamphetamine treatments of hyperactivity: are there true nonresponders? *Psychiatry Res*, 36:141–55.

Emslie GJ, Rush AJ, Weinberg WA et al. (1997) A double-blind, randomized, placebo-controlled trial of fluoxetine in children and adolescents with depression. *Arch Gen Psychiatry*, 54:1031–37.

Emslie GJ, Heiligenstein JH, Wagner KD et al. (2002) Fluoxetine for acute treatment of depression in children and adolescents: a placebo-controlled, randomized clinical trial. *J Am Acad Child Adolesc Psychiatry*, 41:1205–15.

Findling RL, McNamara NK, Branicky LA, Schluchter MD, Lemon E, Blumer JL (2000) A double-blind pilot study of risperidone in the treatment of conduct disorder. *J Am Acad Child Adolesc Psychiatry*, 39:509–16.

Flament MF, Rapoport JL, Berg CJ et al. (1985) Clomipramine treatment of childhood obsessive-compulsive disorder. A double-blind controlled study. *Arch Gen Psychiatry*, 42:977–83.

Freeman MP, Stoll AL (1998) Mood stabilizer combinations: a review of safety and efficacy. *Am J Psychiatry*, 155(1):12–21.

Gabbard G (2000) Psychoanalysis and psychoanalytic psychotherapy. In: Sadock BJ, Sadock VA (eds) *Kaplan and Sadock's Comprehensive Textbook of Psychiatry, volume II*, 7th edn. Philadelphia, Lippincott Williams & Wilkins, 30.1, pp. 2076–8.

Gardiner P, Wornham W (2000) Recent review of complementary and alternative medicine used by adolescents. *Curr Opin Pediatr*, 12:298–302.

Garland EJ, Behr R (1996) Hormonal effects of valproic acid? *J Am Acad Child Adolesc Psychiatry*, 35(11):1424–5.

Geller DA, Biederman J, Stewart SE et al. (2003) Which SSRI? A meta-analysis of pharmacotherapy trials in pediatric obsessive-compulsive disorder. *Am J Psychiatry*, 160:1919–28.

Geller B, Cooper TB, Sun K et al. (1998) Double-blind and placebo controlled study of lithium for adolescent bipolar disorders with secondary substance dependency. *J Am Acad Child Adolesc Psychiatry*, 37:171–8.

Gittelman-Klein R, Klein DF (1973) School phobia: diagnostic considerations in the light of imipramine effects. *J Nerv Ment Dis*, 156:199–215.

Gracious BL, Findling RL, Seman C, Youngstrom EA, Demeter CA, Calabrese JR (2004) Elevated thyrotropin in bipolar youths prescribed both lithium and divalproex sodium. *J Am Acad Child Adolesc Psychiatry*, 43(2):215–20.

Greenhill LL (2003) Assessment of safety in pediatric psychopharmacology. *J Am Acad Child Adolesc Psychiatry*, 42:625–6.

Greenhill LL, Halperin JM, Abikoff H (1999) Stimulant medications. *J Am Acad Child Adolesc Psychiatry*, 38(5):503–12.

Greenhill LL, Pliszka S, Dulcan MK et al. (2002) American Academy of Child and Adolescent Psychiatry. Practice parameter for the use of stimulant medications in the treatment of children, adolescents, and adults. *J Am Acad Child Adolesc Psychiatry*, 41 (Suppl 2):26S-49S.

Grigsby RK (2002) Consultation with foster care homes, group homes, youth shelters, domestic violence shelters, and big brothers and big sisters programs. In: Lewis M (ed.) *Child and Adolescent Psychiatry: A Comprehensive Textbook*, 3rd edn. Philadelphia, Lippincott Williams & Wilkins, pp. 1393–7.

Gutgesell H, Atkins D, Barst R et al. (1999) AHA Scientific Statement: Cardiovascular Monitoring of Children and Adolescents Receiving Psychotropic Drugs. *J Am Acad Child Adolesc Psychiatry*, 38:1047–50.

Guy W (ed.) (1976) *ECDEU Assessment Manual for Psychopharmacology: Publication ADM 76–338*. Washington, DC, US Department of Health, Education, and Welfare, pp. 534–7.

Hazell P, O'Connell D, Heathcote D, Robertson J, Henry D (1995) Efficacy of tricyclic drugs in treating child and adolescent depression: a meta-analysis. *Br Med J*, 310:897–901.

Hendren RL, Hamaran S (2003) Clinical assessment of children and adolescents treated pharmacologically. In: Martin A, Scahill L, Charney DS, Leckman JF (eds) *Pediatric Psychopharmacology: Principles and Practice*. New York, Oxford University Press, pp. 399–403.

Heyman I, Santosh P (2003) Pharmacological and other physical treatments. In: Rutter M, Taylor E (eds) *Child and Adolescent Psychiatry*, 4th edn. Massachusetts, Blackwell Science Ltd, pp. 998-1018.

Hughes CW, Emslie GJ, Crismon ML et al. (1999) The Texas Children's Medication Algorithm Project: report of the Texas Consensus Conference Panel on Medication Treatment of Childhood Major Depressive Disorder. *J Am Acad Child Adolesc Psychiatry*, 38:1442–54.

Isojarvi JIT, Laatikainen TJ, Pakarinen AJ et al. (1993) Polycystic ovaries and hyperandrogenism in women taking valproate for epilepsy. *New Engl J Med*, 329:1383–8.

Jacobs BW (2003) Individual and group therapy. In: Rutter M, Taylor E (eds) *Child and Adolescent Psychiatry*, 4th edn. Massachusetts, Blackwell Science Ltd, pp. 983–97.

Jensen PS, Bhatara VS, Vitiello B, Hoagwood K, Feil M, Burke LB (1999) Psychoactive medication prescribing practices·for U.S. children: gaps between research and clinical practice. *J Am Acad Child Adolesc Psychiatry*, 38(5):557–65.

Johnston HF (1999) More on valproate and polycystic ovaries. *J Am Acad Child Adolesc Psychiatry*, 38(4):354.

Josephson AM (2002) Family therapy. In: Lewis M (ed.) *Child and Adolescent Psychiatry: A Comprehensive Textbook*, 3rd edn. Philadelphia, Lippincott Williams & Wilkins, pp. 1036–54.

Kafantaris V, Coletti DJ, Dicker R, Padula G, Kane JM (2001) Adjunctive antipsychotic treatment of adolescents with bipolar psychosis. *J Am Acad Child Adolesc Psychiatry*, 40:1448–56.

Kafantaris V, Coletti DJ, Dicker R, Padula G, Kane JM (2003) Lithium treatment of acute mania in adolescents: a large open trial. *J Am Acad Child Adolesc Psychiatry*, 42(9):1038–45.

Kazdin AE (2000a) Introduction. In: *Psychotherapy for Children and Adolescents: Directions for Research and Practice*. New York, Oxford University Press, pp. 3–16.

Kazdin AE (2000b) The effects of psychotherapy: current status of the evidence. In: *Psychotherapy for Children and Adolescents: Directions for Research and Practice*. New York, Oxford University Press, pp. 55–71.

Kazdin AE (2000c) The effects of psychotherapy: empirically supported treatments. In: *Psychotherapy for Children and Adolescents: Directions for Research and Practice*. New York, Oxford University Press, pp. 72–88.

Kazdin AE (2000d) Treatments that work: illustrations of exemplary research. In: *Psychotherapy for Children and Adolescents: Directions for Research and Practice*. New York, Oxford University Press, pp. 89–107.

Keller MB, Ryan ND, Strober M et al. (2001) Efficacy of paroxetine in the treatment of adolescent major depression: a randomized, controlled trial. *J Am Acad Child Adolesc Psychiatry*, 40:762–72.

Kiser LJ, Heston JD, Pruitt DB (2002) Child and adolescent partial hospitalization and ambulatory behavioral health services. In: Lewis M (ed.) *Child and Adolescent Psychiatry: A Comprehensive Textbook*, 3rd edn. Philadelphia, Lippincott Williams & Wilkins, pp. 1083-91.

Klein DF, Mannuzza S, Chapman T, Fyer AJ (1992) Child panic revisited. *J Am Acad Child Adolesc Psychiatry*, 31:112–16.

Koller E, Malozowski S, Doraiswamy PM (2001) Atypical antipsychotic drugs and hyperglycemia in adolescents. *J Am Med Assoc*, 286:2547–8.

Kowatch RA, Suppes T, Carmody TJ et al. (2000) Effect size of lithium, divalproex sodium, and carbamazepine in children and adolescents with bipolar disorder. *J Am Acad Child Adolesc Psychiatry*, 39:713–20.

Kumra S, Jacobsen LK, Lenane M et al. (1998) Case series: spectrum of neuroleptic-induced movement disorders and extrapyramidal side effects in childhood-onset schizophrenia. *J Am Acad Child Adolesc Psychiatry*, 37:221–7.

Leonard HL, March J, Rickler KC, Allen AJ (1997) Pharmacology of the selective serotonin reuptake inhibitors in children and adolescents. *J Am Acad Child Adolesc Psychiatry*, 36:725–36.

Lewis M, Summerville JW, Graffagnino PN (2002) Residential treatment. In: Lewis M (ed.) *Child and Adolescent Psychiatry: A Comprehensive Textbook*, 3rd edn. Philadelphia, Lippincott Williams & Wilkins, pp. 1095–103.

Loring DW, Meador KJ (2001) Cognitive and behavioral effects of epilepsy treatment. *Epilepsia*, 42(Suppl 8):24–32.

Malekoff A (1997) *What's so special about group work? An introduction to tradition and theory* in *Group Work with Adolescents*. New York, The Guildford Press, pp. 31–52.

Malone RP, Delaney MA, Luebbert JF, Cater J, Campbell M (2000) A double-blind placebo-controlled study of lithium in hospitalized aggressive children and adolescents with conduct disorder. *Arch Gen Psychiatry*, 57(7):649–54.

March JS, Biederman J, Wolkow R et al. (1998) Sertraline in children and adolescents with obsessive-compulsive disorder: a multicenter randomized controlled trial. *J Am Med Assoc*, 280:1752–6.

March JS, Wells K (2003) *Combining pharmacotherapy and psychotherapy: an evidence-based approach*. In: Martin A, Scahill L, Charney DS, Leckman JF (eds) *Pediatric Psychopharmacology: Principles and Practice*. New York, Oxford University Press, pp. 426–43.

McClellan JM, Werry JS (2003) Evidence-based treatments in child and adolescent psychiatry: an inventory. *J Am Acad Child Adolesc Psychiatry*, 42:1388–400.

McClellan J, Werry J (1997) Practice parameters for the assessment and treatment of children and adolescents with bipolar disorder. *J Am Acad Child Adolesc Psychiatry*, 36(Suppl 10):157S-76S.

McCracken JT, Biederman J, Greenhill LL et al. (2003) Analog classroom assessment of a once-daily mixed amphetamine formulation, SLI381 (Adderall XR), in children with ADHD. *J Am Acad Child Adolesc Psychiatry*, 42:673–83.

McCracken JT, McGough J, Shah B et al. (2002) Research Units on Pediatric Psychopharmacology Autism Network. Risperidone in children with autism and serious behavioral problems. *New Engl J Med*, 347:314–21.

Michelson D, Allen AJ, Busner J et al. (2002) Once-daily atomoxetine treatment for children and adolescents with attention deficit hyperactivity disorder: a randomized, placebo-controlled study. *Am J Psychiatry*, 159:1896–901.

Michelson D, Faries D, Wernicke J et al. (2001) Atomoxetine ADHD Study Group. Atomoxetine in the treatment of children and adolescents with attention-deficit/hyperactivity disorder: a randomized, placebo-controlled, dose-response study. *Pediatr*, 108:E83.

The MTA Cooperative Group (1999) A 14-month randomized clinical trial of treatment strategies for attention-deficit/hyperactivity disorder (ADHD). *Arch Gen Psychiatry*, 56:1073–86.

Mufson L, Dorta KP (2003) Interpersonal psychotherapy for depressed adolescents. In: Kazdin AE, Weisz JR (eds) *Evidence-Based Psychotherapies for Children and Adolescents*. New York, The Guildford Press, pp. 148–64.

Nemeroff CB, DeVane CL, Pollock BG (1996) Newer antidepressants and the cytochrome P450 system. *Am J Psychiatry*, 153:311–20.

Oransky I (2003) FDA questions antidepressant safety for children. *Lancet*, 362(9395):1558.

Pande AC, Crockatt JG, Janney CA, Werth JL, Tsaroucha G (2000) Gabapentin in bipolar disorder: a placebo-controlled trial of adjunctive therapy. Gabapentin Bipolar Disorder Study Group. *Bipolar Disorders*, 2(3 Pt 2):249–55.

Pappadopulos E, Macintyre II JC, Crismon ML et al. (2003) Treatment recommendations for the use of antipsychotics for aggressive youth (TRAAY) Part II. *J Am Acad Child Adolesc Psychiatry*, 42(2):145–61.

Pappadopulos E, Macintyre II JC, Crismon ML et al. (2001) American Academy of Child and Adolescent Psychiatry. Practice parameter for the assessment and treatment of children and adolescents with schizophrenia. *J Am Acad Child Adolesc Psychiatry*, 40(Suppl 7):4S-23S.

Pelham WE, Gnagy EM, Burrows-Maclean L et al. (2001) Once-a-day Concerta methylphenidate versus three-times-daily methylphenidate in laboratory and natural settings. *Pediatr*, 107:E105.

Petti TA, Kronnennberger WG (2002) Cognitive therapies. In: Lewis M (ed.) *Child and Adolescent Psychiatry: A Comprehensive Textbook*, 3rd edn. Philadelphia, Lippincott Williams & Wilkins, pp. 1015–23.

Pine DS (2002) Treating children and adolescents with selective serotonin reuptake inhibitors: how long is appropriate? *J Child Adolesc Psychopharm*, 12:189–203.

Pliszka SR, Greenhill LL, Crismon ML et al. (2000a) The Texas Children's Medication Algorithm Project: Report of the Texas Consensus Conference Panel on Medication Treatment of Childhood Attention-Deficit/Hyperactivity Disorder. Part I. Attention-deficit/hyperactivity disorder. *J Am Acad Child Adolesc Psychiatry*, 39(7):908–19.

Pliszka SR, Greenhill LL, Crismon ML et al. (2000b) The Texas Children's Medication Algorithm Project: Report of the Texas Consensus Conference Panel on Medication Treatment of Childhood Attention-Deficit/Hyperactivity Disorder. Part II: Tactics, attention-deficit/hyperactivity disorder. *J Am Acad Child Adolesc Psychiatry*, 39:920–7.

Popper CW (1995) Combining methylphenidate and clonidine: pharmacologic questions and news reports about sudden death. *J Child Adolesc Psychopharmacol*, 5:157–166.

Post RM, Ketter TA, Pazzaglia PJ et al. (1996) Rational polypharmacy in the bipolar affective disorders. *Epilepsy Res*, 11(Suppl):153–80.

Ratzoni G, Gothelf D, Brand-Gothelf A et al. (2002) Weight gain associated with olanzapine and risperidone in adolescent patients: a comparative prospective study. *J Am Acad Child Adolesc Psychiatry*, 41:337–43.

The Research Unit on Pediatric Psychopharmacology Anxiety Study Group (2001) Fluvoxamine for the treatment of anxiety disorders in children and adolescents. *New Engl J Med*, 344:1279–85.

Riddle MA, Reeve EA, Yaryura-Tobias JA et al. (2001) Fluvoxamine for children and adolescents with obsessive-compulsive disorder: a randomized, controlled, multicenter trial. *J Am Acad Child Adolesc Psychiatry*, 40:222–9.

Riddle MA, Scahill L, King RA et al. (1992) Double-blind, crossover trial of fluoxetine and placebo in children and adolescents with obsessive-compulsive disorder. *J Am Acad Child Adolesc Psychiatry*, 31:1062–9.

Ritvo RZ, Ritvo S (2002) Psychodynamic psychotherapy. In: Lewis M (ed.) *Child and Adolescent Psychiatry: A Comprehensive Textbook*, 3rd edn. Philadelphia, Lippincott Williams & Wilkins, pp. 974–83.

Rockland LH (1989a) What is psychodynamic supportive psychotherapy? In: *Supportive Therapy: A Psychodynamic Approach*. New York, Basic Books, Inc., pp. 2–11.

Rockland LH (1989b) Indications and contraindications. In: *Supportive Therapy: A Psychodynamic Approach*. New York, Basic Books, Inc., pp. 58–71.

Rockland LH (1989c) Mechanisms of therapeutic action. In: *Supportive Therapy: A Psychodynamic Approach*. New York, Basic Books, Inc., pp. 237–52.

Rushton A, Minnis H (2003) Residential and foster family care. In: Rutter M, Taylor E (eds) *Child and Adolescent Psychiatry*, 4th edn. Massachusetts, Blackwell Science Ltd, pp. 359–72.

Rutter M, Taylor E (2003) Clinical assessment and diagnostic formulation. In: Rutter M, Taylor E (eds) *Child and Adolescent Psychiatry*, 4th edn. Massachusetts, Blackwell Science Ltd, pp. 18–31.

Ryan ND, Bhatara VS, Perel JM (1999) Mood stabilizers in children and adolescents. *J Am Acad Child Adolesc Psychiatry*, 38(5):529–36.

Schachter HM, Pham B, King J, Langford S, Moher D (2001) How efficacious and safe is short-acting methylphenidate for the treatment of attention-deficit disorder in children and adolescents? A meta-analysis. *Can Med Assoc J*, 165:1475–88.

Schou M (1997) Forty years of lithium treatment. *Arch Gen Psychiatry*, 54(1):9–13.

Schreter RK (2003) Economic issues in child and adolescent psychiatry. In: Wiener JM, Dulcan MK (eds) *Textbook of Child and Adolescent Psychiatry*, 3rd edn. Washington DC, American Psychiatric Press, pp. 57–67.

Schur SB, Sikich L, Findling RL et al. (2003) Treatment recommendations for the use of antipsychotics for aggressive youth (TRAAY). Part I: A review. *J Am Acad Child Adolesc Psychiatry*, 42:132–44.

Schwab-Stone ME, Henrich C, Armbruster P (2002) School consultation. In: Lewis M (ed.) *Child and Adolescent Psychiatry: A Comprehensive Textbook*, 3rd edn. Philadelphia, Lippincott Williams & Wilkins, pp. 1361–2.

Siennick SE, Jensen PS (2003) Treatment recommendations for the use of antipsychotics for aggressive youth (TRAAY). Part II. *J Am Acad Child Adolesc Psychiatry*, 42:145–61.

Silva RR, Campbell M, Golden RR, Small AM, Pataki CS, Rosenberg CR (1992) Side effects associated with lithium and placebo administration in aggressive children. *Psychopharmacol Bull*, 28:319–326.

Silva RR, Munoz DM, Alpert M, Perlmutter IR, Diaz J (1999) Neuroleptic malignant syndrome in children and adolescents. *J Am Acad Child Adolesc Psychiatry*, 38:187–94.

Snyder R, Turgay A, Aman M, Binder C, Fisman S, Carroll A (2002) Risperidone Conduct Study Group. Effects of risperidone on conduct and disruptive behavior disorders in children with subaverage IQs. *J Am Acad Child Adolesc Psychiatry*, 41:1026–36.

Spencer T, Biederman J, Wilens T, Harding M, O'Donnell D, Griffin S (1996) Pharmacotherapy of attention-deficit hyperactivity disorder across the life cycle. *J Am Acad Child Adolesc Psychiatry*, 35:409–32.

Steiner H, Redlich AD (2002) Child psychiatry and juvenile court. In: Lewis M (ed.) *Child and Adolescent Psychiatry: A Comprehensive Textbook*, 3rd edn. Philadelphia, Lippincott Williams & Wilkins, pp. 1417–25.

Strober M, Morrell W, Burroughs J et al. (1988) A family study of bipolar I disorder in adolescence: early onset of symptoms linked to increased familial loading and lithium resistance. *J Affect Disord*, 15:255–268.

Tonks A (2002) Withdrawal from paroxetine can be severe, warns FDA. *Br Med J*, 324:260.

US Food and Drug Administration (FDA) (2004) Labeling Change Request Letter for Antidepressant Medications, http://www.fda.gov/cder/drug/antidepressants/SSRIlabelChange.htm.

Velosa JF, Riddle MA (2000) Pharmacologic treatment of anxiety disorders in children and adolescents. *Child Adolesc Psychiatric Clin N Am*, 9:119–33.

Vitiello B, Jensen PS (1997) Medication development and testing in children and adolescents: current problems, future directions. *Arch Gen Psychiatry*, 54:871–876.

Vitulano LA, Tebes JK (2002) Child and adolescent behavior therapy. In: Lewis M (ed.) *Child and Adolescent Psychiatry: A Comprehensive Textbook*, 3rd edn. Philadelphia, Lippincott Williams & Wilkins, pp. 998–1115.

Wagner KD, Ambrosini P, Rynn M et al. (2003) Sertraline. Pediatric Depression Study Group: Efficacy of sertraline in the treatment of children and adolescents with major depressive disorder: two randomized controlled trials. *J Am Med Assoc*, 290:1033–41.

Wagner KD, Weller EB, Carlson GA et al. (2002) An open-label trial of divalproex in children and adolescents with bipolar disorder. *J Am Acad Child Adolesc Psychiatry*, 41:1224–30.

Walter G, Rey JM, Ghaziuddin N (2003) Electroconvulsive therapy and transcranial magnetic stimulation. In: Martin A, Scahill L, Charney DS, Leckman JF (eds) *Pediatric Psychopharmacology: Principles and Practices*. New York, Oxford University Press, pp. 377–86.

Waslick B, Greenhill LL (2003) Attention-deficit/hyperactivity disorder. In: Weiner JM, Dulcan MK (eds) *Textbook of Child and Adolescent Psychiatry*, 3rd edn. Washington DC, American Psychiatric Press, p. 494.

Weiner JM (2002) Mental health delivery services for children and adolescents. In: Lewis M (ed.) *Child and Adolescent Psychiatry: A Comprehensive Textbook*, 3rd edn. Philadelphia, Lippincott Williams & Wilkins, p. 1336.

Wernicke JF, Kratochvil CJ (2002) Safety profile of atomoxetine in the treatment of children and adolescents with ADHD. *J Clin Psychiatry*, 63(Suppl 12):50–5.

Werry JS, Andrews LK (2002) Psychotherapies: a critical overview. In: Lewis M (ed.) *Child and Adolescent Psychiatry: A Comprehensive*

Textbook, 3rd edn. Philadelphia, Lippincott Williams & Wilkins, pp. 1078–83.

West SA, Keck Jr, PE McElroy SL et al. (1994) Open trial of valproate in the treatment of adolescent mania. *J Child Adolesc Psychopharmacol*, 4:263–7.

Williams DT (2003) Hypnosis. In: Weiner JM, Dulcan MK (eds) *Textbook of Child and Adolescent Psychiatry*, 3rd edn. Washington DC, American Psychiatric Press, pp. 1043–54.

Wolraich ML, Greenhill LL, Pelham W et al. (2001) Randomized, controlled trial of oros methylphenidate once a day in children with attention-deficit/hyperactivity disorder. *Pediatr*, 108:883–92.

Woolston JL (2002) Psychiatric Inpatient Services. In: Lewis M (ed.) *Child and Adolescent Psychiatry: A Comprehensive Textbook*, 3rd edn. Philadelphia, Lippincott Williams & Wilkins, pp. 1091–5.

Woolston JL (1999a) Combined pharmacotherapy: pitfalls of treatment. *J Am Acad Child Adolesc Psychiatry*, 38:1455–7.

Woolston JL (1999b) Case study: carbamazepine treatment of juvenile-onset bipolar disorder. *J Am Acad Child Adolesc Psychiatry*, 38(3):335–8.

Zellman GL, Fair CC (2002) Preventing and reporting abuse. In: Myers JEB, Berliner L, Briere J, Hendrix CT, Jenny C, Reid TA (eds) *The APSAC Handbook on Child Maltreatment*, 2nd edn. Thousand Oaks, SAGE Publications, pp. 461–75.

Zigler EF, Finn-Stevenson M, Tanner EM (2002) National policies for children, adolescents, and families. In: Lewis M (ed.) *Child and Adolescent Psychiatry: A Comprehensive Textbook*, 3rd edn. Philadelphia, Lippincott Williams & Wilkins, pp. 1340–1.

Chapter 5

American Academy of Child and Adolescent Psychiatry (1999a) Practice parameters for the assessment and treatment of children, adolescents, and adults with autism and other pervasive developmental disorders. *J Am Acad Child Adolesc Psychiatry*, 38(Suppl):32S-54S.

American Academy of Child and Adolescent Psychiatry (1999b) Summary of the practice parameters for the assessment and treatment of children, adolescents, and adults with mental retardation and comorbid mental disorders. *J Am Acad Child Adolesc Psychiatry*, 38:1606–10.

American Psychiatric Association (APA) (1994) *Diagnostic and Statistical Manual of Mental Disorders*, 4th edn. Washington DC, American Psychiatric Association.

American Psychiatric Association (1980) *Diagnostic and Statistical Manual of Mental Disorders*, 3rd edn. Washington DC, American Psychiatric Association.

Amir RE, Van den Veyver IB, Wan M, Tran CQ, Francke U, Zoghbi HY (1999) Rett syndrome is caused by mutations in X-linked MECP2, encoding methyl-CpG binding protein 2. *Nature Genet*, 23:185–8.

Anonymous (1998) Auditory integration training and facilitated communication for autism. American Academy of Pediatrics. Committee on Children with Disabilities. *Pediatr*, 102:431–3.

Aylward GP (1997) Conceptual issues in developmental screening and assessment. *J Dev Behav Pediatr*, 18:240–9.

Baieli S, Pavone L, Meli C, Fiumara A, Coleman M (2003) Autism and phenylketonuria. *J Autism Dev Disord*, 33:201–4.

Bailey A, Bolton P, Butler L et al. (1993) Prevalence of the fragile X anomaly amongst autistic twins and singletons. *J Child Psychol Psychiatry*, 34:673–88.

Bailey A, Le Couteur A, Gottesman I et al. (1995) Autism as a strongly genetic disorder: evidence from a British twin study. *Psychol Med*, 25:63–77.

Bailey DB, Mesibov GB, Hatton DD, Clark RD, Roberts JE, Mayhew L (1998) Autistic behavior in young boys with fragile X syndrome. *J Autism Dev Disord*, 28:499–508.

Baird G, Charman T, Cox A et al. (2001) Current topic: screening and surveillance for autism and pervasive developmental disorders. *Arch Dis Childhood*, 84:468–75.

Baron-Cohen S, Wheelwright S, Cox A et al. (2000) Early identification of autism by the Checklist for Autism in Toddlers (CHAT). *J Roy Soc Med*, 93:521–5.

Baron-Cohen S, Allen J, Gillberg C (1992) Can autism be detected at 18 months? The needle, the haystack, and the CHAT. *Br J Psychiatry*, 161:839–43.

Batshaw ML (1993) Mental Retardation. *Pediatr Clin N Am*, 40:507–21.

Baumgardner TL, Reiss AL, Freund LS, Abrams MT (1995) Specification of the neurobehavioral phenotype in males with fragile X syndrome. *Pediatr*, 95:744–52.

Bayley, N (1993) *Bayley Scales of Infant Development*, 2nd edn. San Antonio, TX, The Psychological Corporation Harcourt Brace Janovich, Inc.

Bellugi U, Bihrle A, Jernigan T, Trauner D, Doherty S (1990) Neuropsychological, neurological and neuroanatomical profile of Williams syndrome. *Am J Med Genet*, (Suppl 6):115–25.

Berument SK, Rutter M, Lord C, Pickles A, Bailey A (1999) Autism screening questionnaire: diagnostic validity. *Br J Psychiatry*, 175:444–51.

Bolton PF, Griffiths PD (1997) Association of tuberous sclerosis of temporal lobes with autism and atypical autism. *Lancet*, 349:392–5.

Bolton P, Macdonald H, Pickles A et al. (1994) A case control family history study of autism. *J Child Psychol Psychiatry*, 35:877–900.

Boyle CA, Decoufle P (1994) Prevalence and health impact of developmental disabilities in UW children. *Pediatr*, 93:399–403.

British Medical Research Council (2000) *Review of Autism Research: Epidemiology and Causes*. British Medical Research Council, London.

Burgemeister BB, Blum LH, Lorge I (1972) *Columbia Mental Maturity Scale*. San Antonio, TX, Psychological Corporation Harcourt Brace Janovich, Inc.

Campbell JM (2003) Efficacy of behavioral interventions for reducing problem behavior in persons with autism: a quantitative synthesis of single-subject research. *Res Dev Disabilities*, 24:120–38.

Campbell M, Anderson LT, Meier M et al. (1978) A comparison of haloperidol and behavior therapy and their interaction in autistic children. *J Am Acad Child Adolesc Psychiatry*, 17:640–55.

Campbell M, Anderson LT, Small AM, Adams P, Gonzalez NM, Ernst M (1993) Naltrexone in autistic children: behavioral symptoms and attentional learning. *J Am Acad Child Adolesc Psychiatry*, 32:1283–91.

Campbell M, Armenteros JL, Malone RP, Adams PB, Eisenberg ZW, Overall JE (1997) Neuroleptic-related dyskinesias in autistic children: a prospective, longitudinal study. *J Am Acad Child Adolesc Psychiatry*, 36:835–43.

Campbell M, Small AM, Collins PJ, Friedman E, David R, Genieser N (1976) Levodopa and levoamphetamine: a crossover study in young schizophrenic children. *Cur Ther Res*, 19:70–86.

Carey T, Ratliff-Schaub K, Funk J, Weinle C, Myers M, Jenks J (2002) Double-blind placebo-controlled trial of secretin: effects on aberrant behavior in children with autism. *J Autism Dev Disord*, 32(3):161–7.

Chakrabarti S, Fombonne E (2001) Pervasive developmental disorders in preschool children. *J Am Med Assoc*, 285:3093–9.

Charman T (2002) The prevalence of autism spectrums disorders: recent evidence and future challenges. *Europ Child Adolesc Psychiatry*, 11:249–56.

Cody H, Pelphrey K, Piven J (2002) Structural and functional magnetic resonance imaging of autism. *Int J Dev Neurosci*, 20:421–38.

Coplan J, Souders MC, Mulberg AE et al. (2003) Children with autistic spectrum disorders. II: Parents are unable to distinguish secretin from placebo under double-blind conditions. *Arch Dis Childhood*, 88:737–9.

Corbett JA (1985) *Mental retardation: Psychiatric aspects.* In: Rutter M, Hersov L (eds) *Child and Adolescent Psychiatry: Modern Approaches*, 2nd edn. Oxford, Blackwell Scientific Publications.

Curry CJ, Stevenson RE, Aughton D et al. (1997) Evaluation of mental retardation: recommendations of a consensus conference: American College of Medical Genetics. *Am J Med Genet*, 72(4):468–77.

Cuskelly M, Dadds M (1992) Behavioral problems in children with Down's syndrome and their siblings. *J Child Psychol Psychiatry*, 33:749–61.

Dosen A (1990) Depression in mentally retarded children and adults. In: Dosen A, Menolascino FJ (eds) *Depression in Mentally Retarded Children and Adults*. Leiden, Logon.

Dykens EM, Cassidy SB (1996) Prader-Willi syndrome: genetic, behavioral and treatment issues. *Child Adolesc Psychiatric Clin N Am*, 5:913–27.

Dykens EM, Kasari C (1997) Maladaptive behavior in children with PWS, Down's syndrome, and nonspecific mental retardation. *Am J Ment Retard*, 102:228–37.

Ehlers S, Gillberg C, Wing L (1999) A screening questionnaire for Asperger syndrome and other high-functioning autism spectrum disorders in school age children. *J Autism Dev Disord*, 29:129–41.

Evangeliou A, Vlachonikolis I, Mihailidou H et al. (2003) Application of a ketogenic diet in children with autistic behavior: pilot study. *J Child Neurol*, 18:113–18.

Famy C, Streissguth AP, Unis AS (1998) Mental illness in adults with fetal alcohol syndrome or fetal alcohol effects. *Am J Psychiatry*, 155:552–4.

Filipek, PA, Accardo PJ, Ashwal S et al. (2000) Practice parameter: Screening and diagnosis of autism: Report of the Quality Standards Subcommittee of the American Academy of Neurology and the Child Neurology Society. *Neurology*, 55:468–79.

Filipek PA, Accardo PJ, Baranek GT et al. (1999) The screening and diagnosis of autistic spectrum disorders. *J Autism Dev Disord*, 29:437–82.

Folstein SE, Sheidley BR (2001) Genetics of autism: complex aetiology for a heterogeneous disorder. *Nature Rev Gen*, 2:943–55.

Fombonne E (1999) The epidemiology of autism: a review. *Psychol Med*, 29:769–86.

Fombonne E (2002) Prevalence of childhood disintegrative disorder. *Autism*, 6:149–57.

Fombonne E (2003) The prevalence of autism. *J Am Med Assoc*, 289:87–9.

Frankhauser MP, Karumanchi VC, German ML, Yates A, Karumanchi SD (1992) A double-blind, placebo-controlled study of the efficacy of transdermal clonidine in autism. *J Clin Psychiatry*, 53:77–82.

Freeman BJ, Ritvo ER, Needleman R, Yokota A (1985) The stability of cognitive and linguistic parameters in autism: a 5 year old study. *J Am Acad Child Adolesc Psychiatry*, 24:459–64.

Fu Y-H, Kuhl DPA, Pizzuti A et al. (1991) Variation of the CGG repeat at the fragile X site results in genetic instability; resolution of the Sherman paradox. *Cell*, 67:1047–58.

Gath A, Gumley D (1986) Behavior problems in retarded children with special reference to Down's syndrome. *Br J Psychiatry*, 149:156–61.

Ghaziuddin M, Ghaziuddin N, Greden J (2002) Depression in persons with autism: implications for research and clinical care. *J Autism Dev Disord*, 32:299–306.

Gillberg C (1998) Chromosomal disorders and autism. *J Autism Dev Disord*, 28:415–25.

Glascoe FP, Byrne KE, Ashford LG, Johnson Kl, Chang B, Strickland B (1992) Accuracy of the Denver-II in developmental screening. *Pediatr*, 89:1221–5.

Gordon CT, State RC, Nelson JE, Hamburger SE, Rapoport JL (1993) A double blind comparison of clomipramine, desipramine, and placebo in the treatment of autistic disorder. *Arch Gen Psychiatry*, 50:441–7.

Gostason, R (1985) Psychiatric illness among the mentally retarded. A Swedish population study. *Acta Psychiatrica Scand*, 70:1–117.

Greenspan SI, Wieder S (1997) Multisystem developmental disorder. In: Greenspan S, Wieder S, Osofsky JK (eds) *Handbook of Child and Adolescent Psychiatry, Volume One*. New York, John Wiley and Sons, Inc.

Grelotti DJ, Gauthier I, Schultz RT (2002) Social interest and the development of cortical face specialization: what autism teaches us about face processing. *Dev Psychobiol*, 40:213–25.

Gresham FM, MacMillan DL (1998) Early intervention project: can its claims be substantiated and its effects replicated? *J Autism Dev Disord*, 28:5–13.

Gualtieri CT, Quade D, Hicks RE, Mayo JP, Schroeder SR (1984) Tardive dyskinesia and other clinical consequences of neuroleptic treatment in children and adolescents. *Am J Psychiatry*, 141:20–3.

Gualtieri CT, Schroeder SR, Hicks RE, Quade D (1986) Tardive dyskinesia in young mentally retarded individuals. *Arch Gen Psychiatry*, 43:335–40.

Hagberg B, Kyllerman M (1983) Epidemiology of mental retardation: a Swedish survey. *Brain Dev*, 5:441–9.

Halsy NA, Hyman SL and the Conference Writing Panel (2001) Measles-mumps-rubella vaccine and autism spectrum disorders: report from the new challenges in childhood immunizations conference convened in Oak Brook Illinois, June 12–13 2000. *Pediatr*, 107:e84.

Harris SL, Handleman JS (2000) Age and IQ at intake as predictors of placement for young children with autism: a four- to six-year follow-up. *J Autism Dev Disord*, 30:137–42.

Haveman MJ (1996) Epidemiological issues in mental retardation. *Curr Opin Psychiatry*, 9:305–11.

Hellings JA, Kelley LA, Gabrielli WF, Kilgore E, Shah P (1996) Sertraline response in adults with mental retardation and autistic disorder. *J Clin Psychiatry*, 57:333–6.

Howlin P, Asgharian A (1999) The diagnosis of Asperger syndrome: findings from a survey of 770 families. *Dev Med Child Neurol*, 41:834–9.

Hunt A, Shepherd P (1993) A prevalence study of autism in tuberous sclerosis. *J Autism Dev Disord*, 23:323–39.

International Molecular Genetic Study of Autism Consortium (1998) A full genome screen for autism with evidence for linkage to a region on chromosome 7q. *Hum Mol Genetics*, 7:571–8.

Jaselskis CA, Cook EH Jr, Fletcher KE, Leventhal BL (1992) Clonidine treatment of hyperactive and impulsive children with autistic disorder. *J Clin Psychopharm*, 12:322–7.

Jellinger KA (2003) Rett syndrome – an update. *J Neur Trans*, 110:681–701.

Kahler SG, Fahey MC (2003) Metabolic disorders and mental retardation. *Am J Med Genet*, 117C:31–41.

Kanner L (1943) Autistic disturbances of affective contact. *Nervous Child*, 2:217–50.

Kaye JA, del Mar Melero-Montes M, Jick H (2001) Mumps, measles, and rubella vaccine and the incidence of autism recorded by general practitioners: a time trend analysis. *Br Med J*, 322:460–3.

Keele DK (1984) The developmentally disabled child: step by step through the workup. *Contemporary Pediatr*, November: 95.

Kemper TL, Bauman M (1998) Neuropathology of infantile autism. *Neuropath Exper Neurology*, 57:645–52.

Kent L, Evans J, Paul M, Sharp M (1999) Comorbidity of autistic spectrum disorders in children with Down syndrome. *Dev Med Child Neurol*, 41:152–8.

King BH, State MW, Shah B, Davanzo P, Dykens E (1997) Mental retardation: a review of the past 10 years. Part I. *J Am Acad Child Adolesc Psychiatry*, 36:1656–63.

Klin A, Jones W, Schultz R, Volkmar F, Cohen D (2002a) Defining and quantifying the social phenotype in autism. *Am J Psychiatry*, 159:985–8.

Klin A, Jones W, Schultz, Volkmar F, Cohen D (2002b) Visual fixation patterns during viewing of naturalistic social situations as predictors of social competence in individuals with autism. *Arch Gen Psychiatry*, 59:809–16.

Knivsberg AM, Reichelt KL, Hoien T, Nodland M (2002) A randomised, controlled study of dietary intervention in autistic syndromes. *Nutr Neurosci*, 5:251–61.

Komen BK, Feldman HM, Handen BL, Janosky JE (1995) Naltrexone in young autistic children: a double-blind placebo-controlled crossover study. *J Am Acad Child Adolesc Psychiatry*, 34:223–31.

Kossoff EH, Pyzik PL, McGrogan JR, Vining EP, Freeman JM (2002) Efficacy of the ketogenic diet for infantile spasms. *Pediatr*, 109:780–3.

Lainhart J, Folstein S (1994) Autism and affective disorders: a review of the literature. *J Autism Dev Disord*, 24, 587–602.

Larson SA, Lakin KC, Anderson L, Kwak N, Lee JH, Anderson D (2001) Prevalence of mental retardation and developmental disabilities: estimates from the 1994/1995 National Health Interview Survey Disability Supplements. *Am J Ment Retard*, 106:231–52.

Leiter RG (1948) *Leiter International Performance Scale*. Wood Dale, IL, Stoelting Co.

Levy SE, Souders MC, Wray J et al. (2003) Children with autistic spectrum disorders. I: Comparison of placebo and single dose of human synthetic secretin. *Arch Dis Childhood*, 88:731–6.

Liss M, Harel B, Fein D et al. (2001) Predictors and correlates of adaptive functioning in children with developmental disorders. *J Autism Dev Disord*, 31:219–30.

Lord C (1995) Follow-up of two-year-olds referred for possible autism. *J Child Psychol Psychiatry Allied Disc*, 36:1365–82.

Lowe TL, Cohen DJ, Miller S, Young JG (1981) Folic acid and B12 in autism and neuropsychiatric disturbances of childhood. *J Am Acad Child Psychiatry*, 20:104–11.

Lowry M, Sovner R (1991) The functional existence of problem behavior: a key to effective treatment. *The Habilitative Mental Health Care Newsletter*, 10:59–63.

Madsen KM, Hviid A, Vestergaard M, Schendel D, Wohlfahrt J, Thorsen P, Olsen J, Melbye M (2002) A population-based study of measles, mumps, and rubella vaccination and autism. *New Engl J Med*, 347:1477–82.

Matson JL, Benavidez DA, Compton LS, Paclawskyj T, Baglio C (1996) Behavioral treatment of autistic persons: a review of research form 1980 to the present. *Res Dev Disabil*, 17:433–65.

McCracken JT, McGough J, Shah B et al. (2002) Research Units on Pediatric Psychopharmacology Autism Network: Risperidone in children with autism and serious behavioral problems. *New Engl J Med*, 347:314–21.

McDougle CJ (1996) A double-blind, placebo-controlled study of fluvoxamine in adults with autistic disorder. *Arch Gen Psychiatry*, 53:1001–8.

McDougle CJ, Brodkin ES, Naylor ST, Carlson DC, Cohen DJ, Price LH (1998) Sertraline in adults with pervasive developmental disorders: a prospective open-label investigation. *J Clin Psychopharm*, 18:62–6.

Menolascino FJ (1983) Overview. In: Menolascino FJ, McCann BM (eds) *Mental Health and Mental Retardation: Bridging the Gap*. Baltimore, University Park Press.

Meyerson MD, Frank RA (1987) Language, speech and hearing in Williams syndrome: interventions approaches and research needs. *Dev Med Child Neurol*, 29:258–70.

Mesibov GB, Schopler E, Schaffer B (1989) Use of the Childhood Autism Rating Scale with autistic adolescents and adults. *J Am Acad Child Adolesc Psychiatry*, 28:538–41.

Moldavsky M, Lev D, Lerman-Sagie T (2001) Behavioral phenotypes of genetic syndromes: a reference guide for psychiatrists. *J Am Acad Child Adolesc Psychiatry*, 40(7):749–61.

Molloy CA, Manning-Courtney P, Swayne S et al. (1989) Lack of benefit of intravenous synthetic human secretin in the treatment of autism. *J Autism Dev Disord*, 32:545–51.

Mostert MP (2001) Facilitated communication since 1995: a review of published studies. *J Autism Dev Disord*, 31:287–313.

Naruse H, Nagahata M, Nakane Y, Shirahashi K, Takesada M, Yamazaki K (1982) A multi-center double-blind trial of pimozide (Orap), haloperidol and placebo in children with behavioral disorders, using crossover design. *Acta Paedopsychiatrica*, 48:173–84.

Nordin V, Gillberg C (1996) Autism spectrum disorders in children with physical or mental disability or both. I: Clinical and epidemiological aspects. *Dev Med Child Neurology*, 38:297–313.

Nordin V, Gillberg C (1998) The long-term course of autistic disorders: update on follow-up studies. *Acta Psychiatrica Scand*, 97:99–108.

Nurmi EL, Dowd M, Tadevosyan-Leyfer O, Haines JL, Folstein SE, Sutcliffe JS (2003) Exploratory subsetting of autism families based on savant skills improves evidence of genetic linkage to 15q11-q13. *J Am Acad Child Adolesc Psychiatry*, 42:856–63.

Osterling J, Dawson G (1994) Early recognition of children with autism: a study of first birthday home videotapes. *J Autism Dev Disord*, 24:247–57.

Osterling J, Dawson G (2000) Brief report: recognition of autism spectrum disorder before one year of age: a retrospective study based on home-videotapes. *J Autism Dev Disord*, 30:157–62.

Osterling JA, Dawson G, Munson JA (2002) Early recognition of 1-year-old infants with autism spectrum disorder versus mental retardation. *Dev Psychopath,* 14(2):239–51.

Page T (2000) Metabolic approaches to the treatment of autism spectrum disorders. *J Autism Dev Disord*, 30:463–9.

Pelios L, Morren J, Tesch D, Axelrod S (1999) The impact of functional analysis methodology on treatment choice for self-injurious and aggressive behavior. *J Appl Behav Anal*, 32:185–95.

Piven J, Harper J, Palmer P, Stephan A (1996) Course of behavioral change in autism: a retrospective study of high IQ adolescents and adults. *J Am Acad Child Adolesc Psychiatry*, 35:523–9.

Piven J, Palmer P, Jacohbi D, Childress D, Arndt S (1997) Broader autism phenotype: evidence from a family history study of multiple-incidence autism families. *Am J Psychiatry*, 154:185–90.

Plomin R, Defries JC (1980) Genetics and intelligence: recent data. *Intelligence*, 4:15–24.

Poustka F, Lisch S (1993) Autistic behaviour domains and their relation to self-injurious behaviour. *Acta Paedopsychiatrica*, 56:69–73.

Prior M (2003) Is there an increase in the prevalence of autism spectrum disorders? *J Paediatr Child Health*, 39:81–2.

Pueschel SM, Bernier JC, Pezzulo JC (1991) Behavioral observation in children with Down's syndrome. *J Ment Deficien Res*, 35:502–11.

Quintana H, Birmaher B, Stedge D, Lennon S, Freed J, Bridge J, Greenhill L (1995) Use of methylphenidate in the treatment of children with autistic disorder. *J Autism Dev Disord*, 25:283–94.

Rapin I (1997) Current concepts: autism. *New Engl J Med*, 337:97–104.

Rapin I (1999) Appropriate investigations for clinical care versus research in children with autism. *Brain Dev*, 21:152–6.

Rimland B (1978) Savant capabilities of autistic children and their cognitive implications. In: Serban G (ed.) *Cognitive Defects in the Development of Mental Illness*. New York, Brunner/Mazel.

Rogers SJ (1998) Empirically supported comprehensive treatments for young children with autism. *J Clin Child Psychol*, 27:167–78.

Rousseau F, Heitz D, Biancalana V et al. (1991) Direct diagnosis by DNA analysis of the fragile X syndrome of mental retardation. *New Engl J Med*, 325:1673–81.

Rumsey JM, Rapoport JL, Sceery WR (1985) Autistic children as adults: psychiatric, social and behavioural outcome. *J Am Acad Child Adolesc Psychiatry*, 24:465–73.

Rumsey JM, Ernst M (2000) Functional neuroimaging of autistic disorders. *Ment Retard Devl Disabil Res Rev*, 6:171–9.

Rutter M, Greenfeld D, Lockyer L (1967) A five to fifteen year follow-up study of infantile psychosis: II. Social and behavioural outcome. *Br J Psychiatry*, 113:1183–99.

Santosh PJ, Baird G (1999) Psychopharmacotherapy in children and adults with intellectual disability. *Lancet*, 354:233–42.

Schultz RT, Gauthier I, Klin A et al. (2000) Abnormal ventral temporal cortical activity among individuals with autism and Asperger syndrome during face discrimination. *Arch Gen Psychiatry*, 57:331–40.

Sigman M (1994) What are the core deficits in autism? In: Broman SH, Grafman J (eds) *Atypical Cognitive Deficits in Developmental Disorders: Implications for Brain Function*. Hilldale, NJ, Lawrence Erlbaum Associates, Inc.

Sigman M, Ruskin E (1999) Continuity and change in the social competence of children with autism, Down syndrome and developmental delays. *Monographs Soc Res Child Dev*, 64:1–130.

Silka VR, Hauser MJ (1997) Psychiatric assessment of the person with mental retardation. *Psychiatric Ann*, 27:162–9.

Simonoff E (1998) Genetic counseling in autism and pervasive developmental disorders. *J Autism Dev Disord*, 28:447–56.

Snow K, Doud LK, Hagerman R, Pergolizzi RG, Erster SH, Thibodeau SN (1998) Analysis of a CGG sequence at the FMR-1 locus in fragile X families and in the general population. *Am J Hum Genet*, 53:1217–28.

Sokol RJ, Miller S, Reed G (1980) Alcohol abuse during pregnancy: an epidemiological study. *Alcohol Clin Exp Res*, 4:135–45.

Sovner R (1986) Limiting factors in the use of DSM-III criteria with mentally ill/mentally retarded persons. *Psychopharm Bull*, 22:1055–7.

Sovner R, Lowry MA (1990) A behavioral methodology in diagnosing affective disorders in individuals with mental retardation. *Rehab Ment Healthcare Newsletter*, 9:55–61.

Sparrow SS, Balla DA, Cicchetti DV (1984) *Vineland Adaptive Behavior Scale, Expanded Form Manual*. Circle Press, MN, American Guidance Services.

Stark JA, Goldsbury T (1990) Quality of life from childhood to adulthood. In: Schalock RL (ed.) *Quality of Life: Perspectives and Issues*. Washington DC, American Association on Mental Retardation.

State MW, King BH, Dykens E (1997) Mental retardation: a review of the past 10 years. Part II. *J Am Acad Child Adolesc Psychiatry*, 36:1664–71.

Streissguth AP, Aase JM, Clarren SK, Randels SP, LaDue RA, Smith DF (1991) Fetal alcohol syndrome in adolescents and adults. *J Am Med Assoc*, 265:1961–7.

Summers JA, Allison DB, Lynch PS, Sandler L (1995) Behaviour problems in Angelman syndrome. *J Intellect Disabil Res*, 39:97–106.

Szatmari P, Jones MB, Zwaigenbaum L, MacLean JE (1998) Genetics of autism: overview and new directions. *J Autism Dev Disord*, 28:351–68.

Szymanski LS, Kiernan WE (1983) Multiple family group therapy with developmentally disabled adolescents and young adults. *Int J Group Psychother*, 33:521–34.

Tanguay P (2000) Pervasive developmental disorders: a 10 year review. *J Am Acad Child Adolesc Psychiatry*, 39:1079–95.

Taylor B, Miller E, Farrington CP et al. (1999) Autism and measles, mumps, and rubella vaccine: no epidemiological evidence for a causal association. *Lancet*, 353(9169):2026–9.

Taylor B, Miller E, Lingam R, Andrews N, Simmons A, Stowe J (2002) Measles, mumps, and rubella vaccination and bowel problems or developmental regression in children with autism: population study. *Br Med J*, 324:393–6.

Thorndike, RL, Hagen EP, Sattler JM (1986) *Guide for Administering and Scoring the Stanford-Binet Intelligence Scale*, 4th edn. Chicago, Riverside Publishing.

Tsai LY (1999) Psychopharmacology in autism. *Psychosomatic Med*, 61:651–65.

Udwin O, Yule W (1991) A cognitive and behavioral phenotype in Williams syndrome. *J Clin Exper Neuropsychol*, 2:232–44.

Unis AS, Munson JA, Rogers SJ et al. (2002) A randomized, double-blind, placebo-controlled trial of porcine versus synthetic secretin for reducing symptoms of autism. *J Am Acad Child Adolesc Psychiatry,* 41:1315–21.

Voigt RG, Dickerson CL, Reynolds AM, Childers DO, Rodriguez DL, Brown FR (2000) Laboratory evaluation of children with autistic spectrum disorders: a guide for primary care pediatricians. *Clin Pediatr*, 39:669–71.

Volkmar R, Cook E, Pomeroy J, Realmuto G, Tanguay P (1999) Summary of the practice parameters for the assessment and treatment of children, adolescents, and adults with autism and other pervasive developmental disorders. *J Am Acad Child Adolesc Psychiatry*, 38:1611–15.

Wang PP, Doherty S, Rourke SB, Bellugi U (1995) Unique profile of visuo perceptual skills in a genetic syndrome. *Brain Cog*, 29:54–65.

Waterhouse L, Fein D, Modahl C (1996) Neurofunctional mechanisms in autism. *Psychol Rev*, 103:457–89.

Wechsler D (1981) *Wechsler Adult Intelligence Scale – Revised*. San Antonio, The Psychological Corporation.

Wechsler D (1991) *Wechsler Intelligence Scale for Children*, 3rd edn. San Antonio, The Psychological Corporation.

Wechsler D (1989) *Wechsler Preschool Primary Scale of Intelligence – Revised*. San Antonio, The Psychological Corporation.

Wenger DA, Coppola S, Liu SL (2002) Lysosomal storage disorders: diagnostic dilemmas and prospects for therapy. *Genet Med*, 4(6):412–19.

Werner E, Dawson G, Osgterling J, Dinno N (2000) Brief report: recognition of autism spectrum disorder before one year of age: a retrospective study based on home videotapes. *J Autism Dev Disord*, 30:157–62.

Wilson K, Mills E, Ross C, McGowan J, Jadad A (2003) Association of autistic spectrum disorder and the measles, mumps, and rubella vaccine: a systematic review of current epidemiological evidence. *Arch Pediatr Adolesc Med,* 157:628–34.

Wing L (1997) The autistic spectrum. *Lancet*, 350:1761–6.

Wing L, Potter D (2002) The epidemiology of autistic spectrum disorders: is the prevalence rising? *Ment Retard Dev Disord Res Rev*, 8:151–61.

Wing L, Attwood A (1987) Syndromes of autism and atypical development. In: Cohen DJ, Donnellan AM (eds) *Handbook of Autism and Pervasive Developmental Disorders*. New York, Wiley.

Chapter 6

American Psychiatric Association (1994) *Diagnostic and Statistical Manual of Mental Disorders (DSM-IV)*, 4th edn. Washington DC, American Psychiatric Press.

Barkley RA (1997) *ADHD and the Nature of Self-Control*. NY, Guilford Press.

Barkley RA (1998) *Attention-Deficit Hyperactivity Disorder: A Handbook for Diagnosis and Treatment*, 2nd edn. NH, Guilford Press.

Broca PP (1863) Localisation des functions cérébrales: siège du langage aricule. *Bulletin de la Société d'Anthropologie de Paris*, 4:200–3.

Cruickshank WM, Bentzen FA, Ratzburg, FH, Tannenhauser, MT (1961) *A Teaching Method for Brain-Injured and Hyperactive Children*. Syracuse NY, Syracuse University Press.

DeFries JC, Gillis JJ (1991) Etiology of reading deficits in learning disabilities: quantitative genetic analyses. In: Obrzut JE, Hynd GW (eds) *Neuropsychological Foundations of Learning Disabilities: A Handbook of Tssues, Methods, and Practice*. San Diego: Academic Press, pp. 29–48.

Fletcher JM, Shaywitz SE, Shaywitz BA (1999) Comorbidity of learning and attention disorders: separate but equal. *Pediatric Clin N Am*, 46:885–97.

Flowers L, Meyer M, Lovato J, Wood F, Felton R (2001) Does third grade discrepancy status predict the course of reading development? *Ann Dyslexia*, 51:49–71.

Flynn JM, Rahbar MH (1994) Prevalence of reading failure in boys compared with girls. *Psychol Schools*, 31:66–70.

Graham S, Harris KR, MacArthur C, Schwartz S (1998) Writing instruction In: Wong B (ed.) *Learning about Learning Disabilities*, 2nd edn. San Diego, Academic Press, pp. 391–424.

Graham S, Schwartz S, MacArthur C (1993) Learning disabled and normally achieving students' knowledge of the writing and the composing process, attitude toward writing, and self-efficacy. *J Learning Disabil*, 26:237–49.

Hoskyn M, Swanson HL (2000) Cognitive processing of low achievers and children with reading disabilities: a selective meta-analytic review of the published iterature. *School Psychol Rev*, 29:102–19.

National Joint Committee on Learning Disabilities (NJCLD) (1988) [Letter from NJCLD to member organizations]. Austin, TX.

Orton S (1937) *Reading, Writing and Speech Problems in Children: A Presentation of Certain Types of Disorders in the Development of the Language Faculty*. NY, Norton.

Osman BB (2000) Learning disabilities and the risk of psychiatric disorders in children and adolescents. In: Greenhill LL (ed.) *Learning Disabilities: Implications for Psychiatric Treatment*. Washington DC, American Psychiatric Press, pp. 1–31.

Reyes M (1991) A process approach to literacy using dialogue journals and literature with second language learners. *Res Teach English*, 25, 291–313.

Rourke BP (1995) *Syndrome of Nonverbal Learning Disabilities: Neurodevelopmental Meanifestations*. NY, Guilford Press.

Share DL, McGee R, Silva PD (1989) I.Q. and reading progress: a test of the capacity notion of I.Q. *J Am Acad Child Adolesc Psychiatry*, 28:97–100.

Shaywitz SE, Escobar MD, Shaywitz BA, Fletcher JM, Makuch R (1992) Evidence that dyslexia may represent the lower tail of a normal distribution of reading ability. *New Engl J Med*, 326:145–50.

Shaywitz SE, Fletcher JM, Holahan JM et al. (1999) Persistence of dyslexia: the Connecticut Longitudinal Study at adolescence. *Pediatr*, 104:1351–9.

Sternberg RJ, Grigorenko EL (2002) Difference scores in the identification of children with learning disabilities: it's time to use a different method. *J School Psychol*, 40:65–84.

Stuebing KK, Fletcher JM, LeDoux JM, Lyon GR, Shaywitz SE, Shaywitz BA (2002) Validity of IQ-discrepancy classifications of reading disabilities: a meta-analysis. *Am Educ Research J*, 39:465–518.

Torgesen JK (1991) Learning disabilities: historical and conceptual issues. In: Wong BYL (ed.) *Learning about Learning Disabilities*. NY, Academic Press, pp. 3–39.

Torgesen JK (1998) Learning disabilities: an historical and conceptual overview. In: Wong B (ed.) *Learning about Learning Disabilities*, 2nd edn. San Diego, Academic Press, pp. 3–34.

US Office of Education (1968) *First Annual Report of the National Advisory Committee on Handicapped Children.* Washington DC, US Department of Health, Education and Welfare.

Vellutino FR, Scanlon DM, Lyon GR (2000) Differentiating between difficult-to-remediate and readily remediated poor readers: more evidence against the IQ-achievement discrepancy definition for reading disability. *J Learning Disabil*, 33, 223–38.

Wernicke, C (1894) *Grundriss der Psychiatrie: psycholphysiologische Eindeitung.* Wiesbaden, Germany.

Wristers KJ, Francis DJ, Foorman BR, Fletcher JM, Swank PR (2002) Growth in precursor reading skills: do low-achieving and IQ-discrepant readers develop differently? *Learning Dis Res Prac*, 17:19–34.

Chapter 7

Adams W (1981) Lack of behavioral effects from Feingold diet violations. *Percept Mot Skills*, 52(1):307–13.

Adler LA, Resnick S, Kunz M, Devinsky O (1995) Open-label trial of venlafaxine in adults with attention deficit disorder. *Psychopharmacol Bull*, 31(4):785–8.

American Psychiatric Association (1980) *Diagnostic and Statistical Manual*, 3rd edn, DSM-III. Washington DC, American Psychiatric Press.

American Psychiatric Association (1986) *Diagnostic and Statistical Manual*, 3rd edn – Revised, DSM-III-R, Washington DC, American Psychiatric Press.

American Psychiatric Association (1994) *Diagnostic and Statistical Manual*, 4th edn, DSM-IV. Washington DC, American Psychiatric Press.

American Psychiatric Association (2000) *Diagnostic and Statistical Manual*, 4th edn – Trace Revision, DSM-IV-TR. Washington DC, American Psychiatric Press.

Anastopoulos AD, Shelton TL, DuPaul GJ, Guevremont DC (1993) Parent training for attention-deficit hyperactivity disorder: its impact on parent functioning. *J Abnorm Child Psychol*, 21(5):581–96.

Antshel KM, Remer R (2003) Social skills training in children with attention deficit hyperactivity disorder: a randomized-controlled clinical trial. *J Clin Child Adolesc Psychol*, 32(1):153–65.

Arnold LE (2000) Methylphenidate vs. amphetamines: comparative review. *J Atten Dis*, 3(4):200–11.

Arnold LE, Pinkham SM, Votolato N (2000) Does zinc moderate essential fatty acid and amphetamine treatment of attention-deficit/hyperactivity disorder? *J Child Adolesc Psychopharmacol*, 10(2):111–7.

Arnold LE, Votolato NA, Kleykamp D, Baker GB, Bornstein RA (1990) Does hair zinc predict amphetamine improvement of ADD/hyperactivity? *Int J Neurosci*, 50(1–2):103–7.

Arnsten AFT, Goldman-Rakic PS (1985) Alpha-2 adrenergic mechanism in prefrontal cortex associated with cognitive decline in aged non-human primates. *Science*, 230:1273–6.

Arnsten AFT, Steere JC, Hunt RD (1996) The contribution of alpha-2 NA mechanism to prefrontal cortical functions: potential significance for attention deficit hyperactivity disorder. *Arch Gen Psychiatry*, 53:448–55.

Barkley RA (2002) Psychosocial treatments for attention-deficit/hyperactivity disorder in children. *J Clin Psychiatry*, 63(Suppl 12):36–43. Review.

Bellinger DC (2004) Lead. *Pediatr*, 113(Suppl 4):1016–22.

Biederman J (1992) New developments in pediatric psychopharmacology. *J Am Acad Child Adolesc Psychiatry*, 31(1):14–15.

Biederman J, Baldessarini RJ, Wright V, Knee D, Harmatz JS (1989) A double-blind placebo controlled study of desipramine in the treatment of ADD. I: Efficacy. *J Am Acad Child Adolesc Psychiatry*, 28(5):777–84.

Biederman J, Faraone SV, Monuteaux MC, Plunkett EA, Gifford J, Spencer T (2003) Growth deficits and attention-deficit/hyperactivity disorder revisited: impact of gender, development, and treatment. *Pediatr*, 111(5 Pt 1):1010–16.

Biederman J, Spencer T, Wilens T (2004) Evidence-based pharmacotherapy for attention-deficit hyperactivity disorder. *Int J Neuropsychopharmacol*, 7(1):77–97. Epub 2004 Jan 21.

Bor W, Sanders MR, Markie-Dadds C (2002) The effects of the Triple P-Positive Parenting Program on preschool children with co-occurring disruptive behavior and attentional/hyperactive difficulties. *J Abnorm Child Psychol*, 30(6):571–87.

Borcherding BG, Keysor CS, Rapoport JL, Elia J, Amass J (1990) Motor/vocal tics and compulsive behaviors on stimulant drugs: is there a common vulnerability? *Psychiatry Res*, 33(1):83–94.

Boris M, Mandel FS (1994) Foods and additives are common causes of the attention deficit hyperactive disorder in children. *Ann Allergy*, 72(5):462–8. Review.

Bradley W (1937) The behavior of children receiving benzedrine. *Am J Psychiatry*, 94:577–85.

Carter CM, Urbanowicz M, Hemsley R et al. (1993) Effects of a few food diet in attention deficit disorder. *Arch Dis Child*, 69(5):564–8.

Casat CD, Pleasants DZ, Schroeder DH, Parler DW (1989) Bupropion in children with attention deficit disorder. *Psychopharmacol Bull*, 25(2):198–201.

Casat CD, Pleasants DZ, Van Wyck Fleet J (1987) A double-blind trial of bupropion in children with attention deficit disorder. *Psychopharmacol Bull*, 23(1):120–2.

Castellanos FX (2002) Proceed, with caution: SPECT cerebral blood flow studies of children and adolescents with attention deficit hyperactivity disorder. *J Nucl Med*, 43(12):1630–3.

Castellanos FX, Acosta MT (2004) The neuroanatomy of attention deficit/hyperactivity disorder. *Rev Neurol*, 38(Suppl 1):131–6.

Castellanos FX, Giedd JN, Elia J et al. (1997) Controlled stimulant treatment of ADHD and comorbid Tourette's syndrome: effects of stimulant and dose. *J Am Acad Child Adolesc Psychiatry*, 36(5):589–96.

Cheon KA, Ryu YH, Kim YK, Namkoong K, Kim CH, Lee JD (2003) Dopamine transporter density in the basal ganglia assessed with [123I]IPT SPET in children with attention deficit hyperactivity disorder. *Eur J Nucl Med Mol Imaging*, 30(2):306–11. Epub 2002 Nov 29.

Cherland E, Fitzpatrick R (1999) Psychotic side effects of psychostimulants: a 5-year review. *Can J Psychiatry*, 44(8):811–13.

Coffey BJ, Biederman J, Geller DA et al. (2000) The course of Tourette's disorder: a literature review. *Harvard Rev Psychiatry*, 8(4):192–8. Review.

Conners CK, Casat CD, Gualtieri CT et al. (1996) Bupropion hydrochloride in attention deficit disorder with hyperactivity. *J Am Acad Child Adolesc Psychiatry*, 35(10):1314–21.

Costello EJ, Mustillo S, Erkanli A, Keeler G, Angold A (2003) Prevalence and development of psychiatric disorders in childhood and adolescence. *Arch Gen Psychiatry*, 60 (8):837–44.

Danckaerts M, Heptinstall E, Chadwick O, Taylor E (2000) A natural history of hyperactivity and conduct problems: self-reported outcome. *Eur Child Adolesc Psychiatry*, 9(1):26–38.

Dunn DW, Austin JK, Harezlak J, Ambrosius WT (2003) ADHD and epilepsy in childhood. *Dev Med Child Neurol*, 45(1):50–4.

Elia J, Gulotta C, Rose SR, Marin G, Rapoport JL (1994) Thyroid function and attention-deficit hyperactivity disorder. *J Am Acad Child Adolesc Psychiatry*, 33(2):169–72.

Faraone SV, Biederman J, Mick E et al. (2000) Family study of girls with attention deficit hyperactivity disorder. *Am J Psychiatry*, 157(7):1077–83.

Fehlings DL, Roberts W, Humphries T, Dawe G (1991) Attention deficit hyperactivity disorder: does cognitive behavioral therapy improve home behavior? *J Dev Behav Pediatr*, 12 (4):223–8.

Fenichel RR (1995) Combining methylphenidate and clonidine: the role of post-marketing surveillance. *J Child Adolesc Psychopharmacol*, 5:155–6.

Findling RL, Schwartz MA, Flannery DJ, Manos MJ (1996) Venlafaxine in adults with attention-deficit/hyperactivity disorder: an open clinical trial. *J Clin Psychiatry*, 57(5):184–9.

Findling RL, Short EJ, Manos MJ (2001) Short-term cardiovascular effects of methylphenidate and adderall. *J Am Acad Child Adolesc Psychiatry*, 40(5):525–9.

Flory K, Lynam DR (2003) The relation between attention deficit hyperactivity disorder and substance abuse: what role does conduct disorder play? *Clin Child Fam Psychol Rev*, 6(1):1–16. Review.

Gadow KD, Sverd J, Sprafkin J, Nolan EE, Grossman S (1999) Long-term methylphenidate therapy in children with comorbid attention-deficit hyperactivity disorder and chronic multiple tic disorder. *Arch Gen Psychiatry*, 56(4):330–6.

Ghaziuddin M, Tsai L, Alessi N (1992) ADHD and PDD. *J Am Acad Child Adolesc Psychiatry*, 31(3):567.

Gittelman R, Eskenazi B (1983) Lead and hyperactivity revisited. An investigation of nondisadvantaged children. *Arch Gen Psychiatry*, 40(8):827–33.

Gomez R, Harvey J, Quick C, Scharer I, Harris G (1999) DSM-IV AD/HD: confirmatory factor models, prevalence, and gender and age differences based on parent and teacher ratings of Australian primary school children. *J Child Psychol Psychiatry*, 40(2):265–74.

Grcevich S (2001) SLI381: a long-acting psychostimulant preparation for the treatment of attention-deficit hyperactivity disorder. *Expert Opin Investig Drugs*, 10(11):2003–11.

Grcevich S, Rowane WA, Marcellino B, Sullivan-Hurst S (2001) Retrospective comparison of Adderall and methylphenidate in the treatment of attention deficit hyperactivity disorder. *J Child Adolesc Psychopharmacol*, 11(1):35–41.

Hauser P, Zametkin AJ, Martinez P et al. (1993) Attention deficit-hyperactivity disorder in people with generalized resistance to thyroid hormone. *New Engl J Med*, 328(14):997–1001.

He Y, Yang X, Xu F (2000) Application of Conners Rating Scales in the study of lead exposure and behavioral effects in children. *Zhonghua Yu Fang Yi Xue Za Zhi*, 34(5):290–3. English abstract.

Hedges D, Reinherr FW, Rogers A, Strong R, Wender PH (1995) An open trial of venlafaxine in adult patients with attention deficit hyperactivity disorder. *Psychopharmacol Bull*, 31(4):779–83.

Hunt RD, Minderaa RB, Cohen DJ (1985) Clonidine benefits children with attention deficit disorder and hyperactivity: report of a double-blind placebo-crossover therapeutic trial. *J Am Acad Child Psychiatry*, 24(5):617–29.

James RS, Sharp WS, Bastain TM et al. (2001) Double-blind, placebo-controlled study of single-dose amphetamine formulations in ADHD. *J Am Acad Child Adolesc Psychiatry*, 40(11):1268–76.

Jensen PS, Hinshaw SP, Kraemer HC et al. (2001) ADHD comorbidity findings from the MTA study: comparing comorbid subgroups. *J Am Acad Child Adolesc Psychiatry*, 40(2):147–58.

Keating GM, McClellen K, Jarvis B (2001) Methylphenidate (OROS formulation). *CNS Drugs*, 15(6):495–500; discussion 501–3.

Kidd PM (2000) Attention deficit/hyperactivity disorder (ADHD) in children: rationale for its integrative management. *Altern Med Rev*, 5(5):402–28. Review.

Kratochvil CJ, Bohac D, Harrington M, Baker N, May D, Burke WJ (2001) An open-label trial of tomoxetine in pediatric attention deficit hyperactivity disorder. *J Child Adolesc Psychopharmacol*, 11(2):167–70.

Krause KH, Dresel SH, Krause J, la Fougere C, Ackenheil M (2003) The dopamine transporter and neuroimaging in attention deficit hyperactivity disorder. *Neurosci Biobehav Rev*, 27(7):605–13. Review.

Krause KH, Dresel SH, Krause J, Kung HF, Tatsch K (2000) Increased striatal dopamine transporter in adult patients with attention deficit hyperactivity disorder: effects of methylphenidate as measured by single photon emission computed tomography. *Neurosci Lett*, 285(2):107–10.

Krummel DA, Seligson FH, Guthrie HA (1996) Hyperactivity: is candy causal? *Crit Rev Food Sci Nutr*, 36(1–2):31–47. Review.

Lahey BB, Loeber R, Burke J, Rathouz PJ, McBurnett K (2002) Waxing and waning in concert: dynamic comorbidity of conduct disorder with other disruptive and emotional problems over 7 years among clinic-referred boys. *J Abnorm Psychol*, 111(4):556–67.

Law SF, Schachar RJ (1999) Do typical clinical doses of methylphenidate cause tics in children treated for attention-deficit hyperactivity disorder? *J Am Acad Child Adolesc Psychiatry*, 38(8):944–51.

MacDonald VM, Achenbach TM (1999) Attention problems versus conduct problems as 6-year predictors of signs of disturbance in a national sample. *J Am Acad Child Adolesc Psychiatry*, 38(10):1254–61.

Manassis K, Monga S (2001) A therapeutic approach to children and adolescents with anxiety disorders and associated comorbid conditions. *J Am Acad Child Adolesc Psychiatry*, 40(1):115–7.

Martinez D, Gelenter J, Abi-Dargham A, vanDyck CH, Kegeles L, Innis RB, Laruelle M (2001) The variable number of tandem repeats polymorphism of the dopamine transporter gene is not associated with significant change in dopamine transporter phenotype in humans. *Neuropsychopharmacol*, 24(5):553–60.

Masi G, Toni C, Perugi G et al. (2003) Externalizing disorders in consecutively referred children and adolescents with bipolar disorder. *Compr Psychiatry*, 44(3):184–9.

McCleary L, Ridley T (1999) Parenting adolescents with ADHD: evaluation of a psychoeducation group. *Patient Educ Couns*, 38(1):3–10.

Mefford IN, Potter WZ (1989) A neuroanatomical and biochemical basis of attention deficit disorder with hyperactivity in children: a defect in tonic adrenalin mediated inhibition of locus ceruleus stimulation. *Med Hypothesis*, 29:33–42.

Michelson D, Faries D, Wernicke J, Kesley D,Kendrick K, Sallee FR, Spencer T (2001) Atomoxetine ADHD Study Group. Atomoxetine in the treatment of children and adolescents with attention-deficit/hyperactivity disorder: a randomized, placebo-controlled, dose-response study. *Pediatr*, 108(5):E83.

Molina BS, Pelham WE Jr (2003) Childhood predictors of adolescent substance use in a longitudinal study of children with ADHD. *J Abnorm Psychol*, 112(3):497–507.

Montiel-Nava C, Pena JA, Barbero I (2003) Epidemiological data about attention deficit hyperactivity disorder in a sample of Marabino children. *Rev Neurol*, 37(9):815–9.

MTA Cooperative Group (2004) National Institute of Mental Health Multimodal Treatment Study of ADHD follow-up: changes in effectiveness and growth after the end of treatment. *Pediatr*, 113(4):762–9.

Nichols SL, Waschbusch DA (2004) A review of the validity of laboratory cognitive tasks used to assess symptoms of ADHD. *Child Psychiatry Hum Dev*, 34(4):297–315.

Olvera RL, Pliszka SR, Luh J, Tatum R (1996) An open trial of venlafaxine in the treatment of attention-deficit/hyperactivity disorder in children and adolescents. *J Child Adolesc Psychopharmacol*, 6(4):241–50.

Overmeyer S, Taylor E (2000) Neuroimaging in hyperkinetic children and adults: an overview. *Pediatr Rehabil*, 4(2):57–70. Review.

Pelham WE, Gnady EM, Burrows-Maclean L et al. (2001) Once-a-day Concerta methylphenidate versus three-times-daily methylphenidate in laboratory and natural settings. *Pediatr*, 107(6):E105.

Pineda D, Ardila A, Rosselli M et al. (1999) Prevalence of attention-deficit/hyperactivity disorder symptoms in 4- to 17-year-old children in the general population. *J Abnorm Child Psychol*, 27(6):455–62.

Pliszka SR (2000) Patterns of psychiatric comorbidity with attention-deficit/hyperactivity disorder. *Child Adolesc Psychiatr Clin N Am*, 9(3):525–40, vii. Review.

Pliszka SR, McCracken JT, Maas JW (1996) Catecholamines in attention-deficit hyperactivity disorder: current perspectives. *J Am Acad Child Adolesc Psychiatry*, 35:264–72.

Popper CW (1997) Antidepressants in the treatment of attention-deficit/hyperactivity disorder. *J Clin Psychiatry*, 58(Suppl 14):14–29; discussion 30–1. Review.

Poulton A, Cowell CT (2003) Slowing of growth in height and weight on stimulants: a characteristic pattern. *J Paediatr Child Health*, 39(3):180–5.

Riccio CA, Reynolds CR, Lowe P, Moore JJ (2002) The continuous performance test: a window on the neural substrates for attention? *Arch Clin Neuropsychol*, 17(3):235–7.

Riddle MA, Nelson JC, Kleinman CS et al. (1991) Sudden death in children receiving Norpramin: a review of three reported cases and commentary. *J Am Acad Child Adolesc Psychiatry*, 30(1):104–8.

Rietveld MJ, Hudziak JJ, Bartels M, van Beijsterveldt CE, Boomsma DI (2003) Heritability of attention problems in children. I: Cross-sectional results from a study of twins, age 3–12 years. *Am J Med Genet*, 117B(1):102–13.

Rowland AS, Lesesne CA, Abramowitz AJ (2002) The epidemiology of attention-deficit/hyperactivity disorder (ADHD) a public health view. *Ment Retard Dev Disabil Res Rev*, 8(3):162–70. Review.

Rubinstein S, Silva LB, Licamele WL (1994) Clonidine for stimulant-related sleep problems. *J Am Acad Child Adolesc Psychiatry*, 33(2):281–2.

Russel VA (2003) Dopamine hypofunction possibly results from a defect in glutamate-stimulated release of dopamine in the nucleus accumbens shell of a rat model for attention deficit hyperactivity disorder – the spontaneously hypertensive rat. *Neurosci Biobehav Rev*, 27(7):671–82. Review.

Rutter M (1982) Syndromes attributed to 'minimal brain dysfunction' in childhood. *Am J Psychiatry*, 139:21–33.

Safer DJ, Malever M (2000) Stimulant treatment in Maryland public schools. *Pediatr*, 106(3):533–9.

Sandyk R (1990) Zinc deficiency in attention-deficit hyperactivity disorder. *Int J Neurosci*, 52(3–4):239–41.

Scahill L, Chappell PB, Kim YS et al. (2001) A placebo-controlled study of guanfacine in the treatment of children with tic disorders and attention deficit hyperactivity disorder. *Am J Psychiatry*, 158(7):1067–74.

Schechter MD, Timmons GD (1985) Objectively measured hyperactivity – I. Comparison with normal controls. *J Clin Pharmacol*, 25(4):269–75.

Simeon Jg, Ferguson HB, Van Wyck Fleet J (1986) Bupropion effects in attention deficit and conduct disorders. *Can J Psychiatry*, 31(6):581–5.

Smith BH, Pelham WE, Evans S et al. (1998) Dosage effects of methylphenidate on the social behavior of adolescents diagnosed with attention-deficit hyperactivity disorder. *Exp Clin Psychopharmacol*, 6(2):187–204.

Spalletta G, Pasini A, Pau F, Guido G, Menghini L, Caltagirone C (2001) Prefrontal blood flow dysregulation in drug naive ADHD children without structural abnormalities. *J Neural Transm*, 108(10):1203–16.

Spencer T, Biederman J, Coffey B, Geller D, Faraone S, Wilens T (2001) Tourette disorder and ADHD. *Adv Neurol*, 85:57–77. Review.

Spencer T, Biederma J, Wilens T, Guite J, Harding M (1995) ADHD and thyroid abnormalities: a research note. *J Child Psychol Psychiatry*, 36(5):879–85.

Stein MA, Blondis TA, Schnitzler ER et al. (1996) Methylphenidate dosing: twice daily versus three times daily. *Pediatr*, 98(4 Pt 1):748–56.

Stein MA, Weiss RE (2003) Thyroid function tests and neurocognitive functioning in children referred for attention deficit/hyperactivity disorder. *Psychoneuroendocrinol*, 28(3):304–16.

Steingard R, Biederman J, Spencer T, Wilens T, Gonzales A (1993) Comparison of clonidine response in the treatment of attention-deficit hyperactivity disorder with and without comorbid tic disorders. *J Am Acad Child Adolesc Psychiatry*, 32(2):350–3.

Swanson JM, Flodram P, Kennedy J et al. (2000) Dopamine genes and ADHD. *Neurosci Biobehav Rev*, 24(1):21–5.

Swanson J, Lerner M, March J, Gresham FM (1999) Assessment and intervention for attention-deficit/hyperactivity disorder in the schools. Lessons from the MTA study. *Pediatr Clin North Am*, 46(5):993–1009.

Swanson JM, Wigal S, Greenhill LL et al. (1998) Analog classroom assessment of Adderall in children with ADHD. *J Am Acad Child Adolesc Psychiatry*, 37(5):519–26.

Thapar A, Holmes J, Poulton K, Harrington R (1999) Genetic basis of attention deficit and hyperactivity. *Br J Psychiatry*, 174:105–11. Review.

Thierry AM, Mantz J, Glowinski J (1992) Influence of dopaminergic and noradrenergic afferents on their target cells in the rat medial prefrontal cortex. *Adv Neurol*, 57:545–54.

Thomson GO, Raab GM, Hepburn WS, Hunter R, Fulton M, Laxen DP (1989) Blood-lead levels and children's behaviour – results from the Edinburgh Lead Study. *J Child Psychol Psychiatry*, 30(4):515–28.

Vaidya CJ, Austin G, Kirkorian G et al. (1998) Selective effects of methylphenidate in attention deficit hyperactivity disorder: a functional magnetic resonance study. *Proc Natl Acad Sci USA*, 95(24):14494–9.

Valentine J, Rossi E, O'Leary P, Parry TS, Kurinczuk JJ, Sly P (1997) Thyroid function in a population of children with attention deficit hyperactivity disorder. *J Paediatr Child Health*, 33(2):117–20.

Vitiello B (2001) Long-term effects of stimulant medications on the brain: possible relevance to the treatment of attention deficit hyperactivity disorder. *J Child Adolesc Psychopharmacol*, 11(1):25–34. Review.

Wechsler D (1974) *Wechsler Intellectual Scale for Children – Revised*. San Antonio, Texas, The Psychological Corporation.

Wechsler D (2004) *Wechsler Intellectual Scale for Children*, 4th edn. San Antonio, Texas, The Psychological Corporation.

Weiss RE, Stein MA, Trommer B, Refetoff S (1993) Attention-deficit hyperactivity disorder and thyroid function. *J Pediatr*, 123(4):539–45.

Wells KC, Pelham WE, Kotkin RA et al. (2000) Psychosocial treatment strategies in the MTA study: rationale, methods, and critical issues in design and implementation. *J Abnorm Child Psychol*, 28(6):483–505.

Wender EH (1986) The food additive-free diet in the treatment of behavior disorders: a review. *J Dev Behav Pediatr*, 7(1):35–42.

Whalen CK, Henker B, Granger DA (1990) Social judgment processes in hyperactive boys: effects of methylphenidate and comparisons with normal peers. *J Abnorm Child Psychol*, 18(3):297–316.

Whitmore EA, Mikulich SK, Thompson LL, Riggs PD, Aarons GA, Crowley TJ (1997) Influences on adolescent substance dependence: conduct disorder, depression, attention deficit hyperactivity disorder, and gender. *Drug Alcohol Depend*, 47(2):87–97.

Wilens TE, Biederman J, Spencer TJ (2002) Attention deficit/hyperactivity disorder across the lifespan. *Ann Rev Med*, 53:113–31. Review.

Winsberg BG, Kupietz SS, Sverg J, Hungund BL, Young NL (1982) Methylphenidate oral dose plasma concentrations and behavioral response in children. *Psychopharmacol (Berlin)*, 76(4):329–32.

Wolraich ML, Greenhill LL, Pelham W et al. (2001) Randomized, controlled trial of oros methylphenidate once a day in children with attention-deficit/hyperactivity disorder. *Pediatr*, 108(4):883–92.

Yusin AS (2004) 2001 American Academy of Pediatrics practice parameter on attention-deficit/hyperactivity disorder. *Pediatr*, 113(2):428–9; discussion 428–9.

Chapter 8

American Psychiatric Association (2000) *Diagnostic and Statistical Manual of Mental Disorders*, 4th edn, revised (DSM-IV-TR). Washington DC, American Psychiatric Press.

Blair RJR, Coccaro E, Connor D et al. (2005) Juvenile maladaptive aggression: a review of the neuroscientific data. *J Am Acad Child Adolesc Psychiatry*, under review.

Brownfield D, Thompson K (2002) Distinguishing the effects of peer delinquency and gang membership on self-reported delinquency. *J Gang Res*, 50:1–10.

Cureton SR (1999) Gang membership: gang formations and gang joining. *J Gang Res*, 48:13–21.

Edens JF, Skeem JL, Cruise KR, Cauffman E (2001) Assessment of 'juvenile psychopathy' and its association with violence: a critical review. *Behav Sci Law*, 19:53–80.

Esbensen F-A, Deschenes EP (1998) A multisite examination of youth gang membership: does gender matter. *Criminol*, 47:799–827.

Garbarino J, Eckenrode J, Barry FD and New York State College of Human Ecology. Family Life Development Center (1997) *Understanding Abusive Families: An Ecological Approach to Theory and Practice*. San Francisco, Jossey-Bass.

Garbarino J, Garbarino AC (1993) *Maltreatment of Adolescents*. Chicago, National Committee to Prevent Child Abuse.

Karnik NS (2004) The social environment. In: Steiner H (ed.) *Handbook of Mental Health Interventions in Children and Adolescents: An Integrated Developmental Perspective*. San Francisco, Jossey-Bass.

Karnik NS, Steiner H (2002) *Adolescence, Incarceration and Experience: Toward a New Theory of Juvenile Psychopathy*. Annual Meeting of the American Academy of Child and Adolescent Psychiatry, San Francisco, CA.

Lock J, Steiner H (1999) Gay, lesbian, and bisexual youth risks for emotional, physical, and social problems: results from a community-based survey. *J Am Acad Child Adolesc Psychiatry*, 38:297–304.

Maxson CL, Whitlock ML, Klein MW (1998) Vulnerability to street gang membership: implications for practice. *The Social Service Review*, 21:70–91.

Raine A (1997) *Biosocial Basis of Violence*. New York, Plenum Press.

Raine A (2002) Biosocial studies of antisocial and violent behavior in children and adults: a review. *J Abnorm Child Psychol*, 30:311–26.

Raine A, Venables PH, Mednick SA (1997) Low resting heart rate at age 3 years predisposes to aggression at age 11 years: evidence from the Mauritius Child Health Project. *J Am Acad Child Adolesc Psychiatry*, 36:1457–64.

Raine A, Yaralian PS, Reynolds C, Venables PH, Mednick SA (2002) Spatial but not verbal cognitive deficits at age 3 years in persistently antisocial individuals. *Dev Psychopathol*, 14:25–44.

Seligman ME, Csikszentmihalyi M (2000) Positive psychology. An introduction. *Am Psychol*, 55:5–14.

Sirpal SK (2002) Familial criminality, familial drug use, and gang membership: youth criminality, drug use, and gang membership-what are the connections? *J Gang Res*, 50:11–22.

Steiner H (1997) Practice parameters for the assessment and treatment of children and adolescents with conduct disorder. *J Am Acad Child Adolesc Psychiatry*, 36(Suppl):122S-39S.

Steiner H (ed.) (2004) *Handbook of Mental Health Interventions in Children and Adolescents: An Integrated Developmental Approach*. San Francisco, CA, Jossey-Bass.

Steiner H, Cauffman E (1998) Juvenile justice, delinquency, and psychiatry. *Child Adolesc Psychiatr Clin N Am*, 7:653–72.

Steiner H, Cauffman E, Duxbury E (1999) Personality traits in juvenile delinquents: relation to criminal behavior and recidivism. *J Am Acad Child Adolesc Psychiatry*, 38:256–62.

Steiner H, Dunne JE (1997) Summary of the practice parameters for the assessment and treatment of children and adolescents with conduct disorder. *J Am Acad Child Adolesc Psychiatry*, 36:1482–5.

Steiner H, Karnik N (2004) Child and adolescent antisocial behavior. In: Sadock BJ, Sadock VA (eds) *Kaplan and Sadock's Comprehensive Textbook of Psychiatry*. Philadelphia, Lippincott Williams & Wilkins.

Steiner H, Saxena K, Chang K (2003) Psychopharmacologic strategies for the treatment of aggression in juveniles. *CNS Spect*, 8:298–308.

Steiner H, Stone LA (1999) Violence and related psychopathology. *J Am Acad Child Adolesc Psychiatry*, 38:232–4.

Tinklenberg JA, Steiner H, Huckaby WJ, Tinklenberg JR (1996) Criminal recidivism predicted from narratives of violent juvenile delinquents. *Child Psychiatry Hum Dev*, 27:69–79.

Winfree LT Jr, Bernat FP, Esbensen F-A (2001) Hispanic and Anglo gang membership in two southwestern cities. *Social Science J*, 49:105–17.

Chapter 9

Achenbach TM, Edelbrock CS (1979) The Child Behavior Profile. II. Boys aged 12–16 and girls aged 6–11 and 12–16. *J Consult Clin Psych*, 47:223–33.

Albano AM, Chorpita BF, Barlow DH (1996) Childhood anxiety disorders. In: Mash EJ, Barkley RA et al. (eds) *Child Psychopathology*. New York, Guilford Press, pp. 196–241.

American Psychiatric Association (1994) *Diagnostic and Statistical Manual of Mental Disorders*, 4th edn (DSM-IV). Washington DC, American Psychiatric Press.

American Psychiatric Association (1986) *Diagnostic and Statistical Manual of Mental Disorders*, 3rd edn, revised (DSM-III-R). Washington DC, American Psychiatric Press.

Anderson JC, Williams S, McGee R et al. (1987) DSM-III disorders in preadolescent children: prevalence in a large sample from the general population. *Arch Gen Psychiatry*, 44:69–76.

Battaglia M, Bertella S, Politi E et al. (1995) Age at onset of panic disorder: influence of familial liability to the disease and of childhood separation anxiety disorder. *Am J Psychiatry*, 152:1362–4.

Baxter L (1999) Functional imaging of brain systems mediating obsessive-compulsive disorder. In: Charney DL, Nessler E, Bunney BS (eds) *Neurobiology of Mental Illness*. New York, Oxford University Press, pp. 534–47.

Beidel D, Morris TL (1995) Social phobia. In: March JS (ed.) *Anxiety Disorders in Children and Adolescents*. New York, Guilford Press, pp. 181–211.

Beidel DC, Turner SM (1988) Comorbidity of test anxiety and other anxiety disorders in childhood. *J Abnorm Child Psychol*, 16:275–87.

Beidel DC, Turner SM, Morris TL (2000) Behavioral treatment of childhood social phobia. *J Consult Clin Psychol*, 68:1072–80.

Bell-Dolan DJ, Last CG, Strauss CC (1990) Symptoms of anxiety disorders in normal children. *J Am Acad Child Adolesc Psychiatry*, 29:259–765.

Benjamin RS, Costello EJ, Warren M (1990) Anxiety disorders in a pediatric sample. *J Anxiety Disord*, 4:293–316.

Bergman RL, Piacentini J, McKracken JT (2002) Prevalence and description of selective mutism in a school-based sample. *J Am Acad Child Adolesc Psychiatry*, 41:938–46.

Berman SL, Weems CF, Silverman WK et al. (2000) Predictors of outcome in exposure-based cognitive and behavioral treatments for phobic and anxiety disorders in children. *Behav Ther*, 31:713–31.

Bernstein GA, Borchardt CM, Perwien AR et al. (2000) Imipramine plus cognitive-behavioral therapy in the treatment of school refusal. *J Am Acad Child Adolesc Psychiatry*, 39:276–83.

Biederman J, Faraone SV, Marrs A et al. (1997) Panic disorder and agoraphobia in consecutively referred children and adolescents. *J Am Acad Child Adolesc Psychiatry*, 36:214–23.

Biederman J, Hirschfeld-Becker DR, Rosenbaum JF et al. (2001) Further evidence of association between behavioral inhibition and social anxiety in children. *Am J Psychiatry*, 158:1673–9.

Biederman J, Rosenbaum JF, Bolduc-Murphy EA (1993) A 3 year follow-up of children with and without behavioral inhibition. *J Am Acad Child Adolesc Psychiatry*, 32:814–21.

Birmaher B, Axelson DA, Monk K et al. (2003) Fluoxetine for the treatment of childhood anxiety disorders. *J Am Acad Child Adolesc Psychiatry*, 42:415–23.

Birmaher B, Khetarpal S, Brent D et al. (1997) The Screen for Child Anxiety Related Emotional Disorders (SCARED) scale construction and psychometric characteristics. *J Am Acad Child Adolesc Psychiatry*, 36:545–53.

Birmaher B, Waterman GS, Ryan N et al. (1994) Fluoxetine for childhood anxiety disorders. *J Am Acad Child Adolesc Psychiatry*, 33:993–9.

Black B (1995) Separation anxiety and panic disorder. In: March JS (ed.) *Anxiety Disorders in Children and Adolescents*. New York, Guilford Press, pp. 212–34.

Black B, Uhde TW (1995) Psychiatric characteristics of children with selective mutism: a pilot study. *J Am Acad Child Adolesc Psychiatry*, 34:847–56.

Bowen RC, Offord DR, Boyle MH (1990) The prevalence of overanxious disorder and separation anxiety disorder: results from the Ontario Child Health Study. *J Am Acad Child Adolesc Psychiatry*, 29:753–8.

Burd L, Kerbeshian L, Wikenheiser M et al. (1986) Prevalence of Gilles de la Tourette syndrome in North Dakota adults. *Am J Psychiatry*, 143:787–8.

Caspi A, Henry B, McGee RO et al. (1995) Temperamental origins of child and adolescent behavior problems: from age three to age fifteen. *Child Dev*, 66:55–68.

Clarke G, Hops H, Lewinsohn PM (1992) Cognitive-behavioral group treatment of adolescent depression: prediction of outcome. *Behav Ther*, 23:341–54.

Costello EJ (1989) Developments in child psychiatric epidemiology. *J Am Acad Child Adolesc Psychiatry*, 28:836–41.

Costello EJ, Angold A, Burns BJ et al. (1996) The great smoky mountain study of youth: goals, designs, methods, and the prevalence of DSM-IIIR disorders. *Arch Gen Psychiatry*, 53:1129–36.

Dadds M, Barrett PM (2001) Practitioner review: psychological management of anxiety disorders in children in childhood. *J Child Psychol Psychiatry*, 42:999–1011.

Dantendorfer K, Prayer D, Kramer J et al. (1996) High frequency of EEG and MRI abnormalities in panic disorder. *Psychiatry Res*, 68:41–53.

Dion Y, Annable L, Sandor P et al. (2002) Risperidone in the treatment of Tourette syndrome: a double-blind, placebo controlled trial. *J Clin Psychopharmacol*, 22:31–9.

Dow SP, Sonies BC, Scheib D et al. (1995) Practical guidelines for the assessment and treatment of selective mutism. *J Am Acad Child Adolesc Psychiatry*, 34:836–46.

Dulcan M, Martini R, Lake M (2003b) Obsessive-compulsive disorder. In: *Concise Guide to Child and Adolescent Psychiatry*. Washington, DC, American Psychiatric Press.

Dummit ES III, Klein RG, Tancer NK et al. (1996) Fluoxetine treatment of children with selective mutism: an open trial. *J Am Acad Child Adolesc Psychiatry*, 35:615–21.

Dummit SE, Klein RG, Tancer NK et al. (1997) Systematic assessment of 50 children with selective mutism. *J Am Acad Child Adolesc Psychiatry*, 36:653–60.

Francis G, Beidel D (1995) Cognitive-behavioral psychotherapy. In: March JS (ed.) *Anxiety Disorders in Children and Adolescents*. New York, Guilford Press, pp. 321–40.

Freud A (1966) Obsessional neurosis: a summary of psychoanalytic views. *Int J Psychoanal*, 47:116–22.

Frick PJ, Siverthorn P, Evans C (1994) Assessment of childhood anxiety using structured interviews: patterns of agreement among informants and association with maternal anxiety. *Psychol Assess*, 6:372–9.

Gaffney GR, Perry PJ, Lund BC et al. (2002) Risperidone versus clonidine in the treatment of children and adolescents with Tourette syndrome. *J Am Acad Child Adolesc Psychiatry*, 41:330–6.

Geller DA, Biederman J, Stewart E et al. (2003) Which SSRI? A meta-analysis of pharmacotherapy trials in pediatric obsessive-compulsive disorder. *Am J Psychiatry*, 160:1919–28.

Gilbert D, Dure L, Sethuraman G et al. (2003) Tic reduction with pergolide in a randomized controlled trial in children. *Neurol*, 60:606–11.

Gittelman R, Klein DF (1984) Relationship between separation anxiety and panic disorder and agoraphobic disorders. *Psychopathol*, 17:56–65.

Goodman WK, Price LH, Rasmussen SA et al. (1989a) The Yale-Brown Obsessive Compulsive Scale. I: Development, use, and reliability. *Arch Gen Psychiatry*, 46:1006–11.

Goodman WK, Price LH, Rasmussen SA et al. (1989b) The Yale-Brown Obsessive Compulsive Scale. II: Validity. *Arch Gen Psychiatry*, 46:1012–16.

Graae F, Milner J (1994) Clonazepam in childhood anxiety disorders. *J Am Acad Child Adolesc Psychiatry*, 33:372- 6.

Greist JH, Bandelow B, Hollander E et al. (2003) WCA recommendations for the long-term treatment of obsessive-compulsive disorder in adults. *CNS Spect*, 8:7–16.

Hayward C, Killen JD, Hammer LD et al. (1992) Pubertal stage and panic attack history in sixth- and seventh-grade girls. *Am J Psychiatry*, 149:1239–43.

Hayward C, Killen JD, Taylor CB (1989) Panic attacks in young adolescents. *Am J Psychiatry*, 146:1061–2.

Jacobs BW (2003) Individual and group therapy. In: Rutter M, Taylor E (eds) *Child and Adolescent Psychiatry*, 4th edn. Massachusetts, Blackwell Science Ltd, pp. 983–97.

Kagan J, Snidman N (1999) Early childhood predictors of adult anxiety disorders. *Biol Psychiatr*, 46:1536–41.

Kashani JH, Orvaschel H (1990) A community study of anxiety in children and adolescents *Am J Psychiatry*, 147:313–18.

Kearney CA, Albano AM, Eisen AR et al. (1997) The phenomenology of panic disorder in youngsters: an empirical study of a clinical sample. *J Anxiety Disord*, 11:49–62.

Kendall PC (1994) Treating anxiety disorders in children: results of a randomized clinical trial. *J Consult Clin Psychol*, 62:100 10.

Kendall PC (1997) Treating anxiety disorders in youth: results of a randomized clinical trial. *J Consult Clin Psychol*, 65:366–80.

Kendall PC, Brady EU, Verduin TL (2001) Comorbidity in childhood anxiety disorders and treatment outcome. *J Am Acad Child Adolesc Psychiatry*, 40:787–93.

Kendall PC, Flannery-Schroeder E (1997) Therapy for youths with anxiety disorders: a second randomized clinical trial. *J Consult Clin Psychol*, 65(3):366–80.

Kendler KS, Neale MC, Kessler RC et al. (1992) The genetic epidemiology of phobias in women: the interrelationship of agoraphobia, social phobia, situational phobia, and simple phobia. *Arch Gen Psychiatry*, 49:273–81.

Klein DF, Mannuzza S, Chapman T et al. (1992) Child panic revisited. *J Am Acad Child Adolesc Psychiatry*, 31:112–16.

Klein RG (1991) Parent-child agreement in clinical assessment in anxiety and other psychopathology: a review. *J Anxiety Disord*, 5:187–98.

Kohn R, Keller MB (2003) Emotional expression of anxiety. In: Tasman A, Kay J, Lieberman J (eds) *Psychiatry*, 2nd edn. Chichester, John Wiley and Sons Ltd, pp. 610–12.

Kristensen H (2000) Selective mutism and comorbidity with developmental disorder/delay, anxiety disorder, and elimination disorder. *J Am Acad Child Adolesc Psychiatry*, 39:249–56.

Krysanski VL (2003) A brief review of selective mutism literature. *J Psychology*, 137:29–41.

Kuikka JT, Pitkanen A, Lepola U et al. (1995) Abnormal regional benzodiazepine receptor uptake in the prefrontal cortex in patients with panic disorder. *Nucl Med Commun*, 16:273–80.

Kutcher SP, Mackensie S (1988) Successful clonazepam treatment of adolescents with panic disorder. *J Clin Psychopharmacol*, 8:299–301.

Labellarte MJ, Ginsburg GS, Walkup JT et al. (1999) The treatment of anxiety disorders in children and adolescents. *Soc Biol Psychiatry*, 46:1567–78.

Last CG (1989) Anxiety disorders of children and adolescence. In: Last CG, Hersen M (eds) *Handbook of Child Psychiatric Diagnosis*. New York, Wiley, pp. 156–69.

Last CG, Perrin S, Hersen M et al. (1992) DSM-III-R anxiety disorders in children: sociodemographic and clinical characteristics. *J Am Acad Child Adolesc Psychiatry*, 31:1070–6.

Last CG, Perrin S, Hersen M et al. (1996) A prospective study of childhood anxiety disorders. *J Am Acad Child Adolesc Psychiatry*, 35:1502–10.

Leckman JF, Harding MT, Riddle MA et al. (1991) Clonidine treatment of Gilles de la Tourette syndrome. *Arch Gen Psychiatry*, 48:324–328.

Leckman J, Peterson B, Cohen D (2002) Tic disorders. In: Lewis M (ed.) *Child and Adolescent Psychiatry: A Comprehensive Textbook*. Philadelphia, Lippincott Williams & Wilkins, pp. 734–44.

Leckman JF, Riddle MA, Hardin MT et al. (1989) The Yale Global Tic Severity Scale: initial testing of a clinician-rated scale of tic severity. *J Am Acad Child Adolesc Psychiatry*, 28:566–73.

Leckman JF, Walker DE, Cohen DJ (1993) Premonitory urges in Tourette syndrome. *Am J Psychiatry*, 150:98–103.

Leckman JF, Weissman MM, Merikangas KR et al. (1985) Major depression and panic disorder. *Psychopharmacol Bull*, 2:543–5.

Leonard HL, Rapoport JL (1991) Separation anxiety, overanxious and avoidant disorder. In: Weiner JM, Dulcan MK (eds) *Textbook of Child and Adolescent Psychiatry*, 3rd edn. Washington DC, American Psychiatric Press, pp. 311–22.

Malizia AL, Cunningham VJ, Bell CJ et al. (1998) Decreased brain GABA (A)-benzodiazapine receptor binding in panic disorder. *Arch Gen Psychiatry*, 55:715–20.

Manassis K, Bardley S, Goldberg S et al. (1994) Attachment in mothers with anxiety disorders and their children. *J Am Acad Child Adolesc Psychiatry*, 33:1106–13.

Manassis K, Bradley S, Goldberg S et al. (1995) Behavioral inhibition, attachment and anxiety in children and mothers with anxiety disorders. *Can J Psychiatry*, 40:87–92.

March JS (1995) Cognitive-behavioral psychotherapy for children and adolescents with OCD: a review and recommendations for treatment. *J Am Acad Child Adolesc Psychiatry*, 34:7–18.

March JS, Parker JD, Sullivan K et al. (1997) The Multidimensional Anxiety Scale for Children (MASC) factor structure, reliability, and validity. *J Am Acad Child Adolesc Psychiatry*, 36:554–65.

Marras C, Andrews D, Sime E, Lang AE (2001) Botulinum toxin for simple motor tics: a randomized, double-blind, controlled clinical trial. *Neurol*, 56:605–10.

Masi G, Toni C, Mucci M et al. (2001) Paroxetine in child and adolescent outpatients with panic disorder. *J Child Adolesc Psychopharmacol*, 11:151–7.

Moreau D, Follet C (1993) Panic disorder in children and adolescents. *Child Adolesc Psychiatr Clin North Am*, 2:581–602.

Morris RJ, Kratochwill TR (1998) Childhood fears and phobias. In: Kratochwill TR, Morris RJ (eds) *The Practice of Child Therapy*, 3rd edn. Needham Heights, MA, Allyn and Bacon, pp. 91–131.

Morrison J, Anders T (1999) Anxiety disorders. In: *Interviewing Children and Adolescents: Skills and Strategies for Effective DSM-IV Diagnosis*. New York, Guilford Press.

Ollendick TH (1983) Reliability and validity of the Revised Fear Survey Schedule for Children (FSSC-R). *Behav Res Ther*, 21:685–92.

Ollendick TH, King NJ (1998) Empirically supported treatments for children with phobic and anxiety disorders: current status. *J Clin Child Psychol*, 27:156–7.

Pimental SA, Chu BC, Robin J et al. (2000) The physiological symptom constellation of youth with generalized anxiety: a preliminary examination. Presented at the 34th Annual Association of Behavior Therapy Convention, New Orleans, LA.

Riddle M (1998) Obsessive-compulsive disorder in children and adolescents. *Br J Psychiatry (Suppl)*:91–6.

Ritvo RZ, Ritvo S (2002) Psychodynamic psychotherapy. In: Lewis M (ed.) *Child and Adolescent Psychiatry: A Comprehensive Textbook*, 3rd edn. Philadelphia, Lippincott Williams & Wilkins, pp. 974–83.

Roy-Byrne P, Wingerson DK, Radant A et al. (1996) Reduced benzodiazepine sensitivity in patients with panic disorder: comparison with patients with obsessive-complusive disorder. *Am J Psychiatry*, 153:1444–9.

Rynn MA, Siqueland L, Rickets K (2001) Placebo controlled trial of sertraline in the treatment of children with general anxiety disorder. *J Am Acad Child Adolesc Psychiatry*, 158:2008–14.

Salee FR, Kurlan R, Goetz CG et al. (2000) Ziprasidone treatment of children and adolescents with Tourette syndrome: a pilot study. *J Am Acad Child Adolesc Psychiatry*, 39:292–9.

Schlagger BL, Mink JW (2003) Movement disorders in children. *Pediatr Rev*, 24:39–51.

Schneier FR, Johnson J, Hornig CD et al. (1992) Social phobia: comorbidity and morbidity in an epidemiological sample. *Arch Gen Psychiatry*, 49:282–9.

Silver AA, Shytle RD, Sheehan KH et al. (2001) Multicenter, double-blind, placebo-controlled study of mecamylamine monotherapy for Tourette disorder. *J Am Acad Child Adolesc Psychiatry*, 40:1103–10.

Silverman WK, Kurtines W, Ginsburg GS et al. (1999a) Treating anxiety disorders in children with group cognitive-behavioral therapy: a randomized clinical trial. *J Consult Clin Psychol*, 67:675–87.

Silverman WK, Kurtines W, Ginsburg GS et al. (1999b) Contingency management, self-control, and education support in the treatment of childhood phobic disorders: a randomized clinical trial. *J Consult Clin Psychol*, 67:675–87.

Simeon JG, Ferguson HB, Knott V et al. (1992) Clinical, cognitive and neurophysiological effects of alprazolam in children and adolescents with overanxious and avoidant disorders. *J Am Acad Child Adolesc Psychiatry*, 31:29–33.

Singer HS, Wendland J, Guiliano J (2001) Baclofen treatment in Tourette syndrome: a double-blind, placebo-controlled crossover trial. *Neurol*, 56:599–604.

Steinhausen HC, Juzi C (1996) Elective mutism: an analysis of 100 cases. *J Am Acad Child Adolesc Psychiatry*, 35, 606–14.

Strauss CC, Last CG (1993) Social and simple phobias in children. *J Anxiety Disord*, 7:141–52.

Sukhodolsky D, Scahill L, Heping Z et al. (2003) Disruptive behavior in children with Tourette syndrome: association with ADHD comorbidity, tic severity, and functional impairment. *J Am Acad Child Adolesc Psychiatry*, 42:98–105.

Swedo SE, Leonard HL, Garvey et al. (1998) Pediatric autoimmune neuropsychiatric disorders associated with streptococcal infections: clinical description of the first 50 cases. *Am J Psychiatry*, 155:264–71.

Swedo SE, Rapaport JL, Leonard H et al. (1989) Obsessive-compulsive disorder in children and adolescents. *Arch Gen Psychiatry*, 46:335–41.

Swerdlow N (2001) Obsessive-compulsive disorder and tic syndromes. *Med Clin N Am*, 85:735–55.

Tourette Syndrome Study Group (2002) Treatment of ADHD in children with tics: a randomized controlled trial. *Neurol*, 58:527–36.

Towbin KE, Riddle MA (2002) Obsessive-compulsive disorder. In: Lewis M (ed.) *Child and Adolescent Psychiatry: A Comprehensive Textbook*, 3rd edn. Philadelphia, Lippincott Williams & Wilkins, pp. 834–47.

Vitiello B, Behar D, Wolfson S et al. (1990) Diagnosis of panic disorder in prepubertal children. *J Am Acad Child Adolesc Psychiatry*, 29:782–4.

Von Korff MR, Eaton WW, Keyl PM (1985) The epidemiology of panic attacks and apenic disorder: results of three community surveys. *Am J Epidemiol*, 122:970–81.

Walkup JT, Labellarte MJ, Riddle MA et al. (2001) Fluvoxamine for the treatment of anxiety disorders in children and adolescents. *New Engl J Med*, 344:1279–85.

Walkup JT, Riddle MA (2003) Childhood disorders: tic disorders. In: Tasman A, Kay J, Lieberman JA (eds) *Psychiatry*, 2nd edn. Chichester, John Wiley and Sons Ltd, pp. 821–41.

Warren SL, Huston L, Egeland B et al. (1997) Child and adolescent anxiety disorders and early attachment. *J Am Acad Child Adolesc Psychiatry*, 36:637–44.

Werry JS (1991) Overanxious disorder: a review of its taxonomic properties. *J Am Acad Child Adolesc Psychiatry*, 30:533–44.

Whitaker A, Johnson J, Shaffer D et al. (1990) Uncommon troubles in young people: prevalence estimates of selected psychiatric disorders in a nonreferred adolescent population. *Arch Gen Psychiatry*, 47:487–96.

Wise SP, Rapoport J (1989) Obsessive-compulsive disorders: is it basal ganglia dysfunction? In: Rapoport J (ed.) *Obsessive-Compulsive Disorder in Children and Adolescents*. Washington DC, American Psychiatric Press, pp. 327–44.

Wright HH, Cuccaro ML, Leonhardt TV et al. (1995) Case study: fluoxetine in the multimodal treatment of a preschool child with Selective Mutism. *J Am Acad Child Adolesc Psychiatry*, 34:857–62.

Chapter 10

Akiskal HS, Downs J, Jordan P, Watson S, Daugherty D, Pruitt DB (1985) Affective disorders in referred children and younger siblings of manic-depressives. Mode of onset and prospective course. *Arch Gen Psychiatry*, 42:996–1003.

Alpert JE, Fava M, Uebelacker LA et al. (1999) Patterns of axis I comorbidity in early-onset versus late-onset major depressive disorder. *Biol Psychiatry*, 46:202–11.

Altshuler LL, Bartzokis G, Grieder T, Curran J, Mintz J (1998) Amygdala enlargement in bipolar disorder and hippocampal reduction in schizophrenia: an MRI study demonstrating neuroanatomic specificity [letter]. *Arch Gen Psychiatry*, 55:663–4.

Altshuler LL, Curran JG, Hauser P, Mintz J, Denicoff K, Post R (1995) T2 hyperintensities in bipolar disorder: magnetic resonance imaging comparison and literature meta-analysis. *Am J Psychiatry*, 152:1139–44.

American Academy of Child and Adolescent Psychiatry (2002) Practice parameters for the use of electroconvulsive therapy with adolescents. *J Am Acad Child Adolesc Psychiatry*, in press.

American Diabetes Association and American Psychiatric Association (2004) Consensus development conference on antipsychotic drugs and obesity and diabetes. *Diabetes Care*, 27:596–601.

American Academy of Child and Adolescent Psychiatry (2004) *AACAP supports stronger warnings not black box for antidepressants.* Press Release, September 28, 2004.

American Psychiatric Association (1994) *Diagnostic and Statistical Manual of Mental Disorders*, 4th edn. Washington DC, American Psychiatric Press.

Andrews JA, Lewinsohn PM (1992) Suicidal attempts among older adolescents: prevalence and co-occurrence with psychiatric disorders. *J Am Acad Child Adolesc Psychiatry*, 31, 655–62.

Angold A, Costello EJ, Erkanli A (1999) Comorbidity. *J Child Psychol Psychiatry*, 40, 57–87.

Angold A, Costello EJ, Worthman CM (1998) Puberty and depression: the roles of age, pubertal status and pubertal timing. *Psychol Med*, 28:51–61.

Asarnow JR et al. (1988) Childhood-onset depressive disorders: a follow-up study of rates of rehospitalization and out-of-home placement among child psychiatric inpatients. *J Affect Disord*, 15:245–53.

Beardslee WR, Versage EM, Gladstone TR (1998) Children of affectively ill parents: a review of the past 10 years. *J Am Acad Child Adolesc Psychiatry*, 37, 1134–41.

Beck A, Beamesderfer A (1974) Assessment of depression: the revised Beck Depression Inventory. *Psychol Measurements Psychopharmacol* 7:151–169.

Biederman J et al. (1991) Evidence of familial association between attention deficit disorder and major affective disorders. *Arch Gen Psychiatry* 48:633–42.

Biederman J, Mick E., Prince J et al. (1999) Systematic chart review of the pharmacologic treatment of comorbid attention deficit hyperactivity disorder in youth with bipolar disorder. *J Child Adolesc Psychopharmacol*, 9:247–56.

Bird HR et al. (1988) Estimates of the prevalence of childhood maladjustment in a community survey in Puerto Rico: the use of combined measures. *Arch Gen Psychiatry*, 45:1078–84.

Birmaher B, Ryan ND, Williamson DE et al. (1996) Childhood and adolescent depression: a review of the past 10 years. Part I. *J Am Acad Child Adolesc Psychiatry*, 35:1427–39.

Birmaher B, Williamson DE, Dahl RE et al. (2004) Clinical presentation and course of depression in youth: does onset in childhood differ from onset in adolescence? *J Am Acad Child Adolesc Psychiatry*, 43:63–70.

Botteron KN, Vannier MW, Geller B, Todd RD, Lee BC (1995) Preliminary study of magnetic resonance imaging characteristics in 8- to 16-year-olds with mania. *J Am Acad Child Adolesc Psychiatry*, 34:742–9.

Breiter HC, Etcoff NL, Whalen PJ et al. (1996) Response and habituation of the human amygdala during visual processing of facial expression. *Neuron*, 17:875–87.

Brent DA (1987) Correlates of the medical lethality of suicide attempts in children and adolescents. *J Am Acad Child Adolesc Psychiatry*, 26:87–91.

Brent DA, Holder D, Kolko D et al. (1997) A clinical psychotherapy trial for adolescent depression comparing cognitive, family, and supportive therapy. *Arch Gen Psychiatry*, 54:877–85.

Brumback RA, Dietz-Schmidt SG, Weinberg WA (1977) Depression in children referred to an educational diagnostic center: diagnosis and treatment and analysis of criteria and literature review. *Disord Nerv Syst*, 38:529–35.

Carlson GA, Kashani JH (1988) Phenomenology of major depression from childhood through adulthood: analysis of three studies. *Am J Psychiatry*, 145:1222–5.

Chang K, Ketter T (2000) Mood stabilizer augmentation with olanzapine in acutely manic children. *J Child Adolesc Psychopharmacol*, 10:45–9.

Chen YW, Dilsaver SC (1996) Lifetime rates of suicide attempts among subjects with bipolar and unipolar disorders relative to subjects with other Axis I disorders. *Biol Psychiatry*, 39:896–9.

Cicchetti D, Toth SL (1998) The development of depression in children and adolescents. *Am Psychol*, 53:221–41.

Clark C, Burge MR (2003) Diabetes mellitus associated with atypical anti-psychotic medications. *Diabetes Technol Ther*, 5:669–83.

Curry JF (2001) Specific psychotherapies for childhood and adolescent depression. *Biol Psychiatry*, 49(12):1091–100.

Dahl RE, Puig-Antich J, Ryan N et al. (1990) EEG sleep in adolescents with major depression: the role of suicidality and inpatient status. *J Affect Disord*, 19, 63–75.

Dasari M, Friedman L, Jesberger J et al. (1999) A magnetic resonance imaging study of thalamic area in adolescent patients with either schizophrenia or bipolar disorder as compared to healthy controls. *Psychiatry Res*, 91:155–62.

Davanzo P, Gunderson B, Belin T et al. (2003) Mood stabilizers in hospitalized children with bipolar disorder: a retrospective review. *Psychiatry Clin Neurosci*, 57:504–10.

DeBellis MD, Dahl RE, Perel JM et al. (1996) Nocturnal ACTH, cortisol, growth hormone, and prolactin secretion in prepubertal depression. *J Child Adolesc Psychopharmacol*, 35:1130–7.

DelBello M, Schwiers M, Rosenberg H, Strakowski S (2002) Quetiapine as adjunctive treatment for adolescent mania associated with bipolar disorder. *J Amer Acad Child Adol Psychiatry*, 41:1216–23.

DelBello MP, Geller B (2001) Review of studies of child and adolescent offspring of bipolar parents. *Bipolar Disord*, 3:325–34.

DelBello MP, Strakowski SM, Zimmerman ME, Hawkins JM, Sax KW (1999) MRI analysis of the cerebellum in bipolar disorder: a pilot study. *Neuropsychopharmacol*, 21:63–8.

Drevets WC, Price JL, Simpson JR et al. (1997) Subgenual prefrontal cortex abnormalities in mood disorders. *Nature*, 386:824–7.

Dulcan M, Lizarralde C (2003) *Helping Parents, Youth, and Teachers Understand Medications for Behavioral and Emotional Problems: A Resource Book of Medication Information Handouts*, 2nd edn. Washington DC, American Psychiatric Press.

Eastgate J, Gilmour L (1984) Long-term outcome of depressed children: a follow-up study. *Dev Med Child Neurol*, 26:68–72.

Ekman P, Oster H (1979) Facial expressions of emotion *Ann Rev Psychol*, 30:527–54.

Emslie GJ, Heiligenstein JH, Wagner KD et al. (2002) Fluoxetine for acute treatment of depression in children and adolescents: a placebo-controlled, randomized clinical trial. *J Am Acad Child Adolesc Psychiatry*, 41(10):1205–15.

Emslie GJ, Kennard BD, Kowatch RA (1995) Affective disorders in children: diagnosis and management. *J Clin Neurol*, 10(Suppl): S42–S49.

Emslie GJ, Mayes TL (1999) Depression in children and adolescents: a guide to diagnosis and treatment. *CNS Drugs*, 11:181–9.

Emslie GJ, Rush AJ, Weinberg WA, Kowatch RA, Carmody T, Mayes TL (1998) Fluoxetine in child and adolescent depression: acute and maintenance treatment. *Depression Anxiety*, 7:32–9.

Emslie GJ, Rush AJ, Weinberg WA et al. (1997a) Double-blind, randomized placebo-controlled trial of fluoxetine in depressed children and adolescents. *Arch Gen Psychiatry*, 54:1031–7.

Emslie GJ, Rush AJ, Weinberg WA et al. (1997b) Recurrence of major depressive disorder in hospitalized children and adolescents. *J Am Acad Child Adolesc Psychiatry*, 36:785–92.

Emslie GJ, Walkup JT, Pliszka SR, Ernst M (1999) Non-tricyclic antidepressants: current trends in children and adolescents. *J Am Acad Ch Adolesc Psychiatry*, 38(5):517–28.

Emslie GJ, Weinberg WA, Rush AJ et al. (1990a) Depressive symptoms by self report in adolescence: phase I of the development of a questionnaire for depression by self report. *J Child Neurol*, 3:114–31.

Emslie GJ, Weinberg WA, Rush AJ et al. (1990b) Children with major depression show reduced rapid eye movement latencies. *Arch Gen Psychiatry*, 47:119–24.

Evans RW, Clay TH, Gualtieri CT (1987) Carbamazepine in pediatric psychiatry. *J Am Acad Child Adolesc Psychiatry*, 26:2–8.

Findling RL, Gracious BL, McNamara NK et al. (2001) Rapid, continuous cycling and psychiatric co-morbidity in pediatric bipolar I disorder. *Bipolar Disord*, 3:202–10.

Findling RL, McNamara NK, Gracious BL et al. (2003) Combination lithium and divalproex sodium in pediatric bipolarity. *J Am Acad Child Adolesc Psychiatry*, 42:895–901.

Fleming JE, Boyle MH, Offord DR (1993) The outcome of adolescent depression in the Ontario child health study follow-up. *J Am Acad Child Adolesc Psychiatry*, 32:28–33.

Fleming JE, Offord DR (1990) Epidemiology of childhood depressive disorders: a critical review. *J Am Acad Child Adolesc Psychiatry*, 571–80.

Frazier J, Meyer M, Biederman J, Wozniak J, Wilens T, Spencer T, Kim G, Shapiro S (1999) Risperidone treatment for juvenile bipolar disorder: a retrospective chart review. *J Am Acad Child Adolesc Psychiatry*, 38:960–5.

Friedman L, Findling RL, Kenny JT et al. (1999) An MRI study of adolescent patients with either schizophrenia or bipolar disorder as compared to healthy control subjects. *Biol Psychiatry*, 46:78–88.

Geller B, Bolhofner K, Craney J, Williams M, Del BM, Gundersen K (2000a) Psychosocial functioning in a prepubertal and early adolescent bipolar disorder phenotype. *J Am Acad Child Adolesc Psychiatry*, 39:1543–8.

Geller B, Zimerman B, Williams M et al. (2000b) Diagnostic characteristics of 93 cases of a prepubertal and early adolescent bipolar disorder phenotype by gender, puberty and comorbid attention deficit hyperactivity disorder. *J Child Adolesc Psychopharmacol*, 10:157–64.

Geller B, Cook EH Jr (1999) Serotonin transporter gene (HTTLPR) is not in linkage disequilibrium with prepubertal and early adolescent bipolarity. *Biol Psychiatry*, 45:1230–3.

Geller B, Cooper TB, Sun K et al. (1998) Double-blind and placebo-controlled study of lithium for adolescent bipolar disorders with secondary substance dependency. *J Am Acad Child Adolesc Psychiatry*, 37:171–8.

Geller B, Craney JL, Bolhofner K, Nickelsburg MJ, Williams M, Zimerman B (2002) Two-year prosepctive follow-up of children with a prepubertal and early adolescent bipolar disorder phenotype. *Am J Psychiatry*, 159:927–933.

Geller B, Luby J (1997) Child and adolescent bipolar disorder: a review of the past 10 years. *J Am Acad Child Adolesc Psychiatry*, 36:1168–76.

Geller B, Sun K, Zimerman B, Luby J, Frazier J, Williams M (1995) Complex and rapid-cycling in bipolar children and adolescents: a preliminary study. *J Affect Disord*, 34:259–68.

Geller B, Tillman R, Craney JL, Bolhofner K (2004) Four-year prospective outcome and natural history of mania in children with a prepubertal and early adolescent bipolar disorder phenotype. *Arch Gen Psychiatry*, 61:459–67.

Goodman SH, Schwab-Stone M, Lahey BB, Shaffer D, Jensen PS (2000) Major depression and dysthymia in children and adolescents: discriminant validity and differential consequences in a community sample. *J Am Acad Child Adolesc Psychiatry*, 39(6):761–70.

Goodyer IM, Ashby L, Altham PME, Vize C, Cooper PJ (1993a) Temperament and major depression in 11–16 year-olds. *J Child Psychol Psychiatry*, 34:1409–23.

Goodyer IM, Cooper PJ, Vize C, Ashby L (1993b) Depression in 11–16-year old girls: the role of past paternal psychopathology and exposure to recent life events. *J Child Psychol Psychiatry*, 34:1103–15.

Goodyer IM (1996) Physical symptoms and depressive disorders in childhood and adolescence. *J Psychosomatic Res*, 41:405–8.

Goodwin FK, Jamison KR (1990) *Manic-Depressive Illness*. New York, Oxford University Press.

Graae F, Tenke C, Bruder G et al. (1996) Abnormality of EEG alpha asymmetry in female adolescent suicide attempters. *Biol Psychiatry*, 40:706–713.

Gur RC, Erwin RJ, Gur RE (1992) Neurobehavioral probes for physiologic neuroimaging studies. *Arch Gen Psychiatry*, 49:409–14.

Harrington R (2003) Affective disorders. In: Rutter M, Taylor E (eds) *Child and Adolescent Psychiatry*, 4th edn. Mullen, Massachusetts, Blackwell Science Ltd, pp. 463–85.

Harrington RC (2000) Childhood depression: is it the same disorder? In: Rapoport J (ed.) *Childhood Onset of 'Adult' Psychiatric Disorder: Clinical and Research Advances*. Washington DC, American Psychiatric Press, pp. 223–44.

Harrington R et al. (1990) Adult outcomes of childhood and adolescent depression. I. Psychiatric status. *Arch Gen Psychiatry*, 47:465–473.

Harrington RC, Rutter M, Weissman M et al. (1997) Psychiatric disorders in the relatives of depressed probands. I. Comparison of prepubertal, adolescent and early adult onset forms. *J Affect Disord*, 42:9–22.

Harrington R, Whittaker J, Shoebridge P (1998) Psychological treatment of depression in children and adolescents. A review of treatment research. *Br J Psychiatry*, 173:291–8.

Hawkins JM (1999) Frontosubcortical neuroanatomy and the continuous performance test in mania. *Am J Psychiatry*, 156:139–41.

Hazell P, O'Connel D, Heathcote D, Henry D (2002) Tricyclic drugs for depression in children and adolescents. *Cochrane Database of Systematic Reviews* (2) CD002317, 2002.

Hovey JD, King CA (1996) Acculturative stress, depression, and suicidal ideation among immigrant and second-generation Latino adolescents. *J Am Acad Adolesc Psychiatry*, 35:1183–92.

Hughes CW, Emslie GJ, Crismon ML et al. (1999) The Texas childhood medication algorithm project: report of the Texas consensus conference panel on medication treatment of childhood major depressive disorder. *J Am Acad Child Adolesc Psychiatry*, 38:1442–54.

Hummel B, Stampfer R, Grunze H et al. (2001) Acute antimanic afficacy and safety of oxcarbazepine in an open trial with on-off-on design. *Bipolar Disord*, 3:43.

Isojarvi JI, Laatikainen TJ, Pakarinen AJ, Juntunen KT, Myllyla VV (1993) Polycystic ovaries and hyperandrogenism in women taking valproate for epilepsy. *New Engl J Med*, 329:1383–8.

Jensen PS, Hoagwood K, Petti T, Burns BJ (1999) Outcomes of mental health care for children and adolescents. *J Am Acad Child Adolesc Psychiatry*, 38:64–71.

Kafantaris V, Coletti DJ, Dicker R, Padula G, Kane JM (2001) Adjunctive antipsychotic treatment of adolescents with bipolar psychosis. *J Am Acad Child Adolesc Psychiatry*, 40:1448–56.

Kafantaris V, Coletti DJ, Dicker R, Padula G, Kane JM (2003) Lithium treatment of acute mania in adolescents: a large open trial. *J Am Acad Child Adolesc Psychiatry*, 42:1038–45.

Kandel DB, Davies M (1986) Adult sequela of adolescent depressive symptoms. *Arch Gen Psychiatry*, 43:255–262, 1986.

Kaplan SJ, Pelcovitz D, Salzinger S et al. (1998) Adolescent physical abuse: risk for adolescent psychiatric disorders. *Am J Psychiatry*, 155:954–9.

Kashani JH, Beck NC, Hoeper EW et al. (1987) Psychiatric disorders in a community sample of adolescents. *Am J Psychiatry*, 144:584–9.

Keck PE Jr (2003) The management of acute mania. *Br Med J*, 327:1002–3.

Keller MB, Baker LA (1991) Bipolar disorder: epidemiology, course, diagnosis, and treatment. *Bull Menninger Clin*, 55:172–81.

Keller MB, Lavori PW, Beardslee WR et al. (1991) Depression in children and adolescents: new data on 'undertreatment' and a literature review on the efficacy of available treatments. *J Affect Disord*, 21:163–71.

Keller MB, Ryan ND, Strober M et al. (2001) Efficacy of paroxetine in the treatment of adolescent major depression: a randomized, controlled trial. *J Am Acad Child Adolesc Psychiatry*, 40:762–72.

Kelsoe JR, Kristbjanarson H, Bergesch P et al. (1993) A genetic linkage study of bipolar disorder and 13 markers on chromosome 11 including the D2 dopamine receptor. *Neuropsychopharmacol*, 9:293–301.

Kessler RC, McGonagle KA, Nelson CB et al. (1994) Sex and depression in the national comorbidity survey. II: Cohort effects. *J Affect Disord*, 30:15–26.

Khouzam HR, El-Gabalawi F (2000) Treatment of bipolar I disorder in an adolescent with olanzapine. *J Child Adolesc Psychopharmacol*, 10:147–51.

Kovacs M (1996) Presentation and course of major depressive disorder during childhood and later years of lifespan. *J Am Acad Child Adolesc Psychiatry*, 35:705–15.

Kovacs M (1981) Rating scales to assess depression in school-aged children. *Acta Paedopsychiatrica* 46:305–15.

Kovacs M, Goldston D (1991) Cognitive and social cognitive development of depressed children and adolescents. *J Am Acad Child Psychiatry*, 30:388–92.

Kovacs M et al. (1984a) Depressive disorders in childhood. I. A longitudinal prospective study of characteristics and recovery. *Arch Gen Psychiatry*, 41:229–37.

Kovacs M et al. (1984b) Depressive disorders in childhood. II. A longitudinal study for the risk of subsequent major depression. *Arch Gen Psychiatry*, 41:643–9.

Kovacs M et al. (1988) Depressive disorders in childhood. III. A longitudinal study of comorbidity with and risk for conduct disorders, *J Affect Disord*, 15:205–17.

Kovacs M, Pollock M (1995) Bipolar disorder and comorbid conduct disorder in childhood and adolescence. *J Am Acad Child Adolesc Psychiatry*, 34:715–23.

Kowatch RA, Bucci JP (1998) Mood stabilizers and anticonvulsants. *Pediatr Clin North Am*, 45:1173–86, ix–x.

Kowatch RA, DelBello MP (2003) The use of mood stabilizers and atypical antipsychotics in children and adolescents with bipolar disorders. *CNS Spect*, 8, 273–80.

Kowatch RA, Suppes T, Carmody TJ et al. (2000) Effect size of lithium, divalproex sodium and carbamazepine in children and adolescents with bipolar disorder. *J Am Acad Child Adolesc Psychiatry*, 39:713–20.

Kowatch RA, Suppes T, Gilfillan SK et al. (1995) Clozapine treatment of children and adolescents with bipolar disorder and schizophrenia: a clinical case series. *J Child Adolesc Psychopharmacol*, 5:241–53.

Lebovitz HE (2003) Metabolic consequences of atypical antipsychotic drugs. *Psychiatr Q*, 74:277–90.

Lewinsohn PM, Klein DN, Seeley JR (1995) Bipolar disorders in a community sample of older adolescents: prevalence, phenomenology, comorbidity, and course. *J Am Acad Child Adolesc Psychiatry,* 34:454–63.

Lewinsohn PM, Rohde P, Klien DN et al. (1999) Natural course of adolescent major depressive disorder. I: Continuing into young adulthood. *J Am Acad Child Adolesc Psychiatry,* 38:56–63.

Lewinsohn PM, Ronde P, Seeley JR (1994) Psychosocial risk factors for future adolescent suicide attempts. *J Consult Clin Psychol,* 62:297–305.

Lewinsohn PM, Ronde P, Seeley JR (1998) Major depressive disorder in older adolescents: prevalence, risk factors, and clinical implications. *Clin Psychol Rev,* 18:765–94.

Manji HK, Zarate CA (2002) Molecular and cellular mechanisms underlying mood stabilization in bipolar disorder: implications for the development of improved therapeutics. *Mol Psychiatry,* 7(Suppl 1):S1–S7.

Marttunen MJ, Henriksson MM, Aro HM, Heikkinen ME, Isometsa ET, Lonnqvist JK (1995) Suicide among female adolescents: characteristics and comparisons with males in the age group 13–22 years. *J Am Acad Child Adolesc Psychiatry,* 34:1297–307.

McCauley E et al. (1993) Depression in young people: initial presentation and clinical course. *J Am Acad Child Adolesc Psychiatry,* 32:714–22.

McCauley E, Myers K (1988) Cognitive attributes of depression in children and adolescents. *J Consult Clin Psychol,* 56:903–8.

Mokros HB, Poznanski EO, Merrick WA (1989) Depression and learning disabilities in children: a test of an hypothesis. *Learning Disabil,* 22:230–3.

Morris JS, Frith CD, Perrett DI et al. (1996) A differential neural response in the human amygdala to fearful and happy facial expressions. *Nature,* 383:812–15.

Nassir Ghaemi S, Ko JY, Katzow JJ (2002) Oxcarbazepine treatment of refractory bipolar disorder: a retrospective chart review. *Bipolar Disord,* 4:70–4.

O'Donovan C, Kusumakar V, Graves GR, Bird DC (2002) Menstrual abnormalities and polycystic ovary syndrome in women taking valproate for bipolar mood disorder. *J Clin Psychiatry,* 63:322–30.

Papatheodorou G, Kutcher SP, Katic M, Szalai JP (1995) The efficacy and safety of divalproex sodium in the treatment of acute mania in adolescents and young adults: an open clinical trial. *J Clin Psychopharmacol,* 15:110–16.

Pavuluri MN, Graczyk PA, Henry DB, Carbray JA, Heidenreich J, Miklowitz DJ (2004) Child- and family-focused cognitive-behavioral therapy for pediatric bipolar disorder: development and preliminary results. *J Am Acad Child Adolesc Psychiatry,* 43:528–37.

Pfeffer CR, Klerman GL, Hurt SW et al. (1991) Suicidal children grow up: demographic and clinical risk factors for adolescent suicide attempts. *J Am Acad Child Adolesc Psychiatry,* 30:609–16.

Pfizer I (2000) FDA Psychopharmacological Drugs Advisory Committee, New York.

Pillai JJ, Friedman L, Stuve TA et al. (2002) Increased presence of white matter hyperintensities in adolescent patients with bipolar disorder. *Psychiatry Res,* 114:51–6.

Pine DS, Cohen P, Gurley D et al. (1998) The risk for early-adulthood anxiety and depressive disorders in adolescents with anxiety and depressive disorders. *Arch Gen Psychiatry,* 55:56–64.

Post RM, Ketter TA, Denicoff K et al. (1996) The place of anticonvulsant therapy in bipolar illness. *Psychopharmacol (Berlin),* 128:115–29.

Post RM, Speer AM, Hough CJ, Xing G (2003) Neurobiology of bipolar illness: implications for future study and therapeutics. *Ann Clin Psychiatry,* 15:85–94.

Post RM, Weiss SRB (1998) Sensitization and kindling phenomena in mood, anxiety, and obsessive-compulsive disorders: the role of serotonergic mechanism in illness progression. *Biol Psychiatry,* 44:193–206.

Poznanski EO, Krahenbuhl V, Zrull JP (1976) Childhood depression: a longitudinal perspective. *J Am Acad Child Psychiatry,* 15:491–501.

Puente RM (1975) In: Birkmayer W (ed.) *Epileptic Seizures – Behaviour – Pain.* University Park Press, Baltimore, pp. 243–52.

Puig-Antich J et al. (1985) Psychosocial functioning in prepubertal major depressive disorders. 1. Interpersonal relationships during the depressive episode. *Arch Gen Psychiatry,* 42:500–7.

Puig-Antich J et al. (1987) Imipramine in prepubertal major depressive disorder. *Arch Gen Psychiatry,* 44:81–9.

Puig-Antich J et al. (1989) A controlled family history study of pubertal major depressive disorder. *Arch Gen Psychiatry,* 46:406–18.

Rao U, Ryan ND, Birmaher B et al. (1995) Unipolar depression in adolescents: clinical outcome in adulthood. *J Am Acad Child Adolesc Psychiatry,* 34:566–78.

Rasgon NL, Altshuler LL, Gudeman D et al. (2000) Medication status and polycystic ovary syndrome in women with bipolar disorder: a preliminary report. *J Clin Psychiatry,* 61:173–8.

Reinecke MA, Ryan NE, DuBois DL (1998) Cognitive-behavioral therapy of depression and depressive symptoms during adolescence: a review and meta-analysis. *J Am Acad Child Adolesc Psychiatry,* 37:26–34.

Renshaw PF, Yurgelun-Todd DA, Tohen M, Gruber S, Cohen BM (1995) Temporal lobe proton magnetic resonance spectroscopy of patients with first-episode psychosis. *Am J Psychiatry,* 152:444–6.

Roberts RE, Chen Y (1995) Depressive symptoms and suicidal ideation among Mexican-origin and Anglo adolescents. *J Am Acad Child Adolesc Psychiatry,* 34:81–90.

Ryan ND (2003) Child and adolescent depression: short-term treatment effectiveness and long-term opportunities. *Int J Methods Psychiatric Res,* 12:44–53.

Ryan ND et al. (1992) Neuroendocrine response to L-5-hydroxytryptophan challenge in prepubertal major depression. *Arch Gen Psychiatry,* 49:843–51.

Ryan ND, Puig-Antich J, Ambrosini P et al. (1987) The clinical picture of major depression in children and adolescents. *Arch Gen Psychiatry,* 44:854–61.

Salee FR, Hilal R, Dougherty D, Beach K, Nesbitt L (1998) Platelet serotonin transporter in depressed children and adolescents: H-paroxetine platelet binding before and after sertaline. *J Am Acad Child Adolesc Psychiatry,* 37:777–84.

Sax KW, Strakowski SM, Zimmerman ME, DelBello MP, Keck PE Jr, Hawkins JM (1999) Frontosubcortical neuroanatomy and the continuous performance test in mania. *Am J Psychiatry,* 156(1):139–41.

Scheffer R, Kowatch R, Carmody T, Rush A (2005) A randomized placebo-controlled trial of Adderall for symptoms of comorbid ADHD in pediatric bipolar disorder following mood stabilization with divalproex sodium. *Am J Psychiatry,* in press.

Shaffer D, Fisher P, Dulcan MK et al. (1996) The NIMH diagnostic interview schedule for children version 2.3 (DISC-2.3) description, acceptability, prevalence rates, and performance in the MECA study. Methods for the epidemiology of child and adolescent mental disorders study. *J Am Acad Child Adolesc Psychiatry*, 35:865–77.

Shafii M, MacMillan DR, Key MP et al. (1996) Noctural serum melatonin profile in major depression in children and adolescents. *Arch Gen Psychiatry*, 53:1009–13.

Siegel JM, Aneshensel CS, Taub B et al. (1998) Adolescent depressed mood in multiethnic sample. *J Youth Adolesc*, 27:413–27.

Silberg J, Pickles A, Rutter M et al. (1999) The influence of genetic factors and life stress on depression among adolescent girls. *Arch Gen Psychiatry*, 56:225–32.

Silberg J, Rutter M, Neale M, Eaves L (2001) Genetic moderation of environmental risk for depression and anxiety in adolescent girls. *Br J Psychiatry*, 179:116–21.

Soares JC, Krishnan KR, Keshavan MS (1996) Nuclear magnetic resonance spectroscopy: new insights into the pathophysiology of mood disorders. *Depression*, 4:14–30.

Soares JC, Mann JJ (1997) The anatomy of mood disorders – review of structural neuroimaging studies. *Biol Psychiatry*, 41:86–106.

Soutullo C, Sorter M, Foster K, McElroy S, Keck P (1999) Olanzapine in the treatment of adolescent acute mania: a report of seven cases. *J Affect Disord*, 53:279–83.

Steingard RJ, Renshaw PF, Yurgelun-Todd D et al. (1996) Structural abnormalities in brain magnetic resonance images of depressed children. *J Child Adolesc Psychopharmacol*, 35:307–11.

Strakowski SM, Del Bello MP, Adler CM, Keck PE Jr (2003) Atypical antipsychotics in the treatment of bipolar disorder. *Exp Opin Pharmacother*, 4:751–60.

Strakowski SM, Del Bello MP, Adler C, Cecil CM, Sax KW (2000) Neuroimaging in bipolar disoders. *Bipolar Disord*, 2:148–64.

Strakowski SM, DelBello MP, Sax KW et al. (1999) Brain magnetic resonance imaging of structural abnormalities in bipolar disorder *Arch Gen Psychiatry*, 56:254–60.

Strakowski SM, DelBello MP, Zimmerman ME et al. (2002) Ventricular and periventricular structural volumes in first- versus multiple-episode bipolar disorder. *Am J Psychiatry*, 159:1841–7.

Strakowski SM, Woods BT, Tohen M, Wilson DR, Douglass AW, Stoll AL (1993) MRI subcortical signal hyperintensities in mania at first hospitalization. *Biol Psychiatry*, 33:204–6.

Strober M et al. (1993) The course of major depressive disorder in adolescents. 1. Recovery and risk of manic switching in a follow-up of psychotic and non-psychotic subtypes. *J Am Acad Child Adolesc Psychiatry*, 32:3442.

Strober M (1998) Mixed mania associated with tricyclic antidepressant therapy in prepubertal delusional depression: three cases. *J Child Adolesc Psychopharmacol*, 8:181–5.

Strober M, Morrell W, Lampert C, Burroughs J (1990) Relapse following discontinuation of lithium maintenance therapy in adolescents with bipolar I illness: a naturalistic study. *Am J Psychiatry*, 147:457–61.

Susman E, Dorn LD, Inoff-Germain G, Nottelmann ED, Chrousos GP (1997) Cortisol reactivity, distress behavior, and behavioral and psychological problems in young adolescents: a longitudinal perspective. *J Res Adolesc*, 7:81–105.

Todd RD, Neuman R, Geller B, Fox LW, Hickok J (1993) Genetic studies of affective disorders: should we be starting with childhood onset probands? *J Am Acad Child Adolesc Psychiatry*, 32:1164–71.

Tohen M, Chengappa KNR, Suppes T et al. (2002) Efficacy of olanzapine in combination with valproate or lithium in the treatment of mania in patients partially nonresponsive to valproate or lithium monotherapy. *Arch Gen Psychiatry*, 59:62–9.

Treatment for Adolescents with Depression Study Team (2004) Fluoxetine, cognitive-behavioral therapy, and their combination for adolescents with depression: Treatment for Adolescents With Depression Study (TADS) randomized controlled trial. *J Am Med Assoc*, 292(7):807–20.

Tutus A, Kibar M, Sofuoglu S et al. (1998) A technetium-99m hexamethyl propylene amine oxime brain single-photon emission tomography study in adolescent patients with major depressive disorder. *Eur J Nucl Med*, 25:601–6.

US Department of Health and Human Services (2001) US Department of Health/NIH.

US Food and Drug Administration (2004) FDA lauches a multi-pronged strategy to strengthen safeguards for children treated with antidepressant medications. *FDA News*, October 15, 2004.

US Food and Drug Administration (2004) Public health advisory: suicidality in children and adolescents being treated with antidepressant medications. *FDA News*, October 15, 2004.

Vostanis P, Feehan C, Grattan E, et al. (1996) A randomized controlled out-patient trial of cognitive-behavioral treatment for children and adolescents with depression: 9 month follow-up. *J Affect Disord*, 40(1–2):105–16.

Wagner KD, Weller E, Biederman J et al. (2002) An open-label trial of divalproex in children and adolescents with bipolar disorder. *J Am Acad Child Adolesc Psychiatry*, 41:1224–30.

Wagner KD, Ambrosini PJ, Rynn M et al. (2003) Efficacy of sertraline in the treatment of children and adolescents with major depressive disorder. *J Am Med Assoc*, 290(8):1033–41.

Wagner KD, Robb AS, Findling R et al. (2001) Citalopram treatment of pediatric depression: results of a placebo-controlled trial. Presented at the American College of Neuropsychopharmacology 40th Annual Meeting, Wailoloa, Hawaii.

Wagner KD, Robb AS, Findling RL, Jin J, Gutierrez MM, Heydorn WE (2004) A randomized, placebo-controlled trial of citalopram for the treatment of major depression in children and adolescents. *Am J Psychiatry*, 161:1079–83.

Weersing VR, Weisz JR (2002) Mechanisms of action in youth psychotherapy. *J Child Psychol Psychiatry Allied Disciplines*, 43(1):3–29.

Weinberg WA, Emslie GJ (1988) Adolescents and school problems: depression, suicide, and learning disorders. In: Feldman RA, Stiffman AR (eds) *Advances in Adolescent Mental Health, Vol. 3: Depression and Suicide*. Greenwich, CT, JAI Press.

Weinberg WA, Emslie GJ (1991) Attention deficit hyperactivity disorder: the differential diagnosis. *J Child Neurol*, 6(Suppl):521–34.

Weinberg WA et al. (1973) Depression in children referred to an educational diagnostic center: diagnosis and treatment. *J Pediatr*, 83:1065–72.

Weinberg WA, Harper CR, Emslie GJ (1994) The effect of depression and learning disabilities on school behavior problems. *Direct Clin Psychol*, 1–21.

Weinberg WA, Harper CR, Emslie GJ (1998) *Weinberg Depression Scale for Children and Adolescents*. Austin, Texas, Pro Ed International Publisher, 1998.

Weinberg WA, McLean A (1986) A diagnostic approach to developmental specific learning disabilities. *J Child Neurol*, 158–72.

Weiss B, Garber J (2003) Developmental differences in the phenomenology of depression. *Dev Psychopathol*, 15:403–30.

Weissman MM, Wolk S, Goldstein RB et al. (1999a) Depressed adolescents grown up. *J Am Med Assoc*, 281:1707–13.

Weissman MM, Wolk S, Wickramaratne P et al. (1999b) Children with prepubertal-onset major depressive disorder and anxiety grown up. *Arch Gen Psychiatry*, 56:794–801.

Weller EB, Weller RA, Rowan AB, Svadjian H (2002) Depressive disorders in children and adolescents. In: Lewis M (ed.) *Child and Adolescent Psychiatry: A Comprehensive Textbook*. Philadelphia, Lippincott Williams & Wilkins, pp. 767–81.

West SA, Keck PEJ, McElroy SL et al. (1994) Open trial of valproate in the treatment of adolescent mania. *J Child Adolesc Psychopharmacol*, 4:263–7.

West SA, McElroy SL, Strakowski SM, Keck PE, Jr, McConville BJ (1995) Attention deficit hyperactivity disorder in adolescent mania. *Am J Psychiatry*, 152:271–3.

West SA, Strakowski SM, Sax KW, McElroy SL, Keck PE, Jr, McConville BJ (1996) Phenomenology and comorbidity of adolescents hospitalized for the treatment of acute mania. *Biol Psychiatry*, 39:458–60.

Wilens TE, Biederman J, Millstein RB, Wozniak J, Hahesy AL, Spencer TJ (1999) Risk for substance use disorders in youths with child- and adolescent-onset bipolar disorder. *J Am Acad Child Adolesc Psychiatry*, 38:680–5.

Williamson DE, Birmaher B, Frank E et al. (1998) Nature of life events and difficulties in depressed adolescents. *J Am Acad Adolesc Psychiatry*, 37:1049–57.

Wood A, Harrington R, Moore A (1996) Controlled trial of a brief cognitive-behavioural intervention in adolescent patients with depressive disorders. *J Child Psychol Psychiatry*, 37(6):737–46.

Woods BT, Yurgelun-Todd D, Mikulis D, Pillay SS (1995) Age-related MRI abnormalities in bipolar illness: a clinical study. *Biol Psychiatry*, 38:846–7.

Wozniak J, Biederman J (1997) Childhood mania: insights into diagnostic and treatment issues. *J Assoc Acad Minor Phys*, 8:78–84.

Wozniak J, Biederman J, Kiely K, Ablon JS, Faraone SV, Mundy E, Mennin D (1995) Mania-like symptoms suggestive of childhood-onset bipolar disorder in clinically referred children. *J Am Acad Child Adolesc Psychiatry*, 34:867–76.

Yurgelun-Todd D, Gruber S, Kanayama W, Baird A, Young A (2000) fMRI during affect discrimination in bipolar affective disorder. *Bipolar Disord*, 2:237–48.

Chapter 11

Agras WS, Rossiter E (1992) Pharmacologic and cognitive-behavioral treatment for bulimia nervosa: a controlled comparison. *Am J Psychiatry*, 149:82–7.

American Psychiatric Association (1994) *Diagnostic and Statistical Manual of Mental Disorders (DSM-IV)*, 4th edn. Washington DC, American Psychiatric Press.

Berkowitz RI et al. (2003) Behavior therapy and sibutramine for the treatment of adolescent obesity: a randomized controlled trial. *J Am Med Assoc*, 289:1805–12.

Branson R et al. (2003) Binge eating as a major phenotype of melanocortin 4 receptor gene mutations. *New Engl J Med*, 348:1096–103.

Carter WP et al. (2003) Pharmacologic treatment of binge eating disorder. *Int J Eating Disord*, 34:S74–S88.

Devlin B et al. (2002) Linkage analysis of anorexia nervosa incorporating behavioral covariates. *Hum Mol Genet*, 11:689–96.

Epstein LH et al. (1990) Ten-year follow-up of behavioral family-based treatment for obese children. *J Am Med Assoc*, 264:2519–23.

Erikson EH (1963) *Childhood and Society*, 2nd edn. New York, WW Norton.

Farooqi IS et al. (1999) Effects of recombinant leptin therapy in a child with congenital leptin deficiency. *New Engl J Med*, 34, 879–84.

Farooqi IS et al. (2003) Clinical spectrum of obesity and mutations in the melanocortin 4 receptor gene. *New Engl J Med*, 348:1085–95.

Fluoxetine Bulimia Nervosa Collaborative (FBNC) Study Group (1992) Fluoxetine in the treatment of bulimia nervosa: a multi-center, placeo-controlled, double-blind trial. *Arch Gen Psychiatry*, 49:139–47.

Garcia VF, Langford L, Inge TH (2003) Application of laparoscopy for bariatric surgery in adolescents. *Curr Opin Pediatr*, 15:248–55.

Goldstein DJ et al. (1995) Long-term fluoxetine treatment of bulimia nervosa. *Br J Psychiatry*, 166:660–6.

Gryboski JD et al. (1968) Eleven adolescent girls with severe anorexia: intestinal disease or anorexia nervosa? *Clin Pediatr*, 7:684–90.

Guedalia JSB et al. (1993) A reversible case of Kluver-Bucy syndrome in association with shigellosis. *J Child Neurol*, 8:313–15.

Hardy BW, Waller DA (1989) Bulimia and opioids: eating disorder or substance abuse? In: Johnson WG (ed.) *Advances in Eating Disorders, Vol 2*. Greenwich, CT, JAI Press.

Harel Z, Biro FM (1994) Hyperthyroidism in an adolescent with bulimia nervosa. *J Adolesc Health*, 15:342–4.

Hill JO et al. (2003) Response to comment on 'Obesity and the environment: Where do we go from here?' *Science*, 301:598.

Kaye WH et al. (2001) Double-blind placebo-controlled administration of fluoxetine in restricting- and restricting-purging-type anorexia nervosa. *Biol Psychiatry*, 49:644–52.

Keel PK et al. (2003) Predictors of mortality in eating disorders. *Arch Gen Psychiatry*, 60:179–83.

Korner J, Leibel RL (2003) To eat or not to eat – how the gut talks to the brain. *New Engl J Med*, 349:926–8.

Kron L et al. (1977) Anorexia nervosa and gonadal dysgenesis: further evidence of a relationship. *Arch Gen Psychiatry*, 34:332–5.

Le Grange D, Lock J, Dymek M (2003) Family-based therapy for adolescents with bulimia nervosa. *Am J Psychother*, 57:237–51.

Lewin K, Mattingly D, Millis RR (1972) Anorexia nervosa associated with hypothalamic tumor. *Br Med J*, 2:629–30.

Lock J (2002) Treating adolescents with eating disorders in the family context. Empirical and theoretical considerations. *Child Adolesc Psychiatr Clin N Am*, 11:331–42.

Malina A et al. (2003) Olanzapine treatment of anorexia nervosa: a retrospective study. *Int J Eating Disord*, 33:234–7.

Marcus MD, Kalarchian MA (2003) Binge eating in children and adolescents. *Int J Eating Disord*, 34:S47–S57.

Mascari MJ et al. (1992) The frequency of uniparental disomy in Prader-Willi syndrome. *New Engl J Med*, 326:1599–607.

McDuffie JR et al. (2002) Three-month tolerability of orlistat in adolescents with obesity-related comorbid conditions. *Obesity Res*, 10:642–50.

Mehler PS (2003a) Osteoporosis in anorexia nervosa: prevention and treatment. *Int J Eating Disord*, 33:113–26.

Mitchell JE, Raymond N, Specker S (1993) A review of the controlled trials of pharmacotherapy and psychotherapy in the treatment of bulimia nervosa. *Int J Eat Disord*, 14:229–47.

Norgren S et al. (2003) Orlistat treatment in obese prepubertal children: a pilot study. *Acta Paediatrica*, 92:666–70.

Ogden CL et al. (2002) Centers for Disease Control and Prevention 2000 growth charts for the United States: Improvements to the 1977 National Center for Health Statistics version. *Pediatr,* 109:45–60.

Pike KM et al. (2003) Cognitive behavior therapy in the posthospitalization treatment of anorexia nerovsa. *Am J Psychiatry*, 160:2046–9.

Rodin GM et al. (1986–7) Eating disorders in female adolescents with insulin dependent diabetes mellitus. *Int J Psychiatry Med*, 16:49–57.

Smith MS, Christie DL (1984) An adolescent with vomiting and weight loss. *J Adolesc Health Care*, 5:279–82.

Stunkard AJ, Allison KC (2003) Binge eating disorder: disorder or marker? *Int J Eating Disord*, 34:S107–S116.

Sugerman HJ et al. (2003) Bariatric surgery for severely obese adolescents. *J Gastrointest Surg*, 7:102–7.

Varadaraj R, Cooper AJ (1986) Addison's disease presenting with psychiatric symptoms [letter]. *Am J Psychiatry*, 143:553–4.

Waller DA et al. (2001) Linkage analysis of anorexia nervosa in a large family with multiple affected individuals. *Am J Med Genet (Neuropsych Genet)*, 105:586.

Waller DA et al. (2003) Three-year follow-up study of children and adolescents with anorexia nervosa initially treated in a continuum of care program. *Eating Disord*, 11:63–72.

Waller DA et al. (1984) Recognizing and managing the adolescent with Kleine-Levin syndrome. *J Adolesc Health*, 5:139–41.

Wilfley DE et al. (2003) The clinical significance of binge eating disorder. *Int J Eat Disord*, 34:S96–S106.

Chapter 12

American Academy of Child and Adolescent Psychiatry (1997) Practice parameter for the assessment and treatment of children and adolescents with bipolar disorder. *J Am Acad Child Adolesc Psychiatry*, 36(Suppl):177S-193S.

American Academy of Child and Adolescent Psychiatry (1998) Practice parameters for the assessment and treatment of children and adolescents with obsessive-compulsive disorder. *J Am Acad Child Adolesc Psychiatry*, 37(Suppl):27S-45S.

American Academy of Child and Adolescent Psychiatry (2004) Practice parameters for the use of electroconvulsive therapy in children and adolescents. *J Am Acad Child Adolesc Psychiatry*, 43(12):1521–39.

American Psychiatric Association (1980) *Diagnostic and Statistical Manual of Mental Disorders*, 3rd edn (DSM-III). Washington DC, American Psychiatric Association.

American Psychiatric Association (1987) *Diagnostic and Statistical Manual of Mental Disorders*, 3rd edn, revised, (DSM-IIIR). Washington DC, American Psychiatric Association.

American Psychiatric Association (1994) *Diagnostic and Statistical Manual of Mental Disorders*, 4th edn (DSM-IV*)*. Washington DC, American Psychiatric Association.

American Psychiatric Association (2000) *Diagnostic and Statistical Manual of Mental Disorders*, 4th edn, text revision (DSM-IV-TR). Washington DC, American Psychiatric Association.

American Psychiatric Association (1997) Practice guideline for the treatment of patients with schizophrenia. *Am J Psychiatry*, 154 (April Suppl).

Bloch Y, Levcovitch Y, Bloch AM, Mendlovic S, Ratzoni G (2001) Electroconvulsive therapy in adolescents: similarities to and differences from adults. *J Am Acad Child Adolesc Psychiatry*, 40(11):1332–6.

Cantor S, Evans J, Pearce J, Pezzot-Pearce T (1982) Childhood schizophrenia: present but not accounted for. *Am J Psychiatry*, 139(6):758–62.

Caplan R, Guthrie D, Foy JG (1992) Communication deficits and formal thought disorder in schizophrenic children. *J Am Acad child Adolesc Psychiatry*, 31:151–9.

Caplan R, Guthrie D, Tang B, Komo S, Asarnow RF (2000) Thought disorder in childhood schizophrenia: replication and update of concept. *J Am Acad Child Adolesc Psychiatry*, 39(6):771–8.

Chambers WJ, Puig-Antich J, Tabrizi MA et al. (1982) Psychotic symptoms in pre-pubertal major depressive disorder. *Arch Gen Psychiatry*, 39:921–7.

Cohen DJ, Towbin KE, Mayes LC, Volkmar FR (1993) Developmental psychopathology of multiplex developmental disorder. In: Friedman SL and Haywood HC (eds) *Developmental Follow-up: Concepts, Genres, Domains, and Methods*. New York, NY, Wiley, pp. 112–32.

Despert L (1942) A comparative study of thinking in schizophrenic children and in children of preschool age. *Nervous Child* 1:189–213.

Egdell HG, Kolvin I (1972) Childhood hallucinations. *J Child Psychol Psychiatry Allied Disciplines*, 13(4):279–87.

Eggers C (1978) Course and prognosis in childhood schizophrenia. *J Autism Child Schizophrenia*, 8:21–36.

Eisner A, McClellan J (1998) Substances of abuse. In: Werry JS, Aman MG (eds) *Practioner's guide to Psychoactive Drugs for Children and Adolescents*, 2nd edn. New York: Plenum, pp. 297–328.

Famularo R, Kinscherff R, Fenton T (1992) Psychiatric diagnoses of maltreated children: preliminary findings. *J Am Acad Child Adolesc Psychiatry*, 31:863–7.

Fink M (2001) ECT has much to offer our patients: it should not be ignored. *World J Biol Psychiatry*, 2(1):1–8.

Galdos P, van Os J (1995) Gender, psychopathology, and development: From puberty to early adulthood. *Schizophrenia Res*, 14(2):105–12.

Garralda ME (1984) Hallucinations in children with conduct and emotional disorders. I: The clinical phenomena. *Psychol Med*, 14(3):589–96.

Garralda ME (1984) Hallucinations in children with conduct and emotional disorders. II: The follow-up study. *Psychol Med*, 14(3):597–604.

Ghaziuddin N, Laughrin D, Giordani B (2000) Cognitive side effects of electroconvulsive therapy in adolescents. *J Child Adolesc Psychopharmacol*, 10(4):269–76.

Gilberg C, Wahlstrom J, Forsman A, Hellgren L, Gillberg JC (1986) Teenage psychoses – epidemiology, classification and reduced optimality in the pre-, peri- and neonatal periods. *J Child Psychol Pscychiatry*, 27:87–98.

Green AI, Canuso CM, Brenner MJ, Wojcik JD (2003) Detection and management of co-morbidity in patients with schizophrenia. *Psychiatric Clin N Am*, 26(1):115–39.

Gross G (1997) The onset of schizophrenia. *Schizophrenia Res*, 28(2–3):187–98.

Hafner H, Nowotny B (1995) Epidemiology of early-onset schizophrenia. *Eur Arch Psychiatry Clin Neuroscience*, 245(2):80–92.

Hughes JR, Hatsukami DK, Mitchell JE, Dahlgren LA (1986) Prevalence of smoking among schizophrenic outpatients. *Am J Psychiatry*, 143:993–7.

Kay SR, Fiszbein A, Opler LA (1987) The Positive and Negative Syndrome Scale (PANSS) for schizophrenia. *Schizophrenia Bull*, 13:261–76.

Klin A, Mayes LC, Volkmar FR, Cohen DJ (1995) Multiplex developmental disorder. *Dev Behav Pediatr*. 16(3):S7–S11.

Klosterkotter J, Ebel H, Schultze-Lutter F, Steinmeyer EM (1996) Diagnostic validity of basic symptoms. *Eur Arch Psychiatry Clin Neuroscience*, 246(3):147–54.

Kobayashi JS (2001) Delirium. In: Jacobson *Psychiatric Secrets*, 2nd edn. Hanley and Belfus.

Kolvin I (1971a) Studies in the childhood psychoses. I. Diagnostic criteria and classification. *Br J Psychiatry*, 118(545):381–4.

Kolvin I, Ounsted C, Humphrey M, McNay A (1971b) Studies in the childhood psychoses. II. The phenomenology of childhood psychoses. *Br J Psychiatry*, 18(545):385–95.

Kopala LC (1996) Spontaneous and drug-induced movement disorders in schizophrenia. *Acta Psychiatrica Scand*, 94:12–17.

Kotsopoulos S (1987) Hallucinating experiences in non-psychotic children. *J Am Acad Child Adolesc Psychiatry*, 26(3):375–80.

Kumra S, Frazier JA, Jacobsen LK et al. (1996) Childhood-onset schizophrenia: a double-blind clozapine-haloperidol comparison. *Arch Gen Psychiatry*, 53:1090–7.

Kumra S, Jacobsen LK, Lenane M (1998) Multidimensionally impaired disorder: is it a variant of very early-onset schizophrenia? *J Am Acad Child Adolesc Psychiatry*, 37(1):91–9.

Kutcher SP (1997a) Psychopharmacologic treatment of acute schizophrenia. In: Kutcher SP (ed.) *Child and Adolescent Psychopharmacology*. Philadelphia, WB Saunders Company, pp. 223–51.

Kydd RR, Werry JS (1982) Schizophrenia in children under 16 years. *J Autism Dev Disord*, 12(4):343–57.

Lewis M (2002) *Child and Adolescent Psychiatry: A Comprehensive Textbook*, 3rd edn. Baltimore, Maryland, Lippincott Williams & Wilkins.

Lieberman J, Jody D, Geisler S (1993) Time course and biological correlates of treatment response in first-episode schizophrenia. *Arch Gen Psychiatry*, 50:369–76.

Lukoff D, Nuechterlein KH, Ventura J (1986) Manual for expanded Brief Psychiatric Rating Scale (BPRS). *Schizophrenia Bull*, 12:594–602.

Marder SR, Essock SM, Miller AL et al. (2002) The Mount Sinai conference on the pharmacotherapy of schizophrenia. *Schizophrenia Bull*, 28(1):5–16.

McGorry PD, McFarlane C, Patton GC et al. (1995) The prevalence of prodromal features of schizophrenia in adolescence: a preliminary survey. *Acta Psychiatrica Scand*, 92(4):241–9.

Miller TJ, McGlashan TH, Woods SW et al. (1999) Symptom assessment in schizophrenic prodromal states. *Psychiatric Q*, 70(4):273–87.

Mueser KT, Yarnold PR, Levinson DF et al. (1990) Prevalence of substance abuse in schizophrenia: demographic and clinical correlates. *Schizophrenia Bull*, 16:31–56.

Naheed M, Green B (2001) Focus on clozapine. *Curr Med Res Opin*, 17(3):223–9.

National Institute of Mental Health (1985) Abnormal Involuntary Movement Scale. *Psychopharmacol Bull*, 21:1077–80.

Norman RM, Malla AK, McLean RS et al. (2002) An evaluation of a stress management program for individuals with schizophrenia. *Schizophrrenia Res*, 58(2–3):292–303.

Rutter M (1972) Childhood schizophrenia reconsidered. *J Autism Childhood Schizophrenia*, 2:315–37.

Taieb O, Flament MF, Chevret S et al. (2002) Clinical relevance of electroconvulsive therapy in adolescents with severe mood disorder: evidence from a follow-up study. *Eur Psychiatry*, 17(4):205–12.

Walter G, Rey JM (2003) Has the practice and outcome of ECT in adolescents changed? Findings from a whole population study. *J ECT*, 19(2):84–7.

Werry JS, McLellan J (1992) Predicting outcome in child and adolescent (early onset) schizophrenia and bipolar disorder. *J Am Acad Child Adolesc Psychiatry*, 31:147–50.

Westin D, Shedler J, Durrett C, Glass S, Martens A (2003) Personality diagnoses in adolescence: DSM-IV Axis II diagnoses and an empirically derived alternative. *Am J Psychiatry*, 160(5):952–66.

Woods SW, Breier A, Zipursky RB et al. (2003) Randomized trial of olanzapine versus placebo in the symptomatic acute treatment of the schizophrenic prodrome. *Biol Psychiatry*, 54(4):453–64.

Yung A, McGorry P, McFarlane C, Jackson H, Patton G, Rakkar A (1996) Monitoring and care of young people at incipient risk of psychosis. *Schizophrenia Bull*, 22:283–303.

Yung AR, Phillips LJ, Yuen HP et al. (2003) Psychosis prediction: 12-month follow-up of a high-risk ('prodromal') group. *Schizophrenia Res*, 60:21–32.

Chapter 13

Albertini RS, Phillips KA (1999) Thirty-three cases of body dysmorphic disorder in children and adolescents. *J Am Acad Child Adolesc Psychiatry*, 38:453–9.

American Psychiatric Association (1994) *Diagnostic and Statistical Manual of Mental Disorders (DSM-IV)*, 4th edn. Washington DC, American Psychiatric Press.

Ayoub CC, Alexander R, Beck D et al. (2002) Position paper: definitional issues in Munchausen by proxy. *Child Maltreatment*, 7:105–11.

Cassar JR, Hales ES, Longhurst JG, Weiss GS (1996) Can disability benefits make children sicker? *J Am Acad Child Adolesc Psychiatry*, 35, 700–1.

Eminson M, Jureidini J (2003) Concerns about research and prevention strategies in Munchausen syndrome by proxy (MSBP) abuse. *Child Abuse Neglect*, 27:413–20.

Fritz GK, Campo JV (2002) Somatoform disorder. In: Lewis M (ed.) *Child and Adolescent Psychiatry: A Comprehensive Textbook*, 3rd edn. Philadelphia, Lippincott Williams & Wilkins, pp. 847–57.

Fritz GK, Fritsch S, Hagino O (1997) Somatoform disorders in children and adolescents: a review of the past 10 years. *J Am Acad Child Adolesc Psychiatry*, 36, 1329–38.

McGuire TL, Feldman KW (1989) Psychologic morbidity of children subjected to Munchausen syndrome by proxy. *Pediatr*, 83:289–92.

Oldershaw L, Bagby RM (1997) Children and deception. In Rogers R (ed.) *Clinical Assessment of Malingering and Deception*. New York, The Guildford Press, pp. 153–66.

Roberts MD (1997) Letter. *J Am Acad Child Adolesc Psychiatry*, 36:579.

Rosenberg DA (2003) Munchausen syndrome by proxy: medical diagnostic criteria. *Child Abuse Neglect*, 27:421–30.

Rubinstein B (1988) Psychological factors influencing medical conditions. In: Kestenbaum CJ, Williams DT (eds) *Handbook of Clinical Assessment of Children and Adolescents*. New York, New York University Press, pp. 771–80.

Stutts JT, Hickson GB (1999) Factitious disorders in children and adolescents. *Ambulatory Child Health*, 5:313–21.

Stutts JT, Hickey SE, Kasdan, ML (2003) Malingering by proxy: a form of pediatric condition falsification. *J Dev Behav Pediatr*, 24:276–8.

Taylor S, Garralda E (2003) Management of somatoform disorder in childhood. *Curr Opin Psychiatry*, 16:227–31.

von Hahn L, Harper G, McDaniel SH, Siegal DM, Feldman MD, Libow JA (2001) A case of factitious disorder by proxy: the role of the health-care system, diagnostic dilemmas, and family dynamics. *Harvard Rev Psychiatry*, 9:124–35.

Wells LA (1996) Functional disorders in children and adolescents: diagnostic considerations. *Mayo Clin Proc*, 71:259–65.

Williams DT, Hirsch G (1988) The somatizing disorders. In: Kestenbaum CJ, Williams DT (eds) *Handbook of Clinical Assessment of Children and Adolescents*. New York, New York University Press, pp. 741–68.

Chapter 14

American Academy of Child and Adolescent Psychiatry (1997) Practice parameters for the assessment and treatment of children and adolescents with substance use disorders. *J Am Acad Child Adolesc Psychiatry*, 36(Suppl):140S–156S.

American Academy of Pediatrics (1988) Evaluation by interview. In: Schonber SK (ed.) *Substance Abuse: A Guide for Health Professionals*. Elk Grove Village, IL, American Academy of Pediatrics.

American Psychiatric Association (1994) *Diagnostic and Statistical Manual of Mental Disorders (DSM-IV)*, 4th edn. Washington DC, American Psychiatric Press.

Jaffe SL (ed.) (1996) Adolescent substance abuse and dual disorders. *Child Adolesc Psychiatric Clin N Am*, 5.

Johnston LD, O'Malley PM, Bachman JG, Schulenberg JD (2004) *Monitoring the Future National Results on Adolescent Drug Use: Overview of Key Findings, 2003*. Bethesda, MD, National Institute of Drug Abuse.

Kandel DB (1975) Stages in adolescent involvement in drug use. *Science*, 190:912–14.

Schwartz RH (2002) Marijuana: a decade and a half later, still a crude drug with appreciated toxicity. *Pediatr*, 109:284–9.

Chapter 15

Abidin RR (1995) *Parenting Stress Index*, 3rd edn. Odessa, FL, Psychological Assessment Resources.

Abramson R, Altfeld S, Teibloom-Mishkin J (2000) *Zero To Three*, 21:11–16.

Achenbach T, Rescorla L (2000) *Child Behavior Checklist for Ages 1½ to 5*. VT, ASEBA.

Ainsworth MDS (1967) *Infancy in Uganda: Infant Care and the Growth of Love*. Oxford, UK, John Hopkins Press.

Ainsworth MS, Blehar MC, Waters E, Wall S (1978) *Patterns of Attachment: A Psychological Study of the Strange Situation*. Oxford, UK, Lawrence Erlbaum.

Als H (1982) *Infant Mental Health Journal*, 3:229–43.

Als H (1984) *Manual for the Naturalistic Observation of Newborn Behavior in Preterm and Full-Term Infants*. Boston, MA, Children's Hospital.

American Psychiatric Association (1994) *Diagnostic and Statistical Manual of Mental Disorders*, 4th edn. Washington DC, American Psychiatric Association.

Bayley N (1993) *Bayley Scales of Infant Development 2*. San Antonio, TX, Psychological Corporation.

Benham AL (2000) In: Zeanah CH Jr (ed.) *Handbook of Infant Mental Health*. The Guilford Press, New York, pp. 249–65.

Blackburn S (1995) *J Obstetr Gynecol Neonatal Nurs*, 24:43–9.

Bowlby J, Robertson J, Rosenbluth D (1952) *Psychoanalytic Study of the Child*, 7:82–94.

Brazelton TB (1973) *Neonatal Behavioral Assessment Scale*. J.B. Lippincott, Philadelphia.

Brazelton TB (1990) *Child Dev*, 61:1661–71.

Brazy JE, Goldstein RF, Oehler JM, Gustafson KE, Thompson RJ Jr (1993) *J Dev Behav Pediatr*, 14:375–80.

Briggs-Gowan MJ, Carter AS (2002) *Brief Infant-Toddler Social and Emotional Assessment (BITSEA) Mannual, Version 2.0*. New Haven, CT, Yale University.

Bronfenbrenner U (1979) *The Ecology of Human Development: Experiments by Nature and Design*. Cambridge, MA, Harvard University Press.

Brooten D, Gennaro S, Brown LP et al. (1988) *Nurs Res*, 37:213–16.

Browne JV, MacLeod A, Smith-Sharp S (1996) *Family-Infant Relationship Support Training*. Denver, CO, Center for Family and Infant Interaction.

Chess S, Thomas A (1991) In: Strelau J, Angleitner A (eds) *Explorations in Temperament: International Perspectives on Theory and Measurement. Perspectives on Individual Differences*. New York, Plenum Press, pp. 15–28.

Cohen LJ, Slade A (2000) In: Zeanah CH Jr (ed.) *Handbook of Infant Mental Health*, 2nd edn.

Coll CG, Magnuson K (2000) In: Shonkoff JP, Meisels SJ (eds) *Handbook of Early Childhood Intervention*, 2nd edn.

Davis L, Mohay H, Edwards H (2003) *J Adv Nurs*, 42:578–86.

DeMier RL, Hynan MT, Hatfield RF, Varner MW, Harris HB, Manniello RL (2000) *J Clin Psychol*, 56:89–100.

Easterbrooks MA (1988) In: Goldberg WA (ed.) *The Transition to Parenthood: Current Theory and Research*.

Eppright TD, Bradley S, Sanfacon JA (1998) *Child Psychiatry and Human Development*, 28:213–22.

Fitzgerald HE, Puttler LI, Mun EY, Zucker RA (2000) In: Osofsky JD, Fitzgerald HE (eds) *WAIMH Handbook of Infant Mental Health*, Vol. 4. New York, John Wiley and Sons, Inc., pp. 124–59.

Fowles ER (1999) *Am J Matern Child Nurs*, 24:287–93.

Fraiberg S, Adelson E, Shapiro V (1975) *J Am Acad Child Psychiatry*, 14:387–421.

Fraiberg S, Fraiberg L (1980) *Clinical Studies in Infant Mental Health: The First Year of Life*. New York, Basic Books.

Frankel KA, Harmon RJ (1996) *J Am Acad Child Adolesc Psychiatry*, 35:289–98.

Frankenburg WK, Dodds J, Archer P et al. (1990) *Denver II Screening Manual*. Denver. CO, Denver Developmental Materials.

Gennaro S (1988) *Nurs Res*, 37:82–5.

Glascoe FP (1997) *Parents' Evaluations of Developmental Status: A Method for Detecting and Addressing Developmental and Behavioral Problems in Children.* Nashville, TN, Ellsworth and Vandermeer Press LLC.

Goldberg S (1979) *Am Sci,* 67:214–20.

Greenspan SI, Wieder S (2003) *Zero To Three,* 24:6–13.

Harmon RJ, Murrow NS (1995) In: MacTurk RH, Morgan GA (eds) *Mastery Motivation: Conceptual Origins and Application.* Norwood, NJ, Ablex Publishing Corporation, pp. 237–56.

Harmon RJ, Riggs PD (1996) *J Am Acad Child Adolesc Psychiatry,* 35:1247–9.

Huberman R, Cahill L, Witt M (2000) In: Goldman HH (ed.) *Review of General Psychiatry.* New York, Lange Medical Books/McGraw-Hill.

Kelly JF, Barnard KE (2000) In: Shonkoff JP, Meisels SJ (eds) *Handbook of Early Childhood Intervention.* Cambridge, UK, Cambridge University Press.

Kempe CH, Silverman FN, Steele BF, Droegemueller W, Silver HK (1962) *J Am Med Assoc,* 181:17–24.

Klinnert MD, Emde RN, Butterfield P, Campos JJ (1986) *Dev Psychol,* 22:427–32.

Kourtis AP (2002) *Drugs,* 62, 2213–20.

LeBuffe PA, Naglieri JA (2002) *Devereux Early Childhood Assessment.* The Devereux Foundation.

Lester BM, Boukydis CFZ, Twomey JE (2000) In: Zeanah CH Jr (ed.) *Handbook of Infant Mental Health.* New York, The Guilford Press, pp. 161–75.

Lester BM, LaGasse LL, Seifer R (1998) *Science,* 282:633–4.

Lester BM, Tronick EZ, LaGasse L et al. (2002) *Pediatr,* 110:1182–92.

Lieberman AF, Silverman R, Pawl JH (2000) In: Zeanah CH Jr (ed.) *Handbook of Infant Mental Health,* 2nd edn.

Lorenz JM, Wooliever DE, Jetton JR, Paneth N (1998) *Arch Pediatr Adolesc Med,* 152:425–35.

Macey TJ, Harmon RJ, Easterbrooks M (1987) *J Consult Clin Psychol,* 55:846–52.

Main M, Solomon J (1986) In: Yogman MW (ed.) *Affective Development in Infancy.*

Maloni JA, Kane JH, Suen LJ, Wang KK (2002) *Nurs Res,* 51:92–9.

Metcalf AW, Rowe J (2000) In: Goldman HH (ed.) *Review of General Psychiatry.* New York, Lange Medical Books/McGraw-Hill, pp. 21–46.

Miceli PJ, Goeke-Morey MC, Whitman TL, Kolberg KS, Miller-Loncar C, White RD (2000) *J Pediatr Psychol,* 25:353–8.

Mullen EM (1991) *The Infant Mullen Scales of Early Learning: Instrument Descriptions.* Cranston, RI, T.O.T.A.L. Child.

National Institute on Drug Abuse (1996) U.S. Department of Health and Human Services, Washington, DC.

Nilsson L, Hamberger L (2003) *A Child is Born.* New York, Delacorte Press.

Olds DL, Robinson J, O'Brien R et al. (2002) *Pediatr,* 110, 486–96.

Pollack H, Kuchuk A, Cowan L et al. (1996) *Brain Behav Immun,* 10:298–312.

Prugh DG (1983) *The Psychosocial Aspects of Pediatrics.* Philadelphia, Lea and Febiger.

Robinson JL, Fitzgerald HE (2002) *Infant Ment Health J,* 23:250–7.

Sameroff AJ, Chandler MJ (1975) In: Horowitz FD (ed.) *Review of Child Development Research,* Vol. 4. Chicago, IL, University of Chicago Press, pp. 187–244.

Sameroff AJ, Fiese BH (2000) In: Shonkoff JP, Meisels SJ (eds) *Handbook of Early Childhood Intervention,* 2nd edn.

Sameroff AJ, MacKenzie MJ (2003) *Zero To Three,* 24:14–22.

Seligman S (2000) In: Zeanah CH Jr (ed.) *Handbook of Infant Mental Health.* New York, The Guilford Press, pp. 211–21.

Shonkoff JP, Phillips DA (eds) (2000) *From Neurons to Neighborhoods: The Science of Early Childhood Development.* Washington DC, National Academy Press.

Shonkoff JP, Phillips DA (2002) *J Am Acad Child Adolesc Psychiatry,* 41:625–6.

Singer LT, Salvator A, Guo S, Collin M, Lilien L, Baley J (1999) *J Am Med Assoc,* 281:799–805.

Sparrow SS, Balla DA, Cicchetti DV (1984) Vineland Adaptive Behavior Scales. Circle Pines, MN, American Guidance Service.

Spitz RA (1946) *Psychoanalytic Study of the Child,* 2:113–17.

Spitz RA, Wolf KM (1946) *Psychoanalytic Study of the Child,* 2:313–42.

Squires J, Bricker D, Twombly E (2002) *The Ages and Stages Questionnaires: Social-Emotional.* Baltimore, MD, Paul H. Brookes Publishing Co.

Streissguth AP (1997) *Fetal Alcohol Syndrome: A Guide for Families and Communities.*

Sullivan PM, Knutson JF (2000) *Child Abuse Neglect,* 24:1257–73.

Tracey N (ed.) (2000) *Parents of Premature Infants: Their Emotional World.*

Weston DR, Thomas J, Barnard KE et al. (2003) *Infant Ment Health J,* 24:410–27.

Winnicott D (1960) Theory of the parent-infant relationship. *Int J Psychoanal,* 41:585–95.

Zeanah CH Jr, Larrieu JA, Heller SS, Valliere J (2000a) In: Zeanah CH Jr (ed.) *Handbook of Infant Mental Health,* 2nd edn.

Zeanah PD, Larrieu JA, Zeanah CH Jr (2000b) In: Zeanah CH Jr (ed.) *Handbook of Infant Mental Health,* 2nd edn.

Zero To Three (1994) *Diagnostic Classification of Mental Health and Developmental Disorders of Infancy and Early Childhood.* Arlington, VA, Zero To Three/National Center for Clinical Infant Programs.

Zero To Three (2003) In: Center P (ed.) *Fact Sheet.* Washington DC, 3.

Zito JM, Safer DJ, dosReis S, Gardner JF, Boles M, Lynch F (2000) *J Am Med Assoc,* 283:1025–30.

Chapter 16

Al-Mateen CS, Afzal A (2004) The Muslim child, adolescent, and family. *Child Adolesc Psychiatric Clin N Am,* 13(1):183–200.

American Academy of Child and Adolescent Psychiatry, Pruitt DB, editor-in-chief (1999) *Your Adolescent.* New York, HarperCollins Publishers.

American Academy of Child and Adolescent Psychiatry, Pruitt DB, editor-in-chief (1998) *Your Child.* New York, HarperCollins Publishers.

American Psychiatric Association (1994) *Diagnostic and Statistical Manual of Mental Disorders,* 4th edn. Washington DC, American Psychiatric Association.

Anders TF (1997) Sleep disorders: infancy through adolescence. In: Weiner JM (ed.) *Textbook of Child and Adolescent Psychiatry,* 2nd edn. Washington DC, American Psychiatric Press, pp. 599–611.

Bimmel N, Juffer F, van Ijzendoorn MH, Bakermans-Kranenburg MJ (2003) Problem behavior of internationally adopted adolescents: a review and meta-analysis. *Harvard Rev Psychiatry,* 11(2):64–77.

Black N (2004) Hindu and Buddhist children, adolescents, and families. *Child Adolesc Psychiatric Clin N Am*, 13(1):201–20.

Boyce WT, Goldstein LH (1999) Critical life events: sibling births, separations, and deaths in the family. In: Levine MD, Carey WB, Crocker AC (eds) *Developmental–Behavioral Pediatrics*, 3rd edn. Philadelphia, W.B. Saunders Company, pp. 141–8.

Carlson EA, Sampson MC, Sroufe LA (2003) Implications of attachment theory and research for developmental–behavioral pediatrics. *J Dev Behav Pediatr*, 24(5):364–79.

Chatoor I (1997) Feeding and eating disorders if infancy and early childhood. In: Weiner JM (ed.) *Textbook of Child and Adolescent Psychiatry*, 2nd edn. Washington, DC, American Psychiatric Press, pp. 527–40.

Chatoor I (2002) Feeding disorders in infants and toddlers: diagnosis and treatment. *Child Adolesc Psychiatric Clin N Am*, 11(2):163–83.

Dell ML (1995) Divorce – are you ready to help? *Contemporary Pediatr*, 12(5):57–66.

Dell ML (2004) Religious professionals and institutions: untapped resources for clinical care. *Child Adolesc Psychiatric Clin N Am*, 13(1):85–110.

Derdeyn AP, Graves CL (1998) Clinical vicissitudes of adoption. *Child Adolesc Psychiatric Clin N Am*, 7(2):373–87.

Derdeyn AP, Lamps CA (2002) Adoption. In: Lewis M (ed.) *Child and Adolescent Psychiatry: A Comprehensive Textbook*, 3rd edn. Philadelphia, Lippincott Williams & Wilkins, pp. 1266–75.

Doka KJ (2004) Grief and bereavement. In: Post SG (editor-in-chief) *Encyclopedia of Bioethics*, 3rd edn. New York, Macmillan Reference USA, pp. 1028–31.

Dowdney L (2000) Annotation: childhood bereavement following parental death. *J Child Psychol Psychiatry*, 41(7):819–30.

Dworkin PH (1999) Behavior problems of toddlers and preschool children. In: Green M, Haggerty RJ, Weitzman M (eds) *Ambulatory Pediatrics*, 5th edn. Philadelphia, W.B. Saunders Company, pp. 404–9.

Fisher M (2003) Functional disorders in children and adolescents. *Clin Family Prac*, 5(2):417–44.

Fowler JW, Dell ML (2004) Stages of faith and identity: birth to teens. *Child Adolesc Psychiatric Clin N Am*, 13(1):17–33.

Givan DC (2004) The sleepy child. *Pediatr Clin N Am*, 51(1):15–31.

Glader L, Rappaport L (2001) Encopresis. In: Stockman JA, Lohr JA (eds) *Essence of Office Pediatrics*. Philadelphia, W.B. Saunders Company, p. 124.

Glaze DG (2004) Childhood insomnia: why Chris can't sleep. *Pediatr Clin N Am*, 51(1):33–50.

Handford HA, Vgontzas AN (2002) Sleep disturbances and disorders. In: Lewis M (ed.) *Child and Adolescent Psychiatry: A Comprehensive Textbook*, 3rd edn. Philadelphia, Lippincott Williams & Wilkins, pp. 876–89.

Hollingsworth LD (1998) Promoting same-race adoption for children of color. *Social Work*, 43(2), 104–16.

Howard BJ (1999) Behavior and development. In: Green M, Haggerty RJ, Weitzman M (eds). *Ambulatory Pediatrics*, 5th edn. Philadelphia, W.B. Saunders Company, pp. 396–404.

Jalkut MW, Lerman SE, Churchill BM (2001) Enuresis. *Pediatr Clin N Am*, 48(6):1461–88.

Josephson AM, Dell ML (2004) Religion and spirituality in child and adolescent psychiatry: a new frontier. *Child Adolesc Psychiatric Clin N Am*, 13(1):1–15.

Kelly JB (1998) Marital conflict, divorce, and children's adjustment. *Child Adolesc Psychiatric Clin N Am*, 7(2):259–271.

Kotagal S (2003) Sleep disorders in childhood. *Neurol Clin N Am*, 9(4):961–81.

Lears MK, Guth KJ, Lewandowski L (1998) International adoption: a primer for pediatric nurses. *Pediatr Nurs*, 24(6):578–86.

Mason TW, Thornton BA (2002) Sleep disorders in children. *Nurs Clin N Am*, 37(4):693–706.

McRoy RG, Grape H (1999) Skin color in transracial and inracial adoptive placements: implications for special needs adoptions. *Child Welfare*, 78(5):673–92.

Meltzer LJ, Mindell JA (2004) Nonpharmacologic treatments for pediatric sleepiness. *Pediatr Clin N Am*, 51(1):135–51.

Mercer JA (2004) The Protestant child, adolescent, and family. *Child Adolesc Psychiatric Clin N Am*, 13(1):161–81.

Mikkelsen EJ (2002) Modern approaches to enuresis and encopresis. In: Lewis M (ed.) *Child and Adolescent Psychiatry: A Comprehensive Textbook*, 3rd edn. Philadelphia, Lippincott Williams & Wilkins, pp. 700–11.

Mitchell MAS, Janista JA (1997a) Health care of the internationally adopted child, part 1: before and at arrival into the adoptive home. *J Pediatr Health Care*, 11:51–60.

Mitchell MAS, Janista JA (1997b) Health care of the internationally adopted child, part 2: chronic care and long-term medical issues. *J Pediatr Health Care*, 11:117–26.

Moncher FJ, Josephson AM (2004) Religious and spiritual aspects of family assessment. *Child Adolesc Psychiatric Clin N Am*, 13(1):49–70.

Murrell K (2004) The Catholic child, adolescent, and family. *Child Adolesc Psychiatric Clin N Am*, 13(1):149–60.

Pelayo R, Chen W, Monzon S, Guilleminault C (2004) Pediatric sleep pharmacology: you want to give my kid sleeping pills? *Pediatr Clin N Am*, 51(1):117–34.

Peterson EA (1997) Supporting the adoptive family: a developmental approach. *Maternal Child Nurs*, 22:147–52.

Pruett MK, Pruett KD (1998) Fathers, divorce, and their children. *Child Adolesc Psychiatric Clin N Am*, 7(2):389–407.

Pruett MK, Hoganbruen K (1998) Joint custody and shared parenting: research and interventions. *Child Adolesc Psychiatric Clin N Am*, 7(2):273–93.

Robson WLM (2001) Enuresis. Advances in Pediatrics, 48:409–38.

Rockney R (1999) Encopresis. In: Levine MD, Carey WB, Crocker AC (eds). *Developmental–Behavioral Pediatrics*, 3rd edn. Philadelphia, W.B. Saunders Company, pp. 413–21.

Roseby V, Johnston JR (1998) Children of Armageddon: common developmental threats in high-conflict divorcing families. *Child Adolesc Psychiatric Clin N Am*, 7(2):295–309.

Rube DM, Kibel N (2004) The Jewish child, adolescent, and family. *Child Adolesc Psychiatric Clin N Am*, 13(1):137–47.

Rudolph CD, Link DT (2002) Feeding disorders in infants and children. *Pediatr Clin N Am*, 49(1):97–112.

Sexson SB (2004) Religious and spiritual assessment of the child and adolescent. *Child Adolesc Psychiatric Clin N Am*, 13(1):35–47.

Shapiro HL (1999) Sleep disorders. In: Levine MD, Carey WB, Crocker AC (eds) *Developmental–Behavioral Pediatrics*, 3rd edn. Philadelphia. W.B. Saunders Company, pp. 422–9.

Sherry SN, Nickman SL (1999) Adoption and foster family care. In: Levine MD, Carey WB, Crocker AC (eds) *Developmental–Behavio-*

ral Pediatrics, 3rd edn. Philadelphia. W.B. Saunders Company, pp. 132–9.

Silverstein DN, Roszia SK (1998) Openness: a critical component of special needs adoption. *Child Welfare*, 78(5):637–51.

Stevenson-Moessner J (2003) *The Spirit of Adoption*. Nashville, TN, Westminster John Knox Press.

Stuber ML, Houskamp BM (2004) Spirituality in children confronting death. *Child Adolesc Psychiatric Clin N Am*, 13(1):127–36.

Stuber ML, Mesrkhani VH (2001) 'What do we tell the children?': understanding childhood grief. *Western J Med*, 174:187–91.

Townsend LL (2000) *Pastoral Care with Stepfamilies*. St. Louis, MO, Chalice Press.

Wallerstein JS (1999) Separation, divorce, and remarriage. In: Levine MD, Carey WB, Crocker AC (eds) *Developmental–Behavioral Pediatrics*, 3rd edn. Philadelphia, W.B. Saunders Company, pp. 149–61.

Wallerstein JS, Corbin SB (1999) The child and the vicissitudes of divorce. In: Lewis M (ed.) *Child and Adolescent Psychiatry: A Comprehensive Textbook*, 3rd edn. Philadelphia, Lippincott Williams & Wilkins, pp. 1275–85.

Walsh T, Menvielle E (1997) Disorders of elimination. In: Weiner JM (ed.) *Textbook of Child and Adolescent Psychiatry*, 2nd edn. Washington DC, American Psychiatric Press, pp. 613–20.

Weller EB, Weller RA, Benton T, Pugh JJW (2002) Grief. In: Lewis M (ed.) *Child and Adolescent Psychiatry: A Comprehensive Textbook*, 3rd edn. Philadelphia, Lippincott Williams & Wilkins, pp. 470–7.

Chapter 17

Admi H (1996) Growing up with a chronic health condition: a model of an ordinary lifestyle. *Qual Health Res*, 6:163–83.

Alderfer MA, Wiebe DJ, Hartmann DP (2001) Social behavior and illness information interact to influence the peer acceptance of children with chronic illness. *Br J Health Psychol*, 6:243–55.

American Psychiatric Association (1994) *Diagnostic and Statistical Manual of Mental Disorders (DSM-IV)*, 4th edn. Washington DC, American Psychiatric Press.

Anthony KK, Gil KM, Schanberg LE (2003) Brief report: parental perceptions of child vulnerability in children with chronic illness. *J Pediatr Psychol*, 28:185–90.

Berry SL, Hayford JR, Ross CK, Pachman LM, Lavigne JV (1993) Conceptions of illness by children with juvenile rheumatoid arthritis: a cognitive developmental approach. *J Pediatr Psychol*, 18:83–97.

Biederman J, Milberger S, Faraone SV, Guite J, Warburton R (1994) Associations between childhood asthma and ADHD: issues of psychiatric comorbidity and familiarity. *J Am Acad Child Adolesc Psychiatry*, 33:842–8.

Blakeney P (1994) School reintegration. In: Tarnowski KJ (ed.) *Behavioral Aspects of Pediatric Burns*. New York, Plenum Press, pp. 217–41.

Boyd-Franklin N, Steiner GL, Boland MG (eds) (1995) *Children, Families, and HIV/AIDS*. New York, Guilford Press.

Brown LK, Bruning K, Fritz GK, Herzog DB (2003) Somatoform disorders. In: Weiner JM, Dulcan MK (eds) *Textbook of Child and Adolescent Psychiatry*. Washington DC, American Psychiatric Publishing, pp. 751–63.

Brown R, Armstrong F, Eckman J (1993) Neurocognitive aspects of pediatric sickle cell disease. *J Learning Disabil*, 26:33–45.

Brown RT, Madan-Swain A (1993) Cognitive, neuropsychological, and academic sequelae in children with leukemia. *J Learning Disabil*, 26:74–90.

Burbach D, Peterson L (1986) Children's concepts of physical illness: a review and critique of the cognitive behavioral literature. *Health Psychol*, 5:307–325.

Cadman D, Boyle M, Szatmari P, Offord DR (1987) Chronic illness disability, and mental and social well-being: findings of the Ontario child health study. *Pediatr*, 79, 805–13.

Centers for Disease Control and Prevention (1999) *HIV/AIDS Surveillance Report*. Midyear edition, 11.

Christian B (2003) Growing up with chronic illness: psychosocial adjustment of children and adolescents with cystic fibrosis. *Ann Rev Nurs Res*, 21:151–72.

Colegrove R, Huntzinger R (1994) Academic, behavioral, and social adaptation of boys with hemophilia/HIV disease. *J Pediatr Psychol*, 19:457–73.

Costello EJ, Edelbrook C, Costello AJ, Dulcan MK, Burns BJ, Brent D (1988) Psychopathology in pediatric primary care; the new hidden morbidity. *Pediatr*, 82:415–24.

Crisp J, Ungerer JA, Goodnow JJ (1996) The impact of experience on children's understanding of illness. *J Pediatr Psychol*, 21:57–72.

Davidow DN (1996) Chronic illness in children and adolescents. In: Parmelee DX (ed.) *Mosby's Neurology Psychiatry Access Series: Child and Adolescent Psychiatry*. St Louis, MO, Mosby-Yearbook Inc., pp. 277–85.

Davis CL, Delamater AM, Shaw KH et al. (2001) Parenting styles, regimen adherence, and glycemic control in 4- to 10-year-old children with diabetes. *J Pediatr Psychol*, 26:123–129.

Eiser C, Morse R (2001) Can parents rate their child's health-related quality of life? Results of a systematic review. *Qual Life Res*, 10:347–57.

Feldman W (1996) Chronic illness in children. In: Haslam RHA, Valletutti PJ (eds) *Medical Problems in the Classroom: The Teacher's Role in Diagnosis and Management*. Austin, Texas, PRO-ED, pp. 115–23.

Fowler MG, Johnson MP, Atkinson SS (1985) School achievement and absence in children with chronic health conditions. *J Pediatr*, 106:683–7.

Garrison WT, McQuiston S (1989) *Chronic Illness during Childhood and Adolescence: Psychological Aspects*. Newbury Park, California, Sage Publications.

Hains AA, Davies WH, Behens D, Biller JA (1997) Cognitive behavioral interventions for adolescents with cystic fibrosis. *J Pediatr Psychol*, 22:669–87.

Havens J, Mellins CA, Hunter JS (2003) Psychiatric aspects of HIV/AIDS in childhood and adolescence. In: Rutter M, Taylor E (eds) *Child and Adolescent Psychiatry*, 4th edn. Mullen, MA, Blackwell Science Publishing, pp. 828–41.

Hindley PA (1997) Psychiatric aspects of hearing impairments. *J Child Psychol Psychiatry*, 38:101–17.

Hindley P, van Gent (2003) Psychiatric aspects of specific sensory impairments. In: Rutter M, Taylor E (eds) *Child and Adolescent Psychiatry*, 4th edn. Mullen, MA, Blackwell Science Publishing, pp. 842–57.

Hobbs S, Sexson S (1993) Cognitive development and learning in the pediatric organ transplant recipient. *J Learning Disabil*, 2:104–13.

Holmes CS, O'Brien B, Greer T (1995) Cognitive functioning and academic achievement in children with insulin-dependent diabetes mellitus (IDDM) *School Psychol Q*, 10:329–45.

Jellinek MS, Murphy JM, Robinson J et al. (1988) Pediatric symptom checklist: screening checklist: screening school-age children for psychosocial dysfunction. *J Pediatr*, 112:201–9.

Jutras S, Morin P, Proulx R, Vinay MC, Roy E, Routhier L (2003) Conception of wellness in families with a diabetic child. *J Health Psychol*, 8:573–86.

Kazak AE, Penati B, Boyer BA et al. (1996) A randomized controlled prospective outcome study of a psychological and pharmacological intervention protocol for procedural distress in pediatric leukemia. *J Pediatr Psychol*, 21:615–31.

Kelly AF, Hewson PH (2000) Factors associated with recurrent hospitalization in chronically ill children and adolescents. *J Paediatr Child Health*, 36:13–18.

Kliebenstein MA, Broome ME (2000) School re-entry for the child with chronic illness: parent and school personnel perceptions. *Pediatr Nurs*, 26:579–83.

Knafl K, Zoeller L (2000) Childhood chronic illness: a comparison of mothers' and fathers' experiences. *J Family Nurs*, 6:287–302.

Knapp P, Harris E (1997) Consultation-liaison in child psychiatry: a review of the past 10 years. I: Clinical findings. *J Am Acad Child Adolesc Psychiatry*, 36:1329–38.

Knapp P, Harris E (1998) Consultation-liaison in child psychiatry: a review of the past 10 years. II: Research and treatment approaches and outcomes. *J Am Acad Child Adolesc Psychiatry*, 37:139–46.

Kyngas HA, Kroll T, Duffy ME (2000) Compliance in adolescents with chronic disease: a review. *J Adolesc Health*, 26:379–88.

Lavigne JV, Faier-Routman J (1993) Correlates of psychosocial adjustment to pediatric physical disorders: a meta-analytic review and comparison with existing models. *Dev Behav Pediatr*, 14:117–23.

Lemanek KL, Kamps J, Chung NB (2001) Empirically supported treatments in pediatric psychology: regimen adherence. *J Pediatr Psychol*, 26:253–75.

Lewis M, Schonfeld D (2002) Dying and death in childhood and adolescence. In: Lewis M (ed.) *Child and Adolescent Psychiatry: A Comprehensive Textbook.* Philadelphia, Lippincott Williams & Wilkins, pp. 1239–45.

Lewis M, Vitulano LA (2003) Biopsychosocial issues and risk factors in the family when the child has a chronic illness. *Child Adolesc Psychiatric Clin N Am*, 12:389–99.

Lightfoot J, Wright S, Sloper P (1999) Supporting pupils in mainstream school with an illness or disability: young people's views. *Child Care Health Dev*, 25:267–83.

Luthar SS, Cicchetti D, Becker B (2000) The construct of resilience: a critical evaluation and guidelines for future work. *Child Dev*, 71:543–62.

Madden SJ, Hastings RP, V'ant Hoff (2002) Psychological adjustment in children with end stage renal disease: the impact of maternal stress and coping. *Child Care Health Dev*, 28:323–30.

Manne S, Duhamel K, Ostroff J et al. (2003) Coping and the course of mother's depressive symptoms during and after pediatric bone marrow transplantation. *J Am Acad Child Adolesc Psychiatry*, 42:1055–68.

Meijer SA, Sinnema G, Bijstra JO, Mellenbergh GJ, Wolters WHG (2000) Social functioning in children with a chronic illness. *J Child Psychol Psychiatry*, 41:309–17.

Meijer SA, Sinnema G, Bijstra JO, Mellenbergh GJ, Wolters WHG. (2002) Coping styles and locus of control as predictors for psychological adjustment of adolescents with a chronic illness. *Soc Sci Med*, 54:1453–61.

Meyer TA, Svirsky MA, Kirk KI, Miyamoto RT (1998) Improvements in speech perception by children with profound hearing loss: effects of device, communication, mode and chronological age. *J Speech Lang Hearing Res*, 41:846–8.

Miller R, Sabin CA, Goldman E et al. (2000) Coping styles in families with haemophilia. *Psychol Health Med*, 3–12.

Moss HA, Bose S, Wolters P, Brouwers P (1998) A preliminary study of factors associated with psychological adjustment and disease course in school-age children infected with immunodeficiency virus. *J Dev Behav Pediatr*, 19:18–25.

Mrazek DA (2002) Chronic pediatric illness and multiple hospitalizations. In: Lewis M (ed.) *Child and Adolescent Psychiatry: A Comprehensive Textbook.* Philadelphia, Lippincott Williams & Wilkins, pp. 1230–8.

Mrazek DA (2003a) Psychiatric aspects of somatic disease. In: Rutter M. Taylor E (eds) *Child and Adolescent Psychiatry.* Mullen, MA, Blackwell Science Publishing, pp. 810–27.

Mrazek DA (2003b) Psychiatric symptoms in patients with asthma causality, comorbidity, or shared genetic etiology. *Child Adolesc Psychiatric Clin N Am*, 12:459–71.

Northam EA, Anderson PJ, Werther GA, Wayne GL, Adler RG, Andrewes D (1998) Neuropsychological complications of IDDM in children 2 years after disease onset. *Diabetes Care*, 21:379–84.

Ogden Burke S, Kauffmann E, LaSalle J, Harrison MB, Wong C (2000) Parents' perceptions of chronic illness trajectories. *Can J Nurs Res*, 32:19–36.

Olson AL, Johnsen SG, Powers LE et al. (1993) Cognitive coping strategies of children with chronic illness. *J Dev Behav Pediatr*, 14:217–23.

Olson AL, Seidler B, Goodman D, Gaelic S, Nordgren R (2004) School professionals' perceptions about the impact of chronic illness in the classroom. *Arch Pediatr Adolesc Med*, 158:53–8.

Ortega AN, Huertas Ramirez R, Rubio-Stipec M (2002) Childhood asthma, chronic illness, and psychiatric disorders. *J Nervous Ment Dis*, 190:275–81.

Packman WL, Crittenden MR, Schaeffer E et al. (1997) Psychosocial consequences of bone marrow transplantation in donor and nondonor siblings. *J Dev Behav Pediatr*, 18:244–53.

Perrin EC, Newacheck P, Pless IB et al. (1993) Issues involved in the definition and classification of chronic health conditions. *Pediatr*, 91:787–93.

Perrin JM, Thyen U (1999) Chronic illness. In: Levine MD, Carey WB, Crocker AC (eds) *Developmental Behavioral Pediatrics.* Philadelphia, WB Saunders, pp. 335–45.

Plante WA, Lobato D, Engel R (2001) Review of group interventions for pediatric chronic conditions. *J Pediatr Psychol*, 26:435–53.

Powers SW (1999) Empirically supported treatments in pediatric psychology: procedure-related pain. *J Pediatr Psychol*, 24:1331–45.

Rapoff MA (1999) Assessing adherence. In: *Adherence to Pediatric Medical Regimens.* New York, Plenum Press, pp. 47–55.

Raymond-Speden E, Tripp G, Lawrence B, Holdaway D (2000) Intellectual, neuropsychological, and academic functioning in long-term survivors of leukemia. *J Pediatr Psychol*, 25:59–68.

Ryan-Wenger NM (1992) A taxonomy of children's coping strategies. *Am J Orthopsychiatry*, 62:256–63.

Sartain SA, Clarke CL, Heyman R (2000) Hearing the voices of children with chronic illness. *J Adv Nurs*, 32:913–92.

Schatz J, Finkle RL, Kellett JM, Kramer JH (2002) Cognitive functioning in children with sickle cell disease: a meta-analysis. *J Pediatr Psychol*, 27:739–48.

Schonfeld DJ (2002) Child's cognitive understanding of illness. In: Lewis M (ed.) *Child and Adolescent Psychiatry: A Comprehensive Textbook*. Philadelphia, Lippincott Williams & Wilkins, pp. 1119–23.

Sexson SB, Dingle AD (2001) Medical disorders. In: Kline FM, Silver LB, Russell SC (eds) *The Educator's Guide to Medical Issues in the Classroom*. Baltimore, Paul H Brookes Publishing Co., pp. 29–45.

Sexson SB, Dingle AD (1997) Medical problems that might present with academic difficulties. *Child Adolesc Psychiatric Clin N Am*, 6:509–22.

Sharpe D, Rossiter L (2002) Siblings of children with chronic illness: a meta-analysis. *J Pediatr Psychol*, 27, 699–710.

Slater J (1994) Psychiatric aspects of organ transplantation in children and adolescents. *Child Adolesc Psychiatric Clin N Am*, 3:557–96.

Slater JA (2002) Psychiatric aspects of cancer in childhood and adolescence. In: Lewis M (ed.) *Child and Adolescent Psychiatry: A Comprehensive Textbook*. Philadelphia, Lippincott Williams & Wilkins, pp. 1135–47.

Stewart JL (2003) Children living with chronic illness: an examination of their stressors, coping responses, and health outcomes. *Ann Rev Nurs Res*, 21:203–43.

Stoddard FJ (2002) Care of infants, children, and adolescents with burn injuries. In: Lewis M (ed.) *Child and Adolescent Psychiatry: A Comprehensive Textbook*. Philadelphia, Lippincott Williams & Wilkins, pp. 1188–208.

Tak YR, McCubbin M (2002) Family stress, perceived social support and coping following the diagnosis of child's congenital heart disease. *J Adv Nurs*, 39:190–9.

Tarnowski K, Brown R (2000) Psychological aspects of pediatric disorders. In: Hersen M, Ammaman R (eds) *Advanced Abnormal Child Psychology*, 2nd edn. Mahway, New Jersey, Lawrence Erlbaum Associates, pp. 131–2.

Tarnowski KJ, Rasnake LK (1994) Long-term psychosocial sequelae. In: Tarnowski KJ (ed.) *Behavioral Aspects of Pediatrics Burns*. New York, Plenum Press, pp. 81–118.

Thies KM, Walsh ME (1999) A developmental analysis of cognitive appraisal of stress in children and adolescents with chronic illness. *Children's Health Care*, 28:15–32.

Thompson RJ, Gustafson KE (1996) *Adaptation to Chronic Childhood Illness*. Washington DC, American Psychological Association.

Vitulano LA (2003) Psychosocial issues for children and adolescents with chronic illness: self-esteem, school functioning and sports participation. *Child Adolesc Psychiatric Clin N Am*, 12:585–92.

Wallender JL, Varni JW (1998) Effects of paediatric chronic physical disorders on child and family adjustment. *J Child Psychol Psychiatry*, 39:29–46.

Wamboldt MZ, Wamboldt FS (2000) Role of the family in the onset and outcome of childhood disorders: selected research findings. *J Am Acad Child Adolesc Psychiatry*, 39:1212–19.

Weinberg NZ, Rahdert E, Colliver JD, Glantz MD (1998) Adolescent substance abuse: a review of the past 10 years. *J Am Acad Child Adolesc Psychiatry*, 37:252–61.

Williams DT, Pleak RR, Hanesian H (2002a) Neurologic disorders. In: Lewis M (ed.) *Child and Adolescent Psychiatry: A Comprehensive Textbook*, 3rd edn. Philadelphia, Lippincott Williams & Wilkins, pp. 755–67.

Williams PD, Williams AR, Graff JC et al. (2002b) Interrelationships among variables affecting well siblings and mothers in families of children with a chronic illness or disability. *J Behav Med*, 25:411–24.

Wolters P, Brouwers P, Moss H (1995) Pediatric HIV disease: effect on cognition, learning, and behavior. *School Psychol Q*, 10:305–28.

Yeh C (2001) Adaptation in children with cancer: research with Roy's model. *Nurs Sci Q*, 14:141–8.

Young AM (1999) Hearing parents adjustment to a deaf child: the impact of a cultural linguistic model of deafness. *J Soc Work Prac*, 13:157–72.

Young B, Dixon-Woods M, Windridge KC, Heney D (2003) Managing communication with young people who have a potentially life threatening chronic illness: qualitative study of patients and parents. *Br Med J*, 326:305.

Chapter 18

Anderson M, Kaufman J, Simon TR et al. (2002) School-associated violent deaths in the United States, 1994–1999. *J Am Medical Assoc*, 286.

Bronfenbrenner U (1986) Ecology of the family as a context for human development: Research perspectives. *Devel Psychol*, 22:723–42.

Comer J (2003) Transforming the lives of children. In: Elias MJ, Arnold H, Steiger-Hussey C (eds) *EQ+IQ=Best Leadership Practices for Caring and Successful Schools*. Thousand Oaks, Corwin.

Erikson EH (1959) Identity and the life cycle. *Psychol Issues* 1:101–72.

Fromme A (1970) Introduction. In: Holt J (ed.) *How Children Fail*. New York, Dell.

Green R-J (1995) High achievement, underachievement, and learning disabilities: a family systems model. In: Ryan BA, Adams GR, Gullotta TO, Weissberg RP, Hampton RL (eds) *The Family-School Connection: Theory, Research, and Practice*. Thousand Oaks, Sage.

Hanson G (1997) The role of the school in the psychotherapy of the child or adolescent. *Child Adolesc Psychiatric Clin N Am*, 6.

Kozol J (1991) *Savage Inequalities*. New York, Crown.

Limber SP (2002) Addressing youth bullying behaviors. In: Fleming M, Towey K (eds) *Education Forum on Adolescent Health, Youth Bullying*. Chicago, The American Medical Association.

Mattison RE (2000) School consultation: a review of research on issues unique to the school environment. *J Am Acad Child Adolesc Psychiatry*, 394(4):402–13.

Olweus D (1993) *Bullying at School: What We Know and What We Can Do*. Oxford, Blackwell.

Rutter M (1980) School influences on children's behavior and development: the 1979 Kenneth Blackfan Lecture, Children's Hospital Medical Center, Boston. *Pediatr*, 65:208–20.

Smith EP, Boutte GS, Zigler E, Finn-Stevenson M (2004) Opportunities for schools to promote resilience in children and youth. In: Maton KI, Schellenbach CJ, Leadbeater BJ, Solarz AL (eds) *Investing in Children, Youth, Families and Communities: Strength-based research and policy*. Washington DC, American Psychological Association.

Chapter 19

References for clinicians

Alan Guttmacher Institute (2002a) *Facts in Brief: Teenagers' Sexual and Reproductive Health*. New York, Alan Guttmacher Institute.

Alan Guttmacher Institute (2002b) *Facts in Brief: Sexuality Education*. New York, Alan Guttmacher Institute.

American Academy of Child and Adolescent Psychiatry (AACAP) (1999) Practice parameters for the assessment and treatment of children and adolescents who are sexually abusive of others. *J Am Acad Child Adolesc Psychiatry*, 38(12):55S–76S.

American Psychiatric Association (2000) *Diagnostic and Statistical Manual of Mental Disorders*, 4th edn. Washington, DC, American Psychiatric Association.

Ammerman SD, Perelli E, Adler N, Irwin CE (1992) Do adolescents understand what physicians say about sexuality and health? *Clin Pediatrics*, 31(10):590–5.

Becker JV, Hunter JA (1993) Aggressive sex offenders. *Child Adolesc Psychiatric Clin N Am*, 2(3):477–87.

Blake SM, Ledsky R, Lehman T, Goodenow C, Sawyer R, Hack T (2001) Preventing sexual risk behaviors among gay, lesbian, and bisexual adolescents: the benefits of gay-sensitive HIV instruction in schools. *Am J Pub Health*, 91(6):940–6.

Bontempo DE, D'Augelli AR (2002) Effects of at-school victimization and sexual orientation on lesbian, gay, or bisexual youths' health risk behavior. *J Adolesc Health*, 30:364–74.

Brown LK, Danovsky MB, Lourie KJ, DiClemente JR, Ponton LE (1997) Adolescents with psychiatric disorders and the risk of HIV. *J Am Acad Child Adolesc Psychiatry*, 36(11):1609–17.

Bullough V (2004) Children and adolescents as sexual beings: a historical overview. *Child Adolesc Psychiatric Clin N Am*, 13:447–59.

Carter D, Al-Mateen C, Brookman RR (1996) Sexuality. In: Parmelee DX, David RB (eds) *Child and Adolescent Psychiatry*. St. Louis, MO, Mosby.

Cass VC (1990) The implications of homosexual identity formation for the Kinsey model and scale of sexual preference. In: McWhirter DP, Sanders SA, Reinisch JM (eds) *Homosexuality/Heterosexuality: Concepts of Sexual Orientation*. New York, Oxford University Press, pp. 239–66.

CDC (2004) Youth Risk Behavior Surveillance – United States, 2003. *MMWR*, May 21, 53(SS-2) Accessed at http://www.cdc.gov/mmwr/PDF/ss/ss5302.pdf on 5–23–04.

CDC-NCHST (2004) Fact sheet – Young People at Risk: HIV/AIDS Among America's Youth. Accessed at http://www.cdc.gov/hiv/pubs/facts/youth.htm on 5–22–04.

Clawson CL, Reese-Webber M (2003) The amount and timing of parent-adolescent sexual communication as predictors of late adolescent sexual risk-taking behaviors. *J Sex Res*, 40(3):256.

Cohen-Kettenis PT, Pfafflin F (2003) *Transgenderism and Intersexuality in Childhood and Adolescence: Making Choices*. Thousand Oaks, CA, Sage Publications.

Coleman E (1987) Assessment of sexual orientation. In: Coleman E (ed.) *Integrated Identity for Gay Men and Lesbians*. New York, Harrington Park Press, p. 9.

DeLamater J, Friedrich WN (1999) Human sexual development. *J Sex Res*, 39(1):10–14.

Denizet-Lewis B (2004) Friends, friends with benefits and the benefits of the local mall. *New York Times Magazine*, May 30. Accessed June 1, 2004 at http://www.nytimes.com/2004/05/30/magazine/30NONDATING.html?th.

Diamond M, Sigmundson HK (1997) Sex reassignment at birth: long-term review and clinical implications. *Arch Pediatr Adolesc Med*, 151:298–304.

DiClemente RJ, Wingood GM, Crosby R et al. (2001) Parental monitoring: association with adolescents' risk behaviors. *Pediatr*, 107(6):1363–8.

DiIorio C, Kelley M, Hockenberry-Eaton M (1999) Communication about sexual issues: mothers, fathers, and friends. *J Adolesc Health*, 24:181–9.

Faulkner AH, Cranston K (1998) Correlates of same-sex sexual behavior in a random sample of Massachusetts high school students. *Am J Pub Health*, 88(2):262–6.

Feldman J, Middleman AB (2002) Adolescent sexuality and sexual behavior. *Curr Opin Obstetr Gynecol*, 14(5):489–93.

Frayser SG (1993) Anthropologic perspective. *Child Adolesc Psychiatric Clin N Am*, 2(3):369–84.

Friedrich WN, Barbaresi WJ (2002) Sexuality. In: Kaye DL, Montgomery, ME, Munson SW (eds) *Child and Adolescent Mental Health*, Philadelphia, PA, Lippincott Williams & Wilkins, pp. 334–49.

Friedrich W, Grambsch P, Damon L et al. (1992) The child sexual behavior: normative and clinical comparisons. *Psychol Assess*, 4(3):303–11.

Friedrich W, Fisher J, Broughton D, Houston M, Shafran C (1998) Normative sexual behavior in children: a contemporary sample. *Pediatr*, 101(4).

Goldman R, Goldman J (1982) *Children's Sexual Thinking*. London, Routledge and Kegan Paul.

Gordon BN, Schroeder CS (1995) *Sexuality: A Developmental Approach to Problems*. New York, Plenum Press.

Harry Benjamin International Gender Dysphoria Association. The Standards of Care for Gender Identity Disorders.

Heiman ML, Leiblum S, Cohen SE, Pallitto LM (1998) A comparative survey of beliefs about 'normal' childhood sexual behaviors. *Child Abuse Neglect*, 22(4):289–304.

Herbert SE (2000) Psychological aspects of sexual differentiation disorders. In: Carpenter SE, Rock J (eds) *Pediatric and Adolescent Gynecology*, 2nd edn. Philadelphia, PA, Lippincott Williams & Wilkins, pp. 102–13.

Herdt G (2001) Social change, sexual diversity, and tolerance for bisexuality in the United States. In: D'Augelli AR, Patterson CJ (eds) *Lesbian, Gay, and Bisexual Identities and Youth: Psychological Perspectives*. New York, Oxford University Press, pp. 267–83.

Imperato-McGinley J, Peterson RE, Gautier T, Sturla E (1979) Androgens and the evolution of male-gender identity among male pseudohermaphrodites with 5(alpha) reductase deficiency. *New Engl J Med*, 300:1233–7.

Joffee A (1999) Introduction to adolescent medicine, Chapter 94. In: McMillan JA, DeAngelis CD, Feigin RD, Warshaw JB (eds) *Oski's Pediatrics: Principles and Practice*, 3rd edn. Philadelphia, PA, Lippincott Williams & Wilkins.

Johnson TC (1993) Assessment of sexual behavior problems in preschool-aged and latency-aged children. *Child Adolesc Psychiatric Clinics N Am*, 2(3):431–49.

Larsson I, Svedin C-G (2002) Sexual experiences in childhood: young adults' recollections. *Arch Sex Behav*, 31(3):263–73.

Lock J (1998) Psychosexual development in adolescents with chronic medical illnesses. *Psychosomatics*, 39(4):340–9.

Lock J (2001) Sexual development and chronic illness. Sexuality Symposium. Presentation at American Psychiatric Association annual meeting.

Lock J, Steiner H (1999) Gay, lesbian, and bisexual youth risks for emotional, physical, and social problems: results from a community-based survey. *J Am Acad Child Adolesc Psychiatry*, 38(3):297–304.

Menvielle E (1998) Gender identity disorder [Comment. Letter]. *J Am Acad Child Adolesc Psychiatry*, 37(3):243–5.

Meyer-Bahlburg HFL (1993) Gender identity development in intersex patients. *Child Adolesc Psychiatric Clin N Am*, 2:501.

Miller KS, Kotchick BA, Dorsey S, Forehand R, Ham AY (1998) Family communication about sex: what are parents saying and are their adolescents listening? *Family Planning Perspectives*, 30(5):218–22, 235.

Minter S (1999) Diagnosis and treatment of gender identity disorder (GID) in children. In: Rottnek M (ed.) *Sissies and Tomboys: Gender Nonconformity and Homosexual Childhood*. New York, New York University Press, pp. 9–33.

Money J, Ehrhardt AA (1972) *Man and Woman, Boy and Girl: The Differentiation and Dimorphism of Gender Identity from Conception to Maturity*. Baltimore, MD, The Johns Hopkins University Press.

Money J, Pranzarone GF (1993) Development of paraphilia in childhood and adolescence. *Child Adolesc Psychiatric Clin N Am*, 2(3):463–75.

Moser C, Kleinplatz PJ, Zuccarini D, Reiner WG (2004) Situating unusual child and adolescent sexual behavior in context. *Child Adolesc Psychiatric Clin N Am*, 13:569–89.

Pleak R (1999) Ethical issues in diagnosing and treating gender-dysphoric children and adolescents. In: Rottnek M (ed.) *Sissies and Tomboys: Gender Nonconformity and Homosexual Childhood*. New York, New York University Press, pp. 34–51.

Ponton LE, Judice S (2004) Typical adolescent sexual development. *Child Adolesc Psychiatric Clin N Am*, 13:497–511.

Reiner WG, Gearhart JP (2004) Discordant sexual identity in some genetic males with cloacal exstrophy assigned to female sex at birth. *New Engl J Med*, 350(4):333–41.

Remez L (2000) Oral sex among adolescents: is it sex or is it abstinence? *Family Planning Perspectives*, 32(6):298–304.

Rosenberg M (2003) Recognizing gay, lesbian, and transgender teen in a child and adolescent psychiatry practice. *J Am Acad Child Adolesc Psychiatry*, 42(12):1517–21.

Rosenfeld AA, Wasserman S (1993) Sexual development in the early school-aged child. *Child Adolesc Psychiatric Clin N Am*, 2(3):393–406.

Rotheram-Borus MJ, Gwadz M (1993) Sexuality among youths at high risk. *Child Adolesc Psychiatric Clin N Am*, 2(3):415–30.

Savin-Williams RC, Cohen KM (2004) Homoerotic development during childhood and adolescence. *Child Adolesc Psychiatric Clin N Am*, 13:529–49.

Schuster MA, Bell RM, Kanouse DE (1996) The sexual practices of adolescent virgins: genital sexual activities of high school students who have never had vaginal intercourse. *Am J Pub Health*, 86(11):1570–6.

Swann SK, Herbert SE (1999) Ethical issues in the clinical treatment of gender dysphoric adolescents. *J Gay Lesbian Soc Serv*, 10(3/4):19–34.

Yates A (2004) Biologic perspectives on early erotic development. *Child Adolesc Psychiatric Clin N Am*, 13:479–96.

Yates A (2002) Childhood sexuality. In: Lewis M (ed.) *Child and Adolescent Psychiatry*, 2nd edn. Philadelphia, Lippincott Williams & Wilkins.

Zucker KJ (2004) Gender identity development and issues. *Child Adolesc Psychiatric Clin N Am*, 13:551–68.

Zucker KJ, Bradley SJ (1995) *Gender Identity Disorder and Psychosexual Problems in Children and Adolescents*. New York, Guilford Press.

Resources for parents

Fairchild B, Hayward N (1989) *Now That You Know: What Every Parent Should Know About Homosexuality*. San Diego, CA, Harcourt, Brace, Jovanovich.

Fenwick E, Smith T (1994) *Adolescence: The Survival Guide for Parents and Teenagers*. New York, Dorling Kindersley, Inc.

Johnson TC (2000) *Understanding Children's Sexual Behaviors: What's Natural and Healthy*. South Pasadena, CA.

Ponton L (2000) *The Sex Lives of Teenagers: Revealing the Secret Lives of Boys and Girls*. New York, Dutton.

Ponton L (2005) *'What Does Gay Mean?' How to Talk With Kids about Sexual Orientation and Prejudice*. National Mental Health Association. Accessed at http://www.nmha.org/whatdoesgaymean/ on 5–17–05.)

Pruitt D (ed.) (2000) *Your Adolescent: Emotional, Behavioral, and Cognitive Development from Early Adolescence Through the Teen Years*. New York, HarperCollins.

Richardson J, Schuster MA (2003) *Everything You Never Wanted Your Kids to Know About Sex (but Were Afraid They'd Ask). The Secrets to Surviving Your Child's Sexual Development From Birth to the Teens*. New York, Three Rivers Press.

Tuerk C, Menvielle E, de Jesus J (2003) *If you are Concerned about your Child's Gender Behaviors: A Guide for Parents*. Children's National Medical Center Outreach Program for Children with Gender Variant Behaviors and their Families, http://www.dcchildrens.com/gendervariance/. (Also available in Spanish.)

Resources for children and adolescents

Bell R et al. (1998) *Changing Bodies, Changing Lives: A Book for Teens on Sex and Relationships*, 3rd edn. New York, Random House.

Bornstein K (1998) *My Gender Workbook*. New York, Routledge.

Gardner-Loulan J, Lopez B, Quackenbush M (1991) *Period*. Volcano, CA, Volcano Press, Inc.

Harrison M (1995) *The Preteen's First Book about Love, Sex, and AIDS*. Washington DC, American Psychiatric Press.

Rench J (1990) *Understanding Sexual Identity: A Book for Gay and Lesbian Teens and Their Friends*. Minneapolis, MN, Lerner Publications Co.

Chapter 20

American Academy of Child and Adolescent Psychiatry (2001) Practice parameter for the assessment and treatment of children and adolescents with suicidal behavior. American Academy of Child and Adolescent Psychiatry, *J Am Acad Child Adolesc Psychiatry*, 40(Suppl 7):24S-51S.

American Psychiatric Association (2000) *Diagnostic and Statistical Manual of Mental Disorders DSM IV-TR*, 4th edn. Washington, DC, American Psychiatric Association.

Apter A, Gothelf D, Orbach I, Weizman R, Ratzoni G, Har-Even D, Tyano S (1995) Correlation of suicidal and violent behavior in different diagnostic categories in hospitalized adolescent patients. *J Am Acad Child Adolesc Psychiatry*, 34(7):912–918.

Ary DV, Duncan TE, Duncan SC, Hops H (1999) Adolescent problem behavior: the influence of parents and peers. *Behav Res Ther*, 37(3):217–230.

Barkley RA (2002) Major life activity and health outcomes associated with attention-deficit/hyperactivity disorder. *J Clin Psychiatry*, 63(Suppl 12):10–5.

Bechara A, Damasio H, Damasio AR, Lee GP (1999) Different contributions of the human amygdala and ventromedial prefrontal cortex to decision-making. *J Neurosci*, 19(13):5473–5481.

Bechara A, Tranel D, Damasio H, Damasio AR (1996) Failure to respond autonomically to anticipated future outcomes following damage to prefrontal cortex. *Cereb Cortex*, 6(2):215–225.

Bhangoo RK, Leibenluft E (2002) Affective neuroscience and the study of normal and abnormal emotion regulation. *Child Adolesc Psychiatr Clin N Am*, 11(3):519–532.

Booth A, Johnson DR, Granger DA, Crouter AC, McHale S (2003) Testosterone and child and adolescent adjustment: the moderating role of parent-child relationships. *Dev Psychol*, 39(1):85–98.

Brent DA, Oquendo M, Birmaher B, Greenhill L, Kolko D, Stanley B, Zelazny J, Brodsky B, Firinciogullari S, Ellis SP, Mann JJ (2003) Peripubertal suicide attempts in offspring of suicide attempters with siblings concordant for suicidal behavior. *Am J Psychiatry*, 160(8):1486–1493.

Cardinal RN, Pennicott DR, Sugathapala CL, Robbins TW, Everitt BJ (2001) Impulsive choice induced in rats by lesions of the nucleus accumbens core. *Science*, 292(5526):2499–2501.

Carlson GA, Mick E (2003) Drug-induced disinhibition in psychiatrically hospitalized children. *J Child Adolesc Psychopharmacol*, 13(2):153–163.

Casey BJ, Castellanos FX, Giedd JN, Marsh WL, Hamburger SD, Schubert AB, Vauss YC, Vaituzis AC, Dickstein DP, Sarfatti SE, Rapoport JL (1997) Implication of right frontostriatal circuitry in response inhibition and attention-deficit/hyperactivity disorder. *J Am Acad Child Adolesc Psychiatry*, 36(3):374–383.

Cloninger CR, Svrakic DM, Bayon C, Przybeck TR (1999) Measurement of psychopathology as variants of personality. In: Cloninger CR (ed.) *Personality and Psychopathology*. American Psychiatric Press, Inc., Washington DC.

Comings DE, Comings BG (1987) A controlled study of Tourette syndrome. II. Conduct. *Am J Hum Genet*, 41(5):742–760.

DeLong GR, Aldershof AL (1987) Long-term experience with lithium treatment in childhood: correlation with clinical diagnosis. *J Am Acad Child Adolesc Psychiatry*, 26(3):389–394.

Dolan M, Park I (2002) The neuropsychology of antisocial personality disorder. *Psychol Med*, 32(3):417–427.

Elliott DS, Tolan PH (1999) Youth violence prevention, intervention, and social policy: an overview. In: Flannery DJ, Huff CR (eds.) *Youth Violence: Prevention, Intervention, and Social Policy*, American Psychiatric Press, Inc., Washington, DC.

Flisher AJ, Kramer RA, Hoven CW, King RA, Bird HR, Davies M, Gould MS, Greenwald S, Lahey BB, Regier DA, Schwab-Stone M, Shaffer D (2000) Risk behavior in a community sample of children and adolescents. *J Am Acad Child Adolesc Psychiatry*, 39(7):881–887.

Fox JA (1996) *Trends in juvenile violence: a report to the United States Attorney General on current and future rates of juvenile offending.* Bureau of Justice Statistics, United States Department of Justice.

Geiger JD, Newsted J, Drongowski RA, Lelli JL (2001) Car surfing: an underreported mechanism of serious injury in children and adolescents. *J Pediatr Surg*, 36(1):232–234.

Healy D (2003) Lines of evidence on the risks of suicide with selective serotonin reuptake inhibitors. *Psychother Psychosom*, 72(2):71–79.

Henggeler SW, Melton GB, Smith LA (1992) Family presentation using multisystemic therapy: an effective alternative to incarcerating serious juvenile offenders. *J Consult Clin Psychol*, 60(6):953–961.

Henggeler SW, Schoenwald SK, Rowland MD, Cunningham PB (2002) *Serious Emotional Disturbance in Children and Adolescents: Multisystemic Therapy*, 1st edn. New York, Guilford Press.

Herpertz SC, Wenning B, Mueller B, Qunaibi M, Sass H, Herpertz-Dahlmann B (2001) Psychophysiological responses in ADHD boys with and without conduct disorder: implications for adult antisocial behavior. *J Am Acad Child Adolesc Psychiatry*, 40(10):1222–1230.

Klein RG, Abikoff H, Klass E, Ganeles D, Seese LM, Pollack S (1997) Clinical efficacy of methylphenidate in conduct disorder with and without attention deficit hyperactivity disorder. *Arch Gen Psychiatry*, 54(12):1073–1080.

Kruesi MJ, Hibbs ED, Zahn TP, Keysor CS, Hamburger SD, Bartko JJ, Rapoport JL (1992) A 2-year prospective follow-up study of children and adolescents with disruptive behavior disorders. Prediction by cerebrospinal fluid 5-hydroxyindoleacetic acid, homovanillic acid, and autonomic measures. *Arch Gen Psychiatry*, 49(6):429–435.

Kuperman S, Stewart MA (1987) Use of propranolol to decrease aggressive outbursts in younger patients. Open study reveals potentially favorable outcome. *Psychosomatics*, 28(6):315–319.

Leibenluft E, Charney DS, Pine DS (2003) Researching the pathophysiology of pediatric bipolar disorder. *Biol Psychiatry*, 53(11):1009–1020.

Li X, Stanton B, Feigelman S (2000) Impact of perceived parental monitoring on adolescent risk behavior over 4 years. *J Adolesc Health*, 27(1):49–56.

Mitchell DG, Colledge E, Leonard A, Blair RJ (2002) Risky decisions and response reversal: is there evidence of orbitofrontal cortex dysfunction in psychopathic individuals? *Neuropsychologia*, 40(12):2013–2022.

Moeller FG, Barratt ES, Dougherty DM, Schmitz JM, Swann AC (2001) Psychiatric aspects of impulsivity. *Am J Psychiatry*, 158(11):1783–1793.

National Institute of Mental Health (2003) Suicide Facts. National Institute of Mental Health.

Olweus D, Mattsson A, Schalling D, Low H (1988) Circulating testosterone levels and aggression in adolescent males: a causal analysis. *Psychosom Med*, 50(3):261–272.

Pappadopulos E, MacIntyre JC II, Crismon ML et al. (2003) Treatment recommendations for the use of antipsychotics for aggressive youth (TRAAY) Part II. 42(2):145–161.

Perrine KR (1991) Psychopathology in epilepsy. *Semin Neurol*, 11(2):175–181.

Petridou E, Zavitsanos X, Dessypris N, Frangakis C, Mandyla M, Doxiadis S, Trichopoulos D (1997) Adolescents in high-risk trajectory: clustering of risky behavior and the origins of socioeconomic health differentials. *Prev Med*, 26(2):215–219.

Pickett W, Garner MJ, Boyce WF, King MA (2002) Gradients in risk for youth injury associated with multiple-risk behaviours: a study of 11,329 Canadian adolescents. *Soc Sci Med*, 55(6):1055–1068.

Pope HG Jr, Kouri EM, Hudson JI (2000) Effects of supraphysiologic doses of testosterone on mood and aggression in normal men: a randomized controlled trial. *Arch Gen Psychiatry*, 57(2):133–140.

Posner MI, Rothbart MK (2000) Developing mechanisms of self-regulation, *Dev Psychopathol*, 12(3):427–441.

Quadrel MJ, Fischhoff B, Davis W (1993) Adolescent (in)vulnerability. *Am Psychol*, 48(2):102–116.

Raine A (1996) Autonomic nervous system factors underlying disinhibited, antisocial, and violent behavior. Biosocial perspectives and treatment implications. *Ann N Y Acad Sci*, 20(794):46–59.

Rubinow DR, Schmidt PJ (1996) Androgens, brain, and behavior. *Am J Psychiatry*, 153(8):974–984.

Schmeck K, Poustka F (2001) Temperament and disruptive behavior disorders. *Psychopathology*, 34(3):159–163.

Steiner H, Saxena K, Chang K (2003) Psychopharmacologic strategies for the treatment of aggression in juveniles. *CNS Spectr*, 8(4):298–308.

Susman EJ, Inoff-Germain G, Nottelmann ED, Loriaux DL, Cutler GB Jr, Chrousos GP (1987) Hormones, emotional dispositions, and aggressive attributes in young adolescents. *Child Dev*, 58(4):1114–34.

Tanev K (2003) Neuroimaging and neurocircuitry in post-traumatic stress disorder: what is currently known? *Curr Psychiatry Rep*, 5(5):369–383.

Taylor MA (1993) *Neuropsychiatric Guide to Modern Everyday Psychiatry*. Free Press, New York, Toronto.

Vitiello B, Stoff DM (1997) Subtypes of aggression and their relevance to child psychiatry. *J Am Acad Child Adolesc Psychiatry*, 36(3):307–315.

Weisfeld G (1999) *Evolutionary Principles of Human Adolescence*. Basic Books, New York.

Weller EB, Rowan A, Elia J, Weller RA (1999) Aggressive behavior in patients with attention-deficit/hyperactivity disorder, conduct disorder, and pervasive developmental disorders. *J Clin Psychiatry*, 60 (Suppl 15):5–11.

Wozniak J, Biederman J (1997) Mania in children with PDD. *J Am Acad Child Adolesc Psychiatry*, 36(12):1646–1647.

Wu Y, Stanton BF, Gilbraith J, Kaljee L, Cottrell L, Li X, Harris CV, D'Alessandri D, Burns JM (2003) Sustaining and broadening intervention impact: a longitudinal randomized trial of 3 adolescent risk reduction approaches. *Pediatr*, 111(1):e32–e38.

Young TL, Zimmerman R (1998) Clueless: parental knowledge of risk behaviors of middle school students. *Arch Pediatr Adolesc Med*, 152(11):1137–1139.

Chapter 21

Ainsworth MDS, Blehar MC, Waters E, Wall S (1978) *Patterns of Attachment: A Psychological Study of the Strange Situation*. Hillsdale, NJ, Erlbaum.

Albus K, Dozier M (1999) Indiscriminate friendliness and terror of strangers in infancy: contributions from the study of infants in foster care. *Infant Mental Health J*, 20:30–41.

American Psychiatric Association (1994) *Diagnostic and Statistical Manual of Mental Disorders*, 4th edn (DSM-IV) Washington, DC, American Psychiatric Association.

Bakermans-Kranenburg MJ, van Ijzendoorn MH, Juffer F (2003) Less is more: meta-analyses of sensitivity and attachment interventions in early childhood. *Psychol Bull*, 129:195–215.

Bender DS, Farber BA, Geller JD (2001) Cluster B personality traits and attachment. *J Am Acad Psychoanal*, 29:551–563.

Boris NW, Zeanah CH (1998) Clinical disturbances of attachment in infancy and early childhood. *Curr Opin Pediatr*, 10:365–368.

Boris NW, Zeanah CH. (1999) Disturbances and disorders of attachment in infancy: an overview. *Infant Mental Health J*, 20:1–9.

Boris NW, Zeanah CH, Larrieu JA, Scheeringa MS, Heller SS (1998) Attachment disorders in infancy and early childhood: a preliminary investigation of diagnostic criteria. *Am J Psychiatry*, 155:295–297.

Bowlby J (1944) Fourty-four juvenile thieves: their characters and home life. *Int J Psychoanal*, 25L:19–52.

Bowlby J (1988) *A Secure Base: Clinical Implications of Attachment Theory*. London, Routledge.

Brisch KH. (2002) *Treating Attachment Disorders: From Theory to Therapy*. New York, Guilford.

Byng-Hall J (1995) Creating a secure family base: some implications of attachment theory for family therapy. *Fam Proc*, 34:45–58.

Cicchetti D, Toth SL, Rogosch FA. (1999) Toddler-parent psychotherapy as a preventive intervention to alter attachment organization in offspring of depressed mothers. *Attach Hum Devel*, 1:34–66.

Cummings M, Cicchetti D (1990) Toward a transactional model of relations between attachment and depression. In: Greenberg MT, Cicchetti D, Cummings M (eds) *Attachment in the Preschool Years: Theory, Research, and Intervention* Chicago, University of Chicago, pp. 339–372

Eyberg S, Boggs S, Algina J (1995) Parent-child interaction therapy: A psychosocial model for the treatment of young children with conduct problem behavior and their families. *Psychopharmacol Bull*, 31:83–91.

Fonagy P (2001) *Attachment Theory and Psychoanalysis*. New York, Other Press.

Fonagy P, Leigh T, Steele M, Steele H, Kennedy R, Mattoon G, Target M, Gerber A (1996) The relation of attachment status, psychiatric classification and response of psychotherapy. *J Consult Clini Psychol*, 64:22–31.

Fraiberg S, Adelson E, Shapiro V (1975) Ghosts in the nursery: A psychoanalytic approach to the problem of impaired infant-mother relationships. *J Am Acad Child Psychiatry*, 14:387–422.

Green J (2003) Are attachment disorders best seen as social impairment syndromes? *Attach Hum Devel*, 5, 259–264.

Guerney BJ. (1964) Filial therapy: description and rationale. *J Consult Clin Psychol*, 28:304–310.

Hall SE (2003) Behavioral and personality characteristics of children with reactive attachment disorder. *J Psychol*, 137:145–163.

Hanson RF, Spratt EG. (2000) Reactive attachment disorder: What we know about the disorder and implications for treatment. *Child Maltreatment*, 5:137–145.

Harlow HF (1961) The development of affectional patterns in infant monkeys. In: Foss BM (ed.) *Determinants of Infant Behavior* (Vol 1) New York, Wiley, pp. 75–97.

Hughes DA (2003) Psychological interventions for the spectrum of attachment disorders and intrafamilial trauma. *Attach Hum Devel*, 5:271–277.

James B (1994) *Handbook for Treatment of Attachment-trauma Problems in Children*. New York, Free Press.

Karen R (1994) *Becoming Attached: Unfolding the Mystery of the Infant-Mother Bond and its Impact on Later Life*. New York, Warner Books.

Keck GC, Kupecky R (1995) *Adopting the Hurt Child*. Colorado springs, CO, Pinon Press.

Kreppner JM, O'Connor TG, Rutter M (2001) Can inattention/over-activity be an institutional deprivation syndrome? *J Abnormal Child Psychiatry*, 29:513–528.

Larner G (1996) Narrative child family therapy. *Fam Proc*, 35:423–440.

Levy TM, Orlans M (1999) Kids who kill. *Forensic Examiner*, March/April, 19–24.

Lieberman AF (2003) The treatment of attachment disorder in infancy and early childhood: Reflections from clinical intervention with later-adopted foster care children. *Attach Hum Devel*, 5:279–282.

Lieberman AF, Zeanah CH (1999) Contributions of attachment theory to infant-parent psychotherapy and other interventions with infants and young children. In: Cassidy J, Shaver P (eds) *Handbook of Attachment*. New York, Guilford, p. 555–574

Lochman JE, Coie JD, Underwood MK, Terry R (1993) Effectiveness of a social relations intervention program for aggressive and nonaggressive, rejected children. *J Consult Clin Psychol*, 61:1053–1058.

Marvin RS, Whelan WF. (2003) Disordered attachments: toward evidence-based clinical practice. *Attach Hum Devel*, 5, 283–288.

Minde K (2003a) Attachment problems as a spectrum disorder: implications for diagnosis and treatment. *Attach Hum Devel*, 5:289–296.

Minde K (2003b) Assessment and treatment of attachment disorders. *Curr Opin Psychiatry*, 16:377–381.

Minnis H (2001) Reactive attachment disorder [Letter to the Editor]. *J Am Acad Child Adolesc Psychiatry*, 40:132.

Minnis H, Keck G (2003) A clinical/research dialogue on reactive attachment disorder. *Attach Hum Devel*, 5:297–301.

O'Connor T, Bredenkamp D, Rutter M (1999) English and Romanian Adoptees (ERA) Study Team. Attachment disturbances and disorders in children exposed to early severe deprivation. *Inf Mental Health J*, 20:10–29.

O'Connor TG, Rutter M (2000) Attachment disorder behavior following early severe deprivation: extension and longitudinal follow-up. *J Am Acad Child Adolesc Psychiatry*, 39:703–712.

O'Connor TG, Zeanah CH (2003) Attachment disorders: Assessment strategies and treatment approaches. *Attach Hum Devel*, 5:223–244.

Richters MM, Volkmar FR. (1994) Reactive attachment disorder of infancy or early childhood. *J Am Acad Child Adolesc Psychiatry*, 33:328–332.

Scott S (2003) Integrating attachment theory with other approaches to developmental psychopathology. *Attach Hum Devel*, 5:307–312.

Sexson SB, Glanville DN, Kaslow NJ. (2001) Attachment and depression: Implications for family therapy. *Child Adolesc Psychiatric Clin N Am*, 10:465–486.

Sheperis CJ, Doggett RA, Hoda NE, Blanchard T, Renfro-Michel EL., Holdiness SH, Schlagheck R (2003) The development of an assessment protocol for reactive attachment disorder. *J Mental Health Counseling*, 25:291–311.

Shields A, Cicchetti D (1998) Reactive aggression among maltreated children: the contributions of attention and emotion dysregulation. *J Clin Child Psychol*, 27:381–395.

Smyke AT, Dumitrescu A, Zeanah CH. (2002) Attachment disturbances in young children. I: The continuum of caretaking casualty. *J Am Acad Child Adolesc Psychiatry*, 41:972–982.

Spitz, R (1947) *Grief: A Peril in Infancy* [Film]. University Park, PA, Penn State Audio Visual Services.

Sund AM, Wichstrom L (2002) Insecure attachment as a risk factor for future depressive symptoms in early adolescence. *J Am Acad Child Adolesc Psychiatry*, 41:1478–1485.

Van Fleet, R (1994) *Filial Therapy: Strengthening Parent-child Relationships through Play*. Sarasota, Professional Resource Press.

Webster-Stratton C, Hammond M (1997) Treating children with early-onset conduct problems: A comparison of child and parent training interventions. *J Consulting Clin Psychol*, 65:93–109.

Wilson SL (2001) Attachment disorders: review and current status. *J Psychol*, 135:37–52.

Yule W (2002) Posts-traumatic stress disorders. In: Rutter M, Taylor E (eds). *Child and Adolescent Psychiatry*, 4th edn. Oxford, Blackwell Science.

Zeanah CH, Smyke AT, Dumitrescu A (2002) Attachment disturbance in young children. II: Indiscriminate behavior and institutional care. *J Am Acad Child Adolesc Psychiatry*, 41:983–989.

Chapter 22

Amaya-Jackson L, Reynolds V, Murray MC et al. (2002) Cognitive-behavioral treatment for pediatric posttraumatic stress disorder: protocol and application in school and community settings. *J Cog Behav Practice* 10:2–35.

American Psychiatric Association (1987) *Diagnostic and Statistical Manual of Mental Disorders*, 3rd edn revised. Washington DC, American Psychiatric Press, pp. 247–251.

American Psychiatric Association (2000) *Diagnostic and Statistical Manual of Mental Disorders*, 4th edn text revision. Washington DC, American Psychiatric Press, pp. 424–432.

Armsworth MW, Holaday M (1993) The effects of psychological trauma on children and adolescents. *J Counseling Devel* 72:49–56.

Arora RC, Fichtner CG, O'Connor F, Crayton JW (1993) Paroxetine binding in the blood platelets of post-traumatic stress disorder patients. *Life Sci* 53:919–928.

Beers SR, De Bellis MD (2002) Neuropsychological function in children with maltreatment-related posttraumatic stress disorder. *Am J Psychiatry*, 159:483–486.

Benkelfat C (1993) Serotonergic mechanisms in psychiatric disorders: New research tools, new ideas. *Int Clin Psychopharmacol* 8 (Suppl 2):53–56.

Berliner L, Saunders B (1996) Treating fear and anxiety in sexually abused children: results of a controlled two-year follow-up study. *Child Maltreatment* 1:294–309.

Birmaher B, Brent D, and the Work Group on Quality Issues (1998) Practice parameters for the assessment and treatment of children and adolescents with depressive disorders. *Am Acad Child Adolesc Psychiatry* 37(Suppl 10):63S-83S.

Blank AS (1993) The longitudinal course of posttraumatic stress disorder. In: Davidson JRT, Foa EB (eds) *Posttraumatic Stress Disorder DSM-IV and Beyond*. American Psychiatric Press I, Washington, DC, pp. 3–22.

Bledsoe BE (2003) Critical incident stress management (CISM) benefit or risk for emergency services? *Prehosp Emergency Care* 7:272–279.

Boney-McCoy S, Finkelhor D (1996) Is youth victimization related to trauma symptoms and depression after controlling for prior symptoms and family relationships? A longitudinal, prospective study. *J Consult Clin Psychol* 64:1406–1416.

Brady K, Pearlstein T, Asnis GM, Baker D, Rothbaum B, Sikes CR, et al. (2000) Efficacy and safety of sertraline treatment of posttraumatic stress disorder: a randomized controlled trial. *J Am Med Assoc*, 283:1837–44.

Bremner JD, Davis M, Southwick SM, Krystal JH, Charney DS (1993) Neurobiology of posttraumatic stress disorder. In: Oldham JM, Riba MB, Tasman A (eds) *In Review of Psychiatry*. Washington, DC, American Psychiatric Press, Inc., pp. 183–205.

Breslau N, Davis GC, Peterson E, Schultz LR (2000) A second look at comorbidity in victims of trauma: the posttraumatic stress disorder-major depression connection. *Biolog Psychiatry*, 48(9):902–909.

Brewin CR, Andrews B, Rose S (2003) Diagnostic overlap between acute stress disorder and PTSD in victims of violent crime. *Am J Psychiatry*, 160:783–785.

Bryant RA, Harvey AG (1997) Acute stress disorder: a critical review of diagnostic issues. *Clin Psychol Rev*, 17:757–773.

Bryant RA, Harvey AG (2002) Delayed-onset posttraumatic stress disorder: a prospective evaluation. *Aust N Z J Psychiatry*, 36:205–209.

Caine RM, Ter-Bagdasarian L (2003) Early identification and management of critical incident stress. *Crit Care Nurse*, 23:59–65.

Carrion VG, Weems CF, Eliez S, Patwardhan A, Brown W, Ray RD, et al. (2001a) Attenuation of frontal asymmetry in pediatric posttraumatic stress disorder. *Biolog Psychiatry*, 50:943–951.

Carrion VG, Weems CF, Ray RD, Glaser B, Hessl D, Reiss AL (2002) Diurnal salivary cortisol in pediatric posttraumatic stress disorder. *Biolog Psychiatry*, 51:575–582.

Carrion VG, Weems CF, Ray RD, Reiss AL (2001b) Toward an empirical definition of pediatric PTSD: the phenomenology of PTSD symptoms in youth. *J Am Acad Child Adolesc Psychiatry* 41:166–173.

Charney DS, Deutch AY, Krystal JH, Southwich SM, Davis M (1993) Psychobiological mechanisms of posttraumatic stress disorder. *Arch Gen Psychiatry* 50:294–305.

Charney DS, Nestler EJ, Bunny BS (1999) *Neurobiology of Mental Illness*. New York, NY, Oxford Press.

Chemtob CM, Narkashima JP, Hamada RS (2002) Psychosocial intervention for postdisaster trauma symptoms in elementary school children. *Arch Pediatr Adolesc Med*, 156:211–216.

Chrousos GP, Gold PW (1992) The concepts of stress and stress system disorders: Overview of physical and behavioral homeostasis. *J Am Med Assoc*, 267:1244–1252.

Clark DB, Lesnick L, Hegedus A (1997) Trauma and other stressors in adolescent alcohol dependence and abuse. *J Am Acad Child Adolesc Psychiatry*, 36:1744–1751.

Cohen JA, and the Work Group on Quality Issues (1998) Practice parameters for the assessment and treatment of children and adolescents with posttraumatic stress disorder. *Am Acad Child Adolesc Psychiatry* 37(Suppl 10):4S-26S.

Cohen JA, Mannarino AP (1993) A treatment model for sexually abused preschool children. *J Interpers Violence*, 8:115–131.

Cohen JA, Mannarino AP (1996) Factors that mediate treatment outcome of sexually abused preschool children. *J Am Acad Child Adolesc Psychiatry*, 35:402–10.

Cohen JA, Mannarino AP (1998a) Factors that mediate treatment outcome of sexually abused preschool children: six- and 12-month follow-up. *J Am Acad Child Adolesc Psychiatry*, 37:44–51.

Cohen JA, Mannarino AP (1998b) Interventions for sexually abused children: initial treatment findings. *Child Maltreatment*, 3:17–26.

Cohen JA, Mannarino AP, Rogal SS (2001) Treatment practices for childhood posttraumatic stress disorder. *Child Abuse Neglect*, 25:123–136.

Croft S, Celano (2005) Management of attachment problems and child abuse and neglect. In: Sexson S (ed.) *Child and Adolescent Psychiatry*. Oxford, Blackwell Publishing.

Davidson JRT, Fairbank JA (1993) The epidemiology of posttraumatic stress disorder. In: Davidson JRT, Foa EB (eds) *Posttraumatic Stress Disorder DSM-IV and Beyond*. Washington, DC, American Psychiatric Press, pp. 147–169.

Davis LV, Carlson BE (1987) Observation of spouse abuse: what happens to the children? *J Interpers Violence*, 2:278–291.

Daviss WB, Mooney D, Racusin R, Ford JD, Fleischer A, McHugo GJ (2000) Predicting posttraumatic stress after hospitalization for pediatric injury. *J Am Acad Child Adolesc Psychiatry*, 39:576–583.

De Bellis MD (2001) Developmental traumatology: the psychobiological development of maltreated children and its implications for research, treatment, and policy. *Devel Psychopathol*, 13:537–561.

De Bellis MD (2003) The neurobiology of posttraumatic stress disorder across the life cycle. In: Soares JC, Gershon S (eds), *The Handbook of Medical Psychiatry*. NY, Marcel Dekker Inc., pp. 449–466.

De Bellis MD, Baum A, Birmaher B, Keshavan M, Eccard CH, Boring AM et al. (1999a) A.E. Bennett Research Award. Developmental traumatology. Part I: Biological stress systems. *Biolog Psychiatry*, 45:1259–1270.

De Bellis MD, Keshavan M, Baum A, Birmaher B, Clark DB, Casey BJ et al. (1999b) A.E. Bennett Research Award. Developmental traumatology. Part I and II: Biological stress systems and Brain development. *Biolog Psychiatry*, 45:1259–1284.

De Bellis MD, Keshavan M, Clark DB et al. (1999c) A.E. Bennett Research Award. Developmental traumatology. Part II: Brain development. *Biolog Psychiatry*, 45:1271–1284.

De Bellis MD, Casey BJ, Dahl R, Birmaher B, Williamson D, Thomas KM et al. (2000) A pilot study of amygdala volumes in pediatric generalized anxiety disorder. *Biolog Psychiatry*, 48:51–57.

De Bellis MD, Chrousos GP, Dorn LD, Burke L, Helmers K, Kling MA et al. (1994a) Hypothalamic-pituitary-adrenal axis dysregulation in sexually abused girls. *J Clin Endocrinol Metab*, 78:249–255.

De Bellis MD, Hall J, Boring AM, Frustaci K, Moritz G (2001a) A pilot longitudinal study of hippocampal volumes in pediatric maltreatment-related posttraumatic stress disorder. *Biolog Psychiatry*, 50:305–309.

De Bellis MD, Keshavan M, Shifflett H, Iyengar S, Beers SR, Hall J, et al. (2002a) Brain structures in pediatric maltreatment-related PTSD: a sociodemographically matched study. *Biolog Psychiatry* 52:1066–1078.

De Bellis MD, Keshavan M, Shifflett H, Iyengar S, Dahl R, Axelson DA et al. (2002b) Superior temporal gyrus volumes in pediatric generalized anxiety disorder. *Biolog Psychiatry*, 51:553–562.

De Bellis MD, Keshavan MS (2003) Sex differences in brain maturation in maltreatment-related pediatric posttraumatic stress disorder. *Special Edition of Neurosciences and Biobehavioral Reviews: Brain Development, Sex Differences, and Stress: Implications for Psychopathology*, 27:103–117.

De Bellis MD, Keshavan MS, Harenski KA (2001b) Case study: anterior cingulate N-acetylasparate concentrations during treatment in a maltreated child with PTSD. *J Child Adolesc Psychopharmacol,* 11:311–316.

De Bellis MD, Lefter L, Trickett PK, Putnam FW (1994b) Urinary catecholamine excretion in sexually abused girls. *J Am Acad Child Adolesc Psychiatry,* 33:320–327.

De Bellis MD, Putnam FW (1994) The psychobiology of childhood maltreatment. *Child Adolesc Psychiatric Clin N Am,* 3:663–677.

Deblinger E, Heflin AH (1996a) *Treating Sexually Abused Children and their Nonoffending Parents: A Cognitive Behavioral Approach.* Thousand Oaks, CA, Sage.

Deblinger E, Heflin AH (1996b) *Cognitive Behavioral Interventions for Treating Sexually Abused Children.* Thousand Oaks, CA, Sage Publications.

Deblinger E, Lippmann J, Steer R (1996) Sexually abused children suffering posttraumatic stress symptoms: initial treatment outcome findings. *Child Maltreatment,* 1:310–324.

Deykin EY, Buka SL (1997) Prevalence and risk factors for posttraumatic stress disorder among chemically dependent adolescents. *Am J Psychiatry,* 154:752–757.

Dodge KA, Frame CL (1982) Social cognitive biases and deficits in aggressive boys. *Child Devel,* 53:620–635.

Doumas D, Margolin G, John RS (1994) The intergenerational transmission of aggression across three generations. *J Fam Violence,* 9:157–175.

Dubner AE, Motta RW (1999) Sexually and physically abused foster care children and posttraumatic stress disorder. *J Consult Clin Psychol,* 67:367–73.

Emslie GJ, Rush AJ, Weinberg WA, Kowatch RA, Hughes CW, Carmody T et al. (1997) A double-bind randomized placebo-controlled trial of fluoxetine in children and adolescents with depression. *Arch Gen Psychiatry,* 54:1031–1037.

Famularo R, Fenton T, Augustyn M, Zuckerman B (1996) Persistence of pediatric post traumatic stress disorder after 2 years. *Child Abuse Neglect,* 20:1245–1248.

Famularo R, Fenton T, Kinscherff R (1993) Child maltreatment and the development of post traumatic stress disorder. *Am J Dis Children,* 147:755 760.

Famularo R, Kinsherff R, Fenton T (1988) Propranolol treatment for childhood posttraumatic stress disorder, acute type. *Am J Dis Children,* 142:1244–1247.

Field T, Seligman S, Scafedi F, Schanberg S (1996) Alleviating posttraumatic stress in children following Hurricane Andrew. *Applied Devel Psychol,* 17:37–50.

Fletcher KE (1996) Childhood posttraumatic stress disorder. In: Mash EJ, Barkley RA (eds) *Child Psychopathology.* New York, Guilford Publications, Inc., pp. 242–276.

Giaconia RM, Reinherz HZ, Silverman AB, Pakiz B, Frost AK, Cohen E (1995) Trauma and posttraumatic stress disorder in a community population of older adolescents. *J Am Acad Child Adolesc Psychiatry,* 34:1369–1380.

Gil E (1991) *The Healing Power of Play.* New York, NY, Guilford Press.

Gould E, Reeves AJ, Graziano MSA, Gross CG (1999) Neurogenesis in the neocortex of adult primates. *Science* 286:548–552.

Gould E, McEwen BS, Tanapat P, Galea LA, Fuchs E (1997a) Neurogenesis in the dentate gyrus of the adult tree shrew is regulated by psychosocial stress and NMDA receptor activation. *J Neurosci* 17:2492–8.

Gould E, Tanapat P, Cameron HA (1997b) Adrenal steroids suppress granule cell death in the developing dentate gyrus through an NMDA receptor-dependent mechanism. *Brain Res. Devel Brain Res* 103:91–3.

Gould E, Tanapat P, McEwen BS, Flugge G, Fuchs E (1998) Proliferation of granule cell precursors in the dentate gyrus of adult monkeys is diminished by stress. *Proc Nat Acad Sci USA,* 95:3168–71.

Green A (1985) Children traumatized by physical abuse. In: Eth S, Pynoos RS (eds) *Post-Traumatic Stress in Children.* Washington, DC, American Psychiatric Press, pp. 133–154.

Harmon RJ, Riggs PD (1996) Clonidine for posttraumatic stress disorder in preschool children. *Am Acad Child Adolesc Psychiatry,* 35:1247–1249.

Harway M, Hansen M (1994) *Spousal Abuse: Assessing and Treating Battered Women, Batterers, and their Children.* Sarasota, FL, Professional Resource Press.

Heim C, Newport DJ, Heit S, Graham YP, Wilcox M, Bonsall R et al. (2000) Pituitary-adrenal and autonomic responses to stress in women after sexual and physical abuse in childhood. *J Am Med Assoc,* 284:592–597.

Herman JL (1993) Sequelae of prolonged and repeated trauma: Evidence for a complex posttraumatic syndrome (DESNOS). In: Davidson JRT, Foa EB (eds) *Post-Traumatic Stress Disorder: DSM-IV and Beyond.* Washington, DC, American Psychiatric Press, pp. 213–228.

Hershorn M, Rosenbaum A (1985) Children of marital violence: A closer look at the unintended victims. *Am J Orthopsychiatry* 55:260–266.

Hill P (2002) Adjustment disorders. In: Rutter M, Taylor E (eds) *Child and Adolescent Psychiatry.* Blackwell Science Ltd, pp. 510–519.

Hillary BE, Schare ML (1993) Sexually and physically abused adolescents: an empirical search for PTSD. *J Clin Psychol,* 49:161–5.

Hinchey FS, Gavelek JR (1982) Empathic responding in children of battered mothers. *Child Abuse Neglect,* 6:395–401.

Horrigan JP (1996) Guanfacine for posttraumatic stress disorder nightmares. *Am Acad Child Adolesc Psychiatry,* 35:975–976.

Johnson JG, Cohen P, Brown J, Smailes EM, Bernstein DP (1999) Childhood maltreatment increases risk for personality disorders during early adulthood. *Arch Gen Psychiatry* 56:600–606.

Kaplan SJ, Pelcovitz D, Salzinger S (1998) Adolescent physical abuse: risk for adolescent psychiatric disorders. *Am J Psychiatry,* 155:954–9.

Kendler KS, Bulik CM, Silberg J, Hettema JM, Myers J, Prescott CA (2000) Childhood sexual abuse and adult psychiatric and substance use disorders in women: an epidemiological and cotwin control study. *Arch Gen Psychiatry,* 57:953–959.

Kessler RC (2000) Posttraumatic stress disorder: the burden to the individual and to society. *J Clin Psychiatry,* 61 (Suppl 5):4–12.

Kessler RC, Sonnega A, Bromet E, Hughes M, Nelson CB (1995) Posttraumatic stress disorder in the national comorbidity survey. *Arch Gen Psychiatry* 52:1048–1060.

Koenen KC, Moffitt TE, Caspi A, Taylor A, Purcell S (2003) Domestic violence is associated with environmental suppression of IQ in young children. *Devel Psychopathol,* 15:297–311.

Kolko DJ (1996) Individual cognitive behavioral therapy and family therapy for physically abused children and their offending parents: a comparison of clinical outcomes. *Child Maltreatment* 1:322–342.

Koluchova J (1972) Severe deprivation in twins: a case study. *J Child Psychol Psychiatry* 13:107–114.

Koluchova J (1976) The further development of twins after severe and prolonged deprivation: A second report. *J Child Psychol Psychiatry,* 17:181–188.

Layne CM, Pynoos RS, Saltzman WR, Arslanagic B, Black MM, Savjak N (2001) Trauma/grief focused group psychotherapy; school based postwar intervention with traumatized Bosnian adolescents. *Group Dynamics* 5:277–290.

Lipschitz DS, Winegar RK, Hartnick E, Foote B, Southwick SM (1999) Posttraumatic stress disorder in hospitalized adolescents: psychiatric comorbidity and clinical correlates. *J Am Acad Child Adolesc Psychiatry* 38:385–92.

Luntz BK, Widom CS (1994) Antisocial personality disorder in abused and neglected children grown up. *Am J Psychiatry,* 151:670–674.

Mannarino AP, Cohen JA, Berman SR (1994) The relationship between preabuse factors and psychological symptomatology in sexually abused girls. *Child Abuse Neglect,* 18:63–71.

March J, Amaya-Jackson L, Murry M, Schulte A (1998) Cognitive-behavioral psychotherapy for children and adolescents with post-traumatic stress disorder following a single incident stressor. *J Am Acad Child Adolesc Psychiatry* 37:585–593.

March JS, Amaya-Jackson L, Terry R, Costanzo P (1997) Posttraumatic symptomatology in children and adolescents after an industrial fire. *J Am Acad Child Adolesc Psychiatry,* 36:1080–1088.

McGloin JM, Widom CS (2001) Resilience among abused and neglected children grown up. *Devel Psychopathol,* 13:1021–1038.

McLeer SV, Callaghan M, Henry D, Wallen J (1994) Psychiatric disorders in sexually abused children. *J Am Acad Child Adolesc Psychiatry* 33:313–319.

McLeer SV, Dixon JF, Henry D, Ruggiero K, Escovitz K, Niedda T, et al. (1998) Psychopathology in non-clinically referred sexually abused children. *J Am Acad Child Adolesc Psychiatry,* 37:1326–33.

Mitchell JT, Dyregrov A (1993) Traumatic stress in disaster workers and emergency personnel: prevention and intervention. In: Wilson J, Raphael B (eds) *The International Handbook of Traumatic Stress Syndromes.* Washington, DC, American Psychiatric Press, pp. 905–914.

Money J, Annecillo C, Kelly JF (1983) Abuse-dwarfism syndrome: after rescue, statural and intellectual catch-up growth correlate. *J Clin Child Psychol,* 12:279–283.

National Research Council (1993) *Understanding Child Abuse and Neglect.* Washington, DC, National Academy Press.

North CS, McCutcheon V, Spitznagel EL, Smith EM (2002) Three-year follow-up of survivors of a mass shooting episode. *J Urban Health,* 79:383–391.

North CS, Nixon SJ, Shariat S, Mallonee S, McMillen JC, Spitznagel EL et al. (1999) Psychiatric disorders among survivors of the Oklahoma City bombing. *J Am Med Assoc,* 282:755–762.

Peled E, Davis D (1995) *Group Work with Children of Battered Women: A Practitioners Guide.* Thousand Oaks, CA, Sage.

Perry BD (1994) Neurobiological sequelae of childhood trauma: PTSD in children. In: Murburg MM (ed.) *Catecholamine Function in Posttraumatic Stress Disorder: Emerging Concepts.* Washington, DC, American Psychiatric Press, Inc., pp. 233–255.

Pitman RK, Sanders KM, Zusman RM, Healy AR, Cheema F, Lasko NB et al. (2002) Pilot study of secondary prevention of posttraumatic stress disorder with propranolol. *Biological Psychiatry* 51:189–192.

Putnam FW (1997) *Dissociation in Children and Adolescents: A Developmental Perspective.* New York, NY, The Guilford Press.

Putnam FW, Peterson G (1994) Further validation of the Child Dissociative Checklist. *Dissociation,* VII:204–211.

Pynoos RS, Eth S (1985) Witnessing acts of personal violence. In: Eth S, Pynoos RS (eds) *Post-Traumatic Stress in Children.* Washington, DC, American Psychiatric Press, pp. 17–43.

Pynoos RS, Eth S (1986) Witness to violence: The child interview. *J Am Acad Child Adolesc Psychiatry,* 25:306–319.

Pynoos RS, Nader K (1988) Psychological first aid and treatment approach to children exposed to community violence: research implications. *J Traumatic Stress Studies,* 1:445–473.

Pynoos RS, Nader K (1989) Children's memory and proximity to violence. *J Am Acad Child Adolesc Psychiatry,* 28:236–241.

Pynoos RS, Nader K (1990) Mental health disturbances in children exposed to disaster: prevention intervention strategies. In: Goldston S, Yager J, Heinicke C, Pynoos RS (eds) *Preventing Mental Health Disturbances in Childhood.* Washington, DC, American Psychiatric Press, pp. 211–233.

Pynoos RS, Nader K (1993) Issues in the treatment of posttraumatic stress disorder in children and adolescents. In: Wilson J, Raphael B (eds) *Issues in the Treatment of Posttraumatic Stress Disorder in Children and Adolescents.* Washington, DC, American Psychiatric Press, Inc., pp. 535–549.

Pynoos RS, Steinberg AM, Wraith R (1995) A developmental model of childhood traumatic stress. In: Cicchetti D, Cohen DJ (eds), *Developmental Psychopathology,* Vol 2. New York, John Wiley and Sons Inc., pp. 72–95.

Reider C, Cicchetti D (1989) Organizational perspective on cognitive control functioning and cognitive-affective balance in maltreated children. *Devel Psychol,* 25:382–393.

Rosenberg DR, Keshavan MS (1998) A.E. Bennett Research Award Toward a neurodevelopmental model of obsessive-compulsive disorder. *Biolog Psychiatry,* 43:623–640.

Sapolsky RM (2000) Glucocorticoids and hippocampal atrophy in neuropsychiatric disorders. *Arch Gen Psychiatry,* 57:925–935.

Saunders BE, Berliner L, Hanson RF (2001) Guidelines for the psycho-social treatment of intrafamilial child physical and sexual abuse. In: Charleston SC (Authors) *Office for Victims of Crime Guidelines.* Funded by the Office of Victims of Crime.

Scheeringa MS, Zeanah CH, Drell MJ, Larrieu JA (1995) Two approaches to the diagnosis of posttraumatic stress disorder in infancy and early childhood. *J Am Acad Child Adolesc Psychiatry* 34:191–200.

Seedat S, Stein DJ, Ziervogel C, Middleton T, Kammer D, Emsley RA (2002) Comparison of response to a selective serotonin reuptake inhibitor in children, adolescents, and adults with PTSD. *J Child Adolesc Psychopharmacol,* 12:37–46.

Silverman RC, Lieberman AF (1999) Negative maternal attributions, projective identifications, and the intergenerational transmission of violent relational patterns. *Psychoanal Dialogues,* 9:161–186.

Southwick SM, Krystal JH, Johnson DR, Charney DS (1992) Neuro-biology of posttraumatic stress disorder. In: Tasman A, Riba AMB (eds) *Review of Psychiatry.* Washington, DC, American Psychiatric Press, Inc., pp. 347–367.

Steinberg AM, Brymer MJ, Decker KB, Pynoos RS (2004) The University of California at Los Angeles Post-traumatic Stress Disorder Reaction Index. *Curr Psychiatry Rep* 6.

Stoddard F, Norman D, Murphy J (1989) A diagnostic outcome study of children and adolescents with severe burns. *J Trauma,* 29:471–477.

Stuber ML, Nader K, Yasuda P, Pynoos RS, Cohen S (1991) Stress response after pediatric bone marrow transplantation: Preliminary results of a prospective longitudinal study. *J Am Acad Child Adolesc Psychiatry,* 30:952–957.

Sulser F (1987) Serotonin-norepinephrine receptor interactions in the brain: implications for the pharmacology and pathophysiology of affective disorders. *J Clin Psychiatry,* 3(Suppl):12–18.

Tanapat P, Galea LA, Gould E (1998) Stress inhibits the proliferation of granule cell precursors in the developing dentate gyrus. *J Devel Neurosci* 16:235–9.

True WR, Rice J, Eisen SA, Heath AC, Goldberg J, Lyons MJ et al. (1993) A twin study of genetic and environmental contributions to liability for posttraumatic stress symptoms. *Arch Gen Psychiatry* 50:257–264.

Urquiza AJ, Mcneil CB (1996) Parent-child interaction therapy: an intensive intervention for physically abusive families. *Child Maltreatment* 1:134–144.

van der Kolk BA, Dreyfuss D, Michaels M, Shera D, Berkowitz R, Fisler R et al. (1994) Fluoxetine in posttraumatic stress disorder. *J Clin Psychiatry,* 55:517–22.

van der Kolk BA, Greenberg MS, Orr SP, Pitman RK (1989) Endogenous opioids, stress induced analgesia, and posttraumatic stress disorder. *Psychopharmacol Bull,* 25:417–421.

van Emmerik AA, Kamphuis JH, Hulsbosch AM, Emmelkamp PM (2002) Single session debriefing after psychological trauma: a meta-analysis. *Lancet* 360:766–771.

Vogel JM, Vernberg RM (1993) Part 1: Children's psychological responses to disasters. *J Clin Child Psychol,* 22:464–484.

Wallerstein JS (1990) Preventive interventions with divorcing families: a reconceptualization. In: Goldston SE, Yager J, Heinicke C, Pynoos RS (eds), *Preventing Mental Health Disturbances in Childhood.* Washington, DC, American Psychiatric Press, pp. 154–174.

Werry JS, Aman MG (1999) *Practitioner's Guide to Psychoactive Drugs for Children and Adolescents* 2nd edn. New York, NY, Plenum Medical Book Company.

Widom CS (1999) Posttraumatic stress disorder in abused and neglected children grown up. *Am J Psychiatry,* 156:1223–1229.

Winston FK, Kassam-Adams N, Vivarelli-O'Neill C, Ford J, Newman E, Baxt C et al. (2002) Acute stress disorder symptoms in children and their parents after pediatric traffic injury. *Pediatr,* 109:e90.

Wolfe DA, Sas L, Wekerle C (1994) Factors associated with the development of posttraumatic stress disorder among victims of sexual abuse. *Child Abuse Neglect,* 18:37–50.

Wolfe J, Charney DS (1991) Use of neuropsychological assessment in posttraumatic stress disorder. Psychological assessment. *J Consult Clin Psychol,* 3:573–580.

Yehuda R, Southwick S, Giller EL, Ma X, Mason JW (1992) Urinary catecholamine excretion and severity of PTSD symptoms in Vietnam combat veterans. *J Nerv Mental Dis,* 180:321–325.

Index

Note: page numbers in *italics* refer to figures, those in **bold** refer to tables.

polycystic ovarian syndrome (PCOS) 151
polysomnography 235
    obstructive sleep apnea 241
pornography, exposure to 290
porphyria, acute intermittent 33, 34
positron emission tomography (PET) 34
    ADHD 93–4
    bipolar disorder 138
post-traumatic stress disorder (PTSD) 321–3
    avoidant symptoms 328–9, 335
    catecholamines 335
    clinical assessment 325–6
    comorbidity 325
    debriefing 329
    developing brain 333
    diagnosis 322, 323
    disruptive disorder comorbidity 110
    dissociative symptoms 328–9, 335
    epidemiology 324–6
    evaluation 327–8, 329–30
    hyperarousal symptoms 329
    intrusive symptoms 328, 334–5
    long-term therapy 332
    long-term therapy-pulsed intervention 331
    medications 334–8
    parents of preterm infants 219
    physiological arousal 335
    prevalence 324
    psychological first aid 329
    psychotic disorder differential diagnosis 172
    re-experiencing symptoms 328, 334–5
    risk factors 325
    risk-taking behavior 305
    serotonin system 334–5
    sexual abuse 330–1
    symptom elucidation 328–9
    treatment 327–8, 329, 330–2
potassium
    anorexia nervosa 156
    bulimia nervosa 159
practitioners 41
Prader–Willi syndrome
    bulimia nervosa differential diagnosis 159
    mental retardation 69
    obesity 161
    PDD 69
pre-adoption period 252–3
pregnancy
    adolescents 295, 296, 297
    history 7
    prevention 296, 301
    substance abuse 219–20
prematurity 204
    developmental assessment 212
    infants at risk 218–19
prenatal development 204
preschool age children
    adoption 253
    chronic illness 265
    divorce impact 245
    history 8
primary care physicians 16–18
    bereavement 259
    learning disorders 89

    role in families of divorce 249
    substance abuse 196–7
probation 43
Procedure Behavior Check List (PBCL) 29
Procedure Behavior Rating Scale (PBRS) 29
processing disabilities 80
propranolol
    post-traumatic stress disorder 337
    risk-taking behaviors 309
protriptyline 242
Prout–Strohmer Emotional Problem Scales (PSAS) 29
pseudohermaphrodites, male 288
psychiatrists, child 41
psychodynamic therapies 43, 44
    anxiety disorder 126
    parenting 46–7
    play therapy for selective mutism 127
psycho-educational interventions
    depressive disorders 146
    psychotic disorders 174
psychological distress 328
psychological factors, risk-taking behavior 307–8
psychological first aid 329
psychological tests 4
    psychotic disorders 169
psychologists 41
psychopathology
    chronic illness 266
    high-risk behavior 304
    risk-taking behaviors 305–6, 308
    transgenderism 299
psychopharmacotherapy 48–56
    ADHD 99–103
    anxiety disorder 126
    chronic illness 277
    conduct disorder 111
    depressive disorders 147–52
    mental retardation 74–5
    PDD 74–5
    post-traumatic stress disorder 334, 335–8
    psychotherapy integration 149–52
    psychotic disorders 173–4
    risk-taking behaviors 309
    tics 130
    use in preschool children 222
psychosis
    infantile 163
    laboratory tests 33
    obsessive–compulsive disorder differential diagnosis 125
    risk-taking behavior 305, 306
    symptoms 164–6
    systemic lupus erythematosus 270
    see also psychotic disorders
psychosocial development
    adoption 254
    chronic illness 266
    Erikson's stages 154, **155**
    non-academic aspects of school 280–4
    school's role 278–85
psychosocial treatment
    ADHD 98
    anxiety disorder 125
    mental retardation 75–6
    PDD 75–6